Audiology
Practice Management

Second Edition

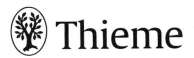

Audiology
Practice Management

Second Edition

Holly Hosford-Dunn, Ph.D.
Managing Member
Arizona Audiology Network, LLC
President
TAI, Inc.
Tucson, Arizona

Ross J. Roeser, Ph.D.
Lois & Howard Wolf Professor in Pediatric Hearing
Executive Director Emeritus
School of Behavioral and Brain Sciences
University of Texas at Dallas/Callier Center for Communication Disorders
Dallas, Texas

Michael Valente, Ph.D.
Professor of Clinical Otolaryngology
Director of Adult Audiology
Division of Audiology
Department of Otolaryngology–Head and Neck Surgery
Washington University School of Medicine
St. Louis, Missouri

Thieme
New York · Stuttgart

Thieme Medical Publishers, Inc.
333 Seventh Ave.
New York, NY 10001

Medical Editor: Birgitta Brandenburg
Vice President, Production and Electronic Publishing: Anne T. Vinnicombe
Production Editor: Molly Connors, Dovetail Content Solutions
Vice President, International Marketing: Cornelia Schulze
Chief Financial Officer: Peter van Woerden
President: Brian D. Scanlan
Compositor: Thomson Digital Services
Printer: Maple-Vail Book Manufacturing Company

Library of Congress Cataloging-in-Publication Data

Audiology. Practice management / edited by Holly Hosford-Dunn, Ross J. Roeser, Michael Valente. — 2nd ed.
    p. ; cm.
Companion v. to: Audiology : diagnosis, and Audiology : treatment.
Includes bibliographical references and index.
ISBN 978-1-58890-511-6 (US : alk. paper) — ISBN 978-3-13-116412-4 (GTV : alk. paper)
    1. Audiology—Practice. I. Hosford-Dunn, Holly. II. Roeser, Ross J. III. Valente, Michael. IV. Title: Audiology practice management.
        V. Title: Practice management.
    [DNLM: 1. Audiology—organization & administration. 2. Practice Management, Medical. WV 270 A912 2007]
RF291.A93 2007
617.8'0068—dc22

                                                    2007028331

Important note: Medical knowledge is ever-changing. As new research and clinical experience broaden our knowledge, changes in treatment and drug therapy may be required. The authors and editors of the material herein have consulted sources believed to be reliable in their efforts to provide information that is complete and in accord with the standards accepted at the time of publication. However, in view of the possibility of human error by the authors, editors, or publisher of the work herein or changes in medical knowledge, neither the authors, editors, nor publisher, nor any other party who has been involved in the preparation of this work, warrants that the information contained herein is in every respect accurate or complete, and they are not responsible for any errors or omissions or for the results obtained from use of such information. Readers are encouraged to confirm the information contained herein with other sources. For example, readers are advised to check the product information sheet included in the package of each drug they plan to administer to be certain that the information contained in this publication is accurate and that changes have not been made in the recommended dose or in the contraindications for administration. This recommendation is of particular importance in connection with new or infrequently used drugs.

Some of the product names, patents, and registered designs referred to in this book are in fact registered trademarks or proprietary names even though specific reference to this fact is not always made in the text. Therefore, the appearance of a name without designation as proprietary is not to be construed as a representation by the publisher that it is in the public domain.

Printed in the United States of America

5 4 3 2 1

US ISBN: 978-1-58890-511-6
GTV ISBN: 978-3-13-116412-4

Contents

Preface to the Second Edition

Harry Truman was a great leader and, some would say, an effective president. However, as is clearly evident in the second edition of our three volumes—*Audiology: Diagnosis, Audiology: Treatment,* and *Audiology: Practice Management*—he was off target when he said, "The only thing new in the world is the history you don't know." Since the publication of the first edition of our series just 7 years ago, there has been not only new information but also new technology, treatments, and trends in practice that have affected audiology in a way that has resulted in all areas of our profession growing exponentially. We now have better diagnostic procedures, more advanced technology and treatment programs, and additional practice strategies that allow audiologists to be more effective in diagnosing and treating their patients.

What's more exciting about the growth in the field of audiology that has occurred in the past few years is that we now have an expanding and maturing educational system for graduate students who choose to spend their lives in the profession. During the preparation of the first edition of our series, the doctor of audiology degree (Au.D.) was new. Yes, in 2000 there were programs in existence, and most universities at the time were in the planning stages of upgrading their programs to the doctoral level. However, at the time it was unclear how this shift in the educational model would impact the profession. Today, according to the Audiology Foundation of America, there are 70 university programs offering the Au.D. degree, 1500 residential students currently enrolled in Au.D. programs, and more than 3725 practicing doctors of audiology. So, we have an expanded body of knowledge that is being consumed by a growing and more sophisticated constituent body of professionals who have dedicated themselves to providing the best diagnosis and treatments to those with hearing disorders using more sophisticated practice procedures. All of these trends point to growth.

A novel thought is to consider the information in these three volumes as a mathematical equation:

$$X = D + T + P$$

where D is diagnosis, T is treatment, P is practice management, and X is the sum of all of the current knowledge in the three represented areas provided by the most knowledgeable experts in their respective fields. That is what we wanted these books to represent.

People don't just decide one day that because there is more information and more individuals to consume it, they will devote a couple years of their lives to putting it together in a bundle of books. The three of us jointly arrived at the decision to publish a second edition of the "trilogy," as it has become known colloquially, because we felt a need to pay back to our profession a modicum of what it has given to us. We each have been very fortunate to be exposed to some of the best mentors, have been provided with tremendous support both psychologically and financially, and have been rewarded greatly in many other ways by being audiologists. We feel that we have been fortunate to practice audiology during the period of growth that the profession has experienced. We want to share those positive experiences with our readers.

We owe a special debt of gratitude to the authors of the chapters in these three volumes, who were willing to contribute their knowledge and experience as well as their valuable time in preparing the material. We thank them not only for all of their hard work and diligence in meeting a demanding publication schedule, but also for their tolerance in putting up with what we considered "constructive editorial comments." We realize that criticism is easy, but it is the science and art that are difficult. They were quite tolerant and gracious.

Finally, Thieme Medical Publishers provided us with the support of Ivy Ip. Ivy was our frontline representative with our authors once they agreed to be part of our team. We thank her for all of her efforts in making the second edition of our books a reality.

Holly Hosford-Dunn—tucsonaud@aol.com
Ross J. Roeser—roeser@utdallas.edu
Michael Valente—valentem@ent.wustl.edu

Preface to the First Edition

This book on the topic of practice management in audiology is one in a series of three texts prepared to represent the breadth of knowledge covering the multi-faceted profession of audiology in a manner that has not been attempted before. The companion books to this volume are titled *Diagnosis* and *Treatment*. In total, the three books provide a total of 73 chapters covering material on the range of subjects and current knowledge audiologists must have to practice effectively. Because many of the chapters in the three books relate to each other, our readers are encouraged to have all three of them in their libraries so that the broad scope of the profession of audiology is made available to them.

A unique feature of all three books is the insertion of highlighted boxes (pearls, pitfalls, special considerations, and controversial points) in strategic locations. These boxes emphasize key points authors are making and expand important concepts that are presented.

The 21 chapters in this book cover or touch on all aspects of audiology practice management. In the first chapter, we define practice management and discuss how it applies to the provision of audiology services. Chapters 2 through 8 present basic and advanced information on fundamental principles of practice management, as they apply to audiology, including: professional education, professional ethics, quality control, principles of outcome measurement, human resource management, marketing principles, and fundamentals of private practice.

Clinical audiology practical topics are reviewed in Chapters 9 through 12. The diverse topics include: interpretation and application of professional Codes of Ethics in audiology, clinical report writing and presentation, infection control, and cerumen management.

Chapters 13 through 18 address a wide variety of business issues including: selecting and designing office space, preparing a business plan, selecting a business type, managerial and financial accounting, functioning in managed-care environments, and responding to managed-care contracting requests for proposals.

Computer technology comprises the final applications section. Chapters 19 and 20 provide extensive explorations of hardware structures and software applications for teaching and administering audiology services. Finally, in Chapter 21, diverse insights into the future of audiology practice management are provided by three leaders from audiology, business, and manufacturing.

The three of us were brought together by Ms. Andrea Seils, Senior Medical Editor at Thieme Medical Publishers, Inc. During the birthing stage of the project Andrea encouraged us to think progressively—out of the box. She reminded us repeatedly to shed our traditional thinking and concentrate on the new developments that have taken place in audiology in recent years and that will occur in the next 5 to 10 years. With Andrea's encouragement and guidance, each of us set out what some would have considered to be the impossible—to develop a series of three cutting-edge books that would cover the entire profession of audiology in a period of less than 2 years. Not only did we accomplish our goal, but as evidenced by the comprehensive nature of the material covered in the three books, we exceeded our expectations! We thank Andrea for her support throughout this 2-year project.

The authors who were willing to contribute to this book series have provided outstanding material that will assist audiologists in-training and practicing audiologists in their quest for the most up-to-date information on the areas that are covered. We thank them for their diligence in following our guidelines for preparing their manuscripts and their promptness in following our demanding schedule.

The consideration of our families for their endurance and patience with us throughout the duration of the project must be recognized. Our spouses and children understood our mission when we were away at editorial meetings; they were patient when we stayed up late at night and awoke in the wee hours of the morning to eke out a few more paragraphs; they tolerated the countless hours we were away from them. Without their support and encouragement we would never have finished our books in the time frame we did.

Finally, each of us thanks our readers for their support of this book series. We would welcome comments and suggestions on this book, as well as the other two books in the series. Our email addresses are below.

Ross J. Roeser—roeser@utdallas.edu
Michael Valente—valentem@ent.wustl.edu
Holly Hosford—Dunn-tucsonaud@aol.com

Contributors

Harvey B. Abrams, Ph.D.
Chief
Audiology and Speech Pathology
   Service
Bay Pines VA Healthcare System
Bay Pines, Florida

A.U. Bankaitis, Ph.D.
Vice President and General Manager
Oaktree Products, Inc.
St. Louis, Missouri

Jane H. Baxter, M.S.
Clinical Audiologist and Owner
Pacific Hearing Service
Menlow Park, California

Joy Colle Benn, M.A., M.B.A.
Tapoco, North Carolina

Darcy Benson, Au.D.
Audiologist
California Hearing Center
San Mateo, California

Theresa Hnath Chisolm, Ph.D.
Professor and Chair
Department of Communication
   Sciences and Disorders
University of South Florida
Tampa, Florida

Deborah W. Clark, M.A.
Clinical Audiologist
Pacific Hearing Service
Menlo Park, California

Teresa M. Clark, Au.D.
Audiologist and Owner
California Hearing Center
San Mateo, California

Robert R. De Jonge, Ph.D.
Department of Communication
   Disorders
Central Missouri State University
Warrensburg, Missouri

Alan L. Desmond, Au.D.
Director
Blue Ridge Hearing and Balance Clinic
Princeton, West Virginia

Kris English, Ph.D.
Associate Professor
University of Pittsburgh
Pittsburgh, Pennsylvania

Robert C. Fifer, Ph.D.
Director of Audiology and
   Speech-Language Pathology
Mailman Center for Child
   Development
University of Miami
Miami, Florida

Kathy A. Foltner, Au.D.
Adjunct Instructor
Department of Communication
   Disorders and Sciences
Rush University Medical Center
Chicago, Illinois
Adjunct Instructor
Pennsylvania College of
   Optometry—School of Audiology
Elkins Park, Pennsylvania
Chief Executive Officer
AuDNet, Inc.
Burnsville, Minnesota

Theodore J. Glattke, Ph.D.
Professor
Department of Speech, Language and
   Hearing Sciences
University of Arizona
Tucson, Arizona

J. Mark Goffinet, M.S.
MidMissouri Audiology
Practice Development Consultant
Phonak
Warrensburg, Missouri

Holly Hosford-Dunn, Ph.D.
Managing Member
Arizona Audiology Network, LLC
President
TAI, Inc.
Tucson, Arizona

Gyl A. Kasewurm, Au.D.
Professional Hearing Services, Ltd
St Joseph, Michigan

Robert J. Kemp, M.B.A.
Founder and Chief Executive Officer
Oaktree Products, Inc.
St. Louis, Missouri

Ross J. Roeser, Ph.D.
Lois & Howard Wolf Professor in
   Pediatric Hearing
Executive Director Emeritus
School of Behavioral and Brain
   Sciences
University of Texas at Dallas/Callier
   Center for Communication
   Disorders
Dallas, Texas

H. Carol Saul, J.D.
Attorney-at-Law
Epstein Becker & Green, P.C.
Atlanta, Georgia

Kathryn L. Shaughnessy, Au.D. , B.S.
Department of Audiology and
   Speech Pathology
University of Memphis
Memphis, Tennessee

Helena Stern Solodar, Au.D.
Audiologist, Co-Founder, Co-Director
Audiological Consultants of Atlanta
Atlanta, Georgia

Kathryn P. Snyder, M.H.A., B.S.
Department of Administration
Mayo Clinic—Jacksonville
Jacksonville, Florida

Wayne J. Staab, Ph.D.
Dr. Wayne J. Staab & Associates
Dammeron Valley, Utah

Robert M. Traynor, Ed.D., M.B.A.
Adjunct Professor of Audiology
University of Florida
Gainesville, Florida

Michael Valente, Ph.D.
Professor of Clinical Otolaryngology
Director of Adult Audiology
Division of Audiology
Department of Otolaryngology–Head
  and Neck Surgery
Washington University School of
  Medicine
St. Louis, Missouri

Kadyn Williams, Au.D.
Audiological Consultants of Atlanta
Atlanta, Georgia

Phillip L. Wilson, Au.D.
Head
Audiology Clinic
School of Behavioral and Brain
  Sciences
University of Texas at Dallas/Callier
  Center for Communication
  Disorders
Dallas, Texas

David A. Zapala, Ph.D.
Assistant Professor
Mayo Medical School
Section of Audiology
Otolaryngology–Head & Neck
  Surgery Audiology
Mayo Clinic
Jacksonville, Florida

Acknowledgments

For the Book Series

The three editors of this book series came together in late 1990. Prior to the first meeting we had all known of each other, but only casually. However, during the first meeting there was an immediate recognition among us that, although we had very different backgrounds and professional orientations, a professional magnetism drew us together. Long hours together flew by during the many sessions where we discussed contents, possible contributors, and logistics.

When asked to produce a second edition, each of us was very reluctant, but agreed because we knew that this would provide us with an opportunity to work together once again. So, strange as it may seem, each of us would like to thank our two other editorial colleagues for making the second edition a reality. We each said that the main reason for taking on this gargantuan task was that we had the support of the two other editors.

Each of us would like to thank the authors for the considerable time and effort they took from their private and professional lives to produce chapters reflecting the highest scholarship.

The staff of Thieme Medical Publishers, Brian Scanlan, President, Birgitta Brandenburg, Editor, and Ivy Ip, Assistant Editor, who worked so many hours during the entire production process deserve special recognition. These key individuals keep the machines running at the Thieme headquarters in the background so that authors and editors can carry out their writing, recruiting, and editorial tasks.

Holly Hosford-Dunn—tucsonaud@aol.com
Ross J. Roeser—roeser@utdallas.edu
Michael Valente—valentem@ent.wustl.edu

For this Book

As primary editor for *Audiology: Practice Management,* I want to thank my coeditors, Ross Roeser and Mike Valente, for their editorial suggestions and advice on many issues in this book. I also want to thank The Computer Guys, Harry and Shaun, who were always there to replace or restore computers, hard drives, motherboards, PC cards, networks, and databases to keep the project going. Sharon K. Hopkins shouldered much of the clinical work while I was otherwise occupied with this book. Finally, my appreciation and thanks to Daniel, Andrew, Hobbes, and O'Dette for 24/7 support throughout the preparation of this book and the trilogy as a whole.

Holly Hosford-Dunn—tucsonaud@aol.com

Chapter 1

What Is Practice Management?

Holly Hosford-Dunn, Ross J. Roeser, and Michael Valente

- ◆ **Defining Practice Management**

  Operational Definition
  Formal Definitions
  Dynamic Model of Audiology Practice Management
  Practice Management Is a Balancing Act

- ◆ **Is Practice Management Necessary?**

  Evolutions and Revolutions
  Frictions Create Dynamic Tensions

- ◆ **How Does Practice Management Work?**

  Using Frictions as Stepping Stones

- ◆ **Management Competencies and Training**

  Areas of Learning
  Human Resource Management

- ◆ **Structure of this Book**
- ◆ **Summary**
- ◆ **Appendix 1–1**

The chapters in this book explore practice management and its application to audiology service delivery. The first edition of this volume marked a departure from previous comprehensive, handbook-type audiology texts, which did not treat practice management as a special topic, if at all. Professional expansion and improvement are manifest as the second edition debuts: the number of audiologists has increased to over 10,000 (see **Fig. 1–1**); doctoral programs in audiology (Au.D.) are proliferating; and audiology is among the "top 10 best professions in the United States," according to *U.S. News and World Report* (Nemko, 2006).

The volumes in this series recognize that today's audiologist must be supported by a training triumvirate of diagnostics, treatment, and practice management. Diagnostic audiology and treatment have been addressed in numerous texts and are fairly well differentiated in most readers' minds, but practice management continues to conjure disparate and confusing images for audiologists on the basis of their individual experiences or lack thereof. The purposes of this volume are to arrive at useful definitions of practice management, develop principles of practice management for audiology, and describe their applications to a comprehensive set of practice environments.

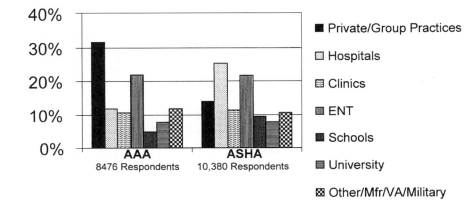

Figure 1–1 Estimates of workforce distribution of audiologists in the United States. Audiologists' work settings are according to membership survey data from the American Speech-Language-Hearing Association (ASHA, 2004a) website and the American Academy of Audiology (AAA; Sullivan, E. Personal communication, March 2, 2007). Mfr, manufacturer; VA, Veterans' Administration.

1

◆ Defining Practice Management

Operational Definition

Audiology is diversifying so rapidly that it is sometimes difficult to recognize the kinship between audiology services performed in one environment versus another or to acknowledge that the audiologists performing the services are products of the same discipline. It is not even clear where and how audiologists work because survey methods cannot stay abreast of rapid shifts in their professional alliances, workplace environments, and workforce employment. For example, **Fig. 1–1** shows U.S. audiology work settings for the memberships of the American Speech-Language-Hearing Association (ASHA) and the American Academy of Audiology (AAA). Six employment categories account for almost 90% of audiologists' work environments. Between professional organizations, members' employment choices are evenly distributed between physician-based clinics, physician-owned private practices, and categories labeled "other," meaning either that the same audiologists belong to two professional organizations or that selection of professional organization is unrelated to work setting for these audiologists. In contrast, private practice audiologists are more than twice as likely to align with AAA as ASHA; the reverse holds true for hospital-based audiologists. This dichotomy is especially interesting in light of another statistic estimating that dispensing audiologists in the United States own 60% of the hearing aid dispensing offices and almost that share of the entire U.S. market (Strom, 2005).

Pearl

- Today's audiologists work in private practices, hospitals, physicians' offices, and newly developing environments.

Survey analyses in the first edition of this book noted that "[o]perationally, the safest conclusion seems to be that today's audiologists are practicing in private practices, hospitals, physicians' offices, or in newly developing environments" (Hosford-Dunn et al, 2000, p. 1). The data in **Fig. 1–1** suggest this statement remains a correct interpretation, but professional migrations, remuneration, and autonomy related to employment selection complicate the development of a comprehensive view of the workforce in our profession.

Moreover, workplace distinctions are becoming blurred as audiologists move into supervisory positions by virtue of their licensure and degrees. It is no longer the case that the professional staff composition of audiology practices, hospitals, or clinics consists of audiologists with varying years of experience supplemented by clerical support. Now, more than 20% of practices employ audiologists and hearing instrument dispensers together, according to one industry survey (Strom, 2005). Fourth-year Au.D. internships are a

Table 1–1 Example of Values and Objectives for an Audiology Organization

Purpose
To maintain or improve the quality of our patients' lives by optimizing their communication ability

Core Values
- Expecting personal best: honest, diligent, always learning
- Teamwork and loyalty
- Our only job is customer service
- Dignity and respect for our patients and each other

new reality for many clinic and hospital settings, as well as in some private practices.

As audiology expands and diversifies, audiologists find themselves working in, directing, or developing a variety of hearing health care organizations over their careers. Whatever the name given, these audiologists are performing practice management. Some audiologists will feel comfortable working in supporting positions in traditional settings, whereas others will push the envelope by bringing strong entrepreneurial forces into practice environments.

In the present milieu, different avenues exist to deliver the tests and services for which audiologists are trained: just as audiologists are unique, so are the organizations they comprise. As examples, hearing health organizations are now categorized according to quantitative measures such as plant or staff size, marketing efforts, service delivery models, treatment outcomes, financial success, staff turnover, and staff credentials. Qualitatively, these same organizations work hard to differentiate themselves by developing objectives and values that define their varying cultures, as shown by the example in **Table 1–1**.

Despite the intentional diversity, these organizations share a common trait: they are all audiology practices that must conform to legal and ethical constraints. Audiologists who participate in or direct these practices must produce in line with organizational objectives; uphold organizational values and encourage similar action by their colleagues; and ensure that individual and organizational efforts are ethical and legal according to state, federal, or professional organization dictates. This formidable array of "musts" is the operational definition of practice management in audiology **(Table 1–2)**.

Operational definitions are based on observation and are helpful in identifying things ("We know it when we see it"). But operational definitions yield little information about the underlying structures and theories that explain how something came to be and how it functions ("What is it?" "How does it work?"). Answering these questions requires formal definitions of practice and management.

Table 1–2 Operational Definition of Audiology Practice Management

Audiologists must produce in line with organizational objectives, uphold organizational values, encourage similar action by their colleagues, and ensure that their individual and organizational efforts are ethical and legal.

Formal Definitions

What Is a Practice?

A practice is a professional organization. Organizations do not have to be professional. Most audiologists work for one organization, belong to several, and interact with many more: universities, audiology clinics, private practices, book clubs, homeowners' associations, alumni groups, and so on. All successful organizations, regardless of how they differ, do a few basic things (Stoner and Wankel, 1986):

♦ *Accomplish objectives* Organizations use human and other resources to achieve goals that would be difficult or impossible to achieve by individuals acting alone.

♦ *Preserve knowledge* Organizations keep records, communicate information, and expand knowledge by developing new or better ways of doing things.

♦ *Provide vocations and avocations* Organizations offer ways of making a living and/or pursuing an area of interest, often serving as a source of personal satisfaction and self-fulfillment.

Audiology practices of all types and sizes satisfy the generic criteria of an organization: set objectives, maintain patient and business records, employ people, and provide settings in which those people can realize personal and professional achievements. More specifically, audiology practices belong to an exclusive subset of professional organizations, along with accounting, medical, legal, and other practices that employ specially licensed and/or credentialed staff. Professional organizations function with special privileges carved out by law (e.g., the right to perform specific procedures and bill for them) and likewise are subject to special scrutiny according to laws and ethical oaths.

Special Consideration

• Professional organizations have special privileges and are subject to special scrutiny.

What Is Management?

In the classic business definition, management is an internal process for achieving organizational objectives:

> Management is the process of planning, organizing, leading, and controlling the efforts of organization members and of using all other organizational resources to achieve stated organizational goals (Stoner and Wankel, 1986, p. 4).

The internal management process is important for maintaining a business, but Drucker (1986) envisions management as a dynamic entity that is more applicable to professional organizations such as audiology practices. Drucker's management model functions in three arenas internal and external to the practice (**Fig. 1–2**):

1. *In the business* Monitoring performance and producing economic results in line with organizational goals

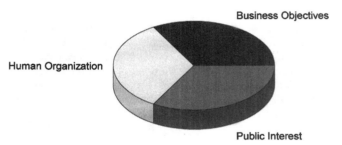

Figure 1–2 Three dimensions of audiology practice management.

2. *In the human organization* Using governance, values, and relationships of power and responsibility to develop, pay, and organize people for productivity

3. *In the dimension of public interest* Developing and using policies to affect the business impact on society and the community (Drucker, 1986)

Dynamic Model of Audiology Practice Management

The operational definition of audiology practice management at the beginning of this section can be segmented into its component parts, using the formal definitions of practices as organizations and management as a dynamic, three-dimensional entity:

1. *In the business* Audiologists must produce in line with organizational objectives.

2. *In the human organization* Audiologists must uphold organizational values and encourage similar action by coworkers in the practice.

3. *In the dimension of public interest* Audiologists must ensure that their individual and organizational efforts are ethical, legal, and positively influence the impact of audiology on society and the community.

This definition leads to important conclusions about successful audiologists, who must use many skills in practice that were not acquired in graduate school. These audiologists function simultaneously on several organizational levels. They are all managers. It is easy to see why Drucker (1986) calls this type of management an "entity." For audiology practices, the management entity is the audiologists, all of whom must manage in the business, in the human organization, and with the public interest in mind.

Practice Management Is a Balancing Act

The constant attention to three management dimensions also makes it easy to understand why Drucker (1986) refers to this type of management entity as "dynamic." Those who have worked in busy clinics or private practices may feel more comfortable describing the dynamic as a circus act. By this analogy, practice management is a balancing act in which managers keep several balls in the air all the time. Good managers do not hesitate to introduce new and different balls to their mix and do not hold on to outmoded balls just because they are in the air. At the same time, they are careful to maintain a balanced mix of balls so that business, human, and public objectives are all well represented. It is a challenging job that never stops—there are always new balls, sometimes many more balls than before, and the balls often appear in groups that threaten to topple the delicate balance of business, human, and public interests. Like other skilled performers, good managers master this never-ending balancing act by virtue of learned competencies and training.

Pearl

- Good managers master the never-ending balancing act by virtue of learned competencies and training.

The motivation of this chapter and others in this volume is to explore and develop principles and applications that help audiologists learn to manage according to the objectives of the three-dimensional model of audiology practice management.

♦ Is Practice Management Necessary?

The short answer to this question is yes. Practice management is necessary everywhere in the audiology profession, all the time. The operational and formal definitions evoke an ideal image of audiology practices as entities that function both as profit-making businesses and community resources by virtue of competent, caring audiologists who exercise solid management and business skills on a daily basis. Simplistically, this image suggests that all audiology practices should function in about the same way, with little need for discussion as to what is "right" or "best." After all, audiologists are trained in accredited institutions with a prescribed curriculum, profitability is an easy concept to grasp, and audiology services improve societal problems. What could be more straightforward than getting paid to provide services that help people improve their hearing or balance? Who needs a manager to do that?

The simplistic ideal does not begin to account for the organizational differences and challenges that exist in audiology. Without active management, differences and disagreements become problems in individual practices, membership organizations, and the profession as a whole. One obvious difference already mentioned is seen in the employment data in **Fig. 1–1**. Private practice emerged as the dominant employment mode in the 1990s, shifting the profession's emphasis away from diagnostic testing and toward hearing aid dispensing. The shift produced many positive changes for the profession and for individual practices, but its repercussions include internecine and external quarrels. Universal agreement does not exist that this shift is in accord with the goals of the audiology profession. Individual practices assume more businesslike profiles when selling hearing aids, some feel to the detriment of professional standing and ethical footing (see discussion of ethics in Chapter 2 of this volume). Brady and Granville (2006) describe a caste system in the

profession in which respect is allocated according to employment or self-employment. Turf disputes surface because audiology dispensing practices must compete with nonaudiology providers and Internet sites for hearing aid sales and with physicians for the entry point of hearing care in health systems. Practice management must address these disagreements as they arise.

Among private practices, another obvious difference causing conflict is that audiologists do not all practice in the same kind of organization. Practices differ by size, legal entity, ownership, objectives, personnel, markets served, and autonomy. The employment situation in audiology is so fluid that no business organizational type dominates. At the time of writing, new types of business organizations are appearing almost out of nowhere, employing audiologists in ways that no one envisioned just 10 years ago. Professional and education organizations are in a similar state of flux, differing in their objectives but all vying for audiologists' membership or enrollment. The success or failure of organizations, from the smallest independent practice to the largest professional association, continues to hinge on how competently the organizations are managed over time as well as how completely they anticipate and meet the needs of their target markets.

Evolutions and Revolutions

The first edition of this book acknowledged the "natural evolution" of organizations, in which fragmentation follows failure to anticipate and serve target markets. From a management perspective, the balancing act fails, and new organizations (and managers) step in to fill the void. These natural evolutions are continuous and occur at all levels of the profession and within individual practices. The evolutions are reflected by changes in the employment settings in which audiologists chose to practice (**Fig. 1–1**), journals read, schools attended, courses offered, services provided, professional memberships renewed or dropped, topics of continuing education selected, technological advances, and so forth. The natural evolutions influence the three dimensions of audiology practice management by effecting many professional changes, including audiology training requirements, credentialing, scope of practice, professional associations, professional autonomy, reimbursement, and work settings.

Pitfall

- Without active management, natural frictions disrupt individual practices and the profession as a whole.

Evolutions occurring simultaneously in other areas affect the internal workings of the audiology profession. Technological advances in automation, for example, threaten to encroach on audiology's diagnostic turf; "disruptive" technologies cause fundamental changes in consumer demand for ear-level communication devices. Other external changes stem from managed care and implementation of the Americans with Disabilities Act in the public arena as well as in service delivery. With these external changes come new questions and challenges to audiology practices: What services are provided and by whom? To whom are they provided? How are services provided? In what setting are they provided? Who is responsible for payment? Who is responsible for billing and collection? External changes also introduce people with different backgrounds into the audiology profession, often in controlling positions.

In all cases, external changes affect the three-dimensional balance of business, human interest, and public interest. In the balancing act analogy, these changes are like new and different balls that either replace or are added to those already in the air. Whether external changes are good or bad for an audiology organization depends on how well and how quickly management integrates the changes and resumes the balancing act at a new equilibrium point. Occasionally, natural evolutions produce so many internal and external changes that a revolution occurs. At such times, professions and organizations must seriously consider redefining business objectives and human organization objectives in ways that affect the public they market to and serve. If consideration prompts action, a revolution occurs. For individual practices, revolutions can be as simple as moving the practice from a hospital setting to a retail mall or as complicated as forming an independent practice association with former competitors or hearing aid dispensers. For the profession, revolutions can be as small as a change in a professional organization's board composition or as large as achieving parity with other health professions via the Au.D. as a first professional degree (Smith and Windmill, 2006). These are the times when practice managers pull all the balls out of the air and start new acts with different balls, or they drop the balls and yield to new managers with different acts.

For example, perhaps the most important and immediate revolution for audiologists is the rapid technology convergence centered on smart phones, ear-level listening devices, Web-based information, and wireless technologies (Dybala, 2006; Hosford-Dunn, 2006). In the final chapter of the first edition of this book (Hosford-Dunn et al, 2000), Skafte anticipated telescoping of the pace of technological change from 25 years to 5 years or less. In the same chapter, Kolind predicted that "we will talk about the twenty-first century as the *knowledge* age, the *networking* age, or the *information* age" (p. 487). The pace of technological change today has overshot Skafte's prediction, especially in the areas of information technology and communications equipment, as predicted by Kolind (Federal Reserve Board, 2006). Audiology's positioning in this new world of enhanced personal listening devices and convergence of hearing aids with popular electronics is not clear, at least to these writers: Will hearing aids become obsolete or remain a niche market for people with severe hearing losses, or will hearing aids morph into a diverse family of multipurpose ear-level devices? Will audiologists retain their preeminence in the dispensing arena as devices become available over the counter, are programmed over the Web, and are purchased for reasons beyond correction of hearing-sensitivity deficits? Will diagnostic evaluations move from traditional audiometric testing to performance-based monitoring and reporting by wearable devices?

Frictions Create Dynamic Tensions

New or unmet needs stimulate change, which produces natural evolutions and revolutions in organizations. In the physical universe, movement from one position to another creates friction, and the same is true of change in organizations. Audiology evolutions and revolutions are generating new needs in the three dimensions of practice management and spawning frictions of all types:

1. *In the business*   Business objectives are commandeering a larger role as audiologists become more entrepreneurial, develop products and patents, attain greater market share, and experience higher revenues and correspondingly greater competitive pressure. "Needs of the business" may clash with "patient-first" professional motives. Depending on how they are addressed by management, such conflicts are also likely to color audiologists' professional relations with suppliers, employers (e.g., universities), other professions, agencies, legal bodies, and, ultimately, other audiologists and audiology organizations.

2. *In the human organization*   Audiologists assume more professional responsibility as practice settings become more independent, as the audiology scope of practice is fully realized, as they assume greater supervisory responsibilities, and as audiology becomes the entry point for hearing health care. At the same time, economic controls may reduce professional autonomy and limit the scope of services and professional "creative" time.

3. *In the dimension of public interest*   As business practices become a greater part of the profile of audiology, professionals becomes more susceptible to the impositions of legal, regulatory, and management bodies, thereby losing considerable autonomy. These frictions affect how audiologists perceive themselves and what they do. Managed care organizations' (MCOs) penetration into audiology is one example. According to an industry survey for 2005 (Strom, 2006), enrollees of MCO/health maintenance organization (HMO) plans comprised 16% of audiologists' hearing aid dispensing revenues in the United States and 18% of their entire consumer base for hearing aid sales. MCO controls on participator enrollment and reimbursement have stimulated strong interest in measuring outcomes of audiology services, especially hearing aid treatment intervention.

Frictions identify potential problems and highlight areas for improvement. They prompt discourse that, at its best, results in a dynamic tension that maintains a forward momentum for audiology practices and the profession. Without friction, the status quo prevails, and the organization languishes while more dynamic organizations step in to fill the void. Back to the balancing act analogy, the performer must always "top" the act with something new and more daring to keep the audience's attention and goodwill. If the act is dull and repetitive, it fails, and the audience goes in search of a better act. Good practice managers understand this analogy and welcome frictions as a means of improving their practices in the eyes of patients, employees, referral sources, and bankers. Examples of issues that cause friction and discussion of how they are handled by practice management are discussed later in this chapter.

This section of the chapter posed the question Is practice management necessary? It concludes as it began, with a definite yes. Audiology is changing rapidly in response to internal and external pressures. In some cases, the changes follow a course of natural evolution as organizations move to accommodate new technologies, new constituents, and demands of the economy and the workforce. Managers are necessary to weigh these changes against the three-dimensional practice management model and decide how and when to adopt the changes for the good of the practices or other organizations. This is the classic balancing act that makes management necessary.

In a few cases, bedrock positions shift, prompting revolution. One need only peruse the first two volumes of this trilogy for evidence that evolution culminating in revolution has been common in the field of diagnostic audiology and hearing aid dispensing over the last 50 years. As for practice management, these are exhilarating yet trying times for audiology practices, associations, and educational organizations (Anderson and Nemes, 2004). Revolution is in the air as doctors of audiology benefit from higher wages/revenues and grapple with greater management responsibilities and ethical demands that come with more vaunted professional status. Henson et al (2006) speculated that increased risks associated with transitions in our profession are creating a new demand among audiologists for business education. They conducted a formal study using a "knowledge gap" metric to assess audiologists' confidence in their understanding of basic business skills and the corresponding values they assigned to those skills. The authors concluded that "[a]udiologists appear to recognize very clearly that they need significant expansion of their business knowledge and skills in order to be successful, compete effectively and make sense of today's complex marketplace" (p. 54). Intriguingly, audiologists identified a greater gap—as much as 87%—for "softer" subjects (marketing, human relationships) than for "harder" subjects (finance, accounting, managerial decision making), suggesting that analytic management skills have a lower designated value in our profession at present.

♦ How Does Practice Management Work?

Many books are dedicated to an analysis of management processes. As editors and audiologists, we do not pretend to know as much about management as these books' experts, nor is this chapter intended to compete with such books. Therefore, the following discussion is practical in nature, eschewing management theories in favor of personal experiences and examples from the audiology profession. Audiologists who are interested in the history of management and synopses of management theories are referred to Chapter 20 in Hosford-Dunn et al (1995).

The following sequential steps are prescribed for starting or redirecting a practice (Hosford-Dunn et al, 1995):

1. Define the business.
   a. Who are the primary and secondary customers?
   b. How are the customers reached?
   c. What do the customers value?

2. Develop a vision of the organization (mission statement and practice philosophy).
   a. Write the purpose.
   b. Write the core values.

3. Identify internal strengths and weaknesses and external opportunities and threats (SWOT).

4. Write specific and measurable goals and objectives.

5. Set strategies outlining plans for achieving goals and objectives.

6. Specify tactics for what will be done by whom and by when to meet objectives.

If one follows these steps in the prescribed order, it becomes clear that practice management is an entity that always exists before creation of the organization that it will subsequently manage. Recall that Drucker (1986) envisions practice management as a dynamic entity. This is an example of why it is dynamic: it plans and creates what it will manage. Of course, not all groups follow the prescribed steps, and not all practice management is dynamic. Organizations can come into being by accident, without any planning. In such cases, practice management is an afterthought. Internal frictions are likely to abound in these chaotic organizations.

Using Frictions as Stepping Stones

In a well-run organization, the SWOT analysis mentioned in step 3 above is the first of many times that practice management brushes up against dynamic tensions. As stated earlier, good practice managers welcome frictions as a means of improving practices. This section looks at a few of these **(Table 1–3)** and examines how they are handled in the three-dimensional, dynamic practice management model.

Table 1–3 Examples of Dynamic Tensions in Audiology Practices

What is taught	What is practiced
What is known	What is implemented
What is complete	What is allowed
What is desirable	What is available
What is recommended	What is affordable or reimbursed
What is a right	What is a privilege
What is an organizational need	What is a patient need
What is necessary	What is sufficient
Practices that are ethical	Practices that are unethical
Outcome measures for counseling	Data for utilization review

What Is Known versus What Is Implemented

In this type of friction, the practice management decision is complicated by too much information rather than not enough information. Clinicians do not use all the information and resources at their disposal to diagnose or treat patients with hearing loss. For instance, it is known from clinical research that multifrequency tympanometry yields more diagnostic information than conventional acoustic immittance, yet multifrequency tympanometry is rarely implemented in clinical practice (Martin et al, 1998). Of course, there are valid reasons for not embracing the routine use of multifrequency tympanometry in clinical practice. Implementation requires replacing existing equipment with new equipment that may be more expensive, larger, and less portable. Practicing audiologists are used to single-frequency immittance, and many do not feel comfortable interpreting results of multifrequency testing. Depending on the patient population, the additional diagnostic information may be more or less helpful to the clinician. Given the known benefits of multifrequency immittance, however, it is likely that it will become the test of choice if/when it is packaged for ease of service delivery (i.e., automated, quick, compact) and interpretation (e.g., automated diagnostic categories).

Here is how the three-dimensional management model works in this example:

1. *In the business*   The organizational objective is to include acoustic immittance as part of every comprehensive audiometry evaluation in a cost-effective manner. Multifrequency immittance equipment will not be purchased for this purpose unless proven to be cost effective.

2. *In the human organization*   The audiologists who perform acoustic immittance tests want equipment that is accessible, rapid, reliable, and results oriented. Management needs input from the audiologists after they have had an opportunity to test the multifrequency immittance equipment in the clinic and compare it with their present equipment. If the audiologists' responses are mixed, management may discuss these ergonomic issues with the equipment manufacturer or supplier.

3. *In the dimension of public interest*   The organization is aware that multifrequency acoustic immittance affords better diagnostic information in some cases. The first step is to estimate differences in diagnostic outcomes for a representative patient sample that would accrue if single-tone immittance were replaced by multifrequency immittance in the clinical protocol, based on outcome measures collected in other practice settings. If outcome differences are deemed clinically significant, the next step is to make the case to consumers in an attempt to influence reimbursement decisions.

Management's role is to balance the information gleaned from the public interest analyses against business objectives and audiologists' needs and to develop an equation in which estimated value to consumers and projected revenue to the business exceed the financial and human costs of new equipment (e.g., purchase price, physical placement and access, training time, test administration time, test interpretation time). A key aspect of dynamic practice management in this example is that it works proactively rather than reactively. The final steps in the human organization and public interest analyses call for management to use clinical data to influence equipment manufacturers' and payers' reimbursement rates. These proactive stances illustrate how practice management works by turning frictions into dynamic tensions that serve to improve and advance the organization in all three dimensions.

Special Consideration

- A key aspect of dynamic practice management is that it works proactively rather than reactively.

Other Issues that Cause Friction

Some of the issues in **Table 1–3** have already been discussed or alluded to in other contexts. For example, in the previous example regarding acoustic immittance, the potential exists for future friction if clinical data support the use of multifrequency tympanometry but managed care refuses to reimburse for that service at a higher rate (friction between what is recommended and what is reimbursed, between what is complete and what is allowed). If that friction arises, it begs the question of whether the better test should be administered to patients even if they cannot pay for it (friction between health care as a right and as a privilege). The audiologists may have concerns that reflect their graduate training in immittance testing (friction between what was taught and what is practiced). Suppose, for example, that the clinical data support the use of multifrequency tympanometry, but the equipment is too expensive to purchase (friction between what is needed and what is available, between organizational needs and patient needs); or suppose that a hearing aid manufacturer offers to purchase the immittance equipment for the practice in return for a minimum of 10 hearing aid orders a month (friction between what is ethical and what is unethical) (Iskowitz, 1998).

The list goes on, even for simple diagnostic examples. One can only imagine the list attached to controversial hearing aid fitting approaches or different balance assessment protocols. Frictions and subfrictions abound, and practice management must anticipate such frictions by using SWOT analyses and by making informed decisions.

◆ Management Competencies and Training

Practice management does not always work. Numerous examples of failed management decisions causing organizational setbacks exist. Practice management does not work in the absence of management competencies. In almost every case, management competencies are not innate but are acquired by training.

Areas of Learning

In the first edition of this book, we surmised that practice management failure stemmed from limitations in graduate education programs and practicum settings: at the time, business and management issues were considered superficially or not included in audiology curricula. The training situation is improving somewhat with the advent of Au.D. programs. Although some programs offer or require nothing beyond a professional practices course, others offer practice management or basic business courses as electives or even required courses. More obligatory business and management training is needed as these programs mature. An example of the underlying mind-set in academic settings may be found in ASHA's most recent scope of practice outline (ASHA, 2004b), which includes a resource bibliography for 13 categories of practice and training. The sole category for business, business practices, has only five references, none more recent than 1997.

Some years ago, ASHA (1995) published curriculum guidelines for practice management that identified six areas of knowledge and skill (see Appendix 1–1):

- Basic management
- Service planning
- Practice, business, and government rules
- Computers and office automation
- Quality improvement issues
- Risk management and professional liability

Over a decade after the ASHA publication, few Au.D. programs have integrated all of these guidelines into their curricula, and no professional organization has updated them.

In anticipation of transitioning to an Au.D. entry-level degree, ASHA (2006) developed new audiology standards and revised its accreditation standards for academic programs (ASHA, 2004c). The new standards do not stipulate course requirements, but they do require unspecified measures of competencies in each standards area. Insofar as this relates to a business management curriculum, Standard IV-B, "Foundations of Practice," states that applicants must "demonstrate acquisition of knowledge" of "supervisory processes and procedures" and "laws, regulations, policies, and management practices relevant to the profession of audiology" (see Sections B-19 and B-20). The fact that the new standards require some demonstration of competencies related to management or business skill has to be taken as an improvement in audiology education.

In audiology, the curricular standards of the Accreditation Council for Audiology Education (ACAE) identify professional responsibilities and values as one of the seven categories in which Au.D. programs must train students and measure their competencies. Included in that category are

- Professional ethics
- Professional, legal, public health, and public policy issues
- Practice management strategies and principles as they apply to audiology

- Business, financial, and reimbursement considerations necessary for operating a practice

Training in these subjects is a good start, but it does not prepare audiologists sufficiently to own or manage private practices or clinics. In the current educational milieu, Henson et al (2006) conclude that "[t]he most obvious implication is the need for dramatically expanded business training and education for audiologists" (p. 54). To address this need, Au.D. programs must incorporate aspects of all eight curricular areas that compose what is considered the common body of knowledge for business: accounting, finance, information systems, law, management, marketing, economics, and quantitative methods.

> **Pitfall**
>
> - Practice management does not work in the absence of management competencies.

Human Resource Management

Audiologists with good professional skills often open practices without first preparing a sufficient business case. Their practices flounder or fail for a variety of reasons, usually related to high overhead, poor organizational skills, poor tax planning, or inadequate or inappropriate marketing.

Some practices, in contrast, flourish, either because of sheer luck or because the audiologists possess innate business acumen. New practices that experience early success, however, often have to deal with problems that arise as a result of human resource mismanagement. As a practice grows, additional audiologists are often hired to handle the workload and increase the bottom line. If a growing staff is not carefully managed, the typical result is high staff turnover with concomitant increases in staff training costs and decreases in productivity. This is not an indictment of audiology practices, but a general observation that human resource management is a rare and highly valuable skill in any organization.

Some audiologists avoid this problem by staying small, rationalizing that the only way to get things done right is to do it themselves. Three practice management problems exist with this approach—one for each of the three practice management dimensions:

1. *In the business*   Organizational growth and profit are limited to the productivity of one audiologist, who must try to see new patients while caring for an ever-growing backlog of patients requiring follow-up care.

2. *In the human organization*   The only asset is the lone audiologist, who runs the risk of burnout as the practice tries to grow in spite of itself.

3. *In the public interest*   Continuity of services to patients depends on the health, age, and motivation of the lone audiologist.

This is negative practice management in action: business trends show negative growth over time; and the value of the practice dies when the audiologist moves on or retires, leaving patients stranded.

All the preceding scenarios are reasons why audiologists must acquire some practice management training and competencies. Training opportunities are present within the profession: continuing education and publications on practice management topics are offered by state and national professional organizations, hearing industry manufacturers, and trade and professional journals. Several Web sites also offer general or audiology-specific management information. This textbook is devoted entirely to practice management education for audiologists.

A readily available option for gaining practice management proficiency is to journey beyond the profession for management training. Audiologists can search out training by enrolling in accounting, business, or computer classes offered by the Small Business Administration, by local colleges or universities, or online at audiologyonline.com and other Web sites.

Yet another option is to go outside the profession to obtain a management team. Arguments exist as to whether this approach yields good or bad management of audiology practices. The arguments are best framed with reference to the three-dimensional model of practice management. On the pro side, outside managers are trained in how to manage businesses and human resources to achieve organizational objectives and optimize productivity. Large audiology practices and professional organizations that employ office managers or management teams with degrees in business administration endorse this approach wholeheartedly (see Kieserman, 1996). Practices of all sizes that outsource some jobs (e.g., payroll accounting, computer support, and marketing) acknowledge the usefulness of the approach without embracing it totally.

On the con side, the competencies of nonaudiology managers usually do not include an appreciation of the "patient-first" training that distinguishes audiology, dentistry, medicine, and so on as health-related professions (Hosford-Dunn, 2006). When one part of three practice management dimensions is diminished, all parts are affected, and the careful balancing act may fail. In this instance, the outside management rightly perceives a fiduciary duty to the organization (e.g., private practice owner, corporate shareholders, and elected officials) and translates this duty into business objectives that audiologists are expected to meet by their daily actions and productivity (emphasis on business organization and directives to human organization). Just as rightfully, the audiologists perceive a fiduciary duty to their patients first and the business second (emphasis on public interest dimension before business organization).

When business objectives are set by outside managers with insufficient regard for professional objectives, the human organization is pulled in two directions and may break down because a patient-first attitude prevails over management's demand for productivity or because audiologists subsume professional responsibility to business demands. Either way, loss of balance places practitioners and organizations at risk: in the former, because the business no longer turns a profit; in the latter, because day-to-day operations may not endure ethical or legal scrutiny. All scenarios point to a failure of practice management.

◆ Structure of this Book

As editors of this volume, we identified certain common frictions seen by us and by the chapter authors, who are themselves competent audiologists trying to grapple with various aspects of practice and management. In most instances, these tensions, as outlined in **Table 1–3**, derive from discussions that surfaced as the authors prepared the various chapters. Their efforts are consistent with one purpose of this volume, which is to respond to these nagging issues with infusions of structured information, much of it integrated from sources outside the discipline and profession of audiology.

These issues were closely coupled to a call for guiding principles for managing our practices. To address this, the book is divided into "Principles" and "Applications" sections, the latter grouped as "Practice Management Applications" and "Business Applications." However, the superficial and near-random consideration of management issues in graduate training noted earlier makes it difficult to arrive at an all-inclusive set of principles, and some readers may take issue with our efforts to categorize chapters. Those authors who agreed to write chapters for the "Principles" section of this volume explore new territory or bring new order to old ground. The latter is exemplified by Theodore J. Glattke's work in Chapter 2. Glattke identifies the "overreaching principles" underlying ethical codes while acknowledging that ethical applications are neither absolute nor agreed upon in our profession. Much new ground is covered in Chapter 3 by Harvey Abrams and Theresa Hnath Chisolm, who introduce the related principles of quality and evidence-based practice. Another common issue is that audiologists have little exposure to other disciplines whose principles form the very core of the business aspects of audiology practices. Many audiologists may find that statement almost nonsensical: how can another discipline form the core of an audiology practice? Chapter 4 by David Allen Zapala, Kathryn L. Shaughnessy, and Ashley Snyder and Chapter 5 by Wayne J. Staab pull together structured principles from public policy, business management, and marketing. These compelling discussions convincingly show that audiologists are not the first managers to encounter thorny personnel issues, discover mentoring, perform needs assessments, or collect and analyze data. It is a humbling and exhilarating experience to realize that audiologists can tap into cohesive theories and well-done research in disciplines much larger and older than audiology, rather than dealing

---

Pearl

- Human resource management is a rare and highly valuable skill in any organization.

with such issues piecemeal and superficially. A closely related issue is that audiologists lack the education and practicum experience in technical, business, and management applications. How can they know what they do not know? Chapter 6 by Teresa M. Clark and Darcy Benson is a remarkably condensed look at the broad range of private practice issues that can and do arise. The chapter belongs in this section because it makes the important point that private practitioners must wear many "hats." Consistent with that principle, this chapter serves as a jumping off point for the rest of the book, which is organized according to practice applications. The "Practice Management Applications" section comprises six chapters addressing issues that arise in most audiology practices. In Chapter 7, Kadyn Williams, Helena Stern Solodar, and H. Carol Saul tackle the legalese of the Health Insurance Portability and Accountability Act (HIPAA). Outcome measures are addressed in Chapter 8 by Abrams and Chisolm. Zapala covers all aspects of documentation in Chapter 9. A. U. Bankaitis and Robert J. Kemp in Chapter 10 and Ross J. Roeser and Philip L. Wilson in Chapter 11 educate readers on the principles of infection control and the characteristics of cerumen, respectively, and proceed to describe clinical procedures for both. The "Practice Management Applications" section ends with new Chapter 12, by Gyl A. Kasewurm and Kris English, who address many of the thorny supervision issues surrounding assistants and fourth-year Au.D. students in clinical practice. This group of chapters is editorially interesting because it illustrates the uneven development of different aspects of audiology practice management and the resulting tensions: some that are done are well documented but controversial (cerumen management), some that are universally accepted to the point that they are de facto principles (infection control), some that enjoy the status of organizational principles but are not implemented consistently (evidence-based practices and outcome measurement), some that are commonplace but lack consensus as to how they should be done (documentation, supervision), and some that have definite rules of implementation but few tools for doing so (HIPAA).

The third section of this volume, "Business Applications," covers a range of topics, underscoring the "many hats" principle of Clark and Benson. The section begins with Kasewurm's explanation of elements that comprise the business plan, in Chapter 13. The new Chapter 14, "Designing Audiology Prac-

tices," by Jane Hildreth Baxter, Deborah W. Clark, and Alan L. Desmond, includes a separate discussion on special considerations for designing a vestibular/balance clinic. Another new chapter, Chapter 15, by Joy Colle Benn and Robert M. Traynor, breathes life into the normally deadly topic of practice accounting. Other menacing but necessary topics for audiologists are Medicare and reimbursement (Chapter 16), covered by Robert C. Fifer, and proposing audiology services to group providers (Chapter 17), covered by Kathy Anne Foltner. Computer principles and applications, relegated to its own section in the first edition, is a bona fide member of the "Business Applications" section in this edition. Chapter 18, by Robert R. De Jonge and J. Mark Goffinet, gives in-depth education and practical tips for almost every conceivable audiology computer application. This final, important chapter should be frequently referenced when reading other chapters in this book.

◆ Summary

Looking toward the future, Hosford-Dunn et al (1995) commented and predicted in a chapter entitled "Audiologists as Managers": "The old-fashioned scope of management to control and monitor is being replaced with new requirements to motivate, train, support, and lead. As audiologists learn and implement modern management concepts, the profession has an opportunity to improve the level of service to patients and become a more vigorous entry point into the health care system" (p. 480). The fact that an entire volume of an audiology series is now dedicated to teaching and implementing practice management marks an important step toward incorporating management principles into audiology training programs and practices. As editors, we have worked closely with all of the authors represented here and have come to believe that the three-dimensional model of practice management is not only exciting and inspirational, but is doable. By learning to be managers and by managing practices well, audiologists have the potential to enhance all aspects of the profession: improve service delivery, empower practitioners, raise profitability, expand market visibility, and increase the satisfaction of both providers and patients.

Appendix 1–1

Guidelines for Education in Practice Management

The Guidelines for Education in Practice Management were prepared by the American Speech-Language-Hearing Association (ASHA) Ad Hoc Committee on Practice Management in Audiology and approved by the ASHA Executive Board (EGB 2–94) and 1994 Legislative Council (LC 8–94). Members of the committee who prepared the guidelines include Holly Hosford-Dunn, chair; Jane H. Baxter; Evelyn Cherow, ex officio; Alan L. Desmond; Gary Jacobson; Jean L. Johnson; and Patty F. Martin. Diane L. Eger, vice president for professional practices (1991–1993), served as monitoring vice president. These guidelines are an official statement of ASHA. They provide guidance on the use of specific practice procedures but are not official standards of the association.

Specific Competency Areas in Practice Management

These areas are directly related to practice management and are suggested for inclusion in a model curriculum for a graduate-level course in practice management in audiology. They are considered the minimum requirements for providing an adequate base of knowledge for managing a practice. Students should be encouraged to take additional classes in cognate areas such as accounting and marketing. Persons managing or directing audiology services should demonstrate knowledge of, and skills in, the following areas:

1. Basic management
   a. Preparation of feasibility studies, market surveys, business plans
   b. Account management, budgeting, billing and collections
   c. Knowledge of financial reports (balance sheet, income statement)
   d. Human resource management/staff recruiting
   e. Knowledge of health care models (e.g., preferred provider organization [PPO], health maintenance organization [HMO], fee for service, sliding scale)
   f. Marketing
   g. Contracts and negotiations
   h. Financial planning/retirement plans

2. Service planning
   a. Physical plant
      i. Site selection
      ii. Equipment selection
      iii. Leasing space and/or equipment
      iv. Automation
   b. Service structure
      i. Record keeping
      ii. Establishing referral networks
      iii. Scheduling patients
      iv. Fee setting

3. Practice, business, and government rules
   a. Americans with Disabilities Act (ADA) accessibility considerations
   b. Federal employment laws
   c. Accreditation requirements (e.g., Joint Commission on Accreditation of Health Care Organizations [JCAHO], ASHA Professional Services Board [PSB], Commission on Accreditation of Rehabilitation Facilities [CARF])
   d. Antitrust regulations
   e. Business entities: tax implication and government reporting regulations
   f. Requirements for nonprofit status
   g. Ethical codes of practice
   h. Licensing requirements

4. Computers and office automation
   a. Diagnostic applications
   b. Data storage/access
   c. Tracking patient outcomes and consumer satisfaction
   d. Professional correspondence
   e. Scheduling and billing
   f. Marketing applications

5. Quality improvement issues
   a. Personnel/leadership training
   b. Client satisfaction/functional assessment
   c. Supervision
   d. Multicultural issues
   e. Professionalism (interactions with competitors, colleagues, associates, agencies)

6. Risk management and professional liability
   a. Insurance
   b. Best practice guidelines and preferred practice patterns
   c. Malpractice trends in the profession
   d. Infection control requirements

Source: American Speech-Language-Hearing Association. (1995). Guidelines for Education in Audiology Practice Management. ASHA, 37 (Suppl. 14); 20.

References

Accreditation Commission for Audiology Education. (2005). Accreditation standards for the doctor of audiology (Au.D.) program. Retrieved June 23, 2006, from http:// www.acaeaccred.org/Documents/ACAE_STANDS_2005r8_05.pdf

American Speech-Language-Hearing Association. (1995). Guidelines for education in audiology practice management. ASHA, 37(Suppl. 14), 20.

American Speech-Language-Hearing Association. (2004a). Audiology survey 2004. Retrieved February 21, 2007, from http://www.asha.org/ NR/rdonlyres/BAC4D9B0-4A5E-483A-A1CE-1015952C83F2/0/04_Audiology_Survey_method. pdf

American Speech-Language-Hearing Association. (2004b). Scope of practice in audiology, 2004–1. Retrieved February 21, 2007, from http://www.asha.org/NR/rdonlyres/036AC2B1-FB02-4124-8709-80881C1079A6/0/v1ScopeofPracticeAudiology.pdf

American Speech-Language-Hearing Association. (2004c). Standards for accreditation of graduate education programs in audiology and speech-language pathology. Retrieved February 21, 2007, from http://www.asha.org/NR/rdonlyres/F6769B82-5583-4978-A6D8-CEC5882A5A4D/0/v1STDAccreditation.pdf

American Speech-Language-Hearing Association. (2006, February 24). 2007 Audiology standards. Retrieved February 21, 2007, from http://www. asha.org/about/membership-certification/certification/aud_standards_new.htm

Anderson, J. J., & Nemes, J. (2004). Lessons from other fields can help audiology complete its transformation. Hearing Journal, 57(10), 28–32.

Brady, J. R., & Granville, Y. (2006). It's time to step up to the plate! Audiology Today, 18(3), 29.

Drucker, P. F. (1986). The practice of management. New York: Harper & Row.

Dybala, P. (2006, March 6). ELVAS sightings—hearing aid or headset? Audiology Online. Retrieved February 16, 2007, from http://www.audiology-online.com/articles/article_detail.asp?article_id=1542

Federal Reserve Board. (2006, January 18). Remarks by Governor Susan Schmidt Bies before the Tech Council of Maryland's Financial Executive Forum, Bethesda, Maryland. Retrieved February 16, 2007, from http://www.federalreserve.gov/boarddocs/speeches/2006/20060118/default.htm

Henson, S., Williamson, S., & Jacques, P. (2006). Business training and education needs of audiology managers. Audiology Today, 18(2), 49–54.

Hosford-Dunn, H. (2006). Integrated Marketing Communications (IMC), Part I - CRM: The Ginsu Knife for Marketing. Audiology Online. Retrieved February 16, 2007, from http://www.audiologyonline.com/articles/article_detail.asp?article_id=1630

Hosford-Dunn, H. L., Dunn, D. R., & Harford, E. R. (1995). Audiology business and practice management. San Diego, CA: Singular Publishing Group.

Hosford-Dunn, H., Roeser, R., & Valente, M. (2000). Audiology: Practice management. New York: Thieme Medical Publishers.

Iskowitz, M. (1998). Manufacturers as partners. Advance for Speech-Language Pathologists and Audiologists, January 26, 13–15, 29.

Kieserman, R. (1996). Hiring administrator can benefit practice. Advance for Speech-Language Pathologists and Audiologists, September 30, 3.

Martin, F. N., Champlin, C. A., & Chambers, J. A. (1998). Seventh survey of audiometric practices in the United States. Journal of the American Academy of Audiology, 9(2), 95–104.

Nemko, M. (2006, January 5). Money: Excellent careers for 2006. U.S. News and World Report. Retrieved June 6, 2006, from http://www.us-news.com/usnews/biztech/articles/060105/5careers_excellent.htm

Smith, M. G., & Windmill, I. M. (2006). A comparison of entrance and graduation requirements for the Au.D. with other first professional degrees. Journal of the American Academy of Audiology, 17(5), 321–330.

Stoner, J. A. F., & Wankel, C. (1986). Management (3rd ed.). Englewood Cliffs, NJ: Prentice-Hall.

Strom, K. E. (2006). The HR 2006 dispenser survey. The Hearing Review. Retrieved from http://www.hearingreview.com/issues/articles/2006-06_11.asp on February 16, 2007

Strom, K. E. (2005). The HR 2005 dispenser survey. The Hearing Review, 12(6), 18–36, 72.

Section I

Principles

Chapter 2

Professional Ethics and Audiology

Theodore J. Glattke

♦ **Ethical Principles in Audiology**
♦ **Ethical Principles of Health-Related Professions**

Nuremberg Code

Belmont Report

♦ **Applying the Principles**
♦ **Summary**

♦ Ethical Principles in Audiology

The professional behavior of audiologists is guided by ideas that stem from customs, laws, regulations, personal values, and ethical codes adopted by professional and lay communities and other organizations. These are mutable forces that are influenced by individual life and community experiences with roots that can be traced to the earliest recorded history. Hinchcliffe (2003) provides a guided tour of issues related to custom, religion, ethics, customary law, which functions to preserve social harmony, and, more formally, the enforceable body of rules known as law that is designed to resolve conflicts. His review is extensive and reaches far beyond narrow professional ethics, as he surveys religious principles ranging from Hinduism to Shintoism, major legal systems, standards writing organizations, and the state of flux that characterizes the status of ethics throughout the world.

As Hinchcliffe notes, a common ethical code for everyone engaged in health care may be desirable to establish important values and create a common ethical context for the provision of care, but it may not be helpful in addressing unanticipated problems (Hinchcliffe, 2003; see also Limentani, 1999).

In audiology, the tremendous expansion of knowledge, communication links, and technology in recent years has created spectacular opportunities to reduce the risk of acquiring hearing loss and to ameliorate the effects of hearing impairment. At the same time, the progress has created ethical dilemmas that were unforeseen a few years ago.

As examples, the combination of newborn hearing screening, DNA analysis, and recent breakthroughs in genetics research provide audiologists with new opportunities and new responsibilities regarding the hearing health care of infants and support of their families. If audiologists are gatekeepers for persons with hearing problems, they must be fully prepared to know when to make referrals for low-incidence problems.

> **Special Consideration**
>
> - If audiologists are gatekeepers, they must be fully prepared to know when to make referrals for low-incidence problems.

Because of recent developments in understanding regarding Jervell and Lange-Neilsen syndrome (Schwartz et al, 2006), for instance, good audiological practice may dictate that infants with congenital hearing loss should be referred for cardiologic studies. The audiologist has access to all of the information needed regarding prevalence of this rare, but often fatal, combination of disorders and may be the first professional in a position to evaluate the need for additional diagnostic studies. Who should make the referral? Should the referral be made only by a physician?

As another example, 40 years ago, cochlear implants were experimental devices, and clinical investigators who were pioneers in the field often encountered palpable professional barriers, often presented under the cover of ethics (Merzenich et al, 1974). Implantation was limited to adults with no usable hearing, and a delay of 2 years between the onset of hearing loss and the implantation was the norm. Today, cochlear implants are performed on infants and young children, "short electrode" implants are being offered to combine artificial electrical stimulation and residual hearing, and it is not unusual to be able to communicate with a cochlear implant user via telephone. Boundaries of the scope of practice of audiology and all professions are pushed by such developments, often long before professional organizations, regulatory agencies, or legislative groups recognize the new landmarks. As a consequence, the rule makers usually find themselves reacting to changes that have occurred in the scope of practice, rather than anticipating changes.

A classic struggle—reacting to rather than anticipating change—was the battle over audiologists' right to dispense hearing aids while conforming to the ethical principles of the American Speech-Language-Hearing Association (ASHA). The prohibition was ultimately eliminated by ASHA's reaction to a U.S. Supreme Court decision that held that prohibition of competition among members of a professional association could not be constrained by the association (ASHA, 1978).

In the United States, three organizations that support the professional activities of audiologists, the Academy of Doctors of Audiologists (ADA), the American Academy of Audiology (AAA), and ASHA, have published codes of ethical behavior (ADA, 2006; AAA, 2006; ASHA, 2003). The respective codes begin with statements of principles that include directives for practitioners.

The ADA (2006) code of ethics states:

Principle I: To protect the welfare of persons served professionally.

Principle II: To maintain high standards of professional competence, integrity, conduct, and ethics.

Principle III: To maintain a professional demeanor in matters concerning the welfare of persons served.

Principle IV: To provide accurate information to persons served and to the public about the nature and management of auditory disorders and about the profession and services provided by its members.

Principle V: To engage in conduct which shall enhance the status of the profession.

Principle VI: To maintain ethical standards and practices of the Academy of Dispensing Audiologists.

The AAA (2006) principles are the following:

Principle 1: Members shall provide professional services and conduct research with honesty and compassion, and shall respect the dignity, worth, and rights of those served.

Principle 2: Members shall maintain high standards of professional competence in rendering services.

Principle 3: Members shall maintain the confidentiality of the information and records of those receiving services or involved in research.

Principle 4: Members shall provide only services and products that are in the best interest of those served.

Principle 5: Members shall provide accurate information about the nature and management of communicative disorders and about the services and products offered.

Principle 6: Members shall comply with the ethical standards of the Academy with regard to public statements or publication.

Principle 7: Members shall honor their responsibilities to the public and to professional colleagues.

Principle 8: Members shall uphold the dignity of the profession and freely accept the Academy's self-imposed standards.

The ASHA (2003) code includes the following:

Principle of Ethics I: Individuals shall honor their responsibility to hold paramount the welfare of persons they serve professionally or participants in research and scholarly activities and shall treat animals involved in research in a humane manner.

Principle of Ethics II: Individuals shall honor their responsibility to achieve and maintain the highest level of professional competence.

Principle of Ethics III: Individuals shall honor their responsibility to the public by promoting public understanding of the professions, by supporting the development of services designed to fulfill unmet needs of the public and by providing accurate information in all communications involving any aspect of the professions, including dissemination of research findings and scholarly activities.

Principle of Ethics IV: Individuals shall honor their responsibilities to the professions and their relationships with colleagues, students and members of allied professions. Individuals shall uphold the dignity and autonomy of the professions, maintain harmonious inter-professional and intra-professional relationships and accept the professions' self-imposed standards.

The ADA code contains a preamble that describes the purpose of the code as providing "the assurance of the highest quality of professional service." The AAA code has no preamble. The ASHA code includes a preamble that identifies the population of practitioners who are responsible for upholding the code. The codes themselves present sets of rules of behavior that follow principles. Under ideal conditions, one could find guidance from these rules that would help determine if a specific action on the part of a member were within the ethical guidelines of the professional group.

None of the professional codes offer discussion about the development or rational basis of the principles, and, as such, they do not present ethical frameworks from which their principles are derived.

This chapter offers information regarding overreaching principles that are recognized as the foundations of the ethical codes of health-related professions. The intent is to provide readers with an analytical framework that will enable them to give thoughtful consideration to professional practice.

Pearl

- According to Annas (2005), "American bioethics is often more pragmatic than principled."

✦ Ethical Principles of Health-Related Professions

Nuremberg Code

The discipline of ethics is as old as recorded history, and, as Gillon (1994) asserts, debates regarding distribution of resources, recognition of patients' rights, and respect for laws/regulations are no closer to resolution today than they were in Aristotle's time. Vanderpool (2002) reminds us that ethical considerations of issues requires some type of framework based on commonly accepted ethical principles. As audiologists are assuming increased responsibilities for audiological diagnosis and treatment of hearing and balance problems experienced by their patients, it is pertinent to consider some history based in allied fields, such as medicine. The modern history of bioethics began at the closing days of World War II. Widespread abuse of persons during the war led to the development of the Nuremberg Code ("Trials of War Criminals," 1949–1953), which articulated 10 principles that must be observed in the conduct of research involving human participants and, by implication, professional interaction with them, as well.

Although the foundation of modern bioethics was forged at Nuremberg, the practical adoption of the kernel elements of the code was slow to arrive in the research and professional practice arenas. As Annas (2005) has noted, "American bioethics is often more pragmatic than principled" (p. 3). This is well illustrated by the history of abuse of patients and others at the hands of professional practitioners and researchers that continued unabated for at least 25 years after publication of the Nuremberg Code.

When discussing concepts related to the protection of clinical patients and others who participate in research projects with students and colleagues, few audience members correctly identify the country that has tolerated the following sorts of activities:

- Infecting children in a residential institution with hepatitis virus (Krugman, 1986)

- Injecting live cancer cells into senile patients (Finn, 1999)

- Denying appropriate treatment to persons with sexually transmitted diseases and lying to them about their medical care (Jones, 1993)

- Inducing orphans to stutter (Dyer, 2001)

The correct answer is the United States of America. In some instances, the abuse was conducted with support from public funds and monitored by federal agencies. Beecher (1966) turned the spotlight on many abuses of patients involved in clinical trials and set the stage for a maturation of ethical principles to address the intimate relationship between professional service provider and patient.

Belmont Report

The National Commission for the Protection of Human Subjects of Biomedical and Behavioral Research was created by the U.S. Congress in 1973. The commission membership was dominated by persons with expertise in theology, philosophy, ethics, and law. A landmark document, commonly known as the Belmont report, was published in 1979 (U.S. Department of Health, Education, and Welfare, 1979). The report first addressed the thorny issue of boundaries between clinical practice and research. Although that boundary may not seem to be an issue for the routine practice of audiology, there are important analogies between that debate and changes in practice that one might choose to make without sufficient evidence in support of the efficacy of the change.

The Belmont report identifies three basic ethical principles: respect for persons, beneficence, and justice.

Respect for Persons

This principle is based on the conviction that individuals should be treated as autonomous agents. Persons who are autonomous are able to participate in deliberation regarding their actions and are capable of acting on the outcome of that deliberation. To adhere to this principle, the audiologist must refrain from interfering with the actions of patients unless there is some compelling reason to do so. In addition, many patients encountered in the practice of audiology may have diminished capacity for self-determination. This may result from mental or physical limitations, immaturity or aging, or economic constraints. These individuals warrant additional protection, perhaps in the form of engagement of an advocate. Audiologists whose practices include the very young and the very old, persons with multiple disabilities, and individuals who are disadvantaged economically will do well to maintain respect for persons as an organizing principle.

Beneficence

The principle of beneficence underlies professional behavior that not only respects patients' decisions and protects them from harm, but also is directed toward securing their well-being. The extensions of this principle lead to the demand that we maximize possible benefits to our patients. Many patients who are in their 7th and 8th decade of life are active, vital, often athletic individuals who have as much interest in knowing where a tennis ball lands as playing a sedate game of cards. Twenty years ago, audiologists might have advised them to remove their hearing aids, to avoid damage due to perspiration, while participating in sports. Today, that is unacceptable. The principle of beneficence dictates that the audiologist learn about patients' desires and needs and do everything possible within the scope of practice to help them maintain their lives as they wish.

Justice

The principle of justice translates to a question of fairness of distribution of resources. As the Belmont report notes, there are several popular approaches to the determination of how benefit may be distributed: (1) each person receives an equal share, (2) each person receives benefits according to need, (3) each person receives benefits in proportion to individual effort, (4) benefits are received by persons according to their societal contributions, and (5) benefits are distributed according to merit. If public funds are used to develop and improve diagnostic tools and therapeutic devices and procedures, the principle of justice fuels debate regarding who receives benefit from the tools, as well as the procedures and the distribution of the devices. The continuum outlined above is accompanied by an increasing responsibility to judge each recipient's position in the society providing the benefit.

An area of concern that stems from the need to apply the principle of justice is centered on the provision of hearing aids to persons who need them. The principle of justice may demand that the system of manufacturing, promotion, federal oversight, and distribution of hearing aids be continuously examined to ensure that resources reach those in need. On one hand, this may involve employing public funding to enable patients to purchase expensive technology. On the other, it may involve removing hearing aids from Food and Drug Administration (FDA) control so that they become essentially over-the-counter products (Boswell, 2003). The combination of over-the-counter and professionally prescribed products is employed in the area of vision health, and the debate regarding treating hearing aids in the same manner promises to be engaging. If only a small proportion of the persons needing hearing aids in the United States (or the world) has access to them, does the audiologist have a role in changing the distribution systems? If so, what is that role? Does the audiologist have a role in protecting the environment from the waste products of the technology? What about recycling of resources? If patients are granted direct access to audiologists through federal or private insurance plans, how will the responsibilities of the audiologist change in terms of overall care of the patients?

Controversial Point

- Does the audiologist have a role in changing the distribution systems for hearing aids?

Nonmaleficence

To this list, Gillon (1994) adds a fourth principle, nonmaleficence. Nonmaleficence obliges every practitioner to advocate only practices well documented as being effective. Ethical practice obligates a practitioner to find the best information available on proposed innovations, to speak out for practices with substantive proof supporting their value, and to strongly question the value of schemes that lack such proof. Charting the best course of action can be difficult. Ross (2006) reminds us that the practice of fitting binaural amplification was, at first, nearly impossible, then thought to be unethical, and finally became the norm. The process

spanned almost 50 years. Upon publication of a landmark study of cochlear implants, Simmons (1966, p. 52) noted, "The chances are small indeed that electrical stimulation of the auditory nerve can ever provide a uniquely useful means of communication." Some 20 years later, Simmons (1985, p. 2) confessed that his frustration was created, in part, by his perception that work in the area of cochlear implants lacked needed support from the scientific community. He noted:

> While skepticism engendered by claimed miracles is healthy, outright denial that a genuine research problem exists is not. While my 1964–65 experiments were in progress I contacted a least six of the most prominent researchers in speech coding, and others in auditory psychophysics. None of these persons were willing or interested in suggesting experiments which might have helped define speech coding strategies for the future. I got the distinct impression, perhaps colored by a little personal paranoia after the first few rejections, that most everyone was either incapable of thinking about the many problems involved or would rather not risk tainting their scientific careers. I do not believe this problem has disappeared completely in the subsequent 20 years.

The time interval between the first explorations of stimulation of the auditory nerve as a means of providing auditory input to persons with hearing loss and approval by the FDA for widespread use of cochlear implants was shorter than the interval described by Ross (2006) for monaural to binaural amplification, but there is much inertia in the scientific, professional, and regulatory systems. Ethical guidelines offered over 30 years ago (Merzenich et al, 1974) continue to evolve and remain the subject of debate, particularly regarding the use of cochlear implants in children (Berg et al, 2005; Lane and Bahan, 1998).

There are many other important examples of the inertia in the basic and clinical sciences. The interval, for example, between von Békésy's initial observations of passive traveling waves and the acceptance that a living ear performs differently than a cadaver ear at low intensities spans more than 50 years. Kemp (2004, 2007) has reviewed the natural history of the interval between initial discovery and clinical acceptance of audiological tools. It is fairly constant for tympanometry, auditory brainstem responses, and otoacoustic emissions: about 25 years.

ASHA (2004) offers some guidelines regarding adoption of new practice strategies. The guidelines include suggestions for types of acceptable evidence and advance the notion that the development of evidence of the efficacy of a clinical practice may require several years of accumulated experience or continuous adjustment in the face of new valid research. For example, an audiologist who decides to incorporate a combination of pure-tone air-conduction thresholds and tympanometric findings but exclude bone-conduction measures from routine practice to increase efficiency should be aware that patients with large vestibular aqueduct syndrome may present with air–bone gaps and normal tympanometric results (Mimura et al, 2005). Undetected, the condition may lead to sudden deafness.

The principle of nonmaleficence may offer the greatest challenge, as practitioners try to balance innovation against accepted practice.

◆ Applying the Principles

Paraphrasing Nuhfer (2001), a clinical practice based on a code of ethics has nothing to do with being preachy or claiming the moral high ground. It has to do with the practical realization that all professionals face difficult situations and need to exercise sophisticated judgment. A functional ethical framework offers a powerful tool—a compass—in carrying out this work. A code of ethics resists yielding to the moment. In work where judgment can be clouded by personal feelings, institutional culture, pressure from authority, fads, or rationalizations, reflection upon each of the four ethical principles described above and a quick review of whether each is violated or honored can help improve the chances of making truly competent decisions.

As Annas (2005, p. 98) notes, the courts have made it clear that the doctor–patient relationship is a fiduciary, or trust, relationship, not an arm's-length business relationship. This means that the audiologist and his or her patient have unequal status and that the audiologist must provide information than enables the patient, not the audiologist, to make a decision on how to proceed. A key element in the relationship is that the patient must be fully informed. Annas (2005) further notes, "Attempts to transform the doctor–patient relationship into a business transaction fundamentally threaten not just . . . professionals but people as patients."

This means, for example, that many common business practices involving incentives from suppliers of goods and services cannot be embraced by the audiologist.

Shinn (2004) reviews this issue in a thoughtful essay that asks if the rules that govern retail sales apply to audiologists. He counters the argument that the professional practice of audiology is simply a business by suggesting that if goods provided by audiologists to their patients are simply retail products, then anyone should be allowed to sell them. He notes that the privileges that professionals enjoy can be retained only if they follow ethical guidelines that hold them apart from the world of free market commerce. The fiduciary link in business is between the organization and its shareholders. Trust between the organization and its customers stems from honesty and integrity, but business organizations do not carry the full burdens of respect for persons, beneficence, justice,

and nonmaleficence. La Puma (1998) says it succinctly: "Doctors care for patients; business people return value."

There is no written guide that will lead the professional through all possible scenarios, but the recently released *Ethics in Audiology* text (Hamill, 2006) provides a glimpse at the scope of the issues confronting the profession. Chapter topics range from child and elder abuse to ethical issues in supervision, practice management, and relationships with hearing instrument manufacturers. The chapter by Fleisher (2006) is especially helpful. It reviews approaches to analyzing ethical dilemmas and provides a foundation for recognizing, analyzing, and making decisions regarding ethical issues. Fleisher outlines five steps, moving from identification of the problem, to data collection, articulation of the issues, deliberation, and, finally, evaluation and reflection.

As a practical matter, ethical issues tend to be reviewed in response to consumer or peer complaints. The professional organizations that involve audiologists support peer review groups that are charged with reviewing individual claims of violations of ethical practice guidelines. The ADA requires that its members report suspected violations to the academy's board of directors. The AAA supports an ethical practice board that receives information about member concerns. ASHA has a board of ethics in place to respond to complaints or concerns regarding its members. In addition, state licensure boards generally have procedures in place to address concerns that may arise regarding any person holding a license to practice professionally. The presence of such bodies is one of the privileges of the profession, but they do not ensure that decisions will be uncontroversial. Ray (2006) reported on the outcome of an interactive session titled "Ethical Practices Board: What Were They Thinking?" held at the 2006 annual meeting of the American Academy of Audiology. Audience members and the members of the Ethical Practice Committee (EPC) voted on several scenarios. The findings reported by Ray indicated that (1) there never was 100% agreement among audience members and (2) discrepancies existed between EPC opinions and those of the majority of the audience.

◆ Summary

It is exciting, yet frustrating, that it is virtually impossible to provide algorithms for the ethical challenges that audiologists may face in their professional lives. A salient feature is that no single act, however well intentioned, will be perceived in a uniform way by all affected parties. The dramatic changes in audiology's ethical landscape that occurred over the past 40 years will no doubt be eclipsed during the next generation, and the profession will be well served if the principles of respect for persons, beneficence, justice, and nonmaleficence continue to be employed to focus professional behavior.

References

Academy of Dispensing Audiologists. (2006). The Academy of Dispensing Audiologists code of ethics. Retrieved April 3, 2006 from http://www.audiologist.org/ about/CodeOfEthics.cfm

American Academy of Audiology. (2006). Code of ethics of the American Academy of Audiology. Retrieved April 3, 2006 from http://www.audiology.org/ about/code.php

American Speech-Language-Hearing Association. (1978). Board moves to change dispensing rules. ASHA, 21, 491–493.

American Speech-Language-Hearing Association. (2003). Code of ethics (revised). ASHA, (Supplement 23), 13–15. Retrieved April 3, 2006 from http:// asha.org/about/ethics/1

American Speech-Language Hearing Association. (2004). Evidence-based practice in communication disorders: An introduction. Retrieved April 3, 2006 from http://asha.org/members/deskref-journals/deskref/default

Annas, G. J. (2005). American bioethics: Crossing human rights and health law boundaries. New York: Oxford University Press.

Beecher, H. K. (1966). Ethics and clinical research. New England Journal of Medicine, 274, 1354–1360.

Berg AL, Herb A., & Hurst M. (2005). Cochlear implants in children: Ethics, informed consent and parental decision making. Journal of Clinical Ethics, 16, 239–250.

Boswell, S. (2003, November 18). Over-the-counter hearing aids: FDA considers two citizens' petitions. The ASHA Leader, pp. 1, 19.

Dyer, J. (2001, June 11). Monster experiment taught children to stutter. San Jose Mercury News, 1a.

Finn, R. (1999). Cancer clinical trials: Experimental treatments and how they can help you. Sebastopol, CA: O'Reilly and Associates.

Fleisher, C. (2006). Approaches to analyzing ethical dilemmas. In T. Hamill (Ed.), Ethics in audiology (pp. 11–25). Reston, VA: American Academy of Audiology.

Gillon, R. (1994). Medical ethics: Four principles plus attention to scope. British Medical Journal, 309, 184–199.

Hamill, T. (Ed.). (2006). Ethics in audiology. Reston, VA: American Academy of Audiology.

Hinchcliffe, R. (2003). Ethics, law and related matters. In L. M. Luxon, J.M. Furman, A. Martini, & D. Stephens (Eds.), Textbook of audiological medicine (pp. 131–147). London: Taylor & Francis.

Jones, J. H. (1993). Bad blood: The Tuskegee syphilis experiment. New York: Free Press.

Kemp, D. (2004, September 26–30). The cochlea and OAEs. Paper presented at the International Congress of Audiology, Phoenix, AZ.

Kemp, D. (2007). Otoacoustic emissions: the basics, the science and the future potential. In M. S. Robinette & T. J. Glattke (Eds.), Otoacoustic emissions: Clinical applications (3rd ed. pp 7–42). New York: Thieme Medical Publishers.

Krugman, S. (1986). The Willowbrook hepatitis studies revisited: Ethical aspects. Reviews of Infectious Diseases, 8, 157–162.

Lane, H., & Bahan, B. (1998). Ethics of cochlear implantation in young children: A review and reply from a deaf-world perspective. Otolaryngology—Head and Neck Surgery, 119, 297–313.

La Puma, J. (1998, July). Understand guiding principles when mixing business, medicine. Managed Care. Retrieved April 3, 2006 from http://www.managedcaremag.com/archives/9807/9807.ethics.shtml

Limentani, A. E. (1999). The role of ethical principles in health care and the implications for ethical codes. Journal of Medical Ethics, 25, 394–398.

Merzenich, M. M., & Sooy, F. (Eds.). (1974). Proceedings of the First International Conference on Electrical Stimulation of the Acoustic Nerve as a Treatment for Profound Sensorineural Deafness in Man. San Francisco: Velo Bind.

Mimura, T., Sato, E., Sugiura, M., Yoshino, T., Naganawa, S., & Kakashima, T. (2005). Hearing loss in patients with enlarged vestibular aqueduct: Air–bone gap and audiological Bing test. International Journal of Audiology, 44, 466–469.

Nuhfer, E. (2001). An ethical framework for practical reasons. The National Teaching and Learning Forum, 10(5), 1–4. Retrieved April 3, 2006 from http:// www.ntlf.com/html/pi/0109/v10n5smpl.pdf

Ray, G. (2006). A question of ethics. Audiology Today, 18(3), 43–45.

Ross, M. (2006). Dr. Ross on hearing loss: Reflections on binaural hearing aid fittings. Rehabilitation Engineering Research Center on Hearing Enhancement. Retrieved April 3, 2006 from http://www.hearingresearch.org/Dr.Ross/Binaural_HA_Fittings.htm

Schwartz, P. J., Spazzolini, C., Crotti, L., et al. (2006). The Jervell and Lange-Nielsen syndrome: Natural history, molecular basis and clinical outcome. Circulation, 113, 783–790.

Shinn, R. (2004). Ethics and audiology. The ASHA Leader, 22, 4–5.

Simmons, F. B. (1966). Electrical stimulation of the auditory nerve in man. Archives of Otolaryngology, 84(1), 2–54.

Simmons, F. B. (1985) History of cochlear implants in the United States: A personal perspective. In R. A. Schindler & M. M. Merzenich (Eds.), Cochlear implants (pp. 1–7). New York: Raven Press.

Trials of war criminals before the Nuremberg military tribunals under Control Council Law No. 10, Vol. 2, Nuremberg, October 1946–April 1949. (1949–1953). Washington, DC: U.S. Government Printing Office.

U.S. Department of Health, Education, and Welfare. (1979). The Belmont report. Retrieved April 3, 2006 from http://ohsr.od.nih.gov/guidelines/belmont.html

Vanderpool, H. Y. (2002). An ethics primer for IRBs. In R. J. Amdur & E. A. Bankert (Eds.), Institutional Review Board: Management and function (pp. 3–8). Sudbury, MA: Jones & Bartlett.

Chapter 3

Quality: The Controlling Principle of Practice Management

Harvey B. Abrams and Theresa Hnath Chisolm

Those of us born shortly after the end of World War II may recall a time when our family doctor made house calls. Following the visit, it was customary for the full payment to be rendered immediately to the physician. Today, of course, it is rare for a doctor to provide treatment in the household and equally as rare for patients to pay for the entire cost of services directly to the provider. How our society has gotten to this point represents a revolution in health care that has occurred within a single generation. The reasons for this revolution and the societal dynamics that have shaped our health care system are many and complex. They include the changing role of women in American society, the increased sophistication of health care, the emergence of medical specialties, the increasing independence of nonphysician specialties, the increased number of health care providers, the demographic shifts of the American population (age, residence, income, distribution of wealth), the rising cost of health care, and the changing cultural precepts concerning aging and dying.

One constant that has persisted throughout these changes has been the continuing effort to improve the quality of the care we provide to our patients. This had been manifested by a drive to improve diagnostic accuracy, treatment efficacy, involvement of the patient and family members in treatment decisions, and decreasing hospital lengths of stay. Just as health care in general has dramatically changed, so has the concept and measurement of quality. Quality, however, is only one of many dimensions of health care that has experienced significant change. To understand the revolution in the health care industry, it may help to understand the forces that drive health care decisions.

In the days when doctors made house calls, the health care industry was provider-driven. The method of payment was fee-for-service, access was provider-controlled, costs were relatively unimportant, and the outcome of the health care episode was the elimination of disease. During the 1970s and 1980s, along with the widespread availability of health insurance, health care became payer-driven. The method of payment was based on new concepts such as diagnosis-related groups (DRGs) and relative value units (RVUs). Access was payer-controlled, costs became very important, and the outcome of the episode was reduced costs. The health care reform initiative begun during President Bill Clinton's first administration has shaped our present system, which can be viewed as consumer-driven. The method of payment is largely based on a risk-adjusted capitation system, access is largely consumer choice, and the outcome is determined by measurements of functional status, quality of life, and consumer satisfaction.

The dimension of quality has also been influenced by the shift of health care from a supply- to a demand-side industry. When the industry was provider-controlled, quality was determined by accreditation and credentialing by an outside review agency or by a board within the hospital. During the payer-driven phase of health care, quality was determined by the institution's self-perception of quality through quality assurance and, later, total quality indices. In a consumer-driven industry, treatment outcomes and measures of consumer satisfaction determine quality. Although continuous quality improvement (CQI) is associated with the payer-driven system, it is a concept that is totally appropriate in any type of health care setting or model. CQI extends beyond a mere measurement of the outcome of the health care episode to all processes and relationships that comprise and finally culminate in some change in the patient's health status.

This chapter will review the recent history of quality measures in health care, the principle concepts of CQI, how CQI is assessed, the emergence of customer service in the health care setting, and some examples of CQI in an audiology setting.

◆ Toward a Description of Quality

In the book *Zen and the Art of Motorcycle Maintenance* (Pirsig, 1984), the narrator, Phaedrus, is eventually driven insane in his attempt to define quality. Early in his intellectual journey, Phaedrus recognizes that quality "is a characteristic of thought and statement that is recognized by a nonthinking process. Because definitions are a product of rigid, formal thinking, quality cannot be defined" (p. 206). Yet Phaedrus understands, as we all do, that, although we may not be able to absolutely define quality, we can recognize it when we see, hear, feel, or experience it. What is it about a piece of music, a painting, a piece of furniture, or an automobile that determines its quality? Can we recognize quality in the service we receive at a store, an auto repair shop, a hospital, or an audiology clinic?

I think most of us will agree that we can recognize quality in the goods and services we receive but that the perception of quality is personal and individualized, or a "characteristic of thought" as Phaedrus observed. To avoid Phaedrus's fate, we will not attempt to define quality broadly but instead attempt to describe it in the narrow arena of health care. To add a measure of safety, we will use the work of others to present a working definition of quality.

The Quality Measurement and Management Project (QMMP) is a hospital industry–sponsored initiative to develop quality monitoring and management tools of

choice for hospitals. In a 1989 publication, James described QMMP health care quality as representing

> an individual's subjective evaluation of an output and the personal interactions that take place as the output is delivered to the individual. It is rooted in that individual's *expectations*, which depend upon the individual's past experiences and individual needs. Quality evaluations therefore arise from, and are part of, an individual's value system. As a value system, quality expectations can be measured and changed through time and through education. They cannot be dictated. (p. 2)

I think Phaedrus would agree.

Pearl
• All members of the organization must reject negativism and the acceptance of errors as just a part of doing business.

◆ The Business of Quality Improvement

The quality concepts and tools currently used in health care have their origins in business, specifically in manufacturing. Perhaps the individual most commonly associated with conceptualizing and applying the concepts of quality to business is W. Edwards Deming. Deming, with advanced degrees in mathematics, engineering, and physics, is often credited with the emergence of postwar Japan as a global powerhouse whose products, particularly electronic and automotive, have been synonymous with quality. He maintained that quality improvement requires a total commitment by everyone within the organization. Deming (1986) articulated his philosophy of quality management through the following 14 points and his seven deadly diseases **(Table 3–1)**:

1. *Create constancy of purpose for the improvement of product and service*   A business must develop a vision for itself that encourages innovation, puts resources into research and education, commits itself to the continuous improvement of services and products, and invests in the maintenance of equipment and other aids to improve production.

2. *Adopt the new philosophy*   All members of the organization must religiously reject negativism and the acceptance of errors.

Table 3–1 Deming's Seven Deadly Diseases

1. Lack of constancy of purpose
2. Emphasis on short-term profits
3. Evaluation by performance, merit rating, or annual review of performance
4. Mobility of management
5. Running a company on visible figures alone
6. Excessive medical costs
7. Excessive costs of warranty, fueled by lawyers who work for contingency fees

3. *Cease dependence on mass inspection* Businesses must reject the practice of inspecting products or services after they are produced. Quality is improved when processes are in place that eliminate errors in the first place.

4. *End the practice of awarding business on the basis of price tag* The low bidder may not produce the best product. Find the best supplier and develop a long-term relationship to ensure the best quality at the best price.

5. *Improve constantly the system of production and service* Quality improvement is a long-term commitment.

6. *Institute training* Employees cannot expect to provide quality products or services if they have not been adequately trained in both their particular job and in the company's commitment to quality.

7. *Institute leadership* Lead by example. Be a coach to your employees.

8. *Drive out fear* Create an environment in which the employees feel safe to question the ways things are done.

9. *Break down barriers between staff areas* Create an environment of teamwork rather than competition among the departments within an organization.

10. *Eliminate slogans, exhortations, and targets for the workforce* Let the workforce create their own slogans.

11. *Eliminate numerical quotas* Workers may feel pressured to meet production quotas at the expense of quality.

12. *Remove barriers to pride of workmanship* Eliminate faulty equipment, defective materials, and counterproductive policies so employees can take pride in the work they accomplish.

13. *Institute a vigorous program of education and retraining* When new methods are introduced, both management and nonmanagement employees must be educated. Training should include statistical methodology and teamwork.

14. *Take action to accomplish the transformation* It takes a dedicated team of top management with a well-defined action plan to lead the quality improvement initiative.

Special Consideration

- "Creating change is how managers break through to new levels of performance; preventing change is how managers control the organization."—J. M. Juran

---

Another quality assurance engineer of note is J. M. Juran. Juran was also instrumental in creating a quality-conscious environment beginning in the 1950s. Such corporations as AT&T, DuPont, and IBM embraced the "Juran trilogy," which stressed the three elements of quality: quality planning, quality control, and quality assurance. Juran (1988) identified eight factors that characterized successful organizations that had made a commitment to improved quality:

1. Senior managers personally led the quality process and served on a quality council as guides.

2. Managers applied quality improvement to businesses and traditional operational processes. These managers addressed internal and external customers.

3. Senior managers adopted mandated, annual quality improvement with a defined infrastructure that identified opportunities to improve and gave clear responsibility to do this.

4. Managers involved all those who effected the plan in the improvement process.

5. Managers used modern quality methodology instead of empiricism in quality planning.

6. Managers trained all members of the management hierarchy in quality planning, quality control, and quality improvement.

7. Managers trained the workforce to participate actively in quality improvement.

8. Senior managers included quality improvement in the strategic planning process.

Another quality improvement consultant was Philip Crosby, who maintained that implementing quality is cost effective. Crosby was the architect of several quality-related concepts, including the quality management maturity grid and the quality improvement process. He coined such phrases as "zero defects" and "right first time." By "zero defects," Crosby did not mean to say that mistakes never happen; rather, he stressed that there is no allowable number of errors built into a product or process. By "right first time," Crosby urged that a group's goal should be to get things right the first time.

Crosby (1979) outlined 14 steps to quality improvement:

1. Management is committed to quality—and this is clear to all.

2. Create quality improvement teams, with representatives from all departments.

3. Measure processes to determine current and potential quality issues.

4. Calculate the cost of poor quality.

5. Raise quality awareness of all employees.

6. Take action to correct quality issues.

7. Monitor progress of quality improvement: establish a zero defects committee.

8. Train supervisors in quality improvement.

9. Hold "zero defects" days.

10. Encourage employees to create their own quality improvement goals.

11. Encourage employee communication with management about obstacles to quality.

12. Recognize participants' efforts.

13. Create quality councils.

14. Do it all over again: quality improvement does not end.

Pearl

- A goal of CQI is to do all things right the first time.

◆ The Health Care Evolution: From Quality Control to Continuous Quality Improvement

The evolution of quality assessment methods in health care has taken about 30 years to reach the point where we now find ourselves. This process is not linear, with one concept discarded as the next is embraced. Rather, concepts build on each other, with one creating the foundation for the next.

Quality Control: Conformance to Specifications

Audiologists are familiar with quality control issues as they apply to the measurements of hearing aids. For example, the American National Standards Institute (ANSI, 2003) specification 53.22–2003 delineates the operating characteristics of hearing aids. The inherent quality of a hearing instrument can be determined by measuring the hearing aid upon receipt from the manufacturer and comparing results with the published specifications. Such measurements allow us to make assumptions regarding the device, although they tell us nothing about the effect of the device on treatment outcome. Similarly, audiologists can measure the quality of equipment and the testing environment by ensuring that each meets published specifications for calibration and ambient noise levels. Again, adherence to such standards ensures a certain level of quality, but it does not ensure a positive treatment outcome, although it eliminates many variables that may decrease the opportunities for patient satisfaction and positive outcome.

Quality Assurance

The origin of quality assurance in health care can be traced to the beginning of the 20th century with the establishments of minimum standards and on-site inspections of hospitals through the American College of Surgeons. The responsibility of inspections and standards development was later assumed by what was then called the Joint Commission on Accreditation of Hospitals (JCAH). The commission was created as a private, nonprofit organization comprised of representatives from large professional associations representing physicians, dentists, and hospitals and was charged with developing standards and accrediting hospitals through a voluntary survey. Accreditation by the JCAH became critical following the creation of Medicare regulations that determined that only accredited hospitals could

be reimbursed through the Medicare program. It was not until the 1980s, however, that the commission's standards began to focus on quality assurance by requiring hospital departments to identify problems through chart audits. In 1987, the organization changed its name to the Joint Commission on Accreditation of Healthcare Organizations (JCAHO) to reflect the need to establish quality care in all settings where health care is provided, including long-term care facilities, rehabilitation units, and outpatient departments. Extending the concept of quality beyond equipment, the JCAHO established standards for each department of the hospital to include standards for leadership, care of patients, training, records, documentation, safety, facility management, and so on. In addition, the commission established specific criteria to assist health care organizations in determining if they were meeting the standards, and if not, what they needed to do to comply.

Through the 10-step monitoring and evaluation process (**Table 3–2**), the JCAHO hoped health care organizations would be able to identify real or potential problems and improve health care quality.

Controversial Point

- It is questionable whether quality can be "assured." Quality can be measured, evaluated, compromised, and improved, but it cannot be guaranteed.

The 10-step program was designed to identify processes that were high volume, high risk, or problem prone; establish some threshold beyond which action would be taken to determine what went wrong; and fix the problem so that performance would remain below that threshold. Each department within the health care facility was responsible for identifying processes that would be reviewed and for establishing these thresholds before action would be taken. As in manufacturing, this is a detection approach (**Fig. 3–1**) that relies on the inspection or examination of services after they have been completed. Often specific individuals are assigned the responsibility of quality assurance through inspection or data review. These inspectors act as screens to ensure a reasonable level of quality.

Table 3–2 Joint Commission on Accreditation of Healthcare Organizations' 10-Step Monitoring and Evaluation Process

1. Assign responsibility.
2. Delineate scope of care.
3. Identify important aspects of care.
4. Identify indicators.
5. Establish thresholds for evaluation improvement.
6. Collect and organize data.
7. Evaluate care.
8. Take action to improve care.
9. Access actions and document.
10. Communicate information.

Source: From Abrams, H. B., & Siferd, S. T. (1994). Total quality improvement: The Department of Veterans Affairs audiology and speech pathology program. Seminars in Hearing, 15 (4), 277–287, with permission.

The Detection Approach

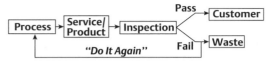

Figure 3–1 The detection approach to quality assurance. (From Abrams, H. B., & Siferd, S. T. (1994). Total quality improvement: The Department of Veterans Affairs audiology and speech pathology program. Seminars in Hearing, 15(4), 277–287, with permission.)

The JCAHO accreditation process has evolved from an inspection process focused on preparation and scores to one that focuses on continuous operational improvement and patient safety. The stated purposes of the most current accreditation process are the following (JCAHO, 2005):

♦ Focuses the survey to a greater extent on the actual delivery of care, treatment, and services

♦ Increases the value and the satisfaction with accreditation among accredited hospitals and their staff

♦ Shifts the accreditation-related focus from survey preparation and scores to continuous operational improvement

♦ Makes the accreditation process more continuous

♦ Increases the public's confidence that hospitals continuously comply with standards that emphasize patient safety and heath care quality

---

Special Consideration

• "[Quality] is the degree to which patient care services increase the probability of desired patient outcomes and reduce the probability of undesired outcomes given the current state of knowledge."—JCAHO definition of quality

---

The Costs of Detection

High quality can be achieved through the detection approach of quality assurance, but only at a high cost. Because problems must be identified to drive an improvement effort, inspectors need to wait before action is taken. Some of the costs associated with the detection approach are

♦ Waste

♦ Time lost for the customer and the department

♦ New or additional material required to repair the problem

♦ Delay in service delivery

♦ Inspection costs

♦ Customer dissatisfaction

The Prevention Approach

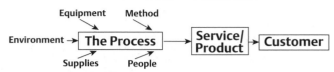

Figure 3–2 The prevention approach to quality assurance. (From Abrams, H. B., & Siferd, S. T. (1994). Total quality improvement: The Department of Veterans Affairs audiology and speech pathology program. Seminars in Hearing, 15(4), 277–287, with permission.)

Case 1 in the Appendix 3–1 presents an example of the detection approach to quality improvement.

Continuous Quality Improvement: The Prevention Approach

The concept of CQI assumes that a process or outcome can always be improved. In contrast to quality assurance, which relies on repeated measures to determine if performance is meeting some predetermined threshold, CQI encourages a preventive approach to identifying and eliminating problems (**Fig. 3–2**). CQI strives to set the bar higher (move the threshold) by improving efficiencies, decreasing costs, improving patient satisfaction, reducing morbidity, reducing lengths of stay, and so on, before the product or service is delivered to the customer. Detecting product or service problems is no longer the responsibility of an inspector, but rather the responsibility of each individual participating in the process. There are costs associated with the prevention approach, however; these include measurement analysis and quality training. These costs can be considered "investment" dollars because continuously increasing quality will ultimately result in less waste and improved patient satisfaction. Case 2 in the Appendix 3–1 is an example of the prevention approach to quality improvement.

The essence of CQI is illustrated in **Table 3–3**. Satisfying the patient should be the unifying principle of everyone in the department. Elimination of waste can be accomplished through several means, including simplification of processes, elimination of duplication, introduction of new technologies, and implementation and expansion of training. The culture must encourage the participation of everyone in the organization. Inherent in this culture is an environment of respect and trust. Chances are, the people who have the solutions are the ones performing the functions. Constructive change and innovation are possible only in an environment of trust. Improving products or systems must be based on data gathered through a formalized approach. This approach should include a clear statement of what needs to be changed and why, how the process is to be changed, how the effects of the change will be measured, and how success will be determined. Decision by assumption cannot succeed.

Table 3–3 The Essence of Continuous Quality Improvement

• Obsession with satisfying customers
• Obsession with eliminating waste
• A culture that encourages ethical, open, respectful, and participative behavior
• Formal systems based on data and continuous improvement

Table 3–4 Berwick's 10 Key Lessons for Quality Improvement

1. Quality improvement tools can work in health care.
2. Cross-functional teams are valuable in improving health care processes.
3. Data useful for quality improvements abound in health care.
4. Quality improvement methods are fun to use.
5. Costs of poor quality are high, and savings are in reach.
6. Involving doctors is difficult.
7. Training needs arise early.
8. Nonclinical processes draw early attention.
9. Health care organizations may need a broader definition of quality.
10. In health care, as in industry, the fate of quality improvement is, first of all, in the hands of leaders.

Pearl

- Doing it right is better than doing it fast.

As discussed earlier, Deming, Juran, and Crosby came out of manufacturing industries, not health care. However, the same principles taught by these individuals have been proven to work in the health care environment. Donald Berwick (Berwick et al, 1990) has adapted industry's quality improvement lessons to health care **(Table 3–4)**. CQI tools, tutorials, and links can be found on the CQI server at http://deming.eng.clemson.edu/. The distinction between quality assurance and quality improvement is illustrated in **Table 3–5**.

Pearl

- "The only performance standard is zero defects."—Philip Crosby

◆ Integrating Quality into Audiologic Practice

Up to this point, I have reviewed the general concepts and philosophies of quality improvement as it applies to organizations in general and to health care facilities in particular. The

Table 3–5 Quality Assurance versus Quality Improvement

Quality Assurance	Quality Improvement
Inspection-oriented (detection)	Planning-oriented (prevention)
Reactive	Proactive
Correction of special causes (individual, machine, etc.)	Correction of common causes (systems)
Responsibility of few	Responsibility of many
Narrow focus	Cross-functional
Leadership may not be vested	Leadership actively leading
Problem solving by authority	Problem solving by employees at all levels

Source: From Koch, M. W. & Fairly, T. M. (1993). Integrated quality management: The key to improving nursing care quality. St. Louis: Mosby-Year Book, with permission.

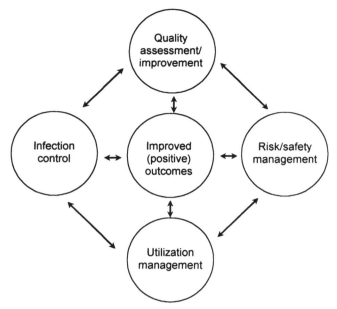

Figure 3–3 Integrated quality improvement model. (From Koch, M. W., & Fairly, T. M. (1993). Integrated quality management: The key to improving nursing care quality. St. Louis: Mosby-Year Book, with permission.)

overall purpose of improved quality is to improve patient outcome. CQI provides us with a process to examine the way we perform care and determine ways of improving that care. In fact, continuous quality improvement requires the integration of information from many sources within the organization. The most important of these are utilization management, patient safety and risk management, workplace safety, and infection control **(Fig. 3–3)**.

Pearl

- "Only positive consequences encourage good future performance."—Kenneth Blanchard

Utilization Management

Utilization management in health care can be defined as "a series of actions to produce a quality health care product in a cost-effective manner while contributing to the overall goals of an institution" (Koch and Fairly, 1993, p. 73). Utilization management is critical in identifying those products and services that result in excessive cost and inefficient delivery of health care. Utilization review examines such things as the appropriateness of admissions, length of stay, use of resources such as laboratory tests and pharmaceuticals, duplication of services, and discharge planning.

Utilization review has been driven, in large part, by the creation of a prospective payment system (PPS) through the development of DRGs. DRGs were developed as a means of grouping patients by lengths of stay, and, hence, resources consumed. Considerations included the patient's principal diagnosis, principal procedure, complications of treatment, any

Table 3–6 Diagnosis-Related Group (DRG) Considerations

- Principle diagnosis
- Principle procedure
- Complications
- Comorbidities
- Age

comorbidity, and the patient's age **(Table 3–6)**. Medicare and private health insurance companies used the DRG system to base their payment to hospitals. Prior to the PPS system, Medicare would reimburse hospitals on a fee-for-service basis. There was no incentive for physicians or hospitals to control costs because those costs would be reimbursed through Medicare or private health insurance. A "capitated" system, which reimburses the hospital a specific amount as a function of diagnosis, regardless of resources consumed, dramatically changed the way the health care industry operates. Naturally, hospitals were under great pressure to examine utilization to ensure that they were not expending more resources than they were recovering. By examining and controlling resources consumed, hospitals could hope not only to recover costs but also to make a profit.

Utilization Review Techniques

There are several ways to analyze utilization management activities:

- *Prospective review* determines the anticipated resources required prior to treatment. Insurance companies exercise this type of review to determine the appropriateness for admission for a particular type of disorder. Often third-party payers will deny coverage for an inpatient procedure requiring admission to a hospital if the same procedure can be performed on an outpatient basis. Health care facilities perform prospective review to determine the ability of a patient to pay for the proposed treatment.

- *Concurrent review* is performed at the time of or within 24 hours of admission to determine the appropriateness of the admission and the anticipated resources required. The facility determines the need for continued stay based on specific criteria as determined by clinical guidelines or by the condition of the patient at the time of review.

- *Retrospective review* takes place after the patient is discharged. The facility can determine the entire costs of the admission episode retrospectively to determine whether criteria for admission, continued stay, use of resources, and practice patterns were appropriate and consistent with the facility's criteria.

- *Focused review* concentrates on a specific issue, such as length of stay, readmission within 72 hours, infection rates, blood usage, and use of ancillary services, which may be of particular concern to the facility. These reviews may be targeted as a result of an internal review (CQI initiative) or an external review (peer review, JCAHO inspection).

Table 3–7 Utilization Management Activities: Outpatient Setting

Assessment
Continuity of care per illness
Patient's/family's ability to follow plan of care
Postdischarge needs

Source: From Koch, M. W., & Fairly, T. M. (1993). Integrated quality management: The key to improving nursing care quality. St. Louis: Mosby-Year Book, with permission.

Utilization Management Criteria

The criteria used to determine the appropriateness of care and resource utilization issues are the responsibility of the particular health care facility **(Tables 3–7** and **3–8)**. Increasingly, however, representatives of specific medical specialties are developing these criteria. The criteria may be based on the diagnosis of the patient, the severity of the illness, the length of stay, or normative or empirically determined data. The development of clinically oriented algorithms, clinical pathways, and practice guidelines, discussed later in this chapter, is providing ways for facilities to determine if they are meeting established criteria, triggering utilization or CQI reviews, and allows for a comparison among groups of health care facilities providing similar services.

Pitfall

- When implementing quality improvement, existing organizational structures may need to be modified, or the development of parallel structures could upset the existing distribution of power throughout the organization and create conflict.

Table 3–8 Utilization Management Activities: Acute Care

Assessment
Admissions
Level of care
Resource use
Need for continued stay
Discharge

Evaluation
Overutilization
Underutilization
Inefficiencies
Lack of cost restraint

Intervention
Problems adversely affecting cost and quality

Discharge Planning
Identifying needs after patient leaves hospital

Source: From Koch, M. W., & Fairly, T. M. (1993). Integrated quality management: The key to improving nursing care quality. St. Louis: Mosby-Year Book, with permission.

Patient Safety and Risk Management

There is no industry in which the cost of error is as extreme as health care. The patient's quality of life, indeed, life itself, is jeopardized when processes fail in a health care setting. The reputation of practitioners and the hospital is at stake, and the economic costs to patient, provider, and facility can be enormous. Indeed, the economic survival of health care facilities rests largely on their ability to provide a safe environment. It is estimated that 44,000 to 98,000 Americans die each year as a result of medical errors (American Hospital Association, 1999). As reported by Kohn et al (2000), more people in the United States die in a given year as a result of medical errors than from motor vehicle accidents, breast cancer, or acquired immunodeficiency syndrome (AIDS; Centers for Disease Control and Prevention, 1999). According to a patient safety in American hospitals report (Health Grades, 2006), 1.24 million total patient safety incidents occurred in almost 40 million hospitalizations in the Medicare population during 2002 through 2004. These incidents were associated with $9.3 billion of excess cost.

Controversial Point

- More people in the United States die in a given year as a result of medical errors than from motor vehicle accidents, breast cancer, or AIDS.

The human and financial consequences of preventable medical errors are so substantial that the Institute for Healthcare Improvement (IHI) has devoted significant resources to identifying the sources of medical errors and proposing innovative solutions to minimize their occurrence. For a detailed description of the problems and solutions associated with preventable medical errors, the reader is referred to the report "To Err Is Human: Building a Safer Health System" (Kohn et al, 2000) and the IHI Web site (http://www.ihi.org/IHI/Topics/PatientSafety/). The IHI launched the 5 Million Lives Campaign (http://www.ihi.org/IHI/Programs/Campaign/), an initiative designed to engage U.S. hospitals in a commitment to implement changes in care proven to improve patient care and prevent avoidable deaths and reduce patient injuries.

The JCAHO has also emphasized patient safety and reduction of medical errors. In 2007, the organization established eight hospital critical access national patient safety goals (NPSGs) applicable to both hospitals and ambulatory care facilities (http://www.jointcommission.org/patientsafety/ nationalpatientsafetygoals/07_hap_cah_npsgs.htm):

1. Improve the accuracy of patient identification

2. Improve the effectiveness of communication among caregivers

3. Improve the safety of using high-alert medications

4. Reduce the risk of health care–associated infections

5. Accurately and completely reconcile medications across the continuum of care

6. Reduce the risk of patient harm resulting from falls

7. Encourage patients' active involvement in their own care as a patient safety strategy

8. The organization identifies safety risks inherent in its patient population

Although the primary benefactor of a safer health care environment is deservedly the patient, the health care organization also benefits. Risk management is the process of making and carrying out decisions that will minimize the adverse effects of accidental losses on an organization (Koch and Fairly, 1993). The driving forces behind the risk management movement occurred primarily in the 1970s and 1980s. These forces included the increasing numbers of malpractice claims, jury awards for malpractice, premiums among health care providers, and the tendency to hold the health care facility (and its stockholders) legally responsible for the actions of its staff. Attempts to limit liability payments at the state level have been largely unsuccessful.

The audiologic community has been fortunate in that malpractice claims have been relatively few, the awards have not been astronomical, and the malpractice premiums have remained reasonable. Historically, our work has not involved disorders for which risky, invasive procedures would pose a significant risk of harm to the patient. However, audiologists have seen their scope of practice widen significantly in recent years with the inclusion of cerumen management, deep canal impression techniques, intraoperative monitoring, and early identification of hearing loss. These expanded procedures and services have created the opportunity for serious mistakes and have exposed the audiologist and the employer to economic liability. Opportunities for economic exposure are associated not only with acts of commission, such as a perforated tympanic membrane following an ear impression, but also with acts of omission, such as neglecting to perform an appropriate diagnostic test or failing to advise patients on the dangers of ingesting batteries.

Risk management and loss avoidance involve several discrete steps (Koch and Fairly, 1993) **(Table 3–9)**.

- *Identify potential exposures to accidental loss* Examine your scope of practice. What services or procedures are provided that pose a risk to the patient? Recall that risk involves not only potential physical harm to the patient but also the potential effects of misdiagnosis. For

Table 3–9 Risk Management Decision Process

- Identify potential exposures
- Examine alternative risk management techniques
- Select the apparently best alternative risk management technique
- Implement the chosen risk management technique
- Monitor the results of the chosen technique

Source: Adapted from Koch, M. W., & Fairly, T. M. (1993). Integrated quality management: The key to improving nursing care quality. St. Louis: Mosby-Year Book.

example, failing to properly diagnose hearing loss in an infant may result in significant speech and language delay, as well as associated "pain and suffering" on the part of the child and parents. High-risk procedures include cerumen management, deep canal impressions, intraoperative monitoring, electrocochleography, and neonatal testing

♦ *Examine alternative risk management techniques associated with these exposures*   Are there techniques, for example, to reduce injury associated with deep canal impression, such as improved illumination, video-otoscopy, vented oto-blocks, lubricated blocks, high-viscosity impression material, or powered syringe? Are methods available to improve the accuracy of diagnosing hearing loss in a neonate population? Is otoacoustic emissions (OAE) the test of choice, or should the clinician use a battery approach including OAE, evoked potentials, and middle ear immittance measures? Are transtympanic electrodes always necessary for measuring the action and summating potentials, or can ear canal electrodes be used with reduced risk at the expense of waveform morphology?

♦ *Select the best risk management technique*   The "best" technique is determined by deciding which technique provides the best result, in terms of accuracy and efficiency, with the least risk. This is not an easy process, sometimes requiring a cost/benefit analysis, where cost is the additional expense associated with reducing risk and benefit is defined as the savings realized by avoiding the financial consequences of risk. An organization may be willing to accept the possibility of an infrequent and less severe loss (in terms of claims) than invest heavily in equipment or personnel to eliminate loss exposure. More often, the "best" techniques are being defined by professional organizations in the form of practice guidelines. These guidelines are often based on current research and represent the state-of-the-art approach for a particular diagnosis or procedure. Some state legislatures have passed laws that protect a practitioner from litigation as long as that person was following current clinical guidelines for that episode of care. A recent example of an evidence-based clinical guideline for audiology is "Guidelines for the audiologic management of adult hearing impairment" (Valente et al, 2006).

♦ *Implement the chosen risk management technique(s)*   Once a decision is made to implement a different protocol to minimize loss exposure, it is important that everyone responsible for delivering audiology services be informed of the change, educated in the new technique(s), if necessary, informed of the implementation date, and held accountable for implementing the technique(s).

♦ *Monitor the results of the chosen technique(s)*   Following implementation of the best technique(s), it is important to establish a monitoring program to ensure that the desired effect has taken place and at the cost anticipated. For example, if the audiology department has decided to purchase a video-otoscope to minimize claims resulting from perforated tympanic membranes and ear canal

hematomas, it is critical to determine if the costs associated with the equipment, training, and implementation have, in fact, reduced the number and severity of claims associated with deep canal impressions. Although video-otoscopy may significantly reduce loss exposure, it is possible that the same results may have been accomplished at a greatly reduced cost with the use of relatively inexpensive vented oto-blocks.

In addition to the establishment of formalized risk management programs by an employer, the individual audiologist has a responsibility to minimize risks to the patient (adapted from Koch and Fairly, 1993):

1. Familiarize yourself with those standards and laws that govern the practice of audiology.

2. Know the policies of your facility and your scope of practice as outlined in your job description.

3. Take responsibility for the education and skills required to perform your particular responsibilities, including new or unfamiliar procedures.

Workplace Safety

A quality work environment is a safe environment. **Table 3–10** lists some common workplace safety concerns associated with health care facilities. Safety can be considered a subset of risk management in the sense that safety policies are put in place to reduce the risk of accidents incidental to the delivery of health care but are not necessarily associated with a particular clinical practice. Accidents are costly in terms of lost productivity, compensation payments, and the retraining of replacement staff. Examples of safety-related issues in the health care arena include electrical safety; the handling and disposal of hazardous materials; spills; needle sticks; maintenance of medical equipment; patient-on-patient, patient-on-staff, and staff-on-staff acts of violence; work-related injuries; and work-related hazardous exposures, including noise.

The Occupational Safety and Health Administration (OSHA) regulates safety in the workplace, and it is the responsibility of the employer to ensure that all applicable laws and regulations are being followed. These include the education of staff, the monitoring of hazards, the provision and maintenance of safety equipment, the health monitoring of employees, and the maintenance of records.

Table 3–10 Workplace Safety Concerns

- Electrical safety
- Hazardous materials
- Spills
- Workplace violence
- Needle sticks
- Work-related injuries
- Work-related exposures (e.g., noise, chemicals)
- Equipment maintenance

JCAHO requires the presence of a safety officer and the establishment of a safety committee to include representatives from administration, clerical, and support services, as well as safety experts. The organization considers risk management and safety to be integral components of a continuous quality improvement program.

Infection Control

Quality management in the health care setting requires an uncompromising commitment to infection control. Perhaps no single issue has focused the attention of health care workers on infection control as has AIDS and the human immunodeficiency virus (HIV). In fact, however, the risk of infection is much greater to the patient than to the health care worker.

Nosocomial Infections

Nosocomial infections, also known as health care–associated infections, are those that occur as a result of hospitalization. Nosocomials include pneumonia, bloodstream infections, surgical wound infections, and urinary tract infections typically associated with long-term catheter use. Patients are ill and often immunocompromised when they enter the hospital; they are in an environment with other individuals who are ill, and have had invasive procedures performed upon them. All of these factors mean that hospitalized patients are at risk for infection. Patients who succumb to nosocomial infections tend to stay longer and require greater resources, increasing the cost of care and jeopardizing a satisfactory outcome.

JCAHO guidelines require an infection control program that includes written policies and procedures for collecting and analyzing data. The health care facility must have a multidisciplinary committee in place to deal with infection control issues. CQI methodology provides an outstanding system for identifying, analyzing, improving processes, and, ultimately, decreasing the rates of infection.

Controversial Point

- In hospitals alone, health care–associated infections (HAIs) account for an estimated 2 million infections, 90,000 deaths, and $4.5 billion in excess health care costs annually (Centers for Disease Control and Prevention, 2006).

◆ Implementing Continuous Quality Improvement

One way quality-related issues are addressed in an organization is through trial and error. Unfortunately, because the causes of and solutions to organizational problems are usually complex, this approach tends to address only the superficial and obvious and fails to resolve the underlying causes of problems. Improvements may occur, but such improvements are not systematic and are rarely continual. Also, because such approaches are often imposed upon the employees by management, the employees have no vested interest in the solution and may be at best unenthusiastic and at worst noncompliant, essentially sabotaging the effort even if the proposed solution is a reasonable one. FOCUS-PDCA provides a strategy that is systematic, involves employees in the process, and allows for continuing improvement.

FOCUS-PDCA

FOCUS-PDCA is a method of quality improvement that uses a systematic approach to analyzing and improving processes. The FOCUS phase of the method is designed to build a knowledge base concerning the process to be improved, including an understanding of how the process is presently operating, what the objective is, and the sources of variation between the existing and desired outcomes. The PDCA phase represents a learning cycle where a plan is conceived and executed, the results are compared with the predicted outcome, and modifications, if needed, are added. Taken together, FOCUS-PDCA is a nine-step process, with each step resulting in sets of data, a plan, or a decision, as illustrated in **Fig. 3–4** (Stolz, 1996).

Pitfall

- FOCUS-PDCA can become an end in itself and replace effective decision making by management even when the cause and solution of a problem are evident.

Step 1. Find a Process to Improve

The purpose of step 1 is to find a process that needs improvement (**Table 3–11**) and to articulate to the employees and management why this is an important process, how it will affect customers, how the process currently performs, and what the objective of the improvement will be. Methods for identifying a process to improve include customer feedback, quality audits and assessments, customer needs analysis, benchmarking, peer review, clinical pathways, and clinical algorithms.

Customer Feedback   Information from patients in the form of complaints or through satisfaction surveys can reveal important deficiencies and opportunities for improvement.

Quality Audits and Assessments   Audits and assessments provide an excellent way of identifying opportunities for improving quality. It is far preferable to identify these opportunities through self-assessment than through an external review where negative findings can jeopardize an institution's credentials and ability to deliver care and stay in business.

JCAHO guidelines provide specific standards against which to compare the organization. A self-audit through a

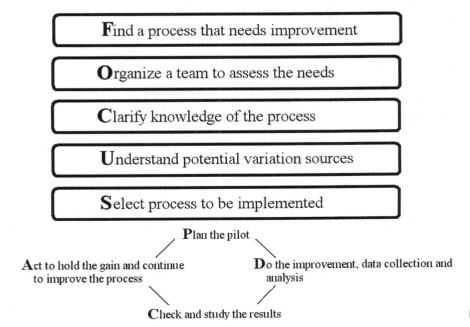

Figure 3–4 The FOCUS-PDCA cycle.

mock survey, prior to a JCAHO inspection, can identify opportunities for improvement while correcting errors that might jeopardize the facility's accreditation.

The Commission on Accreditation of Rehabilitation Facilities (CARF, 2005) has established standards for rehabilitation programs and facilities. There are specific standards for audiology services if they are provided as part of a rehabilitation program. A review of these standards may reveal a process in need of improvement.

The American Speech-Language-Hearing Association (ASHA, 2005) has published standards for quality indicators for professional service programs in audiology and speech-language pathology. Included in the standards are elements related to the purpose and scope of services, service delivery, program operations, program evaluation and performance improvement, and ethics.

Pitfall

- Do not plan and develop strategic initiatives entirely on the results of a focus group. The group may not reflect the opinions of your market. Confirm focus group data with market surveys.

Table 3–11 Methods for Finding a Process to Improve

- Customer feedback
- Quality audits and assessments
- Customer needs analysis
- Benchmarking
- Peer review
- Clinical pathways
- Clinical algorithms

The Malcolm Baldrige National Quality Award program of the National Institute of Standards and Technology (NIST, 2005) was established by Congress in 1987 to recognize U.S. organizations for their achievements in quality and performance and to raise awareness about the importance of quality and performance excellence as a competitive edge. The award is not given for specific products or services. In October 2004, President George W. Bush signed into law legislation that authorized the NIST to expand the program to include nonprofit and government organizations. The NIST began to solicit applications from nonprofit organizations in 2006 for a pilot program, with awards commencing in 2007. The Baldrige performance excellence criteria are a framework that any organization can use to improve overall performance. Seven categories make up the award criteria:

- *Leadership* Examines how senior executives guide the organization and how the organization addresses its responsibilities to the public and practices good citizenship

- *Strategic planning* Examines how the organization sets strategic directions and how it determines key action plans

- *Customer and market focus* Examines how the organization determines requirements and expectations of customers and markets; builds relationships with customers; and acquires, satisfies, and retains customers

- *Measurement, analysis, and knowledge management* Examines the management, effective use, analysis, and improvement of data and information to support key organization processes and the organization's performance management system

- *Human resource focus* Examines how the organization enables its workforce to develop its full potential and how the workforce is aligned with the organization's objectives

♦ *Process management*   Examines aspects of how key production/delivery and support processes are designed, managed, and improved

♦ *Business results*   Examines the organization's performance and improvement in its key business areas: customer satisfaction, financial and marketplace performance, human resources, supplier and partner performance, operational performance, and governance and social responsibility. The category also examines how the organization performs relative to competitors.

As with other audits, the self-assessment, which is accomplished in preparation for the application and site visit, can have very important diagnostic information to the institution for the purposes of quality improvement. Many states and large organizations have created their own version of the Baldrige award, such as the Governor's Sterling Award in the state of Florida and the Secretary of Veterans Affairs Robert W. Carey Quality Award in the Department of Veterans Affairs (VA).

Pearl

- "Benchmarking stimulates innovation and creativity by helping the organization remove self-imposed barriers to greater performance" (Gift, 1996, p. 255).

Customer Needs Analysis   This is a formal, systematic exploration and analysis of customer expectations as driven by the customer's hierarchy of needs and described in the customer's own words (Young, 1996). Such an analysis can effectively reveal problems within the organization that are not necessarily apparent to the management or clinical staff. Identification of customer needs can be achieved through the use of several tools:

1. *Focus group*   A forum of customers who communicate their needs, expectations, concerns, and preferences to the organization. Often, the group dynamics allow for the exchange of information that might not otherwise be communicated in a survey or personal interview format.

2. *Surveys*   Questionnaires designed to solicit information concerning customer needs. It is important to provide open-ended questions so as not to limit the responses of the individual. Survey information can be collected through the mail or over the telephone.

3. *Personal interviews*   Allow for greater flexibility for gathering information in terms of the time, location, or length of questioning. Some individuals may feel more comfortable and be more responsive in a one-on-one situation as opposed to a group situation.

Benchmarking   Another effective method of finding a process to improve is benchmarking, the process of finding the best practices and implementing them in an organization. Gift (1996) describes four types of benchmarking:

1. *Internal*   This involves studying similar practices among different departments or individuals within the same organization. For example, an audiology department may want to benchmark its customer service practices against the radiology department, which has been recognized as a leader in customer service.

2. *Competitive*   This type of benchmarking involves comparing a process or function within an organization with that of a competitor in the community, or with one who shares the same market.

3. *Functional*   This involves comparing a function within an organization with a similar function in an entirely different industry. For example, a hospital may benefit from benchmarking its admissions process against the reservations processes of hotels, airlines, or rental car companies.

4. *Collaborative*   This type of benchmarking involves collaborating with several organizations that provide the same services, identifying best practices within the group, then comparing and benchmarking these best practices against the best practices of external organizations.

Peer Review   Opportunities for improvement can be found by establishing a system of peer review. Such a system involves identifying an individual or group of individuals who are assigned the responsibility of reviewing processes or records of others in the same profession, that is, peers. For example, an audiology program may enlist the assistance of an audiologist working outside the organization to review a sample of records to determine if accepted clinical practices have been followed for the appropriate referral of neonates for additional testing. This method is particularly effective when a department consists of a small number of clinicians who may feel uncomfortable reviewing each others' work, or if the department head has clinical responsibilities and a review of that person's work by individuals he or she supervises would be awkward.

Clinical Pathways   Clinical pathways have been described as an optimum sequencing and timing of interventions of health care providers for a particular diagnosis or procedure, designed to minimize delays and resource utilization and to maximize quality (Coffey et al, 1992). Such pathways are developed either by the facility or by professional associations. Often the services of specialties such as audiology are included within the clinical pathways of a particular diagnosis or procedure. For example, the timing of OAE testing might be described in the clinical pathway for postnatal care in a hospital. If the audiology department is unable to meet these guidelines consistently, resulting in increased lengths of stay or discharge prior to the test, the process of providing OAE testing will have to be reviewed.

Clinical Algorithms Clinical algorithms are systematically developed statements designed to assist practitioner and patient decisions about appropriate health care for specific clinical circumstances. They provide clear, concise formulas and visual detail of the care plan. They can approve the quality of care and decrease costs by guiding clinicians toward standardization and clinically optimal, cost-effective strategies, and by facilitating valid measures of clinical process and outcomes (Kleeb, 1996). Clinical algorithms can be developed by the health care facility, but because they tend to involve specific diagnoses and treatment plans, they are often formulated by a task force and published by a professional association for use by practitioners. Using the previous example, a clinical algorithm developed for neonatal hearing testing would include criteria for testing, pass/fail criteria, referral options, and follow-up requirements. The algorithm might be developed as a visual flow chart, with decision trees indicating the direction of the process at any point. The algorithm may represent the standard of care for neonatal testing throughout the country against which the practice of any specific program can be compared. According to Kleeb (1996), algorithms have the following benefits. They

♦ Provide a method for involving clinicians in clinical quality improvement efforts and give them an opportunity to gain insight into previously unknown practice variations

♦ Offer a way to scrutinize clinical information, which allows for easy isolation of clinical decisions

♦ Provide the foundation for problem identification and improvement opportunities

♦ Act as a visual representation of the care plan and difficult decision-making processes

♦ Reduce variation in practice and improve care through a series of step-by-step recommendations

♦ Provide a forum for education, debate, and conflict resolution

♦ Improve the morale of clinicians by demonstrating commitment to deliver the highest quality of clinical care possible

Special Consideration

• The development of pathways and algorithms are often labor-intensive, time-consuming, and may initially lead to higher costs associated with the implementation of quality improvement ideas.

Step 2. Organize a Team that Knows the Process

Once an opportunity for process improvement is found from one or more of the methods described in step 1, the purpose of step 2 is to organize a team to assess the needs, first, by identifying a group of people familiar with the process, then bringing them together, providing them with the necessary resources, and allowing them to examine the problem and recommend specific actions to improve the process. Stolz (1996) describes the following actions involved in organizing the quality improvement team:

♦ Ensuring appropriate representation of all parts of the process between the boundaries named

♦ Identifying the process owner, or the person with authority and responsibility for leading the improvement effort

♦ Identifying sources of technical or educational support, often a facilitator/adviser

♦ Identifying the leadership liaison responsible for helping align the improvement effort with other, often larger organizational priorities and for securing necessary resources

♦ Formulating a plan or road map for the improvement effort

♦ Determining how those engaged in making improvements will work together, including roles, responsibilities, and expectations

♦ Initiating methods to keep others in the organization informed of progress and to promote learning

An essential part of this step is to develop a charter describing the purpose of the team, goals, membership, meeting times, roles of the members, and rules for interaction to ensure a civil and constructive exchange of ideas. The charter is developed and agreed upon by all members of the team.

Pearl

• When organizing a quality improvement team, involve the people who are most familiar with the process identified for improvement. These are usually front-line employees, not managers and supervisors.

Step 3. Clarify Current Knowledge of the Process

To improve a process, it is imperative that there be an accurate assessment of how the current process operates. Step 3 is designed to ensure that all members of the quality improvement team have a complete and shared understanding of the way things are currently being done. An effective tool for step 3 is flowcharting. Flowcharting allows the members of the group to describe each step of the process as a logical and visual progression of events. It also may identify opportunities for immediate improvement, such as eliminating obvious redundancies or unnecessary steps. If published clinical algorithms exist for this process, the group can identify where the current process deviates from accepted clinical practice. In the absence of published algorithms, the group will determine how the current flow needs to change to improve the quality of the process—a quicker return appointment for hearing aid fittings, for example, or a faster response rate to provide baseline examinations for patients on potentially cochleotoxic drugs.

Step 4. Understand the Source of Variation in the Process

The improvement team cannot simply recommend changes to the existing process based on what they assume will result in the greatest improvement. Changes that may appear to be intuitively reasonable may, in practice, be counterproductive. Step 4 allows the team members to examine and understand the types and sources of variation in the process by studying the performance of the process over time and identifying which factors within the process have a strong influence on the outcome most important to the customer (Stolz, 1996). The following actions are recommended as part of this step (Stolz, 1996):

♦ Reviewing customer requirements and judgments of quality

♦ Gathering and analyzing data on process performance variation over time

♦ Removing or incorporating special causes to make the process stable over time

♦ Identifying, gathering, and analyzing data on factors within the system of common causes that have a significant influence on the process outcome

As part of the data gathering, the group will need to agree on what and how the data will be measured, who will collect the data, and how long the data will be gathered.

Pitfall

• Take care not to tackle processes that are too complex or beyond the control of the quality improvement team. This will lead to frustration and reluctance to participate in future quality improvement efforts.

Step 5. Select the Process to Be Implemented

Following an analysis of the data in step 4, step 5 requires the group members to list, prioritize, and select the changes most likely to result in a significant quality improvement. The choice of which change to select may not necessarily be based on effectiveness alone. The cost of implementing the change as compared with the amount of predicted benefit should be considered as well. Costs may be associated with additional personnel, equipment, structural changes, overtime, contracting, and so on. Following a decision concerning the planned changes, the group enters into the second phase of the quality improvement process: the PDCA cycle.

Step 6. Plan the Pilot

At this point in the process, the quality improvement team needs to plan how the changes identified in the above step will be implemented and how the effects of those changes will be measured. The actions associated with this step include (Stolz, 1996)

♦ What the change is in terms that are easily understood

♦ Who is responsible for implementation

♦ Who must be informed and/or trained

♦ Where the pilot test will be held

♦ When it will begin

♦ How long it will last

♦ What the implementation requirements, such as communication, equipment, and training, are and how will they be addressed

Step 7. Do the Improvement, Data Collection, and Analysis

This is the point at which the team implements a quality improvement plan and measures the results. Actions associated with this step include (Stolz, 1996)

♦ Preparing workers and the work environment for the process change

♦ Implementing the change and conducting work accordingly

♦ Observing and documenting the effects of the change

♦ Observing for, documenting, and addressing, as appropriate, surprises or unforeseen circumstances such as failures or deficiencies in planning and implementation and changes in the organization that could affect the process under study

Step 8. Check and Study the Results

Step 8 involves reviewing the results to see if the implemented change had the desired and anticipated effects. Actions included in this step involve comparing the outcome before the changes were implemented with those achieved after implementation. The team needs to understand the causes of any failures that may have occurred and, conversely, to be able to explain why outcomes exceeded the predicted results.

Step 9. Act to Hold the Gain and to Continue to Improve the Process

Recall that FOCUS-PDCA is a method for implementing continuous quality improvement. It is not enough to demonstrate that the implemented changes had a positive result. The team must take action to ensure that realized gains continue to occur and to examine methods to improve outcome even further. Actions associated with this step include (Stolz, 1996)

Table 3–12 FOCUS-PDCA Tools

Cause-and-effect diagram	An illustration representing an identified problem (effect) and the possible contributing factors (causes)
Flowchart	A simple illustration of the steps involved in a process, usually represented chronologically
Gantt chart	A time table displaying action items, assignments, and time frames for completion
Pareto diagram	A vertical bar graph developed through brainstorming or existing data to help identify those issues that represent the greatest problems associated with a process
Run chart	A line graph representing the occurrence of an event over time; useful in monitoring the results of a new or modified procedure
Control chart	Similar to a run chart but with a statistically determined upper and/or lower limit to identify critical variations in a process
Scatter plot	A plot of data points often representing two variables that may help to identify relationships between those variables
Histogram	A bar chart that displays the frequency at which particular events occur

♦ *Anchoring the benefit and extending the gain* Make changes to organization policies and procedures, implement training programs, and develop a mechanism for monitoring the long-term effects of the change.

♦ *Acting to continue making improvements* Review the initial list of potential changes (step 5), implement another pilot study, and find another process to improve.

♦ *Adapt the change* Modify the change if it appears that an improved outcome will result.

♦ *Abandon the change* Select another change from the list if the assumptions on which the predicted change were based proved to be in error.

A list of tools commonly used as part of the FOCUS-PDCA process is listed in **Table 3–12**.

♦ Customer Service

An audiology program that is committed to quality improvement is passionate and uncompromising in its commitment to customer service (**Table 3–13**). Industry recognizes the

Table 3–13 Customer Service: Critical Factors

- Customer feedback and information management
- Leadership
- Strategic planning
- Continuous improvement
- Empowerment and accountability
- Education, training, and staff development
- Reward and recognition
- Communication
- Patient-centered culture

importance of customer service in a competitive marketplace where the customer has many choices and loyalty is no longer a motivating factor in the customer's purchasing decisions.

What is customer service? We recognize good and poor service when we encounter it. We recognize it in the businesses we use and in the businesses we are in. Customer service is simply a measure of the degree of caring communicated by the people, processes, and environment in the organization, whether that organization consists of one person or 100,000.

Who are your customers? Almost all businesses have both internal and external customers. Your internal customers are the people you report to in an organization and the people who report to you. They are other members of the organization on whose support you depend, both administratively and clinically. External customers are the people who refer patients to you, the vendors you depend upon, your banking and business associates, and, most importantly, your patients.

Pearl

- Okyakusama wa kamisama desu.—"The Customer Is God."

Critical Success Factors for Outstanding Customer Service

Customer Feedback and Information Management

Feedback and information from customers are designed to inform the organization of customers' expectations and needs. These expectations drive the identification of other organizational information needs that support improving customer service. One strategy that can improve an organization's ability to perform is to involve and listen to its customers through the types of customer feedback methods described earlier in this chapter. Good customer feedback and information management systems are used to support managerial, operational, financial, performance improvement, and clinical decision making.

Leadership

Leadership has overall responsibility for planning and directing an organization's activity. In this context, it refers to top and middle management, such as department and section heads and supervisors. Middle managers are key individuals in achieving customer goals. A key responsibility of leadership is to use customer input and assessments to evaluate available resources and to set priorities. The leadership team must model its commitment to customer service and support staff in complying with customer requirements appropriately. The principal duty of leadership is to ensure that daily work is aligned with the organization's strategic direction and that all efforts remain patient centered.

Strategic Planning

Strategic planning includes using information derived from the community and customer feedback and information systems, as well as the organization's mission and vision. The resource deployment process involves how an organization allocates, aligns, and integrates major resources (e.g., human resources, capital, information, and technologies) into its strategies to meet its customers' needs and expectations, as well as the organization's own goals and mission. This convergence of an organization's major resources using a systems approach is essential to achieving sustainable performance improvements.

Process of Continuous Improvement

Customer-focused continuous improvement is a data-driven process planned by leadership to accomplish the strategic goals of the organization. It is achieved through teams of individuals who work day to day on the processes that produce the organization's services and products.

Empowerment and Accountability

Excellent organizations accomplish good customer service by allowing and encouraging all levels of staff to meet or exceed customer needs and expectations. It applies not only to direct customer interactions but also to the day-to-day operation of processes. Successful empowerment of staff requires an understanding that they know what they can do and that they feel that their actions will be valued by their colleagues and supported by all levels of leadership within the organization. Accountability refers to defining and communicating customer service expectations to employees and ensuring that expectations are met through the establishment of customer service performance standards, for example. **Table 3–14** gives examples of role changes made by management in an environment that empowers staff members.

Table 3–14 Management's Role Changes in an Empowered Environment

From	To
Commander	Coach, facilitator
Controller	Leader
Individualist	Team builder
Internally competitive	Cooperative
Withholding	Open, explaining
Owner mentality	Trustee mentality

Education, Training, and Staff Development

Education, training, and staff development are ongoing processes used to develop customer-focused knowledge, skills, and attitudes of employees. Organizations that are known for their excellent customer service are also known for investing substantial resources to ensure that staff members are competent to do their job and are skilled in providing customer service.

Reward and Recognition

Reward and recognition systems are generally extrinsic methods developed by organizations to enhance employees' feelings of satisfaction with their work. It is important to realize, however, that satisfaction with work is inherently an individual employee's perception and feelings about work and the environment. The intrinsic rewards are more closely aligned with the culture and values of an organization than its formal reward and recognition systems. It is essential that formal reward and recognition processes and programs be aligned with both the values and strategic goals of a patient-centered culture. Reward systems that promote customer service ensure that performance ratings and bonuses are at least partially based on serving customers well. They also reward teams rather than individuals. Customer service organizations are characterized by a variety of creative methods of recognition that are clearly tied to meeting customer needs and expectations.

Communication

Customer-focused organizations have and use multiple methods of communicating with customers, stakeholders, the community, and each other. Both formal and informal methods of communication abound. Effective communication builds commitment, investment, and ownership toward the principles of customer service.

Patient-Centered Culture

Most importantly, organizations that are outstanding in customer service have a patient-centered culture. Culture refers to the way people interact, communicate, and behave based on a shared system of values, beliefs, mores, and attitudes. These organizations put patients'/customers' needs at the very center of what they do. They continuously and consistently adopt the patients' perspective. Their highest priority strategic goals come from identified customer needs and expectations. For instance, continuity, coordination of care, and emotional support have been identified by patients as areas that need improvement. This has led many organizations to implement a patient-centered primary care model. They focus on understanding a patient's experience with illness and health care. Everyone must be involved in making the culture a primary and legitimate expression of the organization's values. Management designs processes and services to meet customer needs, not employee or service needs.

Building Customer Loyalty

In a highly competitive environment in which consumers are becoming more educated about the marketplace and will seek out the best service for the lowest cost, how can a business create an environment where the customer wants to return? Heil et al (1995) describe six challenges of revolutionary service that, if successfully met, will help an organization develop a loyal customer base by adding value to every aspect of the customer relationship.

Challenge 1. Make an Emotional Connection

Giving customers a quality product or service at a fair price meets only customers' minimum expectations. To develop loyalty, we have to make an emotional connection with our customers. That means bringing humanity back into the workplace, showing empathy, and providing a personal touch with every customer contact.

Challenge 2. Attack the Structures

Do our structures make sense to our customers? Do our policies, procedures, and decisions add value for our customers, or do they make it more difficult to do business with us? Current structures were designed to get current results. If we want dramatically different results tomorrow, we will have to redesign our structures.

Challenge 3. Align Structures with Words

Are we walking the talk? Practices that undermine employees' efforts to build customer loyalty will make everyone cynical. Ensure that employees have been trained adequately, have enough information, and that all procedures exist to give customers the best service possible.

Challenge 4. Know Your Customer

One size fits one, not all. We must improve at understanding our customers, their preferences and needs, and their reasons for choosing to do business with us to personalize our relationship with them. What high- and low-tech methods can we use to gather customer data?

Challenge 5. Make Recovery Strategic

Relationships are tested when times are tough, not when everything is going smoothly. When we've made a mistake or a customer wants a customized product or service, it is our opportunity to demonstrate our true colors. Are our policies and procedures limiting or enhancing our abilities to recover from mistakes?

Challenge 6. Service Is Reselling

There is no more "old business." Whether we've had a customer relationship for 10 days or 10 years, every time that customer chooses to do business with us, he or she should be recognized for that choice. The business we get from now on is brand new. We need to change our focus from recruiting new customers to retaining the customers we already have.

Service Recovery

Heil et al (1995) describe the importance of recovering from mistakes. The techniques associated with this type of recovery are often referred to as service recovery. The *VA Handbook* (Department of Veterans Affairs, 2004) describes service recovery as a four-step process that

- Identifies a service expectation that was not met
- Effectively resolves service problems
- Classifies the root cause(s)
- Yields data that can be integrated with other sources of performance measurement to assess and improve the system

Service recovery entails making a person "feel whole" by staff demonstration of politeness, concern, and candor. It is taking a negative experience and turning it into a positive and memorable one. It is a second chance, so it must be done right the second time. Those organizations truly committed to customer service see complaints as a significant opportunity to improve processes and build customer loyalty. Suggested techniques for service recovery are listed in **Table 3–15** and include the following:

- *Remain calm* Patients who are ill or in pain may have little tolerance for what they perceive is poor service. If you are the target of their anger or frustration, remain calm and do not become hostile or defensive. When you remain calm in the face of adversity, you exercise a critical interpersonal skill.

Table 3–15 Ten Steps to Successful Service Recovery

1. Remain calm
2. Stop, look, listen
3. Accept anger
4. Accept responsibility
5. Refer
6. Ask questions
7. Restate
8. Respond
9. Agree
10. Develop solutions
11. Exceed expectations
12. Personalize
13. Thank

♦ *Stop, look, and listen*   Stop what you are doing, even if busy. Look at the person; make eye contact. Let him or her know you are engaged in the conversation. Listen to what is being said and communicate your empathy with facial expressions and occasional nods.

♦ *Accept anger*   Anger is a common expression of frustration. Allow the patient to vent the emotion.

♦ *Accept responsibility*   Do not immediately pass off a complaint by saying, "That's not my job," even if the problem is not within your area of responsibility. From the patient's viewpoint, you are a representative of the organization that has caused a problem. Become an advocate for the patient, not the organization. Assist the patient with identifying the individual or department that will be most effective at resolving the complaint.

♦ *Refer*   Make certain that the person to whom you refer the patient is the appropriate individual. The patient's frustration will only grow if he or she is passed on to the wrong person or department.

♦ *Ask questions*   Engage the patient in direct, open-ended questions that will help you to define the specifics of the problem, for example, "What is the problem?" "Where did it happen?" "What can I do to resolve this situation to your satisfaction?"

♦ *Restate*   If the situation is complicated, be sure that you understand the problem by restating your interpretation of the events and by asking for confirmation.

♦ *Respond*   Act quickly. A visual confirmation that you take the problem seriously by taking notes or making a phone call will reassure the patient that something is being done.

♦ *Agree*   Try to find something in the person's remark with which you agree. Emphasizing what you have in common, even if it is relatively unimportant, can eliminate an argument.

♦ *Develop solutions*   If a single solution to the problem is obvious, implement it. If you have the opportunity to develop several alternative solutions, allow the person to make a choice. The opportunity to choose a plan of action most suitable to the individual's needs invariably forces him or her to be reasonable.

♦ *Exceed expectations*   Don't promise anything you may not be able to deliver. Your effectiveness in handling complaints is based on honestly stating what can reasonably be done. Let the patient know what to expect, and whenever possible exceed those expectations.

♦ *Personalize*   Introduce yourself to the patient and learn the person's name. For many, it is difficult to remain angry when you show you care enough about an individual to know his or her name.

♦ *Thank*   If possible, thank the patient for bringing the problem to your attention. Often the problem is systemic and has occurred in the past but has never been brought to your attention. Communicating an attitude that you sincerely appreciate knowing about such problems will encourage the person to feel more satisfied about the way in which it is handled.

Customer Service Self-Assessment

The following self-assessment may be helpful in identifying opportunities in your organization for improving customer service.

♦ Do you reward behavior in others that would further support customer service standards?

♦ Do you know how others view you and your behavior in relation to furthering effective customer service?

♦ How do you determine customer service expectations?

♦ Do you compare or benchmark yourself to others?

♦ Do you view customer complaints as problems or opportunities for improvement?

♦ Does your organization make it easy for employees to solve problems?

♦ In what ways do you communicate and explain the mission, vision, and values of your organization to employees?

♦ What methods do you use to reinforce positive customer service?

♦ Are you measuring what you want repeated in your organization? Are you communicating these expectations to your employees?

♦ Do you set aside time each week to solicit feedback from patients, employees, and visitors?

♦ Do you walk around the department on a regular basis?

♦ Do you personally participate in employee orientation?

♦ Do you personally participate in CQI training?

♦ Are you or have you ever been a member of a process action or quality improvement team?

♦ Do you personally review summary data related to customer service? Can you name any actions taken recently as a result of such a review?

♦ Can you name a time recently when you have encouraged a staff member to "take a risk" or recognized one who did?

◆ Treatment Outcome as an Indication of Quality Improvement

All of the concepts discussed to this point, from the integration of continuous quality principles to customer service, are designed to improve the outcome associated with the patient's episode of care. Managed care firms, insurers, government agencies, and our patients are justifiably demanding that our interventions make meaningful differences. It is these meaningful differences that we commonly refer to as treatment outcomes, and it is these outcomes that we can point to as the fruit of our continuous quality improvement labors.

In an attempt to demonstrate effective treatment outcomes, the entire health care industry, including audiology, has developed an impressive array of outcome measures. Unfortunately, the proliferation of these tools has created confusion concerning the terminology and appropriate utilization of these instruments. The result is that we do not always measure what we think we are measuring. There are several outcomes that audiologists are interested in assessing. These include impairment, activity limitations, participation restrictions, satisfaction, and quality of life. Each of these has measuring instruments that are specific to that domain. Although some of these terms are used (and misused) interchangeably, they do have distinct meanings and measuring instruments that are unique to that domain. Because of the complexities associated with the issue of outcome measures and the emerging importance of accountability in the profession, the topic of outcomes is addressed more completely in Chapter 8 in this volume.

◆ Integrating Quality into Clinical Training: The 4th-Year Experience

The concept of quality is as integral to education as it is to health care. Just as quality of care in the health care arena can be described as the degree to which health services for individuals and populations increase the likelihood of desired health outcomes and are consistent with current professional knowledge, quality of education can be described as the degree to which learning for individuals and populations increases the likelihood of desired educational outcomes and is consistent with current professional knowledge. Perhaps there is no greater challenge in the education of audiologists today than in ensuring the quality of the 4th-year clinical educational experience.

As Wilson (2003) pointed out, currently, there is no mechanism by which the quality of 4th-year clinical experiences is assessed. The need for establishing clear standards was exhorted by the members of the Big 10 consensus group ("Big Ten Consensus Statement," 2003). The group agreed that specific guidelines were needed for the inclusion of a clinical practicum site in an audiology educational program and that these guidelines should consider issues such as accreditation by appropriate bodies, number and adequacy of preparation of the clinical staff who would be responsible for the students' supervision, consistency with the amount of

supervision provided, and the willingness of clinical staff to engage in formative assessment of student learning outcomes.[1] The importance of the 4th-year doctorate in audiology (Au.D.) experience and the concerns raised regarding a lack of criteria for assessing its quality led the American Academy of Audiology (AAA), with support from the AAA Foundation and the VA, to sponsor the Consensus Conference on Issues and Concerns Related to the 4th-Year Au.D. Student, in January 2004 (Mashie and Mendel, 2005). The result of the conference, which was attended by more than 115 individuals from some 35 universities, private practices, VA medical centers, educational audiology, pediatric tertiary care centers, corporate and network audiologists, and Au.D. students, was, again, the highlighting of the need for standards for the preceptor and the externship site.[2] Specific recommendations regarding standards included (1) that the qualifications of the preceptor exceed state licensure and voluntary entry-level certification and that the preceptor should be able to demonstrate competency in scope of practice and supervision of externs; and (2) that the externship site (whether involving sequential or simultaneous rotations at multiple sites or at one site) be able to document staffing, depth and breadth of clinical experiences, physical environment, compliance with applicable state and federal regulations, time for learning, complementary activities, and a willingness to participate in the evaluation of student competencies.

Pearl

- The widely used quality improvement principles found in health care and business readily lend themselves to application in the higher education arena.

Although it is clear that there is a need for determining the quality of 4th-year experiences in audiology education, the actual mechanism by which this will be done has not yet been determined. In fact, at the first Audiology Education Summit, which occurred in January 2005, it was agreed that the quality of external practicum sites was critical to the training of audiologists. Further discussion, however, was needed regarding how to recognize and possibly "accredit" quality clinical sites. Indeed, the second Audiology Education Summit, in February

---

[1] Formative assessment is conducted while an educational event or procedure is ongoing. The purpose of formative assessment is to monitor students' acquisition of knowledge and skills during educational preparation and is designed to help students and instructors to systematically track and document progress toward the attainment of learning outcomes (Rassi, 1998).

[2] The term *preceptor* was adopted at the Consensus Conference on Issues and Concerns Related to the 4th-Year AuD Student (Mashie and Mendel, 2005) to refer to the licensed audiologist providing clinical education to the *extern,* which was the term designated for the student. *Externship* was adopted as the appropriate term for long-term clinical training outside the university.

2006, focused on this and other issues related to the 4th-year Au.D. experience. Although summit attendees were able to agree on several essential qualities for preceptors, including a desire to teach and mentor student clinicians, having the necessary interpersonal, communication, and counseling skills for mentoring students, and a clear understanding of the needs and role of a student clinician, it was also agreed that a method for evaluating supervisory skills needed to be developed. The summit participants also found as essential the use of formalized assessment tools that would allow for communication between externs and preceptors, which could be used to evaluate both students and the practicum sites.

Formative assessments of students, the use of formalized assessment tools, and the possibility of accrediting clinical educational sites all provide mechanisms that will allow for continuous quality improvement in the education of future doctors of audiology. Indeed, as Rassi (1998) points out, the widely used quality improvement principles found in health care and business readily lend themselves to application in the higher education arena. Assessing the outcomes of student learning and preceptor effectiveness in 4th-year placements is critical to the provision of a quality educational experience. Just as the preceptors and clinical sites should continually assess the ability of students to demonstrate their knowledge and skills in engaging in clinical activities, with ever-growing independence and competence, the continuous assessment of clinical teaching effectiveness, by both self- and external review, encourages ongoing adjustments that can serve to improve the teaching-learning process.

♦ Summary

In this chapter, the concepts of quality improvement in a health care setting have been reviewed. The reason quality remains a controlling principle of practice management is that it is infused, knowingly or unknowingly, in every aspect of what we do as health care providers. From the moment we open our doors in the morning to the time we shut off the lights in the evening, the effectiveness of the care we provide to our patients is determined by the investment in quality we place in our planning, staff, resources, education, equipment, customer service, marketing, physical plant, and networking. Committing yourself and your practice to an ethic of excellence, however, will not be enough. You will need to discover ways to continue to improve the quality of your practice.

Appendix 3–1

Case Studies

Case 1: Detection Approach to Quality Improvement

The owner of a busy multioffice audiology practice in a large metropolitan area in the Southwest established a threshold that 90% of all hearing aids will be delivered to the patients within 14 calendar days of the audiologic examination. Once a month, the owner would review all records to determine if the threshold had been surpassed. For most months, the performance level was acceptable, with ~91 to 94% of instruments delivered within an acceptable time frame. During those periods when performance fell below 90%, no specific reason (office, clinician, manufacturer, etc.) could be identified.

♦ What are the costs associated with this approach?

♦ Is 90% an acceptable criterion? Why not 85%, 95%, 100%?

♦ Is 14 days an acceptable criterion?

♦ How can performance improve if the threshold is rarely crossed?

♦ Is the owner necessarily the best individual to make these measurements? Should others be involved?

♦ How can opportunities for improvements be identified using this approach?

♦ How does this approach maximize patient satisfaction?

Case 2: Prevention Approach to Quality Improvement

In response to periodic patient complaints and increasing competition in the community, the owner in case 1 determines that the existing 14-day time frame for delivering hearing aids is no longer appropriate. The owner appreciates the complexity of the business and the many separate processes that culminate in the final delivery of the hearing aid. She appoints a team consisting of the appointment clerk, an audiologist, and the business manager to review all processes involved and to recommend improvements that will decrease the delivery time to no more than 7 calendar days.

♦ What are the advantages of appointing a team to identify solutions as opposed to having the owner of the practice develop solutions?

♦ How can this approach prevent problems from occurring as opposed to detecting them after the fact?

♦ How can this approach maximize patient satisfaction?

♦ Might the team benefit from training in CQI techniques?

♦ What should the role of the owner be as the team analyzes the processes and develops recommendations?

♦ What should the role of the remaining staff be during this process?

References

Abrams, H. B., & Siferd, S. T. (1994). Total quality improvement: The Department of Veterans Affairs audiology and speech pathology program. Seminars in Hearing, 15(4), 277–287.

American Hospital Association. (1999). Hospital statistics. Chicago: Author.

American National Standards Institute. (2003). Specification of hearing aid characteristics (ANSI S3.22–2003). New York: Acoustical Society of America.

American Speech-Language-Hearing Association. (2005). Quality indicators for professional service programs in audiology and speech-language pathology. Retrieved April 27, 2007 from http://www.asha.org/NR/rdonlyres/6FFAAB77-CC9E-4DE9-9B4C-F887202B45BA/0/v1CD_quality_indicators.pdf

Barlow, N, Bentler, R., Blood, I., Corney, A., Chambers, R, et al (2003). Big ten consensus statement regarding the future of audiology education. Audiology Today, 15(5), 46–48.

Berwick, D. M., Godfrey, A. B., & Roessner, J. (1990). Curing health care: Strategies for quality improvement. San Francisco: Jossey-Bass.

Centers for Disease Control and Prevention. (2006). Retrieved April 25, 2007 from http://www.cdc.gov/ncidod/dhqp/healthDis.html

Coffey, R. J., Richards, J. S., Remmert, C. S., LeRoy, S. S., Schoville, R. R., & Baldwin, P. J. (1992). An introduction to critical paths. Quality Management in Health Care, 1(1), 45–54.

Commission on Accreditation of Rehabilitation Facilities. (2005). The 2005 medical rehabilitation standards manual. Tucson, AZ: CARF International.

Crosby, P. B. (1979). Quality is free: The art of making quality certain. New York: McGraw-Hill.

Deming, W. E. (1986). Out of the crisis. Cambridge: Massachusetts Institute of Technology, Center for Advanced Engineering Study.

Gift, R. G. (1996). Benchmarking in today's management methods. In. R. G. Gift & C. F. Kinney (Eds.), Today's management methods: A guide for the health care executive. Chicago: American Hospital Publishing.

Gift, R. G., & Kinney, C. F. (Eds.). (1996). Today's management methods: A guide for the health care executive. Chicago: American Hospital Publishing (pp. 245–261).

Health Grades. (2006). Health Grades quality study: Third annual patient safety in American Hospitals study. Retrieved April 25, 2007 from http://www.healthgrades.com/media/dms/pdf/patientsafetyinAmericanHospitals Study2006.pdf

Heil, G., Tate, R., & Parker, T. (1995). Revolutionary service: Building customer loyalty one customer at a time. Des Moines, IA: Excellence in Training Corp.

James, B. C. (1989). Quality management for health care delivery. Chicago: The Hospital Research and Education Trust.

Joint Commission on Accreditation of Healthcare Organizations. (2005). Comprehensive accreditation manual for hospitals: The official handbook. Oakbrook Terrace, IL: Author.

Juran, J. M. (1988). Juran on planning for quality. New York: The Free Press.

Kleeb, T. (1996). Pathways and algorithms in today's management methods. In R.G. Gift & C. F. Kinney (Eds.), Today's management methods: A guide for the health care executive. Chicago: American Hospital Publishing (pp. 187–207).

Koch, M. W., & Fairly, T. M. (1993). Integrated quality management: The key to improving nursing care quality. St. Louis: Mosby-Year Book.

Kohn, L., Corrigan, J., & Donaldson, M. (2000). To err is human: Building a safer health system. Washington, DC: National Academy Press.

Mashie, J., & Mendel, L. L. (2005). The AuD externship experience: Summary document from the Consensus Conference on Issues and Concerns Related to the 4th Year AuD Student. Retrieved April 30, 2007 from http://www.capcsd.org/proceedings/2005/toc2005.html

National Institute of Standards and Technology. (2005). Baldrige national quality program. Retrieved April 27, 2007 from http://www.quality.nist.gov/

Pirsig, R. M. (1984). Zen and the art of motorcycle maintenance. New York: William Morrow.

Rassi, J. A. (1998). Outcome measurement in universities. In C. M. Frattali (Ed.), Measuring outcomes in speech-language pathology. New York: Thieme Medical Publishers (pp. 177–502).

Stolz, P. K. (1996). FOCUS-PDCA in today's management methods. In R. G. Gift & C. F. Kinney (Eds.), Today's management methods: A guide for the health care executive. Chicago: American Hospital Publishing (pp. 223–244).

Thomas, E. J., Studdert, D. M., Newhouse, J. P., et al. (1999). Costs of medical injuries in Utah and Colorado. Inquiry, 36, 255–264.

U.S. Department of Veterans Affairs. (2004, February 4). Service recovery in the Veterans Health Administration (VHA Handbook 1003.2, transmittal sheet). Washington, DC: Author.

Valente, M., Abrams, H., Benson, D., Chisolm, T., Citron, D., Hampton, D., & Loavenbruck, A. (2006). Guidelines for the audiologic management of adult hearing impairment. Retrieved April 21, 2007 from http://www.audiology.org/NR/rdonlyres/5DE475B4-58I3-40P7-934E-584AC11EABE9/0/haguidelines.pdf

Wilson, R. H. (2003). Issues and concerns for the 4th year AuD student. Audiology Today, 15, 1, 12.

Young, J. O. (1996). Customer needs analysis in today's management methods. In R. G. Gift & C. F. Kinney (Eds.), Today's management methods: A guide for the health care executive. Chicago: American Hospital Publishing.

Chapter 4

Human Resources Management in Audiology

David A. Zapala, Kathryn L. Shaughnessy, and Kathryn P. Snyder

Think of the last satisfying job you held. What made it satisfying? Chances are your satisfaction revolved around one of three factors. It could have been that you enjoyed your coworkers as interesting people, as effective teammates, or both. It could have been that you enjoyed the job. Either it was something you were good at, it helped you develop in some way, you were challenged, or you made a difference. Perhaps it was all of these. Very likely, the business that employed you was successful. There is little satisfaction working on a sinking ship.

Now think of that job again. Were the factors that contributed to your satisfaction the consequence of chance or planning? If you believe it was chance, consider yourself lucky to have stumbled upon a fortunate capricious moment in the history of that business. If you believe there was some planning, consider yourself very lucky indeed. Study that experience and learn from it. The best organizations strive to create situations where smart, industrious, capable individuals are organized into teams focused on successfully meeting the demands of the enterprise. This takes thoughtful planning and execution.

Whenever individuals unite to work toward a common goal, they can be seen as resources that should be organized and managed wisely. This concept applies not only to business concerns but also to professionals and their organizations. The principle message of this chapter is that, as professionals, each of us is a resource that contributes to the collective health of the discipline and profession of audiology. How we contribute forges our individual and collective future in the service of persons with hearing impairment.

This chapter approaches human resources management from a broad perspective. Specifically, human resources management is discussed from the point of view of the individual professional, the employer, and the profession. Human resources problems, particularly when they involve employer–employee relationships, are complex and best managed by professionals in the area of human resources and law. The approach taken here is to present the principal themes that run throughout one's professional life and to point out potential roadblocks to the advancement of the individual and profession.

◆ Self-Management

Most audiologists have three professional relationships: with their patient, their profession, and their employer. In this section, factors that affect these relationships are presented from the point of view of the individual audiologist.

Relationship with the Patient: Personal and Professional Propriety

Any professional who offers his or her service to the community holds a trust. Professional status implies that, in a given area of enterprise, laypersons cannot reasonably obtain the expertise held by professionals, and may not be able to act in their own best interest without the assistance of one more knowledgeable (Fox and Battin, 1978; Pellegrino, 2002). Because the consumer must rely on the judgment of the professional, the professional holds a fiduciary responsibility to the consumer. That is, the professional is expected to act in a manner that is in his or her client's or patient's best interest. It is the professional's expertise and fiduciary relationship that are purchased by the patient, not just a product or service.

From the profession's prospective, audiologists do not treat disease with medication or surgery. We improve people's ability to function or communicate in the face of impaired hearing or balance largely by changing the behavior of those we help. Audiologist-directed behavior change can only occur when the practitioner is perceived as holding a high standard for personal propriety and professional knowledge. It stands to reason, then, that these attributes are important assets for all audiologists.

Professionals are held to a higher standard of conduct than others in the workforce, primarily because of their fiduciary responsibilities to those whom they serve. Most licensure statutes have sections detailing standards for personal propriety and ethical behavior. An example of such a section is shown in **Table 4–1**. These statutes are designed to protect the public from professionals who have poor character and are thus unworthy of the public trust. They are based on the assumption that the individual who is worthy of professional status will stand a test of good citizenship. So, for example, most statutes specifically require that the professional be free of felony conviction, have no evidence of fraudulent activities, and be in general good moral standing as judged by peers. Most statutes also require the applicant to follow a professional code of ethics. These are typically modeled after the codes of pertinent professional organizations, such as the American Academy of Audiology (AAA), the American Board of Audiology (ABA), and the American Speech-Language-Hearing Association (ASHA). (See Appendix I in this volume.)

Employers and other accrediting agencies may require higher minimum standards of good citizenship. For example, many agencies receive government funds and must provide evidence of a drug-free environment (Drug-Free Workplace Act of 1988; see Whiting, 2005). In passive enforcement, a drug-related arrest may be enough for disciplinary action. In active enforcement, random tests may be required. Other requirements might include standards to ensure against sexual harassment, gender, or cultural or racial discrimination, or set minimum requirements for employee health status or credit worthiness (Paulson, 2003; Whiting, 2005).

Professional propriety refers to actions involved in professional practice. The ASHA Certification of Clinical Competence and the American Board of Audiology's board certification program require that the professional maintain minimum standards in the areas of professional propriety, experience, and knowledge. These are embodied in both organizations' codes of ethics.

Standards imposed by employers and other agencies are not the only ones to which the professional must subscribe. What might a patient expect from an audiologist in terms of personal propriety and ethical behavior? What would we expect from our colleagues? From the patient's perspective, Bendapudi et al (2006) systematically reviewed patient attitudes and expectations about their health care providers. They developed the following list of desirable behaviors or attributes for health care providers:

Humane   Caring and wants what is best for the patient

Personal   Interested in the patient as a person and interacts with the patients in a personal way

Empathetic   Tries to understand how the patient is feeling emotionally and physically

Table 4–1 Ethical and Personal Proprietary Standards

Section 21. Subject to the due process requirements of the Uniform Administrative Procedures Act, compiled in Title 4, Part 5, any person registered under this part may have his license denied, revoked or suspended for a fixed period to be determined by the council for any of the following causes:

1. Conviction of an offense involving moral turpitude. The record of such conviction, or certified copy thereof from the clerk of the court where such conviction occurred, or by the judge of such court, is sufficient evidence to warrant revocation or suspension;

2. Securing a license under this part through fraud or deceit;

3. Unethical conduct, gross and/or repeated acts of ignorance or insufficiency in the conduct of his practice;

4. Knowingly practicing while suffering with a contagious or infectious disease;

5. Use of a false name or alias in the practice of his profession; and

6. Violating any of the provisions of this part.

Source: From Tennessee Code Annotated, Title 63, Chapter 17, Part 2, Section 21.

Respectful   Takes patient input seriously and is respectful of his or her time

Thorough   Determined and complete

Forthright   Speaks to the patient in understandable terms

Confident   Assuring

These behaviors can be reduced to three principles. Health care providers are expected to deliver empathetic care, demonstrate personal integrity, and work to preserve the personal autonomy of the patient or client. Empathetic care means the ability to understand the patient's circumstance as if it were one's own (empathy) and have compassion for the patient (humane, personal). Integrity means the ability to be truthful (forthright) and to act consistently with a moral and ethical code. Preservation of personal autonomy means including patients as active participants in their own care (respectful). To include patients as participants in the treatment process, they must be informed of treatment options, participate in the selection of their treatment, hold some responsibility for compliance with the treatment plan, and participate in the assessment of treatment outcomes (Beuf, 1979; Inlander et al, 1988).

Delivering care based on these principles is harder than it seems. The process starts with a commitment to basic values, self-evaluation, and a desire to improve. Issues of integrity become more complex as one ventures further into the field of audiology. For example, are professionals showing integrity when they accept gifts from manufacturers? Are they always on time and focused when they see patients? The wise professional is always vigilant for signs of self-delusion, substandard care, and potential conflicts of interest. This is necessary to maintain his or her fiduciary responsibility to patients. (For further discussion, see Chapter 2 in this volume and the AAA's guidelines [Hamill, 2006].)

This is not a chapter about ethics. However, a profession is made up of individual practitioners. We are defined as much by the actions of our peers as by our own actions or those of our professional societies. In the long term, an individual's personal and professional propriety is recognizable in the marketplace and contributes to the perception of the profession as a whole.

Pearl

- "Patients don't much care about what you know until they know that you care."—Anonymous

---

Relationship with the Profession: Personal Growth

Most audiologists selected their profession out of a strong desire to help others. Audiology is a young, dynamic, growing field with plenty of opportunities to learn more or improve outcomes. Often the same desire to help propels the accomplished practitioner to innovate or master a new area. Thus, it is not surprising that audiologists feel a need and an obligation for continuing education and self-development.

The process of planning for continued growth begins soon after the audiologist leaves graduate school. Typically,

at some point during the 4th year externship experience, the new audiologist begins a process of self-evaluation. The extern may find several areas where his or her clinical skills or knowledge base fall short. Although this can leave the new audiologist feeling inadequately trained and frustrated, it heralds the beginning of the next stage in self-development. It is only through honest self-evaluation that the audiologist can prioritize deficient areas and plan for further education and skill development. Later, when the audiologist has developed clinical acumen, this same process of self-assessment will spark efforts to broaden and diversify areas of expertise. The process continues throughout one's professional life—always with the goal of improving one's ability to contribute to the health and well-being of the community.

Audiologists have several tools with which to develop their knowledge base and clinical skills. Professional journals are available in audiology, medicine, and the basic sciences. Textbooks and formal continuing education coursework can improve the didactic knowledge of the audiologist. Web-based continuing education opportunities, including services such as Audiology Online (www.audiologyonline.com) and virtual seminars (e.g., the AAA's continuing education page: www.audiology.org/professional/ce), as well as library services (e.g., the Dome: www.comdisdome.com), have greatly increased the availability of continuing education experiences. The habit of reading professional literature and completing coursework starts in graduate school and continues throughout one's professional life. No better way to develop the knowledge base of the practitioner exists.

Developing clinical skills often takes more than didactic instruction. Three powerful methods are available to help improve clinical skills: (1) outcome measurement and evidence-based practice development, (2) structured formal case presentations, and (3) mentorship.

Outcome measurement and evidence-based practice development are addressed elsewhere in this book (see Chapter 8). Briefly, one cannot improve if one does not measure current performance. The discipline required to track outcomes is the necessary first step toward self-improvement in the clinical realm.

A structured formal case presentation involves offering details on a difficult or interesting case to a group of peers. The role of the presenter in "case staffing" is to outline the case information in the most efficient way possible in an effort to highlight the clinician's decision making. The role of the peer group is to listen respectfully and to offer insight into how the case could have been managed better. This is not an adversarial situation. The presenter must be willing to take some criticism as a price of improved clinical decision making. The listeners must be tactful enough to offer suggestions in a helpful manner. For this to work, a bond of trust must exist between a group of colleagues dedicated to improving clinical efficacy. When care is taken to maintain this bond of trust, routine staffing can be the best way to sharpen clinical judgment. An example of a case presentation is shown in **Table 4–2**.

Mentorship is vital to the life of any discipline or profession. Mentoring is a relationship in which individuals in

Table 4–2 Example of a Case Presentation, with Headings Added to Highlight the Structure

1. Who (demographics) has what chief complaints (when possible, note onset and progression of symptoms; separate medical from auditory/communicative)

A 7-week-old infant was seen in follow-up after failing an otoacoustic emission (OAE) hearing screen before discharge and again 4 weeks after discharge. Test results obtained at 4 weeks suggest a strong chance of sensorineural hearing loss. This is the first birth in a young family (mother and father are 19 and 21 years old, respectively). Good extended family support is present. However, the mother's parents are not supportive of her efforts to follow up with the audiologic evaluations to date. No risk factors were associated with the birth; specifically, no history of hearing loss was present in any of the known family members. The family was sent to our clinic to confirm or refute the results of the referring hospital and, if necessary, to develop a management plan for the family.

2. Background and related information

At the 4-week visit, OAE were absent to 80 dB peak equivalent sound pressure level (pe SPL) clicks (transient evoked otoacoustic emission [TEOAE], ILO88, quick screen differential mode). An auditory brainstem response (ABR), obtained at the 4-week visit, demonstrated click-evoked responses down to 40 dB normalized hearing level (nHL) in the right ear, and 55 dB nHL in the left ear. High-frequency tympanometry yielded patterns consistent with the Vanhuyse model at 220 Hz and 1000 Hz (Y, G, B) in both ears. In addition, an ipsilateral acoustic reflex was measured in the left ear at 95 dB.

3. Subjective and objective assessment

Parents present with sleeping child. No physical sign of cranial facial malformation is present. TEOAE were absent in the left ear, and a possible emission was detected in the 700 Hz region (signal-to-noise ratio [SNR] 4 dB; absolute level –10 dB SPL) distortion product otoacoustic emissions (DPOAE) were absent between 1000 and 8000 Hz (L1/L2: 65:55 dB, F1/F2: 1.2:4.0 points/octave) bilaterally. DPOAE were present between 1000 and 1500 Hz using 70:70 (L1/L2) primaries in the right ear. They were absent in the left ear. ABR was identical to prior study, except I obtained a threshold of 35 dB on the right side (latency prolonged). Otologic evaluation: no middle ear effusion, normal infant head and neck inspection; need to rule out congenital hearing loss.

4. Assessment/impressions (information that is dictating your management)

  a. Suspect at least mild sensorineural hearing loss bilaterally, greater in the left ear
  b. Communicatively significant?
  c. At risk for progressive hearing loss
  d. Parent anxiety with family members that may impede further compliance

5. Management plan and outcome

I told the parents that I was reasonably sure that a hearing loss was present. However, I am not sure that it is great enough to warrant the use of hearing aids at the present. I told them I would present this in staffing and call them with our conclusions. I am not sure they will return.

6. Problems (best to list in order of importance; your colleagues may modify the list)

  a. I am not sure whether this is communicatively significant. Should I initiate an early intervention program or just monitor hearing?
  b. Do I have enough information?
  c. Parents are now less sure of the diagnosis and may not remain compliant.

the midpoints of their careers aid individuals in the earlier stages of their careers (Mathis and Jackson, 2000; Rall and Brunner, 2006). This is a personal relationship in which clinicians with knowledge in a given area help other audiologists or students acquire that knowledge. They help by offering guidance in the development of new skills, provide personal feedback about the audiologist's progress, and provide a glimpse of the lifestyle that might be enjoyed once a new area is mastered. Audiologists play the role of mentee or mentor many times in the course of their career. Not only do less experienced individuals benefit, but mentors enjoy sharing their wisdom (Mathis and Jackson, 2000.) In many ways, it is this collegial sharing that keeps the profession vital.

The ABA (www.americanboardofaudiology.org) has formalized mentorship, continuing education, and professional development ladders through its board certification program. By providing a structured process for continued improvement, the board certification program offers a systematic approach to lifelong learning and improvement of the profession.

Pitfall

- On occasion, an audiologist graduates with the misunderstanding that it is not necessary to continue the path of self-learning taught in graduate school. Nothing could be further from the truth. Self-learning must continue throughout one's professional life just to maintain minimal standards.

In discussing self-development within the professional arena, it is easy to end with issues of continuing education and skill development. However, audiology is not practiced in a vacuum. Political and legislative initiatives often promote or threaten our ability to practice independently. As members of a profession, we have a responsibility to be informed and act proactively to protect and strengthen our right to practice. More on this topic will be offered later in this chapter.

Relationship with an Employer: Being Managed

Accepting a job offer requires commitment and investment for the employee and the employer. From the latter's view, the audiologist will "cost" a significant amount of time and money for training, orientation, and continuing education. Furthermore, he or she will cost a salary plus 30 to 75% in indirect costs (Whiting, 2005). The employer is gambling that the ultimate contribution the audiologist makes to the business exceeds the hiring costs. It is easy to see why the employer would expect a commitment from the audiologist to constantly improve performance.

From the audiologist's point of view, employment offers a venue for practicing audiology and contributing to the health and well-being of the community. It is also an opportunity to exchange clinical service for financial reward, professional growth, and career advancement. When audiologists become employees, they take on a set of responsibilities and allegiances to the employer, along with fiduciary responsibilities to the patient. In most cases, employer allegiances are not in conflict with the audiologist's fiduciary responsibilities or his or her obligations to the profession. However, incongruent allegiances can occur. It is important for the audiologist to remember that, as a licensed professional, he or she will always be ethically and often legally bound to honor his or her fiduciary responsibility to patients, even when this is not honored by the employer.

Consider a hypothetical example. An audiologist, employed by a nonaudiologist, fits a hearing aid that ultimately is returned for credit. The employer does not honor the required refund. The patient has the recourse to complain to the licensing board against the audiologist, who may be held responsible for the refund. The fiduciary relationship is between the audiologist and the patient, not the nonaudiologist employer. Thus, it is always best to discover these incongruent allegiances before accepting employment. The only way to accomplish this is for the applicant to consider his or her own obligations and allegiances beforehand and be able to explore the mission, goals, and methods of the organization with which employment is sought.

Allegiance to an employer is dictated in part by the nature of the employment relationship. Audiologists may be hired as independent contractors, technical service providers, or part- or full-time employees. When audiologists are hired as independent contractors, they have a more distant relationship to the employer. They may be paid more than a full-time employee, but they are essentially self-employed and are responsible for self-employment tax. The employer has no obligation to the contractor, does not contribute to the contractor's income tax responsibilities, and provides no benefits. The allegiance to the employer in this case is driven solely by the audiologist's prerogatives. Independent contractors will be discussed in greater detail in the following sections.

Technical service providers are employed by an agency, which in turn contracts with a client service provider. For example, an audiology group may hire an audiologist and send him or her to several otolaryngologists' offices to cover clinics. The audiologist holds an allegiance to the audiology group as an employer. Holding the interests of each otolaryngology office in mind, the audiologist would also consider the needs of each client, but only to the extent that this is in the interest of the audiology group.

Part- and full-time employees share more of a stake in the success of the employer. Full-time employees in particular may feel a greater allegiance to their employer, as their own career development is tied more closely to the success of the practice.

How important are these allegiances, and how do they affect one's behavior? Three factors bear on these questions. First, the audiologist is always responsible for protecting his or her fiduciary relationship with patients. Second is the issue of personal propriety. If one agrees to work in a certain situation, it is best to show integrity and perform the job to the best of one's abilities. The third factor is the legal doctrine called "employment at will." The employment-at-will doctrine is incorporated into the laws of most states and gives the employer the right to fire an employee without cause unless the employee's civil rights have been violated (Burrows, 2006; Hosford-Dunn et al, 1995; Whiting, 2005). By design, this gives the employer the upper hand when dealing with the performance of an employee.

Ideally, both the employer and the employee share the same mission and in the successive achievements of the practice. However, even when good alignment exists between the mission, goals, and methods of the employing agency and the audiologist, conflicts in perceived obligations may occur. No perfect rule exists for settling these disagreements. In general, a professional's first obligation is his or her fiduciary responsibility to patients. The next obligation is to stay within the bounds of legal and ethical professional practice. The final obligation is to the employer.

What should an employer expect when hiring an audiologist? A good starting place is found in Chial's (1998) 25 points for developing professionalism **(Table 4–3)**. Graduate students at various universities are presented with this list at the start of their clinical experiences. It lays a good foundation for future professional development.

◆ Human Resources Issues in Practice Management

The career paths of many audiologists eventually lead to management positions or private practice. Every audiologist/manager wants to create an innovative, high-quality audiology service. Experienced managers realize that their ability to accomplish this depends little on their own personal clinical acumen. Instead, it is the ability to attract, develop, and keep a skilled, motivated, energetic group of workers (audiologists and others) who are aligned with the goals of the organization. This working definition is the heart of human resources (HR) management (Podmoroff, 2005). Many texts on HR management focus on the bewildering

Table 4–3 Professionalism

Audiology is a professional discipline. Professions require certain behaviors of their practitioners. Professional behaviors (which may or may not directly involve other people) have to do with professional tasks and responsibilities, with the individuals served by the profession, and with relations with other professions. Included among professional tasks are education and training. The following convey expectations about the behaviors of those who seek to join this profession.

1. You show up.
2. You show up on time.
3. You show up prepared.
4. You show up in a frame of mind appropriate to the professional task.
5. You show up properly attired.
6. You accept the idea that "on time," "prepared," "appropriate," and "properly" are defined by the situations, by the nature of the task, or by another person.
7. You accept that your first duty is to the ultimate welfare of the persons served by your profession and that "ultimate welfare" is a complex mix of desires, wants, needs, abilities, and capacities.
8. You recognize that professional duties and situations are about completing tasks and about solving problems in ways that benefit others, either immediately or in the long term. They are not about you. When you are called on to behave as a professional, you are not the patient, the customer, the star, or the victim.
9. You place the importance of professional duties, tasks, and problem solving above your own convenience.
10. You strive to work effectively with others for the benefit of the person served. This means you pursue professional duties, tasks, and problem solving in ways that make it easier (not harder) for others to accomplish their work.
11. You properly credit others for their work.
12. You sign your work.
13. You take responsibility for your actions, your reactions, and your inaction. This means you do not avoid responsibility by offering excuses, by blaming others, by emotional displays, or by helplessness.
14. You do not accept professional duties or tasks for which you are personally or professionally unprepared.
15. You do what you say you will do, by the time you said you would do it, and to the degree of quality you said you would do it.
16. You take active responsibility for expanding the limits of your own knowledge, understanding, and skill.
17. You vigorously seek and tell the truth, including those truths that may be less than flattering to you.
18. You accept direction (including correction) from those who are more knowledgeable or more experienced. You provide direction (including correction) to those who are less knowledgeable or less experienced.
19. You value the resources required to perform duties, tasks, and problem solving, including your time and that of others.
20. You accord respect to the values, interests, and opinions of others that may differ from your own, as long as they are not objectively harmful to the persons served.
21. You accept the fact that others may establish objectives for you. Although you may not always agree with those goals or may not fully understand them, you will pursue them as long as they are not objectively harmful to the persons served.
22. When you attempt a task for the second time, you seek to do it better than you did the first time. You revise the ways you approach professional duties, tasks, and problem solving in consideration of peer judgments of best practices.
23. You accept the imperfections of the world in ways that do not compromise the interests of those you serve.
24. You base your opinions, actions, and relations with others on sound empirical evidence and on examined personal values consistent with the above.
25. You expect all the above from other professionals.

Source: Adapted from Chial, M. (1998). Viewpoint: Conveying expectations about professional behavior. Audiology Today, 10(4), 25, with permission.

array of laws, standards, and tasks that must be addressed by large corporations. To be sure, HR management complexities increase with the size of the employing agency, but the heart of the task remains the same.

Pearl

- The heart of HR management is the ability to attract, develop, and keep a skilled, motivated, energetic group of workers who are aligned with the goals of the organization.

Attracting, developing, and keeping a skilled workforce is basic to the success of any company. Staff turnover is directly related to job satisfaction, which in turn reflects the degree to which an employee's expectations are met. Dissatisfied employees are more likely to leave, increasing training costs and making it more difficult to maintain consistent, high-quality service (Mathis and Jackson, 2000; Podmoroff, 2005; Whiting, 2005). Turnover in audiologic practices is costly. Successful audiologists are highly trained and establish close, trusting relationships with their patients. When they leave an organization, their technical expertise and personal relationships are lost. So, from a patient care perspective, it is important to maintain a stable, skilled workforce.

The other part of the heart of HR management is maintaining a motivated group of workers who are aligned with the goals of the organization (DuBrin, 2002; Labovitz and Rosansky, 1997; Podmoroff, 2005). This is a leadership function. An often-quoted adage is "You manage supplies and equipment, you lead people." To do this, an organization's leadership must communicate its mission and goals in a way that inspires understanding and commitment in its membership (Bick, 1997; Levine and Crom, 1995). Communication is important to ensure that the right people focus on the right tasks at the right time (Belker and Topchik, 2005; Podmoroff, 2005; Schlesinger et al, 1992). Therefore, good HR management includes the communication of information that motivates and directs the activities of the workforce.

How does one attract and develop a skilled, motivated group of audiologists and keep them aligned with the goals of the organization? This discussion will focus on three critical areas: organization and staff planning, attracting and hiring staff members, and developing and retaining a competent staff.

Organization and Staff Planning

Before anyone can be hired, the potential employer must define who is needed to perform what tasks. This process starts by examining the organizational model defined in the business plan. The organizational model answers the "form follows function" edict. That is, one first defines the functions that must be achieved by the organization, then one designs an organizational model that can achieve those functions efficiently and effectively (Belker and Topchik, 2005; Mathis and Jackson, 2000; Schlesinger et al, 1992). The model defines the following six form/function issues:

◆ Key tasks and processes that must be accomplished to provide targeted services

◆ Positions within the organization and the skills required for each position to ensure completion of assigned tasks

◆ Organizational structure that (1) allocates responsibilities, activities, and authority to individuals and (2) coordinates these individuals with others in the organization. Typically, the model is mapped as an organizational chart with clear functional lines of authority established.

◆ Performance-appraisal system to provide feedback to each person about his or her efforts to achieve the tasks and processes of their position

◆ Reward system, including pay, benefits, and intangibles such as status, career development opportunities, and the chance to contribute to an important objective

◆ Selection and development system for attracting and training employees

The organizational plan defines each position in an organization by the key processes and tasks performed and how those relate to the mission of the organization (Belker and Topchik, 2005; Carnegie, 1995).

Organizational Structure and Job Descriptions

The organizational plan usually identifies two different types of associates. First, a set of outside consultants provides needed skills to the organization. These typically include an accountant, attorney, banker, financial planner, insurance agent, and perhaps a bookkeeper, collection agency, and computer consultant. They are typically identified as management consultants within the business plan of the organization (Hosford-Dunn et al, 1995; Paulson, 2003). The business plan may or may not identify the management consultants by name. Their importance rests in what skills they bring to the enterprise, although individuals with a good reputation can make the organization look more attractive to potential investors.

Employees constitute the second set of associates. Job positions, responsibilities, and competencies follow from the organizational model and are used to create job descriptions for each position in the organization. The job description outlines responsibilities and duties of each position. It should also define performance standards and expectations, and how these will be measured.

In a solo audiology practice, the organizational model is very simple: all jobs fall within the job description of the owner, who is self-motivated and intrinsically aligned with the goals of the organization. As the practice grows, audiologists, support personnel, and other professionals may be hired. In these small organizations, one manager can use face-to-face communication to direct, monitor, and coordinate the activities of others. At some point, growth forces a formal structure for communication and decision-making authority purposes. This occurs because informal communication systems break down with growth. A single manager can no longer deal with everyone on a one-on-one basis. Charismatic workers may informally take on leadership functions and make decisions that may not be compatible with the mission and goals of the organization. For these reasons, it is wise to develop an organizational model and staff plan that address the six form/function issues presented in the last section regardless of the size of the organization. Clearly establishing a chain of command between job positions will define the flow of information and decision-making prerogatives. This information needs to be communicated formally through an organizational diagram and specific job descriptions to avoid misunderstanding.

The job description is the central tool for documenting the role, responsibilities, performance expectations, and location in the chain of command for each position within an organization. Typical items for a job description include the following:

Job title One or two identifying words, such as audiologist or business manager

Job statement A sentence or two that defines how a person in this position contributes to the goals of the organization

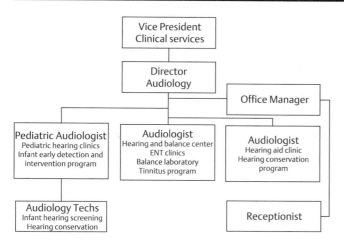

Figure 4–1 Organizational chart of a hospital-based audiology department. ENT, ear, nose, and throat.

Major/minor duties The major aspects of the job that relate the skills of the individual, with performance standards and expectations for the position. An example for a receptionist might be "Greets patients cheerfully."

Relationships This delineates the organizational structure and chain of command. For example, a supervisor may oversee the performance of several individuals and report to a director.

Qualifications This specifies the minimum educational and licensure requirements, experience level, physical abilities, travel demands, and other prerequisites to qualify for the position.

A sample organizational diagram and job description are presented in **Fig. 4–1** and Appendix 4–1 at the end of this chapter, respectively. Hosford-Dunn et al (1995) and Welch and Fowler (1994) also offer sample job descriptions for independent practices and large clinics, respectively.

An entire organization can be structured using this approach (Fine, 1999). When implemented successfully, each employee understands his or her responsibilities and performance expectations, how decisions are made and by whom, and how information should flow through the organization. From clearly defined job descriptions, the manager can define and measure the important aspects of an individual's job performance. This is critical for providing accurate feedback on performance (Carnegie, 1995; Schlesinger et al, 1992). It is also helpful for determining whether poor performance is due to an employee motivation problem, a skill deficit, or an overall problem with the process (Levine and Crom, 1995; Podmoroff, 2005). Finally, a rigorously defined job description and performance appraisal system help protect the employer from litigation when an employee is discharged for inadequate job performance (Whiting, 2005; Wolper, 2004).

Regulatory Considerations in Employer–Employee Relationships

Several legal doctrines and federal mandates define the employer–employee relationship. This section will review some of the more commonly applied rules of employment. However, this review is not comprehensive, nor is it meant to replace legal or professional counsel. The reader is cautioned to seek the services of a competent HR professional before employing individuals in a private practice.

Employment-at-Will Doctrine

"Employment at will" refers to the common law doctrine that holds that either an employer or an employee can terminate an employment relationship at any time, and for any reason, or for no reason at all. Although this is generally true, Whiting (2005) identifies several exceptions to the employment-at-will doctrine.

♦ Written or implied contracts may stipulate that termination can only occur for "good cause" or "just cause." This is a common policy in large organizations or in some union contracts. An audiologist may or may not be offered an employment contract, depending on the organization's staffing plan. If neither a written nor implied contract is in force, employment is "at will."

♦ Violations of public policy may limit employment-at-will prerogatives. For example, discharging an employee would be illegal if the discharge were based on the employee's race, gender, age, national origin, religion, physical handicap, mental disability, marital status, or union activity.

♦ An employer may inadvertently lose the employment-at-will prerogative when discipline is inconsistently applied and results in the perception that discrimination has taken place. For example, if other employees perceive that one employee is able to arrive late for work without reprimand, they may feel discriminated against on the basis of race, gender, age, and the like, when they are reprimanded or discharged for a similar behavior. The result can be litigation and loss of the employer's employment-at-will prerogative with other employees if the court sides with the discharged employee. Therefore, it is important to develop, communicate (verbally and in writing), and enforce policies and procedures consistently.

♦ Another way an employer may inadvertently lose the employment-at-will prerogative is by implying permanent employment. For example, statements such as "During your probationary period, you may be discharged for any reason" may be taken to mean that a higher standard than employment at will is in place after the probationary period. Similarly, offering a "yearly salary" may be interpreted that employment is for a year period. Such misunderstandings imply a promise for continuing employment. The result can be litigation when an employee is discharged and loss of the employer's employment-at-will prerogative with other employees if the court sides with the employee.

Because of these potential problems, it is wise to provide written notification that employment is at will and may be terminated by either the employee or employer at any time, for any reason or no reason at all, without cause or notice (Whiting, 2005). This is best accomplished within the context of an employment agreement.

Employment Agreements

It may be that an audiologist enters into a formal contract when he or she accepts a position. This is sometimes called an employment agreement or service contract (Desmond, 1994; Hosford-Dunn et al, 1995). Such a contract defines whether the employee is "at will" and describes the compensation package, termination provisions, restrictive provisions, time to be devoted to the business, vacation and sick days, and any fringe benefits that will be provided. Restrictive provisions are designed to protect the employer. Typical restrictive provisions include (1) noncompete/nonsolicitation clauses, (2) patient and practice confidentiality clauses, and (3) antiprivacy clauses. Noncompete/nonsolicitation clauses ensure that while the employee works for the business and for some time after termination, the employee will not interfere with the practice's patients or contracts (Hosford-Dunn et al, 1995).

Patient and practice confidentiality clauses protect patient information and trade secrets, such as pricing, contractual and vendor relationships, business strategies, and methods of business. Antiprivacy clauses protect against the theft of intellectual property, such as computer programs, forms, and correspondence (Hosford-Dunn et al, 1995).

Two factors should be considered when developing protective provisions. First, they must be specific and fair. Noncompete and nonsolicitation clauses need to have a limited scope. They must apply to a reasonable geographical region and must restrict competition for a reasonable time period. "Reasonable" is typically defined in regional court cases and may vary from state to state. Consequently, it is important to have these clauses and all aspects of the employment agreement reviewed by an attorney who is familiar with local standards (Whiting, 2005).

The second consideration is that enforcement of restrictive provisions is not automatic. Rather, violations must be adjudicated through civil litigation. If the restrictive provisions are considered unfair to the employee, they may be unenforceable by legal decree. Hosford-Dunn et al (1995) recommend that a "comprehensive severability clause" be incorporated into employment agreements. This clause protects the remaining scope of a set of restrictive provisions if one part of the agreement is disallowed by legal decree.

Other Laws and Regulations that Impact the Employer–Employee Relationship

Sexual Harassment

Employers have the responsibility to maintain a workplace that is free from sexual harassment, discrimination, or intimidation of any form (Whiting, 2005; Wolper, 2004).

Also, employees are held responsible if they knew of sexual harassment and made no effort to stop it. Larger organizations are required to have a written policy banning sexual harassment. However, as a preventive measure, all organizations should have these policies in writing, and they should be communicated to all employees. Training of all employees, especially managers and supervisors, is stressed by legal experts. The employer should act promptly to investigate sexual harassment and punish the identified harassers to aid in their defense (Mathis and Jackson, 2000). Furthermore, employers may be held vicariously liable for the actions of subordinates in the organization if written policies are not enforced (Mathis and Jackson, 2000; Whiting, 2005).

Wrongful Discharge

Several common law doctrines may also lead to litigation on the basis of "wrongful discharge." Wrongful discharge occurs when the implied covenant to act in "good faith and fair dealing" is breached by the employer, and by doing so, the employee is damaged. Five common causes of this type of common law tort are as follows:

- Breach of implied contract
- Workers' compensation retaliation
- Invasion of privacy
- Fraudulent misrepresentation
- Defamation

Breach of implied contract was discussed in the section describing employment at will and will not be reviewed here. Workers' compensation retaliation may occur when an employee is injured on the job and starts collecting workers' compensation. The company then discharges the individual to avoid making the compensation payments. In this situation, the injured worker can claim workers' compensation retaliation and sue for lost wages and other damages. Invasion of privacy occurs when an employee's name, likeness, private information, or information that places the employee in a false light is released to the public without consent.

The remaining two causes of tort action require special attention because they may be more commonly encountered in organizations similar to audiology practices. Fraudulent misrepresentation occurs when an employer makes representations that are known to be false, to induce an employee to take certain action, and the employee acts on these representations to his or her detriment. For example, if a potential employer attempts to induce an applicant to accept a job offer by promising the potential for a long-term career with the organization when the true aim is to simply hire the applicant for a short-term purpose, the employer is guilty of fraudulent misrepresentation. For this reason and for the purpose of protecting employment-at-will prerogatives, it is wise to describe honestly and explicitly the expected employment arrangement in the form of an employment agreement.

Defamation occurs when publishing or providing information about someone that is false and injures that person's reputation. Two types of defamation are libel and slander. Libel refers to written defamatory statements, and slander denotes spoken defamation. Defamation may occur when making statements about an individual's performance, character, or ethics, as might occur during a performance review, discharge interview, or reference check. In general, the following must occur for a prima facie case of defamation:

1. A false or derogatory statement is made about a person.

2. The statement was "published" to a third person.

3. The statement caused actual damage, or the statement falls into a "defamation per se" category, which presumes harm and permits the award of damages without proof of actual injury.

In professional circles, it is common to receive requests for employment or character references. It is important to carefully choose the information given out for these references. Any negative statement may lead to the loss of a significant and potentially profitable career goal. Such a loss can be considered actual damage and result in litigation. In general, the truth is a defense against defamation. However, one must go to court to prove the truth, which is costly and time consuming. Furthermore, although the truth is the best defense against a defamation suit, it is always difficult to prove an opinion. If a reference is to be given, stick to facts that are documented unambiguously in the employee's record. Alternately, many organizations have chosen a policy of providing limited information for employment references (Desmond, 1994; Whiting, 2005). Many provide only a simple verification of employment statement.

Pitfall

- *Example of defamation* "She was a good employee. However, she liked to party too much and frequently arrived late to work."

- *Analysis* "Party too much" is an opinion about the cause of a behavior about which the employer may have no direct knowledge. Better to note that the employee was counseled about being late for work after checking the employee's record and finding a signed, written tardiness warning.

Obviously, several pitfalls can be encountered when entering into an employer–employee relationship. Several actions can protect the employer from the deleterious effects of litigation. It is important to communicate (preferably in writing) the nature of the employment arrangement, performance expectations, and applicable rules and regulations to avoid misunderstandings (Hosford-Dunn et al, 1995; Paulson, 2003). Consistency and fairness in enforcing rules and regulations are also important (Whiting, 2005). HR professionals insist on a policy and procedure manual to formalize the employer–employee relationship (Paulson, 2003). Given the cost of legal action, it is always advisable to have HR and legal professionals review the organizational plan before it is in place and when conflicts arise.

Other Regulations Affecting the Employer–Employee Relationship

Several other laws and regulations commonly affect the employer–employee relationship. These are summarized in **Table 4–4**. Review of these laws and regulations is beyond

---

Table 4–4 Summary of Major Laws and Regulations Affecting Human Resources Management*

Law or Regulation	Summary
Wages, Hours, and Conditions of Employment	
Fair Labor Standards Act (FLSA)	Sets minimum wage standards, overtime pay rules, record-keeping requirements, and child labor restrictions.
Walsh-Healey Public Contracts Act	Employers with certain government supply contracts must pay time and a half to employees working more than 40 hours per week.
McNamara-O'Hara Service Contract Act (MOSCA)	Employers with certain government service contracts must pay specified minimum hourly rates and fringe benefits.
Davis-Bacon Act	Employers with certain government public works contracts must pay specified minimum hourly rates and fringe benefits.
Family and Medical Leave Act (FMLA) and the Health Insurance Portability and Accountability Act (HIPAA)	Mandates that an employer must extend health care coverage to employees after they leave an organization.
Worker Adjustment and Retraining Notification Act (WARN)	As of 1988 it is required that most employers give 60 days notice if a mass layoff or facility closing is to occur.
Employment Practices	
Title VII of the Civil Rights Act of 1964	Prohibits discrimination because of race, color, national origin, religion, sex, pregnancy (including childbirth or related condition).
Title I of the Americans with Disabilities Act of 1990	Prohibits discrimination in terms, conditions, and privileges of employment against individuals with disabilities who, with or without reasonable accommodation, can perform essential functions of job.
Section 1981, Title 42 U.S.C. (Civil Rights Act of 1966)	Prohibits racial and ethnic bias in employment.

(Continued)

Table 4–4 *(Continued)*

Law or Regulation	Summary
Executive Order 11246	For government contractors, requires antidiscrimination clause in contract plus written affirmative action plan for single contract of $50,000+ and 50+ employees.
Age Discrimination in Employment Act (ADEA)	Prohibits age discrimination in employment, including benefits, for employees 40 or older. Specifically, most employees cannot be forced to retire at any age.
Older Workers Benefit Protection Act (OWBPA)	Passed in 1990, this act requires equal treatment for older workers in early retirement or severance situations. It includes specific criteria that must be met when older workers sign waivers agreeing not to sue for age discrimination.
Equal Pay Act of 1963 (EPA)	Prohibits pay differentials on basis of sex in substantially equal work requiring skill, effort, and responsibility under similar working conditions. No exemption for executive, administrative, professional, and outside sales employees.
Rehabilitation Act of 1973, Section 503	Requires affirmative action and nondiscrimination in employment of handicapped persons.
Rehabilitation Act of 1973, Section 504	No discrimination against, denying benefits to, or exclusion from participation, including employment, of any qualified handicapped individual.
Employee Polygraph Protection Act of 1988 (EPPA)	Generally prohibits the use of "lie detectors" and lie detector results in private employment. Limited exemptions apply for certain internal investigations.
Federal Military Selective Service Act	Gives employees returning from U.S. military service the same wages, benefits, and rights as the employee would have received had he or she not left. Discrimination against reservists barred.
Jury System Improvement Act	Provides that an employer cannot discharge, or threaten to discharge, an employee for serving on a federal jury.
Vietnam Era Veteran Readjustment Assistance Act	Requires affirmative action regarding Vietnam-era veterans and disabled veterans.
Immigration Reform and Control Act of 1995 (IRCA)	Prohibits hiring of illegal aliens. Requires verification and record keeping of work authorization documents.
Drug-Free Workplace Act of 1988	Establishes drug-free awareness program and makes good faith effort to carry out; requires penalties or rehabilitation for employees convicted of workplace drug offenses.
Department of Transportation Drug Testing Regulations	Requires employers to conduct drug tests of certain employees in compliance with strict regulations; to provide education and minimal Employee Assistance Programs (EAPs).
Worker Adjustment and Retaining Notification Act (WARN)	With some exceptions, requires 60-day notice to employees and state and local governments before layoffs of 50 or more employees.
Taxes, Insurance, and Employee Benefits	
Social Security Act (FICA)	As of 1992, employer and employee each must contribute 7.65% of wages up to $55,500 and 1.45% on excess up to $130,200. Withholding required. Wage base subject to annual adjustment.
Federal Unemployment Tax Act (FUTA)	Must contribute 0.8% (varies with credits for participation in state unemployment programs) up to $7000 of each employee's wages.
Employee Retirement Income Security Act of 1974 (ERISA)	Requires extensive pension and welfare plan reporting, plus disclosure to plan participants and beneficiaries; minimum participation vesting and funding standards for pension plans, including profit-sharing plans; plan termination insurance for pension plans.
Consolidated Omnibus Budget Reconciliation Act of 1985 (COBRA)	Requires provision of continuation coverage under employer's group health plan to employees, spouses, and/or dependent children on the occurrence of specified events, including termination of employment or reduction in hours.
Labor Relations	
Health Maintenance Organization Act (HMO)	Specific employers must offer membership in a qualified HMO if available where employees live.
National Labor Relations Act (NLRA)	Covers employee rights to engage in protected concerted activity and organize or decertify union.
Railway Labor Act	Regulates co-union elections/mandatory dispute-resolution processes.
Occupational Safety and Health Act (OSHA)	Employer must furnish safe employment according to designated workplace standards; record keeping; no retaliation against employees for exercising rights.
Consumer Credit Protection Act, Title III (Federal Wage Garnishment Law)	Restricts garnishment w/holding to 25% or less of disposable income. Allows larger deduction for support or alimony garnishment. No discharge for one or more garnishments of one debt.
Fair Credit Reporting Act	Discloses to applicants/employees intent to use investigative consumer report and, on request, nature/scope of investigation. Must inform applicant/employee if credit report is related to adverse action and disclose credit agency.
State Laws and Regulations	
State labor regulations	Provide for workers' compensation benefits after a work-related injury.
State licensure acts	Provide the definition of the profession and the legal right to practice.

* Listing is not complete, and not all listed laws may apply to a specific organization. Seek professional advice before acting on this information.

the scope of this text. Moreover, some only impact organizations that employ more than a certain minimum number of employees. Consultation with HR and legal professionals is strongly encouraged to understand how these regulations might affect an individual practice situation.

Regulations that Impact the Right to Practice

Several other regulations may impact the staff and organizational plan. First, most states have licensure requirements for an individual to practice as an audiologist. State licensure agencies are listed in Appendix 4–2 of this chapter. Associated with licensure are the rules and regulations for the legal practice of audiology. Verification of license status is certainly an important requirement when employing a potential staff member. Furthermore, the rules and regulations for legal practice of audiology must be understood and followed. This is particularly important for sites that might participate in 4th year clinical externships. The types of activities a 4th year student can perform vary from state to state, depending on licensure rules and regulations.

Finally, depending on the venue, voluntary standards may apply. For example, the Commission on Accreditation of Rehabilitation Facilities (CARF) accredits rehabilitation agencies, the Joint Committee on Accreditation of Healthcare Organizations (JCAHO) accredits hospital and other health care organizations, and the ASHA Professional Services Board (PSB) accredits agencies that provide speech-language or hearing services. Compliance with the standards of these agencies is often required by third-party payers. All of these agencies have rules and regulations that may impact how audiologists perform their professional tasks.

Attracting and Hiring Staff Members

Once the organizational structure and job descriptions are in place, a great deal of detail is known about the type of person best suited for each position in the organization. Assuming that the organization has a need and can financially support adding a new employee, the next task is finding that best person for the position. How a candidate is selected depends on the position to be filled, the current job market, and the current needs of the business (Podmoroff, 2005).

Hiring or Contracting

One of the first decisions to be made when filling a position is whether the position should be full time and permanent. Full-time, permanent employment requires a great deal of commitment on the part of the employer. Employees receive pay and benefits regardless of changes in the organization's profitability (Paulson, 2003). This level of commitment may not be reasonable, particularly in the case of small or start-up organizations and particularly when the position is not one involved in direct patient care. Creative and fair alternatives to full-time positions exist.

Secretarial and support staff are not directly involved with patient care. Furthermore, their skills are commonly available in the job market. Consequently, secretarial and support staff might be better outsourced to an employment

agency (Hosford-Dunn et al, 1995; Paulson, 2003). The agency hires the person, pays all employment taxes and benefits, and then contracts that person to the business as a temporary employee. The cost per hour may be greater than if the support person were a full-time employee. However, no commitment exists on the part of the clinic to keep the contract employee. Furthermore, the level of commitment made by the contract employee may be greater than a full-time associate. This is because the contract employee's continued employment is directly related to the employer's day-to-day satisfaction with his or her job performance (Paulson, 2003).

In some circumstances, audiologists can be engaged as contractors. This model is more common in larger cities where more than one practice may have a need for audiology services on an "as-needed" basis. If the audiologist is holding himself or herself out as an independent contractor, great care must be taken to ensure that Internal Revenue Service (IRS) regulations are not broken (Desmond, 1994). If a contract is written that defines the audiologist as an independent contractor, and the IRS finds that the person did not meet the requirements of independent contractor status, the organization may be responsible for back taxes and penalties (Paulson, 2003). Consultation with the organization's attorney and accountant is necessary before entering into this type of relationship. Further information can be obtained from IRS publication 937.

Special Consideration

- Independent contractor status is appealing to many audiologists who wish to develop an independent practice. In contracting audiology services to physicians, these audiologists are able to develop a stable income stream while developing other referral sources. However, care must be exercised to ensure that the contracting audiology services qualify under IRS rules for independent contractor status. Do audiologists schedule or otherwise direct their activities with sufficient independence to meet minimum IRS requirements for independent contractor status? Review of IRS publication 937 with a knowledgeable tax consultant is recommended before entering into these relationships.

Hiring Employees

In general, hiring an employee involves six steps: (1) determining what is needed, (2) employee recruiting, (3) prescreening and reference checking, (4) interviewing and testing, (5) selecting the applicant, and (6) orientation.

Determining Exactly What Is Needed By having up-to-date organizational and staff plans, the job description and requisite skills have been defined. These help define a "candidate profile" or the minimum requirements for a position

(Whiting, 2005; Yate, 2006). Other factors may also influence this profile. For example, each organization has a culture or personality, and each position in the organization may be more particularly suited to people with a specific temperament (Yuill, 2003). It takes a great deal of work to develop or analyze the behavioral patterns, values, and attitudes that members use to guide organizational life (Kilpatrick and Johnson, 1999; Schlesinger et al, 1992). Candidates who share these attitudes and temperaments likely will "fit in" better and are thus more attractive to the hiring organization.

Pitfall

- Looking for an ideal candidate.

Employee Recruiting   Recruiting professional employees has become much easier with the advent of the Internet and career-specific Web sites. More traditional recruiting methods, such as networking, advertising, using employment agencies, and using walk-ins, are still options (Hosford-Dunn et al, 1995), particularly when hiring support staff. However, even here, Internet-based classified ads are commonly available through local media (often under the banner of a local newspaper), greatly improving recruiting efficiency.

Networking involves communicating the availability of a job position to individuals likely to encounter qualified applicants. Professional colleagues, local educational institutions, the alma maters of current staff members, Internet list servers and professional sites, and industry contacts (hearing aid manufacturers, equipment and service representatives) are productive contacts for this purpose. The value of networking from a recruitment point of view varies. In some cases, associates familiar with your needs and work style may find the right person with little expense to the company.

Advertising available positions is sometimes an effective tool. The strategy for advertising depends on the relative scarcity of the qualified candidates in the local job market. In general, advertisements should be designed to appeal to candidates with the personality and job skills that are being sought. When advertising for support staff, the response is sometimes overwhelming. Consequently, the ad needs to state job specifications clearly to discourage unqualified respondents. They should not violate Equal Employment Opportunity Commission (EEOC) guidelines (see the EEOC Web site: http://www.eeoc.gov/). Specifically, they should not specify gender, race, age, religious affiliation, or physical or mental health as a condition for employment (Podmoroff, 2005; Whiting, 2005). Although the EEOC is a federal agency, each state has its own Human Rights Commission. Specific guidelines may vary on a state-by-state basis. Because of this, the services of an HR expert are helpful in questionable cases.

Placing help wanted ads in local or regional newspapers or on Internet sites can be an effective means of filling support positions. It is less successful for finding audiologists unless there is a large number of audiologists in the area. In these situations, the advantage of advertising in the mass media must be weighed against the disadvantage of giving competitors information about the organization's staffing situation. Blind advertisements do not identify the practice and use the publication's address or a post office box to receive correspondence. The value of placing a blind ad is that the practice does not reveal its intentions to potential competitors (Hosford-Dunn et al, 1995).

Recruiting audiologists has become much easier with the advent of the Internet and career-specific Web sites. For example, ASHA (www.asha.org) and AAA (www.audiology.org) have Web pages directed at advertising available positions. Industry trade journals, such as *Advance* magazine (www.advanceweb.com) and *The Hearing Journal* (www.thehearingjournal.com), have Web as well as print-based classified sections. In most cases, résumés are available so that potential recruits can be screened before formal contact is made. National publications and trade journals (e.g., *Audiology Today, The Hearing Journal,* and *Hearing Review*) are also helpful. However, print methods are much slower than Web-based options. Publication lead times can be as long as 90 days.

National and state conventions are also good places to look for potential applicants. Extern positions available to 4th year students in doctor of audiology (Au.D.) programs are best promoted by posting position-available announcements on the National Association of Future Doctors of Audiology (NAFDA; www.nafda.org) Web site and at regional universities. In the near future, there may be a national match program for this purpose.

Filling audiology positions can be a lengthy process. Once someone responds to a national ad, travel time will be required for interviewing. If the job offer is accepted, time for relocating and obtaining appropriate licensure may be needed. Consequently, unless someone local is interested in the position, finding an experienced audiologist can take many months (Hosford-Dunn et al, 1995). Moreover, the more technical the position or the more experience required, the longer it may take to fill the position.

State and federal employment agencies often maintain lists of unemployed workers in the area according to job category (Paulson, 2003). This can be a rich source of applications for nonprofessional positions. In some cases, tax benefits and other inducements may be available if a long-term unemployed worker is hired from one of these lists. However, care must be taken to ensure that the potential employee has the skills necessary to fulfill the job requirements.

There are also private agencies that will search and do the initial screening of candidates. They are most effective in filling jobs requiring special or professional skills. Private employment agencies are appealing because if they do not have the right person to fill the position, they will go out and find such people. However, they can be expensive, usually 10 to 30% of the first year's salary.

Occasionally, a résumé will appear serendipitously when a position is available. Although this can save an incredible amount of time when the applicant is well qualified, this is obviously not a good staffing strategy to use.

Practice building requires a more active commitment on the part of the manager to ensure the right person is hired for the job. Nevertheless, when an unsolicited résumé is sent to an organization, it is good form to respond to it in writing. If a position is available, this can be pointed out, and the applicant can enter the prescreening process. If no positions are available, a letter should still be written, to acknowledge the job seeker as a colleague, wish him or her well, guide the individual to other job openings, and incorporate him or her into the practice's network (Hosford-Dunn et al, 1995).

Prescreening and Reference Checking   Before time is spent interviewing, a system for prescreening applicants should be undertaken. Several prescreening tools are available. The simplest is a résumé review with transcripts and letters of recommendation (Desmond, 1994; Podmoroff, 2005). For nonprofessional positions, résumés may not be all that informative, and the employer may feel overwhelmed with the number of seemingly qualified candidates. In such cases, it is helpful to use a telephone prescreening interview before an application is accepted. During the telephone interview, the following questions should be asked:

- Where does the applicant work currently?

- If not now employed, where did the applicant work last?

- How long did the applicant work there?

- Why did the applicant leave?

- What did the applicant do?

- What was the applicant's rate of pay?

This line of questioning is repeated until it is established that the applicant does or does not have the prerequisite qualifications for the job. Very little information about the job requirements should be provided during the prescreening interview. This limits the applicant's ability to tell the interviewer that he or she had a specific skill, solely on the basis that the interviewer stated that was a skill that was desirable. If the applicant is not qualified for the position, the conversation should be terminated by explaining that "we are looking for someone else whose background and qualifications more closely meet our requirements." The advantage of the strategy is that nonqualified applicants are not given an opportunity to set the stage for litigation if that is their objective (Whiting, 2005).

Prescreening is also necessary when filling professional positions. As mentioned before, résumés, personal and professional references, employment histories, and license status are helpful tools in assessing minimum qualifications. Because of the threat of lawsuits, written references seldom contain negative information (see "Defamation" section). However, carefully thought out telephone interviews with reference sources can yield information that might not have been put in writing (Desmond, 1994). One question that may elicit good information is, Would you rehire this person? Sometimes, a failure to respond to this question is as meaningful as a response.

At this stage of prescreening, another advantage to blind advertisements becomes apparent. Applicants can be screened on the basis of résumé information and references before learning the potential employer's identity. This strategy may also decrease the organization's exposure to litigation (Whiting, 2005).

Interviewing and Testing   This section will review the major steps in the interview process. The first step is to prepare well for the interview. Review the job description for accuracy. Prepare your questions in advance, and ensure that the process and questions are applied consistently across all candidates (see **Table 4–5** for examples of open-ended questions). EEOC

Table 4–5   Selected Examples of Open-Ended Questions for Interviewing

Area	Example Questions
Communication skills	Tell me about a time when you had to use speaking skills to make a point that was important to you.
	Give me an example of a time when you built motivation among subordinates and what rewards you got out of that experience.
Problem-solving skills	Give me an example of when you had to make a quick decision.
	Describe a situation when several coworkers were angry about a company policy. What did they do? What did you do? Why?
Organizational skills	How did you set priorities for your staff in previous jobs? How did you update them?
	Let's suppose you could devise a procedure that would get your work done in an hour less a day. How would you spend that extra time?
Customer service	Give me an example of when you had to be flexible and creative to meet new customer requirements.
	What are some of the behaviors and attitudes you want your staff to practice to ensure excellent customer service?
Leadership skills	In past supervisory roles, how many employees did you supervise? In what areas?
	How did you deal with employee conflict?
	What type of employee behavior makes you angry?
	What's your philosophy in dealing with low morale of staff?

(Continued)

Table 4–5 *(Continued)*

Area	Example Questions
Audiology specific	Why did you choose to become an audiologist? What is the most difficult clinical case you have experienced? What is the most rewarding thing you have done as an audiologist? What aspect or job in audiology really gets you excited? What do you like to do?

regulations and the Americans with Disabilities Act prohibit questions about race, age, religion, marital status, child care arrangements, transportation, or handicap status (Paulson, 2003; Whiting, 2005). To be safe, questions that may be construed as discriminatory should be avoided, regardless of the intent. **Table 4–6** presents some examples of legal and problematic questions.

The purpose of the initial preemployment interview is to discover information about the applicant that is not on his or her résumé or application. The purpose is not necessarily to tell the applicant about the job or the organization. Behavioral interviewing is used by many premier organizations. This is an interview in which applicants give examples of how they have handled situations in the past. The following questions may be asked in this type of interview:

♦ How have you handled a situation in which coworkers were not contributing to the mission of the company?

♦ How did you choose your approach?

♦ How did your coworkers react? (Mathis and Jackson, 2000)

Several books are available that provide a good overview of other interviewing techniques, objectives, and pitfalls (see, e.g., Podmoroff, 2005; Yate, 2006).

It is advisable to have more than one person interview viable candidates. Part of the interview process is to determine how well the applicant's personality matches the culture of the organization. Furthermore, interviews for professional positions can be quite intense. It helps to break the interview up into smaller segments to decrease the stress level of candidates and give them time to loosen up. Finally, the time commitment shown by the organization is a sign of respect to the applicant.

It is also important to prepare applicants for the interview. Let them know before they arrive what the interview schedule will be like. This is particularly important when interviewing for professional positions. Start the interview with courteous and friendly small talk to relax candidates. Explain the hiring process early in the interview. Specifically, explain when they can expect to hear if the position is offered and set a deadline beyond which they can conclude someone else has been selected. From then on, the goal is for the applicant to do all of the talking. Following the "80–20 rule," the interviewer should talk 20% of the time and listen 80% of the time (Podmoroff, 2005; Whiting, 2005; Yate, 2006).

The interviewer will want to determine candidates' knowledge bases; ability to think on their feet; their level of maturity and self-awareness; their motivations, values, and attitudes; their ability to handle stress; and their overall ability to contribute to the organization. Remembering the 80–20 rule, preselect open-ended questions that relate directly to written job requirements. When more than one person is involved as an interviewer, it is helpful to assign specific areas of assessment to each interview. For example, one audiologist might probe the candidate's knowledge

Table 4–6 Selected Examples of Interview Questions that Could Be or Are Discriminatory under United States Law

Category	Questions that Should Be Posed Only in Specific Situations	Questions that Should Not Be Posed
Citizenship or national origin	Can you show proof of your eligibility to work in the United States? Are you fluent in any language other than English? (Ask only if it applies to the job being sought)	Are you a United States citizen? Were you born here?
Religion or political beliefs	Will the work hours, as described, pose any problem for you? (You may inquire about weekend availability only if it is required for the job being sought.)	What is your religion? Which church do you attend? What are your religious holidays?
Race	None	
Sexual identity	Have you worked or attended school under another name?	Are you male or female? Have you ever been married?
Family status	Do you have any responsibilities that conflict with job attendance or travel requirements? (If you ask this, you must ask it of all applicants.)	Are you married? What is your spouse's name? What is your maiden name? Do you have any children? Are you pregnant? What are your child care arrangements?

Source: http://interview.monster.com/archives/attheinterview/ (retrieved May 7, 2006) and http://www.eeoc.gov. Retrieved May 7, 2006.

base in auditory diagnostics and pediatric patient care. Another might look for computer skills and the ability to fit programmable hearing aids. Again, each area of inquiry should relate directly to the written job description.

When interviewing for support positions, it may be helpful to formally test the candidate's ability to perform specific tasks. Typing, math, filing tests, or observation of computer use can access specific clerical skills. Professional skills can be observed by having the audiologist work with a patient (Desmond, 1994). If formal testing is used, it is a good strategy to start with less expensive tests first. If an applicant fails one of the less expensive tests, the evaluation process can stop before unnecessary expenses are incurred (Paulson, 2003; Whiting, 2005).

Under certain highly restricted conditions, applicants may be asked to take sample health examinations.* These examinations are obtained to ensure that the applicant has no communicative diseases. The results cannot be used as grounds for not hiring. Rather, reasonable accommodations must be made. Applicants may also take a urine test to determine substance use or abuse. Audiologic practices often operate in proximity to other health care providers. It is detrimental to the practice's reputation if an employee or associate is suspected of or caught abusing substances illegally in the medical environment (Hosford-Dunn et al, 1995).

When the interview is completed, the interviewee should be given a chance to ask questions. These are often just as informative as formal responses. One difficult question to answer involves salary. Early in the search process, it may be more productive to ask, "How much money are you looking for?" At the conclusion of the interview, you may want to provide serious candidates with a ballpark salary range. Always thank the applicant and document the highlights of the interview (Whiting, 2005).

Background investigations usually take place at this point in the interview process. There is some cost as well as time involved, but it is generally worth the effort, as some applicants could misrepresent their qualifications. One way to protect against résumé fraud and false credentials is to check references and request verification of credentials. The following sources are often used to check a potential employee's background:

♦ Academic transcripts

♦ Prior work references

♦ Credit checks

♦ Law enforcement records (Mathis and Jackson, 2000)

---

* Title 1 of the Americans with Disabilities Act (ADA) places severe restrictions on the use of health examinations in the screening and hiring process. Preoffer examinations are prohibited. ADA does not prohibit voluntary tests. An offer may be contingent on satisfactory results of a medical examination. However, the results cannot be used to withdraw the offer unless they show that the potential employee is unable to perform tasks required of the job. ADA includes people with acquired immunodeficiency syndrome (AIDS), human immunodeficiency virus (HIV), and rehabilitated drug abusers in its definition of "disabled." The ADA does not require, however, that employers hire persons who are known drug users or who have contagious diseases (Jenkins, 1999).

It is not uncommon for applicants who have not been offered a position to call back just to confirm the decision. In these cases, it is important to tell them that somebody else was selected "whose background and qualifications more closely matched our requirements." Telling them why they were not hired or answering questions about what they could have done differently or better may expose the organization to litigation if the applicant perceives discrimination (Paulson, 2003; Whiting, 2005).

Selecting the Candidate   When the top candidates have been selected, the most promising prospect is generally brought in for a final interview. This is the final opportunity to make sure that the candidate is the right person for the position. Whiting (2005) suggests that this is the time to describe the job fully to the applicant. This "job preview" presents the applicant with a realistic description of the job situation, including any positive and negative aspects. The applicant should have a good understanding of the positive attributes of the organization and its mission, the importance of the job to the organization, and how his or her background and qualifications qualify the candidate for the position. The applicant also needs to know to whom he or she will be reporting, advancement opportunities, and any fringe benefits. In this way, the potential employee understands the terms and benefits of employment.

A tentative salary and benefit package may be presented. However, the position might not be formally offered until a few days after the interview. The final interview is designed to provide just enough information to ensure that the candidate can make an informed judgment about the position's desirability. Making that judgment should take some time. Moreover, the organization has a psychological advantage if it is seen as having other selection options (Hosford-Dunn et al, 1995). Making an offer at the final interview may show desperation and decrease the perceived value of the offer. Podmoroff (2005) suggests making the offer 24 hours after the final interview if all goes well.

Special Consideration

• Firing an employee is traumatic for both the organization and the employee. Keeping an employee who is not producing is demoralizing to employees who are dedicated and hard working. No manager who has gone through firing an employee is capricious in how he or she chooses new employees. Hire well.

Compensation levels vary from one community to another and also according to current market conditions. The practice must determine the current market conditions and make an appropriate offer. Additional negotiations are not uncommon before the practice and the candidate agree to a final package (Hosford-Dunn et al, 1995).

Once the applicant accepts the offer of employment, the employer is required under federal law to check for alien status (Hosford-Dunn et al, 1995; Whiting, 2005). The new

Table 4–7 List of Acceptable Documents for Establishing Identity and/or Employment Eligibility

Documents that Establish Identity	Documents that Establish Employment Eligibility	Documents that Establish Both
1. U.S. passport (unexpired or expired)	1. Driver's license or identification card issued by a state or outlying possession of the United States, provided it contains a photograph or information such as name, date of birth, sex, height, eye color, and address	1. U.S. Social Security card issued by the Social Security Administration (other than a card stating it is not valid for employment)
2. Certificate of U.S. citizenship (INS Form N-560 or N-561)		2. Certification of birth abroad issued by the Department of State (Form FS-545 or Form OS-1350)
3. Certificate of naturalization (INS Form N-550 or N-570)		3. Original or certified copy of birth certificate issued by a state, county, municipal authority, or outlying possession of the United States bearing an official seal
4. Unexpired foreign passport, with 1-551 stamp or attached	2. Identification card issued by federal, state, or local government agencies or entities provided it contains a photograph or information such as name, date of birth, sex, height, eye color, and address	
5. INS Form 1-94 indicating unexpired employment authorization		4. Native American tribal document
6. Alien registration receipt card with photograph or permanent resident card (Form 1-151 or 1-551)	3. School identification card with a photograph	5. U.S. citizen identification card (INS Form 1-197)
7. Unexpired temporary resident card (INS Form 1-688)	4. Voter's registration card	6. Identification card for use of resident citizen in the United States (INS Form I-179)
8. Unexpired employment authorization card (INS Form I-688A)	5. U.S. military card or draft record	7. Unexpired employment authorization document issued by the INS (other than those listed under column 1)
9. Unexpired reentry permit (INS Form 1-327)	6. Military dependent's identification card	8. Completed Employment Eligibility Verification form (Form I-9) if hired
10. Unexpired refugee travel document (INS Form 1-571)	7. U.S. Coast Guard Merchant Mariner card	
11. Unexpired employment authorization document issued by the INS that contains a photograph (INS Form 1-688B)	8. Native American tribal document	
	9. Driver's license issued by a Canadian government authority	
	For persons less than age 18 who are unable to present a document listed above:	
	10. School record or report card	
	11. Clinic, doctor, or hospital record	
	12. Day care or nursery school record	

Note: Employers may terminate an employee who fails to produce the required document(s), or a receipt for a replacement document(s) (in the case of lost, stolen, or destroyed documents), within 3 business days of the date employment begins. However, employers must apply these practices uniformly to all employees. Employees must present original documents. The only exception is an employee may present a certified copy of a birth certificate. For more detailed information on employment eligibility verification, see http://uscis.gov/graphics/howdoi/faqeev.htm. INS, Immigration and Naturalization Service.

employee must complete a form I-9 (employment eligibility verification). Depending on the employee's citizenship status, the new employee must either demonstrate proof of U.S. citizenship or provide one or more of the following: (1) a certification of naturalization, (2) an alien registration card, or (3) a current Immigration and Naturalization Service (INS) employment authorization with proper passport identification, depending on immigration status. A list of acceptable documents for establishing identity and/or employment eligibility is shown in **Table 4–7**. Please note that INS requirements may change quickly depending on the security risks of the country. It is always advisable to obtain a current opinion from a legal or HR specialist with any question about employment eligibility verification.

In addition, the employer must establish the employee's tax status. For federal and state income taxes, this is determined from the employee's responses on IRS Form W-4. The organization will also need to determine Social Security, Medicare, Federal Unemployment, and State Unemployment withholding. The organization's accountant will help set up the employee's tax and benefit withholding.

Orientation Period   In many organizations, the first few months of employment are described as a "probationary period." The implication is that the employee is being evaluated during this period and may be discharged if performance is unsatisfactory. Many HR specialists advocate against this term because it implies that employment-at-will status will change after the employee finishes the probationary period (Whiting, 2005). Rather than placing an employee on "probation," they suggest providing an "orientation period." The orientation period focuses on developing the new employee, without implying a promise of "permanent" employment after the period has passed.

The goal of the orientation period is to familiarize the new employee to the organization with the responsibilities of his or her position. This starts with an explanation of the values and mission statement of the organization (Whiting, 2005). Every other aspect of the organization should be presented in terms of how each relates to the mission of the organization. Understanding the values and mission of the organization will help new members approach their job tasks in a way that is congruent with the current objectives of the organization.

The orientation process starts on the first day. Several administrative topics must be covered early in the process. These include an orientation to payroll practices, company policies and procedures, the daily routine, employee relation's policies, and employee benefits (Whiting, 2005). In health care settings, additional information may be disseminated. These include Health Insurance Portability and Accountability Act (HIPAA) standards and procedures, infection control procedures, Occupational Safety and Health Administration (OSHA) safety programs, and procedures for dealing with medical emergencies if medically frail patients are to be seen. No employee can assimilate all this information at once, and some will not ask many questions. This information should be in written form so that the employee can refer to specific areas as needed (Paulson, 2003).

Orientation procedures must also clearly define the vital processes and outcomes for which the employee is responsible and any quality indicators that may be used to measure job performance. Examples may include audiologist's ratings on patient satisfaction surveys, length of time per evaluation, or number of hearing aid returns per number sold. Careful orientation procedures help maintain employees' confidence, communicate and reinforce practice policies and procedures, and address positive and negative behavior. Employee confidence and satisfaction will increase as the knowledge of the job expectations is communicated and reinforced (Belker and Topchik, 2005; Hosford-Dunn et al, 1995; Welch and Fowler, 1994).

Many organizations provide a mentor to the new employee early in the orientation process. The mentor's role is to help the new employee in his or her new surroundings and answer simple questions in the absence of the supervisor. Mentors also help demonstrate the performance expectations of the organization. For example, new audiologists may need help formatting reports and correspondence or determining when clinical policy may call for a specific evaluation or referral. Most of these issues should be addressed in a protocol manual to ensure uniformity of quality service across practitioners (see the next section on staff training). Nevertheless, such manuals cannot address all the contingencies that might be encountered in clinical practice. In these cases, the judgment of an experienced clinician can go a long way in promoting the new employee's clinical skill and confidence.

Occasionally, it becomes apparent that the new employee is not well suited to the tasks of his or her position. In these cases, it is better to let the employee go early in the orientation process (Hosford-Dunn et al, 1995; Whiting, 2005). Discharging a marginal employee well past the orientation period is more stressful because he or she has settled in to the job.

Developing and Retaining a Competent Staff

One of the attractions of a career in audiology is the fact that the profession is dynamic and growing. Consequently, an audiologist's skills and the venues in which one may practice are in constant evolution. Continued training and education, both self and organization directed, is vital to developing and maintaining a competent audiology staff. The obligation of the audiologist to maintain a regimen for self-development was addressed earlier in this chapter. This section will focus on the organization's interest in the development of a competent staff.

From a service organization's point of view, survival depends on the ability to deliver high-quality services consistently and as cost-effectively as possible. Consistently delivering a high-quality service requires that individual audiologists within the organization hold to a common standard of quality for each service delivered. Moreover, as professionals, most audiologists recognize the obligation to contribute to the mission of the organization by seeking to enhance the quality and efficiency of the services they provide through the organization. Thus, the organization must have some system to coordinate and train new audiologists to meet existing quality standards and to foster innovations that improve quality or efficiency. (For a full discussion of this topic, see Chapter 3 in this volume.)

Training to Meet Existing Requirements

The first step in developing a competent audiologic staff occurs when the organization hires the best applicant. Once hired, the new audiologist learns the administrative aspects of the position. Orientation to the technical and clinical aspects of a practice may require more time. Audiology is very equipment dependent. Larger clinics may have several different pieces of equipment that accomplish the same task (e.g., there may be more than one type of auditory evoked potential system). Clinical information management systems have increased in both complexity and power with the integration of newer computer systems (see Chapters 9 and 18 in this volume). Thus, the orientation process must result in proficiency in the use of clinical equipment, clinical test techniques, assessment protocols for various patient types (basic comprehensive examinations, tinnitus and balance assessments, infant and pediatric assessments, etc.), and information management systems for audiologic services (documentation of clinical encounters, test forms, reports and letters to referral sources, outcome assessment results, billing, scheduling, etc.).

In large clinics, the orientation to the technical and clinical aspects of practice is formalized (Zapala, 1996). First, most facilities have protocols established for each test or test battery used by the clinic. Each test protocol documents the applicable patient selection criteria, the data collection method, reporting procedure, and expected cross-checks. A sample protocol is shown in **Table 4–8**. The formal process of assessing competency begins with an initial skills assessment. Here, the new audiologist demonstrates that he or she has the skill to perform each test by either performing the test under supervision or showing that he or she performed the test in the past at an appropriate level of competence. A sample form for cataloging clinical skills is shown in Appendix 4–3 at the end of the chapter.

Once clinical skills are cataloged, a personal plan for development may be established. This plan identifies deficits in the audiologist's clinical armamentarium and prioritizes which skills should be developed first. This process need

Table 4–8 Sample Clinical Protocol

Department of Audiology Protocol		INDEX: **Tech27765** **DPOAE**	
☐ Administrative ✓ Technical ☐ Office Procedure		DATE: PAGE:	REPLACES 06/22/2007 | 01/30/1996 1 of 1 | 1 of 2
Originator	Chief of audiology		
Subject	Procedure 27765, DPOAE Infant Hearing Screen		
Purpose	To detect hearing impairments greater than 40 dB HL in newborns that may significantly impede natural speech, language, and cognitive development		
Patient selection	Newborns and infants < 6 months of age who are at low risk for central forms of hearing loss and are able to rest quietly for the screening procedure		
Protocol	1. Instrument: GSI 60 DPOAE system 2. Data: DPOAE are obtained from primaries at 1500, 2000, 3000, and 4000 Hz (geometric mean frequency.) L1/L2 65 to 55 dB SPL in the ear canal, F1/F2 ratio 1:2. Maximum permissible ear canal level in the region of the expected primary is 15 dB peak SPL. A minimum of 60 frames must be averaged. A DP is present when the SNR is 13 dB. 3. Method: The ear canal is inspected, and a probe is inserted so that no acoustic leak from the ear canal and no evidence of an occluded probe port are present. Either a sequential or a simultaneous presentation mode is acceptable. 4. Validation: By either cross-check or retest		
Reporting	"Pass": Three of four expected DPs detected with amplitudes > 5 dB SPL in at least one ear with an acceptable SNR. "Refer": Any nonpass test.		
Expected cross-checks	None as a screening procedure		
Additional cross-checks	TEOAE, ABR, tympanometry if middle ear effusion suspected		
	Alterations in protocol or reporting must be documented on screening form with explanation of how procedures varied and why alteration was necessary.		

ABR, auditory brainstem response; DP, directional preponderance; DPOAE, distortion product otoacoustic emission(s); GSI, Grason-Stadler Inc.; HL, hearing level; SNR, signal-to-noise ratio; SPL, sound pressure level; TEOAE, transient evoked otoacoustic emission(s).

not be restricted to new audiologists. Many clinics have established these systems as part of a yearly performance appraisal. Some accreditation agencies, such as the Joint Commission on Accreditation of Healthcare Organizations (JCAHO), require yearly competency evaluations as well. The value of the yearly evaluation goes beyond satisfying external requirements. A yearly evaluation helps focus the audiologist and the organization on the long-term development of the individual, the organization, and the profession. Further recognition of formal mastery helps bolster the sense of accomplishment of the individual and identifies potential mentors for other less experienced staff members. Finally, if a career ladder is to be developed (e.g., recognition of a senior audiologist with mastery of a wide range of skills), formal assessment of competency is invaluable.

Clinical Case Staffing The ability to perform a test does not necessarily imply good patient care. Audiologic patient care involves the diagnosis and management of auditory-based functional deficits, patient education, and the art of directing patients to act in their own best interests. Within this context, accurate test performance comprises a small part of clinical practice. How does one evaluate or, more importantly, enhance patient care abilities? One tool is the practice of case staffing. Case staffing is a peer review process in which an audiologist formally presents a case and seeks advice from colleagues (see **Table 4–2**). Assessment choices, treatment plans, and outcomes are discussed. If necessary, literature reviews and outside mentors are consulted to improve the breadth of the learning experience. The peers award the presenting audiologist a score for the quality of the patient care provided. Each audiologist maintains a casebook documenting every case presented and the peer-awarded score. At the end of the year, this information is also used to establish the audiologist's competency. The expectation is that every year the casebook will document how the audiologist is managing cases of increasing complexity with improving outcomes.

Three advantages exist to staffing cases formally:

1. Accomplishment in specific aspects of patient care is documented for accreditation purposes. This is a necessary task in some practice environments but is not an adequate justification for the practice.

2. Practitioners are reinforced for being responsible for patient outcomes.

3. All the participants learn to think in terms of quality care and patient outcomes. The group comes to consensus about what constitutes quality patient care. In this sense, staffing can be a real team-building activity.

Staffing is difficult to do when interpersonal relationships are not open and honest in the office. Ideally, one chooses to staff those cases that were problematic. Lack of trust or respect among staff members can lead to personal attacks during staffing. This must be strongly discouraged. The ethic should be that case presentations are a professional exercise. Personal differences should be left at the door. Thus, to use this important tool, a professional culture conducive to this activity must prevail within the organization. The concept of the professional culture will be discussed in the following section.

Performance Appraisal   Performance appraisal can refer to two separate processes. In the first, an individual's performance is monitored, and constructive feedback is given, with the goal of improving performance. This is the leadership function that optimally instructs, motivates, and directs the activities of employees. Optimal ongoing performance appraisals correct deficit performance while leaving employees feeling that they have self-direction, they are competent, and they are contributing to a worthy goal (Byham and Cox, 1998). More often than not, it is these feelings that lead to employee commitment and longevity (Labovitz and Rosansky, 1997).

Pearl

- Correct errors in private with prior warning and reward in public with prior announcement.

The second type of performance appraisal is more problematic. In larger organizations, a yearly performance appraisal process is often tied to merit-based pay increases (Cascio, 2003; DuBrin, 2002). Giving merit raises on the basis of performance may make intuitive sense. However, some see problems with this type of reward system. W. Edwards Deming, a leader in the total quality movement, believed such appraisals were devastating to organization performance and individual achievement (Walton, 1986). The problem, in Deming's view, was that, in most organizations, factors that affect individual performance were beyond the control of the individual. Rather, they reflected problems in the process or systems that underpinned performance. This is not to say that individuals do not make choices and are sometimes not productive. Rather, the focus should be on ensuring that employees are properly trained and are in an environment that promotes quality before too much focus is placed on individual ability.

It is not always obvious how to improve systems or processes, particularly when the processes have not changed in several years. One method of determining whether a process can be improved is by benchmarking for best practices. The concept behind benchmarking is simple. An organization, in this case an audiology department, compares its productivity against other departments with similar circumstance. If areas exist in which the audiology department's performance does not compare favorably, a process or system may need to be improved. Benchmarking is a way of identifying what is possible for an organization. However, it should not be used to define what individuals

can do unless all process issues have been solved. For further discussion of benchmarking, see Chapters 3 and 8 in this volume.

Individual performance appraisals are a fact of life for many audiologists. Those that are performed well help the audiologist see personal growth opportunities and new development challenges. Constant feedback about growth and performance on a daily basis is key to ensuring that performance appraisals are a positive experience. If a surprise deficit area is seen on an annual performance review, the supervisory and leadership process has failed (Belker and Topchik, 2005; Walton, 1986). Barring unforeseen surprises, the evaluation should review the employee's abilities and performance (which should be readily apparent from the casebook), adherence to the value system of the organization, growth over the year, and areas of weakness or areas where new skills can be obtained.

When Performance Flounders   Discipline is the process used to train, correct, and mold behavior. It is the basis for giving continued feedback to employees about their performance. Whiting (2005) identifies two types of discipline. Negative discipline emphasizes punishment for breaking rules. Positive discipline assumes that employees are adults who have self-respect and a desire to do what is expected of them. As long as a rule has been communicated to such employees and that rule is perceived to be reasonable, employees will generally obey the rule (DuBrin, 2002; Levine and Crom, 1995; Wolper, 2004).

When performance flounders, the supervisor should first assess whether a problem exists with a procedure or the knowledge base of the employee (Belker and Topchik, 2005; Byham and Cox, 1998; Walton, 1986). If this is the case, retraining or redesigning the work process should solve the problem. If this is not the case, and the employee repeatedly demonstrates that he or she will not change inappropriate work behaviors, formal corrective action is required.

For corrective action to be effective, employees must first know what is expected of them and why. Policies, procedures, rules, and regulations must be communicated to employees, preferably in writing. Furthermore, employees must believe that the expectations of the organization are reasonable. Consequently, it is important that employees understand why the policies and procedures are in place (Belker and Topchik, 2005; Walton, 1986; Whiting, 2005).

Traditionally, corrective action has been based on the concept of progressive discipline (Mathis and Jackson, 2000; Whiting, 2005). Typically, four levels of progressive discipline exist: verbal warnings, written warnings, suspension, and discharge. In general, the first time an employee commits a minor rule violation, a friendly reminder or warning is all that is necessary. A written warning is given to an employee who commits a more serious violation or who fails to improve after repeated verbal warnings. Written warnings should contain the following information:

- The reason for the disciplinary action
- Date of the disciplinary action

- Action to be taken
- Description of the incident causing the disciplinary action
- What will happen if the employee violates the rule again
- What the employee agrees to do to correct his or her behavior
- A place for the employee to sign and date the form
- A place for the supervisor to sign and date the form

Written warnings should be placed in the employee's personnel file.

Suspension, with or without pay, is usually reserved for employees who commit very serious violations of the rules or have committed repeated violations with written warnings. Whiting (2005) recommends that it is wise to have more than one manager in the meeting when the suspension is given, and it is desirable to suspend with pay. Suspending without pay seldom results in improved performance. The employee should be charged with deciding whether he or she wants to return to work the following day. The employee should understand that everyone must follow the rules and that no exception will be given. If the employee decides to stay after this type of ultimatum, it is more likely that he or she will attempt to be compliant.

The final step in progressive discipline is discharge. A constructive discharge occurs when management creates a situation in which the employee is not able to exercise free choice when deciding whether to resign. In some cases, a constructive discharge leaves the employee eligible for benefits that he or she may not obtain if fired (Whiting, 2005).

Before offering a constructive discharge or terminating an employee, the following questions should be addressed:

- Was there a written rule or regulation covering the type of activity for which the employee is being discharged?
- Was the employee informed about these rules and regulations, either through written or verbal communications?
- Have these rules been administered in a fair and consistent manner?
- Is there adequate written documentation in the form of written disciplinary actions to support the discharge?
- Has there been a fair investigation of the facts surrounding the case to ensure that the manager was aware of all of the possible circumstances?
- Has the employee been presented with an opportunity to present his or her side of the story?
- Have the employee's past record and time of service been considered?
- Is it fair to the organization and the employee to terminate employment?
- Would it seem fair to a judge?

If all of these questions can be answered yes, the employee should probably be discharged. Whenever possible, it is best to review each case with the personnel department or a consulting HR specialist to ensure that no legal exposure to the termination is present. Employees should be paid for all hours worked up until the time they are terminated. They also have a right to continue their group insurance under the Consolidated Omnibus Budget Reconciliation Act of 1986 (COBRA) as long as they are not discharged for gross misconduct (e.g., theft, fraud, embezzlement, or physical assault).

If it is determined that an employee should be discharged, the supervisor should conduct a discharge interview. Whiting (2005) recommends that at least two managers or, in small practices, the owner and an unbiased witness be present for the interview. The interview should last no more than 2 or 3 minutes. The supervisor should explain that it is necessary to terminate the employee and briefly give the reason why. The procedure for obtaining the final paycheck should be explained. The employee should be escorted to his or her work area to clean up the desk and then escorted to the door. It is good form to wish him or her well in the future. Most discharged employees are not bad people. They were simply hired for the wrong job. Nevertheless, firing an employee is traumatic for both the organization and the employee. No manager who has gone through this process is capricious in how he or she chooses new employees.

The Special Case of the Au.D. Student Externship

Offering an Au.D. student an externship presents unique opportunities and challenges. For the student, it offers experiences, acculturation, and a vehicle for academic instructors and practicing professionals to interact. However, there are important issues to consider when offering an externship experience. The purpose of the 4th year externship is to provide students with opportunities to "practice" in real-world settings under the supervision of experienced audiologists. This activity is more than simply observing clinical activities. As agents of the sponsoring sites and receiving benefit (experience) from the relationships with the sponsors, students may be considered employees, even if they are not paid. This is an area of controversy at the time of writing.

In many practice settings, the student externship experience is treated as equivalent to the clinical fellowship experience developed for master's level graduates. The tendency is to consider the extern as an employee rather than a student. In fact, the actual relationship between the student extern and the facility offering the clinical externship experience may not be clear-cut. Clearly, if externs are paid a salary, they will be considered employees. If externs are paid a stipend (payment offered to offset the expenses incurred for going to the externship site, irrespective of any time or "work" accomplished), they still may be considered employees from a liability and medical malpractice perspective. For example, the student extern is on site in a professional role with the consent of the owner and supervising audiologist. Any harm caused by the student while on the premises or under the direction of the externship site opens the site to liability exposure. Students and universities may offer malpractice insurance. However, sponsoring externship sites need to review their own insurance policies to ensure coverage for student-related activities. Student and university-based malpractice policies may not automatically cover the supervising externship site in all situations, particularly if culpability for harm can be ascribed to "inadequate" supervision.

Beyond this, salary or stipend payment must still be considered income and may be subject to income tax and Federal Insurance Contributions (FICA), or Social Security, withholding. Other forms of insurance, such as workers' compensation and disability, may be required, depending on whether the student is considered an employee by the state and, ultimately, the courts. Even if the student is not paid and is not considered an employee, the sponsoring site may still need insurance coverage for any harm that may come to the student while he or she is on the premises. Each site should investigate its insurance coverage to ensure that students in training are covered.

♦ Ownership of the Profession

The saying "All ships rise at high tide" means that when times are good, everyone prospers, so all have an obligation to work for good times. The same principle applies to audiology. Audiology is both a discipline and a profession. Both require good stewardship. All audiologists and hearing scientists have an obligation to support the development of the discipline and the profession for the sake of the persons with hearing impairment and the future of the profession. The following sections suggest ways in which the practitioner can support both the profession and the discipline.

Minding the Discipline

The profession of audiology is founded on the bedrock of basic and applied science. A healthy scientific discipline provides the theories that underpin new understandings of clinical problems and new treatments. Audiologists are well trained in the scientific underpinnings of the profession in graduate school. In practice, a strong background in clinical research is essential to the evaluation of new technologies and clinical methods that inevitably evolve. Without this knowledge, clinicians might become overly influenced by manufacturers' claims rather than the best clinical evidence and optimum clinical outcomes. The first obligation to the profession, then, is to keep current in the scientific discipline that underpins the profession.

A second way to help maintain a healthy scientific discipline is to support those individuals and institutions that contribute to the discipline. This may include lobbying for increased funding from the National Institutes of Health, participating in a clinical trial evaluating a new device or equipment, or simply helping to enroll subjects in a graduate student's research project. Collaborations between clinicians and researchers are vital for both groups. Clinicians benefit from the repeated exposure to basic science practices. Researchers benefit from exposure to common clinical problems that can be better managed with new data, information, or theory. All of us as owners of the profession share the responsibility to our patients to promote the art and science of audiology. We should always look for ways to innovate, collaborate, and share our knowledge with others.

Developing the Profession

Unlike a discipline, which can be understood from a completely scholarly viewpoint, a profession is defined within the context of the marketplace. From this perspective, the profession is the translation of the knowledge base of the discipline into goods or services that are valued by the market. Two attributes are commonly ascribed to a profession. First, the market perceives that part of the value of an individual practitioner's goods or services is a by-product of considerable training and specialized study. Second, the market perceives that all practitioners of the profession have a common identity, share a common level of training and study, and offer a high minimum level of quality in the goods or services offered.

Professional status offers several advantages to its members. First, individual practitioners share the market's value of their services without each individual first developing a reputation. Second, professions are more able to capture markets because they can promote the relationship between their group identity and the value of their goods or services. Third, following the saying "All ships rise at high tide," the group affiliation that is part of professional status allows members to work as a group to promote common interests. As such, they truly become a human resource.

The value of professional status is determined by market perceptions. Consequently, professionals invest in efforts that enhance the value of their services in the market and promote the association between high value and professional affiliation. These activities are often accomplished through professional organizations.

Professional organizations perform at least one of three core functions: they facilitate the development and dissemination of new knowledge to their membership, they offer a vehicle for self-policing by establishing guidelines for entry into the profession and determination of what is and what is not acceptable professional practice, and they protect the interests and enhance the position of the profession within the marketplace.

Facilitating the development and dissemination of new knowledge to their membership helps the profession develop more efficient and effective goods and services. Self-policing helps maintain the quality of goods and services provided by the profession. Both these functions enhance the perceived value of the profession within the market. Protecting the interests and position of the profession within the marketplace involves ensuring that the market has optimum exposure and access to the profession. All three functions are often accomplished within the same organization. So, for example, members of professional audiology organizations (e.g., AAA, ABA, ADA, ASHA) may be grappling with the acceptance of a new clinical technique, lobbying for a new licensure law, establishing practice guidelines, promoting the profession to third-party payers, and disciplining a member for an ethics violation.

Except in very restrictive circumstances, membership in a professional organization is voluntary. Achieving the objectives of the organization (and the goals of the profession) requires an investment of financial support, time, effort, and involvement on the part of the membership. This is a professional obligation, particularly in view of the benefits afforded to the practitioner if the organization enhances the perception of the profession of audiology within the marketplace.

Acculturation

Many professions develop a sense of responsibility for participation in the profession through a process of acculturation. In this use of the term, *acculturation* means maintaining a culture among professionals that promotes the health of the profession. For example, most professional schools (medical, legal, and military schools in particular) maintain close relationships with their practitioners. It is not uncommon for practitioners to sponsor social activities with students for the sole purpose of helping new members in training to network. These social activities help the students identify clinical mentors and establish professional bonds that build group cohesion. Later, these relationships foster diplomacy in solving internal controversies and promote united action when there is an external threat to the profession.

Audiology also has several vehicles for professional acculturation. ASHA, AAA, and ADA, for example, have affiliated student organizations. Most state organizations promote student participation through reduced membership fees and special clinical forums. Individual practitioners support the process by taking students in clinical fellowship and 4th year Au.D. externship positions. All of these activities acculturate new members into the profession.

The National Association of Future Doctors of Audiology (NAFDA), founded by students, also has a role in developing group cohesion between student experiences and professional practice groups. NAFDA is truly an amazing organization. Typically, it is the experienced professionals (faculty members and practitioners) who create vehicles for acculturation. In the case of NAFDA, the students filled a void not met by faculty members and practitioners. NAFDA members sit on many of the professional organization's boards and hold their own

conventions, typically in concert with other professional organizations.

The value of acculturation extends beyond initial entry into the profession. Audiologists often compete with each other in professional practice. Competition can be a positive influence in that the search for a competitive advantage can lead to improvements in service delivery. Competition can also have a negative effect when the importance of maintaining a healthy profession gives way to issues of commerce. When competitive pressures break down professional relationships, the parties are trading the future of the profession for short-term gain. This is never a good trade.

Pearl

- Acculturation promotes diplomacy in solving internal controversies and united action when an external threat to the profession is present. Because these are vital to the survival of the profession, each member is responsible for developing collegial interpersonal relationships with other members of the profession.

By working to build positive relationships and sharing innovations with colleagues, the overall knowledge base of the profession grows. Furthermore, when outside forces threaten the professional prerogatives of audiology, members are more likely to become involved for the common good. One approach to promote this type of collegiality is taken by the American College of Surgeons. Fellowship in this prestigious organization requires that the potential members subscribe to the fellowship pledge (**Table 4–9**).

By subscribing to this oath, the American College of Surgeons promotes an ethic of placing the patient and the profession ahead of commerce. This ethic creates a heritage or standard that ensures the health of the profession. A similar pledge has been proposed for audiologists (Steiger et al, 2002; see **Table 4–10**).

Professional organizations ideally serve as a vehicle for establishing and maintaining professional relationships within audiology. They help organize and act in ways that are in our own professional interest. However, for various reasons, organizations do not always rise to meet their

---

Table 4–9 American College of Surgeons' Fellowship Pledge

Recognizing that the American College of Surgeons seeks to exemplify and develop the highest traditions of our ancient profession, I hereby pledge myself, as a condition of Fellowship in the College, to live in strict accordance with its principles and regulations.

I pledge myself to pursue the practice of surgery with honesty and to place the welfare and the rights of my patient above all else. I promise to deal with each patient as I would wish to be dealt with if I was in the patient's position, and I will set my fees commensurate with the services rendered. I will take no part in any arrangement, such as fee splitting or itinerant surgery, which induces referral or treatment for reason other than the patient's best welfare.

Upon my honor, I declare that I will advance my knowledge and skills, will respect my colleagues, and will seek their counsel when in doubt about my own abilities. In turn, I will willingly help my colleagues when requested.

Finally, I solemnly pledge myself to cooperate in advancing and extending the art and science of surgery by my Fellowship in the American College of Surgeons.

Source: Fellowship pledge, American College of Surgeons, n.d., with permission.

Table 4–10 The Proposed Doctor of Audiology Oath

As a doctor of audiology, I pledge to practice the art and science of my profession to the best of my ability and to be ethical in conduct. I will respect and honor my teachers, and also those who forged the path I freely follow. According to their example, I will continue to expand my knowledge and improve my skills.

I will collaborate with my fellow audiologists and other professionals for the benefit of our patients.

I will, to the best of my ability and judgment, evaluate, manage, and treat my patients.

I will willingly do no harm, but rather always strive to provide care according to the standards of the profession.

I will act to the benefit of those needing care, striving to see that none go untreated.

I will practice when competent to do so, and refer all others to practitioners capable of providing care in keeping with this Oath.

I will aspire to personal and professional conduct free from corruption.

I will keep in confidence all information made known to me about my patients.

As a doctor of audiology, I agree to be held accountable for any violation of this Oath and the ethics of the profession. While I keep this Oath unviolated, may it be granted to me to enjoy life and the practice of the art and science of audiology, respected by all persons, in all times.

Source: From Steiger, J., Saccone, P., & Freeman, B. (2002, September–October). A proposed doctoral oath for audiologists. Audiology Today, pp. 12–14.

responsibility to the profession. It falls to the professionals who make up the membership to ensure that the organization's governance acts in the profession's best interests.

Participation in state and local organizations is often overlooked and yet vital to the profession. State-level organizations deal with licensure and other right-to-practice legislation. These are the factors that directly affect the day-to-day practice of audiology. Membership rosters for most state organizations are small. Typically, a small group of dedicated audiologists are expected to do the work of the profession. It often cannot be done. It is vital to participate in state-level organizations, if for no other reason than to develop and protect audiology's scope of practice. No one else will protect our interests in our absence.

Controversial Point

- Most issues involving the right to practice, such as licensure, scope of practice, minimum qualifications to practice, and, increasingly, provider reimbursement issues, are decided on the state level. Yet membership in state professional organizations is low relative to national organizations. It may be wiser to invest more in state organizations to promote changes at the state level than to expect national organizations to influence decisions that are decided at the state level.

◆ **Summary**

This chapter has dealt with HR issues from a very broad prospective. On the micro level, audiology is a high-technology endeavor. Successful practice requires that the individual master complex assessment and management tools. However, we are about human perception and communication. Our contribution is not our machinery. Rather, the difference between a good audiology practice and a great practice is the "high touch" or "human factor." Wise stewardship is necessary to capitalize on the human potential of our profession. As professionals, we are responsible for our own development and the promotion of our discipline and profession. Without this, we cannot maintain our fiduciary responsibilities to our patients. It is hoped that this chapter has presented some principles that will aid in this endeavor.

On the macro level, audiology is young and still growing. We have matured into a doctoral-level profession. However, we will face many issues and threats, both internal and external, which will impact our long-term future. It will become increasingly important for us to develop and maintain a cohesive group culture. This starts with an ethic that promotes the development of the profession and discipline, places the patient and the profession before commerce, reinforces respect for colleagues, and promotes coordinated action to advance the initiatives of the profession and those it would serve.

Appendix 4–1

Example of Job Description for Audiologist

Job title: Audiologist

Department: Audiology-Hearing and Balance Center

Supervisor: Director of Audiology

Job summary: The audiologist is responsible for evaluating, treating, and counseling with the pediatric, adult, or geriatric patient with hearing disorders in accordance with professional and corporate quality standards. Models appropriate behavior as exemplified in corporate value system and the operating mission, which reflects commitment to total quality improvement.

Job functions (major and minor duties):

1. Conducts hearing and balance evaluations for inpatients and outpatients, including neonates, pediatric patients, adolescents, adults, and geriatric patients, and assesses the history, medical diagnosis, social, and communicative condition of the patient through testing and interview to establish a basis for patient treatment (type I services)

    a. Through history, interview, and formal diagnostic testing, characterizes the perceptual abilities and physiological state of the auditory system in neonatal, pediatric, adult, and geriatric patients

    b. Understands otologic and neurologic diagnostic processes well enough to obtain audiologic information that will help the physician distinguish between competing etiological entities in a given patient

    c. Generates written communications for treating physicians that are timely, clear, and succinct

    d. Understands the theory behind established clinical protocols and can modify diagnostic procedures to meet the needs of the patient/customer without sacrificing test reliability or validity

    e. Has expertise in at least two of the following areas and provides inservice and professional training in same: infant and pediatric audiology, diagnostic audiology, forensic and occupational audiology, amplification and aural rehabilitation, balance and spatial orientation

    f. Provides all services with a caring, empathetic manner, holding to the highest professional, ethical, and legal standards

2. Determines patient's perceptual and communicative needs and formulates, implements, and measures the efficacy of an audiologic rehabilitation treatment plan (type II service)

    a. Interprets the results of hearing evaluation data within the context of the patient's perceptual, social, and communicative needs; identifies deficit areas; and communicates this information clearly to the patient as the first step in rehabilitation

    b. Together with the patient and significant others, develops a rational treatment and monitoring plan, including the use of amplification, assistive listening devices, aural rehabilitation, and counseling as indicated

    c. Demonstrates knowledge of current amplification technologies, fitting practices, and validation procedures

    d. Monitors treatment effectiveness and modifies treatment plans when necessary for optimal treatment outcomes

    e. Develops and assesses impact of family-based education to facilitate carryover of new skills into everyday environments

3. Together with other audiology staff members, develops methods to identify hearing-impaired patients in the hospital and community and facilitates community awareness of hearing impairment and its management (type III service)

    a. Uses basic and advanced diagnostic technologies to screen the hearing of at-risk populations

    b. Develops and maintains data management systems to facilitate efficient follow-up of at-risk patients

    c. Presents information within the community to promote awareness of hearing impairment and its management

    d. Participates in studies designed to assess the effectiveness of hearing screening programs

    e. Develops new methods and systems to promote hearing health care within the hospital and community

4. Promotes professional practice of all members of the departmental care team

    a. Supports the team concept among all staff; participates in mutual problem solving to achieve positive outcomes and improve quality of services; documents incidents of critical nature; participates in departmental meetings

    b. Demonstrates initiative in identifying opportunities for self-development and enhancement of professional competency through self-study, on-the-job training, and attending professional meetings

    c. Demonstrates effective customer relations skills, promotes a positive work environment, and contributes to the overall team effort

    d. Participates in quality monitoring and evaluation activities and implements measures to ensure that hospital, Joint Commission on Accreditation of Healthcare Organizations (JCAHO), and other quality standards are met

    e. Works together with audiology, other department staff, and administration in sharing and giving information and support as needed in a manner of dignity, respect, and helpfulness as exemplified in the corporate value system, total quality improvement (TQI) process, and the organization's mission statement

5. Performs other job functions as needed

6. Acts in a manner consistent with the following value system:

    a. Demonstrates dedication to quality

        ◆ Makes effort to do each job function correctly

        ◆ Keeps persons informed who should and need to be informed

        ◆ Takes responsibility for problems, questions, or issues and makes effort to solve or get someone who can, rather than passing on the problem

        ◆ Identifies barriers to efficiency and effectiveness in own job, department, or other areas and suggests ways to improve

    b. Demonstrates dedication to fairness

        ◆ Treats others with dignity and respect

        ◆ Promotes cooperation and teamwork among coworkers

        ◆ Works and behaves in a manner that does not create problems or provoke negative reactions from others

        ◆ Demonstrates support of corporate and department policies to ensure consistency of impact on others

    c. Demonstrates dedication to customer service (internal or external)

        ◆ Provides quick service

        ◆ Is polite in interactions, which includes body language and tone of voice

        ◆ Demonstrates a concerned and caring attitude

- ♦ Communicates needed information to those who need to know
- ♦ Provides clean environment that gives appearance of professionalism
- ♦ Provides a quiet atmosphere by low-key interactions demonstrating a professional demeanor in the work unit and in any affiliated facility
- ♦ Takes initiative to offer assistance when needed
- ♦ Takes initiative to coach fellow associates to appreciate and demonstrate customer-focused behaviors
- ♦ Goes beyond the specific demands of his or her job to serve the customer better
- ♦ Stays focused on the customer as long as needed

d. Demonstrates dedication to integrity

- ♦ Is honest in all interactions
- ♦ Demonstrates a work ethic that is exemplified by reporting to work on time, not taking excessive breaks, working until end of shift, and not wasting time
- ♦ Is honest in time card and time off reporting
- ♦ Reports own errors to correct problems and develop trust
- ♦ Demonstrates behavior that is consistent with the American Speech-Language-Hearing Association (ASHA) and American Academy of Audiology (AAA) codes of ethics

Personal contacts:

Internal: The audiologist has daily contact with associates, supervisors, and managers in audiology, in other areas of rehabilitation services, and in other hospital departments, such as nursing floors.

External: The audiologist has daily contact with physicians, patients, and patients' family members.

Supervision given: Lead responsibilities are to direct and to monitor performance of audiometric technicians as assigned by director.

Physical demands/conditions: Exposure to patient body fluids; ability to react quickly to emergency situations; ability to read and write to communicate both orally and in writing with other individuals; normal vision, including peripheral vision; occasional travel within the region; some lifting of equipment weighing up to 35 lb

Minimum qualifications:

1. a. Possession of a current license to practice in the state of Tennessee as an audiologist (master's degree required for licensure)

   b. Possession of current certificate of clinical competence in audiology from ASHA, or current board certification from AAA or equivalent

2. Knowledge of audiology methods and techniques in two or more of the following areas (2 years' experience desirable): industrial audiology; pediatric audiology, including hearing aid fitting, aural rehabilitation, and community-based programming; infant hearing assessment, including otoacoustic emissions and evoked potentials; educational audiology, including assessment and management of auditory language/learning disabled children; advanced differential diagnostic testing of otologic and neurological patients; assessment of spatial orientation, including electronystagmography (ENG), rotational tests, posturography, and behavioral assessment

3. Ability to understand and prepare moderately complex written materials, such as patient records

4. Prepared by education, training, or experience to work with the adult, geriatric, pediatric, or neonatal patient

5. Ability to communicate verbally with associates, physicians, and other outside professionals

6. Ability to work without close supervision and to exercise independent judgment

7. Ability to organize multiple tasks and projects and maintain control of work flow

Appendix 4–2

Regulatory Agencies for Speech-Language Pathology and Audiology

The following is a listing of the agencies that regulate speech-language pathologists and audiologists through state licensure, certification, or registration. In some states, different boards regulate the dispensing of hearing aids. For an up-to-date list of regulatory agencies; please check the American Academy of Audiology Web site (http://audiology.org) or the Audiology Foundation of America Web site (http://audfound.org).

Alabama

Alabama Board of Examiners for Speech Pathology
and Audiology
P.O. Box 304760
Montgomery, AL 36104
Phone: 334–269–1434
Fax: 334–834–6398

Alaska

Division of Occupational Licensing
P.O. Box 110806
Juneau, AK 99811–0806
Phone: 907–465–2695
Fax: 907–465–2974

Arizona

Arizona Department of Health Services
Office of Special Licensing
150 North 18th, Suite 460
Phoenix, AZ 85007
Phone: 602–364–2050
Fax: 602–364–4769

Arkansas

Board of Examiners for SP and AUD
101 East Capitol, Suite 211
Little Rock, AR 72201
Phone: 501–682–9180
Fax: 501–682–9181

California

Speech-Language Pathology and Audiology Board
1422 Howe Avenue, Suite 3
Sacramento, CA 95825–3204
Phone: 916–263–2666
Fax: 916–263–2668

Colorado

Audiologists and Hearing Aid Providers Registration
1560 Broadway, Suite 1545
Denver, CO 80202
Phone: 303–894–2464
Fax: 303–894–7885

Connecticut

SLP and Audiology Licensure
Department of Public Health
410 Capitol Avenue, MS #12APP
P.O. Box 340308
Hartford, CT 06134–0308
Phone: 860–509–7560
Fax: 860–509–8457

Delaware

Audiology, SLP, and Hearing Aid Dispensing Board
Canon Building, Suite 203
861 Silver Lake Boulevard
Dover, DE 19904
Phone: 302–744–4504
Fax: 302–739–2711

Florida

Board of Speech-Language Pathology and Audiology
4052 Bald Cypress Way, Bin C06
Tallahassee, FL 32399
Phone: 850–245–4444, ext. 3456
Fax: 850–921–6184

Georgia

Board of Examiners for Speech-Language Pathology
   and Audiology
237 Coliseum Drive
Macon, GA 31217
Phone: 478–207–1670
Fax: 478–207–1676

Hawaii

Board of Speech Pathology and Audiology
Department of Commerce and Consumer Affairs
P.O. Box 3469
Honolulu, HI 96801
Phone: 808–586–2698
Fax: 808–586–2689

Illinois

Illinois Department of Professional Regulations
320 West Washington Street
Springfield, IL 62786
Phone: 217–782–8556
Fax: 217–782–7645

Indiana

Indiana Speech-Language Pathology and Audiology Board
Indiana Health Profession Service Bureau
402 West Washington Street, Room W066
Indianapolis, IN 46204–2758
Phone: 317–234–2064
Fax: 317–233–4236

Iowa

State Board of SLP and Audiology Examiners
Bureau of Professional Licensure
Lucas State Office Building
321 East 12th Street, 5th Floor
Des Moines, IA 50319–0075
Phone: 515–281–4408
Fax: 515–281–3121

Kansas

Kansas Department of Health and Environment
Health Occupations Credentialing
1000 SW Jackson, Suite 200
Topeka, KS 66612–1365
Phone: 785–296–1240

Kentucky

Kentucky Board of Speech-Language Pathology and
   Audiology
P.O. Box 1360
Frankfort, KY 40602–1360
Phone: 502–564–3296, ext. 240
Fax: 502–564–4818

Louisiana

Louisiana Board of Examiners for Speech-Language
   Pathology and Audiology
18550 Highland Road, Suite B
Baton Rouge, LA 70809
Phone: 225–756–3480
Fax: 225–756–3472

Maine

Board of Examiners on Speech Pathology
   and Audiology
35 State House Station
Augusta, ME 04333
Phone: 207–624–8603
Fax: 207–624–8637

Maryland

Maryland Board of Examiners for Audiology,
    Hearing Aid Dispensers, and Speech-Language
    Pathologists
4201 Patterson Avenue
Baltimore, MD 21215
Phone: 410–764–4725
Fax: 410–358–0273

Massachusetts

Massachusetts Board of Speech-Language
    Pathology and Audiology
239 Causeway Street, Suite 500
Boston, MA 02114
Phone: 617–727–3071
Fax: 617–727–2669

Michigan

Bureau of Health Professions
P.O. Box 30670
Lansing, MI 48909–8170
Phone: 517–335–0918
Fax: 517–373–2179

Minnesota

Minnesota Department of Health
Speech-Language Pathology and Audiology
    Advisory Council
85 East Seventh Place
St. Paul, MN 55164
Phone: 651–282–5629
Fax: 651–282–5628

Mississippi

Mississippi State Department of Health, Professional
    Licensure
570 East Woodrow Wilson Drive
Jackson, MS 39216
Phone: 601–576–7260
Fax: 601–576–7267

Missouri

Missouri Board of Registration for the Healing Arts
Advisory Commission of Professional Speech-Language
    Pathologists and Audiologists
3605 Missouri Boulevard
Jefferson City, MO 65102
Phone: 573–751–4117
Fax: 573–751–3166

Montana

Board of Speech-Language Pathologists and Audiologists
301 South Park, 4th Floor
Helena, MT 59620
Phone: 406–841–2385 or 406–841–2300
Fax: 406–841–2305

Nebraska

Board of Audiology and Speech-Language Pathology
P.O. Box 94986
301 Centennial Mall South
Lincoln, NE 68509
Phone: 402–471–2299
Fax: 402–471–3577

Nevada

Nevada State Board of Examiners for Audiology and Speech
    Pathology
P.O. Box 70550
Reno, NV 89570–0550
Phone: 775–857–3500
Fax: 775–857–2121

New Hampshire

New Hampshire Board of Hearing Care Providers
8 Fillmore Road
Portsmouth, NH 03801
Phone: 603–433–7512
Fax: 603–271–4141

New Jersey

Audiology and Speech-Language
Advisory Committee
124 Halsey Street, 6th Floor
Newark, NJ 07102
Phone: 973–504–6390
Fax: 973–648–3355

New Mexico

SLP, AUD and Hearing Aid Dispensers
Practices Board
P.O. Box 25101
Santa Fe, NM 87504
Phone: 505–476–7098
Fax: 505–476–7094

New York

New York State Board for Speech-Language
    Pathology and Audiology
Education Building, 2nd Floor
West Wing
Albany, NY 12234
Phone: 518–474–3817, ext. 100
Fax: 518–486–4846

North Carolina

North Carolina Board of Examiners for Speech-Language
    Pathology and Audiology
P.O. Box 16885
Greensboro, NC 27416
Phone: 336–272–1828
Fax: 336–272–4353

North Dakota

Board of Examiners on Audiology and SLP
Bureau of Educational Services and Applied Research
P.O. Box 7189
Grand Forks, ND 58202–7189
Phone: 701–777–4421
Fax: 701–777–4365

Ohio

Board of SLP and Audiology
77 South High Street, 16th Floor
Columbus, OH 43266
Phone: 614–466–3145
Fax: 614–995–2286

Oklahoma

State Board of Examiners for SLP and Audiology
P.O. Box 53592
Oklahoma City, OK 73152
Phone: 405–840–2774
Fax: 405–843–3489

Oregon

Board of Examiners for Speech-Language Pathology
    and Audiology
800 NE Oregon Street, Suite 407
Portland, OR 97232
Phone: 503–731–4050
Fax: 503–731–4207

Pennsylvania

Board of Examiners for Speech-Language
    and Hearing
Bureau of Professional and Occupational Affairs
P.O. Box 2649
Harrisburg, PA 17105–2649
Phone: 717–783–1389
Fax: 717–787–7769

Rhode Island

Board of Examiners in SLP and Audiology
Rhode Island Department of Health
3 Capitol Hill, Room 104
Providence, RI 02908–5097
Phone: 401–222–2828
Fax: 401–277–1272

South Carolina

South Carolina Board of Examiners in Speech
    Pathology and Audiology
P.O. Box 11329, Suite 101
Columbia, SC 29211
Phone: 803–896–4650
Fax: 803–896–4719

South Dakota

South Dakota Board of Hearing Aid Dispensers
    and Audiologists
135 East Illinois, Suite 214
Spearfish, SD 57783
Phone: 605–642–1600
Fax: 605–642–1756

Tennessee

State Board of Communication Disorders
    and Sciences
Speech Pathology and Audiology
425 5th Avenue N, 1st Floor
Nashville, TN 37247
Phone: 615–532–3202, ext. 25132
Fax: 615–741–7698

Texas

State Board of Examiners for SLP and Audiology
1100 West 49th Street
Austin, TX 78756–3183
Phone: 512–834–6627
Fax: 512–834–6786

Utah

Speech-Language Pathology and Audiology
Licensing Board
P.O. Box 146741
Salt Lake City, UT 84114–6741
Phone: 801–530–6632
Fax: 801–530–6511

Vermont

Vermont Department of Education
120 State Street
Montpelier, VT 05620–2501
Phone: 802–828–2445

Virginia

State Board of Audiology and Speech Pathology
6606 West Broad Street, 4th Floor
Richmond, VA 23230–1717
Phone: 804–662–7390
Fax: 804–662–9523

Washington

Board of Hearing and Speech
Department of Health
1300 SE Quince Street
P.O. Box 47869
Olympia, WA 98504–7869
Phone: 360–236–4914
Fax: 360–236–2406

West Virginia

Board of Examiners for SLP and AUD
HC 78, Box 9A
Troy, WV 26443
Phone: 304–473–4289
Fax: 304–462–5482

Wisconsin

Council on SLP and Audiology
Department of Regulation and Licensing
P.O. Box 8935
Madison, WI 53708–8935
Phone: 608–266–2811
Fax: 608–261–7083

Wyoming

Board of Speech-Language Pathology and Audiology
2020 Carey Avenue, Suite 201
Cheyenne, WY 82002
Phone: 307–777–6529
Fax: 307–777–3508

Regulatory Agencies for Hearing Aid Dispensing

This is a listing of agencies that regulate the dispensing of hearing aids. In some states, hearing aid dispensing by audiologists and nonaudiologists is regulated by the state board. In other states, hearing aid dispensing by these groups is regulated by different boards. This listing is for hearing aid dispensing only.

Alabama

Licensed Audiologists and Nonaudiologists
Hearing Instrument Dealer's Board
 400 South Union Street, Suite 445
Montgomery, AL 36104
Phone: 334–242–1925
Fax: 334–834–6398

Alaska

Licensed Audiologists and Nonaudiologists
Division of Occupational Licensing
Hearing Aid Dealer Section
P.O. Box 110806
Juneau, AK 99811–0806
Phone: 907–465–2695
Fax: 907–465–2974

Arizona

Licensed Audiologists and Nonaudiologists
Arizona Department of Health Services
Office of Special Licensing
150 North 18th Avenue, Suite 460
Phoenix, AZ 85007
Phone: 602–364–2079
Fax: 602–364–4769

Arkansas

Licensed Audiologists
Board of Examiners for SP and AUD
101 East Capitol, Suite 211
Little Rock, AR 72201
Phone: 501–682–9180
Fax: 501–682–9181

Nonaudiologists
Board of Hearing Aid Dispensers
305 North Monroe
Little Rock, AR 72205
Phone: 501–663–5869
Fax: 501–663–6359

California

Licensed Audiologists and Nonaudiologists
Hearing Aid Dealers' Examining Committee
1420 Howe Avenue, Suite 12
Sacramento, CA 95825–3230
Phone: 916–263–2288
Fax: 916–920–6377

Colorado

Licensed Audiologists and Nonaudiologists
Audiologists' and Hearing Aid Dealers' Registration
1560 Broadway, Suite 1545
Denver, CO 80202
Phone: 303–894–2464

Connecticut

Licensed Audiologists
SLP and Audiology Licensure
Department of Public Health
410 Capitol Avenue, MS #12APP
P.O. Box 340308
Hartford, CT 06134–0308
Phone: 860–509–7560
Fax: 860–509–8457

Nonaudiologists
Board of Hearing Aid Dispensers
401 Capitol Avenue, MS# 12APP
P.O. Box 340308
Hartford, CT 06134

Delaware

Licensed Audiologists and Nonaudiologists
Audiology, SLP, and Hearing Aid Dispensing Board
Division of Professional Regulation
P.O. Box 1401
Dover, DE 19903
Phone: 302–739–4522, ext. 215
Fax: 302–739–2711

Florida

Licensed Audiologists
Board of SLP and Audiology
Department of Professional Regulation
1940 North Monroe
Tallahassee, FL 32399–0778
Phone: 850–488–0595
Fax: 850–921–5389

Nonaudiologists
Board of Hearing Aid Specialists
4025 Bald Cypress Way, Bin #C-08
Tallahassee, FL 32399
Phone: 850–245–4444
Fax: 850–921–5389

Georgia

Licensed Audiologists
Board of Examiners for Speech-Language
    Pathology and Audiology
237 Coliseum Drive
Macon, GA 31217
Phone: 478–207–1300
Fax: 478–207–1699

Nonaudiologists
Board of Hearing Aid Dealers and Dispensers
237 Coliseum Drive
Macon, GA 31217
Phone: 478–207–1686
Fax: 478–207–1699

Hawaii

Licensed Audiologists and Nonaudiologists
Licensure Branch of HADs and Fitters
Professional and Vocational Licensing Division
P.O. Box 3469
Honolulu, HI 96801
Phone: 808–586–3000

Illinois

Licensed Audiologists and Nonaudiologists
Board for Hearing Aid Dispensers
Consumer Protection Program
Department of Public Health
Division of Health Assessment and
    Screening, 2nd Floor
535 West Jefferson Street
Springfield, IL 62761
Phone: 217–782–4733

Indiana

Licensed Audiologists and Nonaudiologists
Committee of Indiana Hearing Aid Dealer Examiners
Health Professions Bureau
402 West Washington Street, Room W041
Indianapolis, IN 46204
Phone: 317–234–2067
Fax: 317–233–4236

Iowa

Licensed Audiologists and Nonaudiologists
Board of Examiners for Hearing Aid Dealers
Department of Public Health
Lucas State Office Building
321 East 12th Street, 5th Floor
Des Moines, IA 50319–0075
Phone: 515–281–4408

Kansas

Licensed Audiologists and Nonaudiologists
Board of Hearing Aid Examiners
600 North St. Francis
P.O. Box 252
Wichita, KS 67201
Phone: 316–264–8870

Kentucky

Licensed Audiologists and Nonaudiologists
Kentucky Licensing Board for Specialists in Hearing Instruments
P.O. Box 1360
Frankfort, KY 40602–1360
Phone: 502–564–3296, ext. 240
Fax: 502–564–4818

Louisiana

Licensed Audiologists
Louisiana Board of Examiners for Speech-Language
    Pathology and Audiology
18550 Highland Road, Suite B
Baton Rouge, LA 70809
Phone: 225–756–3480
Fax: 225–756–3472

Nonaudiologists
Board of Hearing Aid Dealers
2205 Liberty Street
Monroe, LA 71211
Phone: 318–362–3014
Fax: 318–362–3019

Maine

Licensed Audiologists and Nonaudiologists
Board of Hearing Instrument Dealers and Fitters
Office of Licensing and Regulation
35 State House Station
Augusta, ME 04333
Phone: 207–624–8603
Fax: 207–624–8637

Maryland

Licensed Audiologists and Nonaudiologists
Maryland Board of Examiners for Audiology,
    Hearing Aid Dispensers, and Speech-Language
    Pathologists
4201 Patterson Avenue
Baltimore, MD 21215
Phone: 410–764–4725
Fax: 410–358–0273

Massachusetts

Licensed Audiologists and Nonaudiologists
Massachusetts Board of Registration of Hearing
    Instrument Specialists
239 Causeway Street, Suite 500
Boston, MA 02114
Phone: 617–727–5339
Fax: 617–727–1627

Michigan

Licensed Audiologists and Nonaudiologists
Consumer and Industry Services
Bureau of Commercial Services
Licensing Division
Board of Hearing Aids
P.O. Box 30018
Lansing, MI 48909
Phone: 517–241–9288
Fax: 517–241–9280

Minnesota

Licensed Audiologists and Nonaudiologists
Health Occupations Programs
Board of Examiners for Hearing Aid Dealers
717 SE Delaware Street
Minneapolis, MN 55440–5620
Phone: 651–282–5620

Mississippi

Licensed Audiologists and Nonaudiologists
Professional Licensure/Hearing Aid Specialists
P.O. Box 1700
Jackson, MS 39215–1700
Phone: 601–576–7260
Fax: 601–987–3784

Missouri

Licensed Audiologists and Nonaudiologists
Board of Hearing Instrument Specialists
P.O. Box 471
Jefferson City, MO 65102
Phone: 573–751–0240
Fax: 573–526–3481

Montana

Licensed Audiologists and Nonaudiologists
Board of Hearing Aid Dispensers
Professional and Occupational Licensing Division
301 South Park
Helena, MT 59602
Phone: 406–841–2395

Nebraska

Licensed Audiologists and Nonaudiologists
Board of Hearing Aid Instrument Dispensers and Fitters
Division of Professional and Occupational Licensure
P.O. Box 94986
Lincoln, NE 68509–5007
Phone: 402–471–2299
Fax: 402–471–3577

Nevada

Licensed Audiologists and Nonaudiologists
Board of Hearing Aid Specialists
3172 North Rainbow, Suite 141
Las Vegas, NV 89108
Phone: 775–226–5716

New Hampshire

Licensed Audiologists and Nonaudiologists
Board of Hearing Aid Dealers
8 Fillmore Road
Portsmouth, NH 03801
Phone: 603–433–7512
Fax: 603–271–4141

New Jersey

Licensed Audiologists and Nonaudiologists
Hearing Aid Dispensers Examining Committee
124 Halsey Street, 6th Floor
Newark, NJ 07102
Phone: 973–504–6331

New Mexico

Licensed Audiologists and Nonaudiologists
SLP, AUD, and HAD Practices Board
Regulation and Licensing Department
P.O. Box 25101
Santa Fe, NM 87504
Phone: 505–476–7100
Fax: 505–827–7095

New York

Licensed Audiologists and Nonaudiologists
New York State Department of State
84 Holland Avenue
Albany, NY 12208
Phone: 518–474–4664

North Carolina

Licensed Audiologists and Nonaudiologists
Hearing Aid Dealers and Fitters Board
401 Overlin Road, Suite 111
Raleigh, NC 27605
Phone: 919–834–0430
Fax: 919–833–9954

North Dakota

Licensed Audiologists and Nonaudiologists
Board of Hearing Instrument Fitters
   and Dispensers
825 25th Street
Fargo, ND 58103
Phone: 701–237–9977

Ohio

Licensed Audiologists
Ohio Board of Speech Pathology
   and Audiology
77 South High Street, 16th Floor
Columbus, OH 43215
Phone: 614–466–3145

Nonaudiologists
Hearing Aid Dealers and Fitters
   Licensing Board
246 North High Street
P.O. Box 118
Columbus, OH 43216
Phone: 614–466–5215
Fax: 614–466–0217

Oklahoma

Licensed Audiologists
State Board of Examiners for SLP and Audiology
P.O. Box 53592
Oklahoma City, OK 73152
Phone: 405–840–2774
Fax: 405–843–3489

Nonaudiologists
Hearing Aid Dealers and Fitters
Department of Health
1000 N.E. 10th Street
Oklahoma City, OK 73117
Phone: 405–721–5243
Fax: 405–721–5286

Oregon

Licensed Audiologists and Nonaudiologists
Hearing Aid Dealers Board
Health Division Licensing Programs
700 Summer Street NE, Suite 100
Salem, OR 97310
Phone: 503–378–8667, ext. 4306
Fax: 503–585–9114

Pennsylvania

Licensed Audiologists and Nonaudiologists
Pennsylvania Department of Health
Hearing Aid Program
132 Kline Plaza, Suite A
Harrisburg, PA 17104
Phone: 717–783–8078
Fax: 717–772–0232

Rhode Island

Licensed Audiologists and Nonaudiologists
Rhode Island Department of Health
3 Capitol Hill, Room 104
Providence, RI 02908–5097
Phone: 401–277–2827
Fax: 401–277–1272

South Carolina

Licensed Audiologists
South Carolina Board of Examiners in Speech
   Pathology and Audiology
P.O. Box 11329, Suite 101
Columbia, SC 29211
Phone: 803–896–4650
Fax: 803–896–4719

Nonaudiologists
Department of Health and Environmental Control
Division of Health Licensing
2600 Bull Street
Columbia, SC 29201
Phone: 803–898–3432
Fax: 803–737–7212

South Dakota

Licensed Audiologists and Nonaudiologists
Board of Hearing Aid Dispensers
P.O. Box 654
Spearfish, SD 57783–0654
Phone: 605–642–1600
Fax: 605–642–1756

Tennessee

Licensed Audiologists and Nonaudiologists
Board of SLP, AUD, and Hearing Aid Dispensers
Board of Communication Disorders and Sciences
287 Plus Park Boulevard
Nashville, TN 37247–1010
Phone: 888–310–4650, ext. 25132
Fax: 888–310–4650, ext. 25132

Texas

Licensed Audiologists
Board of Examiners for SLP and Audiology
1100 West 49th Street
Austin, TX 78756–3183
Phone: 512–834–6627
Fax: 512–834–6677

Nonaudiologists
Board of Examiners in the Fitting and Dispensing of
    Hearing Instruments
1100 West 49th Street
Austin, TX 78756
Phone: 512–834–6784
Fax: 512–834–6677

Utah

Licensed Audiologists and Nonaudiologists
Bureau Manager Health Professional Licensing
P.O. Box 45805
160 East 300 South
Salt Lake City, UT 84144
Phone: 801–530–6628
Fax: 801–530–6511

Vermont

Licensed Audiologists and Nonaudiologists
Office of Professional Regulation
Hearing Aid Dispensers Advisors
109 State Street
Montpelier, VT 05609–1101
Phone: 802–828–2191

Virginia

Licensed Audiologists and Nonaudiologists
Department of Professional and Occupational Regulation
3600 West Broad Street
Richmond, VA 23230
Phone: 804–367–8544
Fax: 804–367–2475

Washington

Licensed Audiologists and Nonaudiologists
Department of Health
Board of Audiology, Speech-Language-Pathology and
    Hearing Instrument Fitters
P.O. Box 47869
Olympia, WA 98504–7869
Phone: 360–236–4916

West Virginia

Licensed Audiologists
West Virginia Board of Examiners for SLP and Audiology
701 Jefferson Road
South Charleston, WV 25309
Phone: 304–558–7886

Nonaudiologists
Board of Hearing Aid Dealers
167 11th Avenue
South Charleston, WV 25303
Phone: 304–542–7595

Wisconsin

Licensed Audiologists and Nonaudiologists
Hearing and Speech Examining Board
Council on SLP and Audiology
Department of Regulation and Licensing
P.O. Box 8935
Madison, WI 53708–8935
Phone: 608–266–2811
Fax: 608–261–7083

Wyoming

Licensed Audiologists and Nonaudiologists
Board of Hearing Aid Specialists
2020 Carey Avenue, Suite 201
Cheyenne, WY 82001
Phone: 307–777–6529

Appendix 4–3

Record of Competency

Department of Audiology

Name:

Job title:

Supervisor

Date:

S.S. #:

Code Key:
P = Reviewed policy
0 = No knowledge/optional skill
1 = Didactic knowledge or procedure
2 = Performs procedure with supervision
3 = Performs procedure independently
4 = Master/mentor: Teaches and assess competency

Modifiers:
NI = Needs improvement
R = Retraining required
N/A = Not applicable
O = Optional skill

Scores are awarded on the basis of case staffing performance or oversight by an audiologist rated as a mentor in the area assessed. For new hires, transfers, and promotions: This record will be administered at the beginning of the departmental orientation. Those items highlighted (*) must be completed prior to the end of the department orientation. Competencies for all staff members will be reevaluated at least annually.

Technical Competencies

Competencies	Date	Code	Initial
I. *Basic comprehensive examination*			
a. Case history			
b. Pure-tone audiometry			
c. Speech recognition testing			
d. Tympanometry			
e. Acoustic reflex testing			
f. Clear statement of clinical impressions			
g. Statement of recommendations			
II. *Cochlear-retrocochlear differential*			
a. PI-PB testing			
b. SSI-PI testing			
c. Acoustic reflex decay testing			
d. UCL			
e. Electrocochleography			
f. ABR-AEPs			
g. MLR-AEPs			
h. Transient otoacoustic emissions			
i. Distortion product otoacoustic emissions			
III. *Brainstem-cerebral differential*			
a. Masking level differences			
b. SSI-ICM			
c. SSI-CCM			
d. Temporal patterns and tonal patterns			
e. SSW			
f. Late and endogenous AEPs			
IV. *Spatial orientation assessments*			
a. ENG—Visual tracking (gaze, saccadic, and smooth pursuit)			
b. ENG—Optokinetic induced eye movements			

Competencies	Date	Code	Initial
c. Spontaneous, positional, and positioning nystagmus assessment			
d. Bithermal caloric testing			
e. Vertical and single eye recording techniques			
f. Assessment of eye movements through Frenzel lenses			
g. Detection of Tullio and Hennabert's signs			
h. Postural sway foam and dome assessments			
i. Bedside evaluation of VOR, VVOR, OPN, pursuit, saccadic eye movements, posture, and head/neck orientation			
j. Development of functional treatment plan			
k. Performs canalith repositioning and monitors effectiveness			
l. Orchestrates multidisciplinary balance rehabilitation treatment programs			
V. *Tinnitus assessment and rehabilitation*			
a. Tinnitus matching			
b. Assessment of residual inhibition			
c. Prescription of maskers			
d. Multidisciplinary management strategies and counseling			
VI. *Special populations*			
a. Nonorganic loss: Stenger tests			
b. Nonorganic loss: Lombard tests			
c. Nonorganic loss: LOT tests			
d. Childhood central auditory abilities: figure–ground assessment			
e. Childhood central auditory abilities: sequential memory assessment			
f. Childhood central auditory abilities: short-term memory assessment			
g. Childhood central auditory abilities: auditory maturity assessment			
h. Childhood educational audiology: academic achievement assessment			
i. Childhood educational audiology: IEP and least restrictive environment			
j. Childhood educational audiology: monitoring IEP implementation			
k. Pediatric audiology: visual reinforcement audiometry			
l. Pediatric audiology: COR play audiometry			
m. Adult audiology: hearing handicap communication assessments			
n. Aural rehabilitation: ASL interpreting			
o. Adult audiology: aural rehabilitation—ALD prescription and dispensing			
p. Aural rehabilitation: hearing aid selection and fitting			
q. Aural rehabilitation: environment adaptation strategies			
r. Electroacoustic assessment and modification of hearing aids			
s. In situ probe measurements			
VII. *Infant hearing assessment*			
a. High-frequency tympanometry			
b. OAE screening			
c. Family contact protocols			
d. AEP assessment of the infant			
VIII. *Hearing conservation programming*			
a. Plan and implement yearly monitoring service			
b. Consult re: management of STS cases			
c. Consult re: selection and verification of hearing protective devices			
d. Plan, implement, and evaluate employee education program			
e. Consult re: ADA and hearing impairment			
IX. *Student/resident instruction*			
X. *Basic computer literacy*			

ABR, auditory brainstem response; ADA, Americans with Disabilities Act; AEP, auditory evoked potential; ALD, assistive listening device; ASL, American Sign Language; CCM, contralateral competing message; COR, conditioned orientation reflex; ENG, electronystagmography; ICM, ipsilateral competing message; IEP, individualized education plan; LOT, lengthened off time test ; MLR, middle latency response; OAE, otoacoustic emission(s); OPN, optokinetic nystagmus test; PB, phonetically balanced; PI, performance intensity; SSI, synthetic sentence identification test; SSW, Staggered Spondee Word test; STS, standard threshold shift; UCL, uncomfortable loudness level; VOR, vestibulo-ocular reflex; VVOR, visual and vestibular ocular reflex

References

Belker, L. B., & Topchik G. S. (2005). The first-time manager. New York: Amacom.

Bendapudi, N. M., Berry, L. L., Frey, K. A., Parish, J. T., & Rayburn, W. L. (2006). Patients' perspectives on ideal physician behaviors. Mayo Clinic Proceedings, 81, 338–344.

Beuf, A. H. (1979). Biting off the bracelet: A study of children in hospitals. Philadelphia: University of Pennsylvania Press.

Bick, J. (1997). All I really need to know in business I learned at Microsoft. New York: Simon & Schuster/Pocket Books.

Burrows, D. L. (2006). Human resource issues: Managing, hiring, firing and evaluating employees. Seminars in Hearing, 27, 5–17.

Byham, W. C., & Cox, J. (1998). Zapp! The lightning of empowerment: How to improve productivity, quality, and employee satisfaction. New York: Fawcett Columbine/Ballantine.

Carnegie, D. (1995). Leadership training for managers: Team building skills for today's quality-conscious organizations. Garden City, NY: Dale Carnegie and Associates.

Cascio, W. F. (2003). Managing human resources: Productivity, quality of work life, profits. Boston: McGraw-Hill/Irwin.

Chial, M. (1998). Viewpoint: Conveying expectations about professional behavior. Audiology Today, 10(4), pp. 2–5.

Desmond, A. (1994). Personnel management. In Development and management of audiology practices: Report by the American Speech-Language-Hearing Association (ASHA) Ad Hoc Committee on Practice Management in Audiology (pp. 67–70). Rockville, MD: American Speech-Language-Hearing Association.

DuBrin, A. J. (2002). The winning edge: How to motivate, influence, and manage your company's human resources. Cincinnati, OH: South-Western.

Fine, S. A. (1999). Functional job analysis a foundation for human resources management. Retrieved from http://0-www.netlibrary.com.uncclc.coast.uncwil.edu/urlapi.asp?action=summary&v=1&bookid=19338

Fox, D., & Battin, R. (1978). Private practice in audiology and speech pathology. New York: Grune & Stratton.

Hamill, T. (2006). Ethics in audiology: Guidelines for ethical conduct in the clinical, educational and research settings. Reston, VA: American Academy of Audiology.

Hosford-Dunn, H., Dunn, D. R., & Harford, E. (1995). Audiology business and practice management. San Diego, CA: Singular Publishing.

Inlander, C., Levin, L., & Weiner, E. (1988). Medicine on trial. Englewood Cliffs, NJ: Prentice Hall.

Jenkins, M. D. (1999). Starting and operating a business in the U.S. Palo Alto, CA: Running R Media.

Kilpatrick, A. O., & Johnson, J. A. (1999). Human resources and organizational behavior: Cases in health services management. Chicago: Health Administration Press.

Labovitz, G., & Rosansky, V. (1997). The power of alignment. New York: John Wiley & Sons.

Levine, S. R., & Crom, M. A. (1995). The leader in you: How to win friends, influence people and succeed in a changing world. New York: Simon & Schuster/Dale Carnegie and Associates.

Mathis, R. L., & Jackson, J. H. (2000). Human resource management. Cincinatti, OH: South-Western College Publishing.

Paulson, E. (2003). The complete idiot's guide to starting your own business (4th ed.). New York: Alpha Books.

Pellegrino, E. D. (2002). Professionalism, profession and the virtues of the physician. Mount Sinai Journal of Medicine, 69, 378–384.

Podmoroff, D. (2005). How to hire, train and keep the best employees for your small business. Ocala, FL: Atlantic Publishing Group.

Rall, E., & Brunner, E. (2006). Mentoring and audiology. Seminars in Hearing, 27, 92–97.

Schlesinger, P. E., Sath, V., Schlesinger, L. A., & Kotter, J. P. (1992). Organization: Text, cases, and readings of the management of organizational design and change (3rd ed.). Homewood, IL: Irwin.

Steiger, J., Saccone, P., & Freeman, B. (2002, September–October). A proposed doctoral oath for audiologists. Audiology Today, pp. 12–14.

Walton, M. (1986). The Deming management method. New York: Perigee Book.

Welch, C., & Fowler, K. (1994). Human resource management. In S. R. Rizzo & M. D. Trudeau (Eds.), Clinical administration in audiology and speech-language pathology (pp. 93–132). San Diego, CA: Singular Publishing Group.

Whiting, R. (2005). Hiring and firing within the law. Carrollton, TX: Whiting and Associates.

Wolper, L. F. (2004). Health care administration: Planning, implementing, and managing organized delivery systems. Boston: Jones and Bartlett Publishers.

Yate, M. (2006). Hiring the best: A manager's guide to effective interviewing (5th ed.). Cincinnati, OH: Adams Media Corp.

Yuill, J. (2003). Six things that challenge—seven things that bring success. Ottawa, Ontario, Canada: On Purpose Publishing

Zapala, D. (1996). Professional issues in hospital practice. Seminars in Hearing, 17(3), 261–274.

Chapter 5

Marketing Principles and Application

Wayne J. Staab

The complexities and volatility of the hearing health care marketplace dictate that marketing must be an ongoing or daily activity. The market is dynamic and ever changing. Too much of today's marketing, unfortunately, is based on the reliance on a hearing aid product or hearing aid technology, assuming that if it can be made a little better, success will inevitably follow. However, without a program to make oneself unique in patients' minds, technological superiority alone does not guarantee success or even a competitive position in the practice of hearing aid dispensing. Even good products will not sell themselves. In the long run, hearing aid patients' needs and desires define the products. As they change, so must the product, because evolving patients demand evolving products. Just as product complexities make it easier to make products different, however, they also make it difficult for patients to understand the differences that do exist. And if the differences do not exist in patients' minds, they do not exist in the marketplace.

Pitfall

- Without a program to make oneself unique in patients' minds, technological superiority alone does not guarantee success or even a competitive position in the practice of hearing aid dispensing.

The ever-changing marketplace presents several challenges: (1) survival in the marketplace as the hearing health care system changes, (2) the perception of the product/service delivered as a commodity for which price is the only distinguishing feature, (3) the inability to define sufficient benefit with amplification to patients having a hearing impairment, and (4) the management of a successful business with the understanding that it involves more than being a skilled audiologist (see Chapter 6 in this volume for related information).

With projections suggesting hearing health care in the United States is a growth industry, competition and consumerism are shifting much of the emphasis of the marketplace away from the system as we know it today, resulting in alternative and nontraditional sites and purveyors. Added to this, and contributing to challenges, are changes in the state of the economy, changes in tax laws and government regulations, investigations by the U.S. Food and Drug Administration (FDA) into hearing aid dispensing practices and pricing, negative media publicity, perceptions on the part of consumers that the only real difference between dispensers is their name, and health care reform proposals that have affected and are expected to continue to affect the stability and growth of the hearing health care industry. A reality check of the significance of good hearing to patients complicates matters further. For example, those who provide services to people having hearing impairment, and for whom providing this care is a livelihood, are often adamant in their belief that hearing is very important. The unfortunate reality is that, to many people with hearing impairment, loss of hearing is not that big a problem. This discrepancy between audiologists' perception of the problem and consumers' reality mandates in large part the necessity for a chapter on marketing.

Controversial Point

- Those who provide services to persons having hearing impairment believe that hearing is very important. The unfortunate reality is that, to many people with hearing impairment, loss of hearing is not that big a problem.

Do these incursions and perceptions suggest that there are negatives only and no opportunities? On the contrary, opportunities exist. As a prime example, the aging of the U.S. population will contribute to the percentage of people having hearing impairment. The number of people age 65 and over accounted for 8.1% of the population in 1950; this number is expected to grow to 20.7% of the total population by 2050, according to the U.S. Census Bureau (2004). Additionally, new computer-based technologies, hearing and hearing aid test equipment, hearing aids, and office automation systems have the potential of contributing to diagnosis, productivity, quality assurance, hearing aid performance, and patient satisfaction. A significant hurdle continues to be the acceptance of and motivation for individuals to act relative to their loss of hearing.

How is the hearing health care professional to meet these challenges and take advantage of opportunities in the short and long run? There is no single answer to this question. However, a rational, market-based response can be made by preparing goals and strategies and then employing the basic precepts embodied in good business planning: know your market; know your market's needs; present appropriate products and services; price according to market conditions; and merchandise, advertise, and sell.

The purpose of this chapter is to explain marketing principles that can be used to bridge the transitions in

meeting the challenges identified and to help narrow the discrepancy between perception and reality in the marketplace. The contents relate more specifically to marketing than to sales principles, explain key marketing concepts, suggest methods to foster practical marketing skills, and provide step-by-step descriptions and analyses of the tools needed to design and implement a complete marketing plan.

◆ Hearing Aid Dispensing as a Business

Despite the "audiology as a profession" rhetoric, it is mandatory to recognize, first of all, that an audiologic practice is a business. Being a professional does not generate business, but business and its subsequent demand can and do create a profession. (A glossary of marketing terms is available in Appendix 5–1.)

Failure to understand and accept these realities can lead to failure, both professional and financial. In their article "The Hearing Aid Office as a Marketing Tool," Jelonek and Staab (1994) suggest that you ask the following practical questions: What do you anticipate in dollars or unit sales? How will you compete against similar competitors, much less with managed care, Internet sales, encroachment by distribution from outside the discipline, a growing number of competitors in a marketplace, and large retail operations? How will your office be different from other dispensing audiology practices in your marketing area? Will you be able to increase your net income 15% or so per year? More specifically, will you be able to survive another 5 years? Will you be financially successful, just comfortable, or out of business? What are the amounts of savings and investments your business must provide for you on the day you retire, and to do this comfortably? Appendix 5–2 can be used to assist you in obtaining an estimate to the last question, which may in turn drive business decisions to provide answers to the other questions. Realize that this is just an estimate and does not take into consideration individual circumstances. A Web search will provide numerous retirement calculations that will result in rather different estimates. If you are fairly young, it would be wise to make such calculations without considering income from Social Security. A more complete ballpark estimate of retirement needs can be obtained from the American Savings Education Council Internet site (http://www.choosetosave.org).

Special Consideration

- Hearing aid dispensing is, first of all, a business. Not understanding and recognizing this can lead to failure, both professional and financial.

With business as a focus, what business concerns are most frequently addressed by today's dispensing audiologists?

Over a 2-year period, during which 18 intensive marketing programs were offered to those dispensing hearing aids, the following list of issues (unranked) was cited most frequently as requiring attention by attendees (Staab and Jelonek, 1994b, 1995b):

- Building revenue
- Generating new patients—expanding markets served
- Generating referrals
- Competing with a referral source
- Competing with price discounters
- Meeting personal financial needs
- Working with health maintenance organizations (HMOs), preferred provider organizations (PPOs), and the like
- Marketing on a limited budget

There is nothing to suggest that these concerns have changed.

Hearing aid dispensing is considered a small business activity. Small businesses (fewer than 500 employees) constitute 99.9% of the businesses in the United States (24.7 million), provide 50.1% of the work force, 39% of all sales, generate 52% of the private sector product, and pay 45% of the total U.S. private payroll (Small Business Notes, 2007). They also have the greatest risk. Statistics indicate that failure correlates with the number of years in business; ~33% fail before the end of the 2nd year, and 44% survive at least 4 years. Data are inconsistent, depending on how *failure* is defined. The Education Foundation of the National Federation of Independent Business (NFIB, 2002) estimates that over the lifetime of a small business, 39% are profitable, 30% break even, 30% lose money, and 1% fall in the "unable to determine" category. Regardless, risk is associated with small business and emphasizes the necessity of a marketing plan to ensure that your practice not only has a start, but survives and grows. The adage "People don't plan to fail, they fail to plan" certainly holds true when it comes to small business success.

The amount of personal financial investment risk, and hence reward, varies with the management structure of the practice. Audiologists working for an ear, nose, and throat (ENT) practice, a public-funded agency, a hospital, or a clinic who have patients referred to them from internal sources for hearing aids and services have considerably less risk (this is not to minimize the risk of job or income loss, etc.). Understandably, the rewards are not as great either because of the reduced financial investment risk involved. Audiologists who put their finances and reputations on the line as free-standing diagnostic and dispensing audiology practices have much greater risk and investment and expect rightly to reap the financial benefits of that risk. Capital equipment purchases, leases, utilities, taxes, time, salaries, and the hearing aids themselves represent substantial financial and personal commitment. Daily concerns center on running the business, the patient base, and cash flow.

◆ Marketing versus Sales

Simply stated, marketing is understanding, and delivering or responding to, consumers' (or, in terms of audiology, patients') needs, whereas sales is providing for the individual company (or audiologist's) financial needs. This distinction is not always as clear in actual practice, but the differentiation must be understood to succeed in business. **Table 5–1**, although generic, suggests strongly the necessity of being aware of patients' needs.

◆ Essential Marketing Skills

The development of marketing skills should be as much a priority as hearing evaluation and hearing aid dispensing skills. The dispensing audiologist must understand the fundamental principles of marketing and have basic marketing skills. According to Stabb and Jelonek (1994a,b), essential skills include how to:

- Set reasonable, achievable marketing and financial goals
- Analyze competitors and patients, and develop competitive marketing offerings and programs that meet patients' needs and wants
- Identify or develop, then utilize, competitive advantages
- Develop a profitable line of products and services that meet patients' needs while ensuring your ability to learn, control, and knowledgeably apply technology
- Competitively and profitably price products and services
- Sell, that is, personally market, products, technologies, and services
- Design a market communications program for current patients, prospective patients, and referral sources
- Market without advertising
- Develop and successfully implement marketing programs

Table 5–1 Why Customers Are Lost

- 1% die
- 4% move
- 9% competitive inroads
- 15% product dissatisfaction
- 67% quit because of an attitude of indifference by someone who works in your office

Source: Epromotional Products and Gifts. (2007). Statistics show the following why customers leave. Retrieved May 15, 2007, from http://www.epromotionalproductsandgifts.com/loyalty.aspx

◆ Marketing Action Plan

Management by crisis is how much of the marketing in audiology practices occurs today. However, crisis management alone cannot and should not dictate the development of sales or promotional programs. Market planning should not be a one-time event initiated with the start-up of a business or the need for a bank loan. Communications and sales programs must reflect the unique demographic character and lifestyle of local populations. It must be recognized that mature populations are not a homogeneous group having uniform needs and purchasing behaviors. To that end, a marketing action plan is needed. Unfortunately, only 50% of audiologists report having a preplanned marketing program (Strom, 2001).

The successful professional must have a marketing action plan that can readily adapt to competitive events or changing patient behavior; it must be dynamic in that it is modified to meet changing market needs. A marketing action plan is a marketing and financial road map of how you are going to get from your current position to your desired destination. It describes how you will allocate scarce resources (time, finances, and personnel) to reach that destination. It outlines strategies and programs that will enable you to traverse a highly competitive landscape. It also should include a method to measure how well the plan's goals were met. **Figure 5–1** illustrates the basic flow of the overall marketing action plan.

As you continue planning, assess the viability of your internalized or written marketing action plan using the following nine-point questionnaire modified from Jelonek and Staab (1994):

1. *Do I have specific quantified goals for the coming year?* Are these goals in terms of sales units, billable revenue, number of patients, growth, and productivity?

2. *Who are my current and prospective patients?* What are their demographics and lifestyles? What will motivate them to purchase hearing aids?

3. *Who are my key competitors?* What marketing actions are they likely to take in the coming year? What are their relative marketing strengths and weaknesses?

4. *What is my competitive advantage?* How am I going to advance or succeed competitively?

5. *How am I going to use technology, products, services, and office equipment to achieve my marketing and financial goals?* Do I have marketing programs organized to take advantage of these features? Do I have procedures and protocols in place that will ensure product performance and patient satisfaction?

6. *Do my pricing and sales strategies reflect competitive actions and positions?* Have I changed these strategies from last year? Am I just copying the actions of my competitors? Do my strategies support the achievement of my goals?

7. *What is my market communications program?* How am I going to communicate with my current patients, prospective patients, and referral sources? What message am I going to give them?

8. *What resources do I have, and how will I allocate them to achieve my goals?* How will I use my money, time, and personnel?

9. *What are the potential barriers to achieving my goals?* Is it the economy, competitors, personal knowledge or skill, or finances? What can I do to eliminate or minimize these barriers?

Having a marketing action plan is essential to your professional survival and continued success. A plan does not have a magical starting date. It can begin January 1 or March 13. The date does not determine its success. The actual development of the plan can be self-directed, guided by outlines or texts, or accomplished via a group seminar. It should, however, be written, because the very act of writing goals, strategies, and tactics is a commitment to their completion.

Market Analysis

Where Is Your Business, and What Is Your Market Potential?

The hearing aid marketplace is an ever-changing entity, and you must be able to adjust your practice rapidly to accommodate the recognized changes. Markets are driven by the relationships and interactions of its players, with no members of the market isolated from the others. This means that what affects one segment of the market is likely to affect your practice as well. This requires an ongoing market analysis (a snapshot of the marketplace at a point in time), which is essential to find new ways to compete and grow an existing practice.

This analysis should provide you with specific answers about what the served market is, as well as about the entire market. Such a review of the general market that you function in and also of your own business should be performed routinely. This can be as sophisticated as you would like, taking as little as a few hours to several days, but should include monitoring of your market in terms of its conditions or trends, growth, stagnation, or decline. Market analysis is used to assist in planning of successful marketing strategies and programs, and to evaluate the performance of your general market plan.

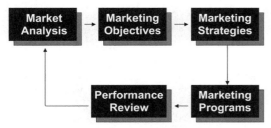

Figure 5–1 Action plan for the marketing process, indicating the flow of events.

Market Analysis (Situational Analysis)

The purpose of market analysis is to determine the status of your practice and where it is going. It is here that an assessment of the market is determined from the market structure (definition, size, and growth), market conditions (economic, social, environmental, and governmental), demographics (age and income), and competition. The worksheet given in Appendix 5–3 can be used to gather such information, but you can make this much more elaborate, if you choose to do so. These data are then used to focus on a segment of the total hearing aid market by offering products and/or services for this segment. It is unrealistic to believe that you will serve the entire market. A market analysis should be done at least annually, or more frequently if market conditions change. Think of market analysis as an annual checkup of the local market that assesses the market environment, the market profile, an analysis of the patient, and a competitive analysis.

Before initiation of a market analysis, the following information should be obtained, limiting the gathering of data to an area approximating 80% from where your patients are expected to come:

♦ *Geographical and population information*   This should consist of such information as zip codes, census data, psychographics, maps covering your market area (to plot competitors, referral sources, etc.), income, age demographics, geographical mix, home or business breakdowns by area, and any other information that allows you to analyze the population within your area.

♦ *Economic information*   This is often found in local newspapers, from the chamber of commerce, banks, local business publications if the area is sufficiently large, and the Internet.

♦ *Competitive information and/or referral sources*   Telephone directories, professional directories, sales representatives, the competition themselves, advertising/promotion, news stories, professional membership lists; state registration or licensing lists, local newspapers, and meetings/conventions are sources of this information.

♦ *Industry information*   Each year hearing aid trade publications provide information about state sales (trends, volume, sources of revenue, and expenditures), sources of competition, pricing, and so on.

♦ *Public and commercial resources*   Many of these resource data sources can be obtained from the public library, Internet, state and local chambers of commerce, government offices, and commercial sources.

Market Definition: Area and Scope of the Market   A simple way to identify your market may be to (1) limit it to the geographical area where your current patient base lives or works (general demographics are available from the public library or from the Internet) or (2) define it by the geographical area from which you are drawing large clusters of new patients (take this from your office visit statistics). When viewed in these ways, your market can be identified by a list of zip codes, cities, or counties (see part 1, Market Definition, Appendix 5–3).

Market Size   The market size is determined generally by summing the population statistics from your market definition (see part 2, Market Size, Appendix 5–3). The actual number of persons with hearing impairment can be calculated as 9.4% of the market size (**Fig. 5–2**). If based on a percentage of the population statistics, is it a percentage of the overall population in your marketing area or a percentage of your served market (**Fig. 5–2**).

An alternative method to market size estimation is to base it on the total number of hearing aids sold within the geographical served area. One method is to guesstimate the monthly unit new sales of hearing aids in competitors' offices based on the number of persons a given office employs (see part 2, Market Size, Appendix 5–3), or based on industry sales per average office (20 units median; Strom, 2004). Another method is to estimate competitors' office unit sales from your unit sales on a per person employed basis. Soliciting comments from manufacturers' representatives can also provide you with ballpark figures. Hearing aid sales by competitive offices could provide insight into the total population served. Realize, however, that ~74% of the sales are binaural, thus reducing the market penetration somewhat (Kochkin, 2005).

Is there an optimum market size at which your practice can exist and grow? There are no data that the author is aware of from the hearing aid industry to this effect. It has been estimated that the dispenser-to-population ratio in the United States is 1:25,972, and the dispenser-to-over 65 population is estimated at 1:3110. Jelonek (1992a) suggested that a population of ~30,000 is sufficient per dispenser, that less than 20,000 is very competitive, and that at 18,000, it is very difficult to survive. What is perhaps more critical are (1) the age and income of the population, (2) the incidence of hearing impairment in the population considered, and (3) the type of marketing program(s) provided, even when faced with a greater number of competitors than the market would seem to support. For example, when comparing cities with populations of 35,000, city A, with 48% of individuals age 65 and older, is likely to support more dispensing operations than city B, with 14% of individuals in that same age group. Keep in mind, also, that, although the hearing aid sales potential is anywhere from 40 to 80% of the hearing-impaired market, industry statistics indicate that the actual market penetration is only ~24% (Kochkin, 2005).

How many hearing aids sold in your market area should be sufficient for your practice? The answer lies in the determination of whether there are enough new units sold within that marketing area to sustain you and your competitors.

Market Growth   Just as important as the market size is the expected growth of the market in question. Is it growing, stable, or shrinking, and by what percent? What are the long-term growth prospects for your market? Is population growth city or county related? Is it due to low- or no-growth policies of local governments? Are you growing more or less than the market? If less, you are losing market share. If

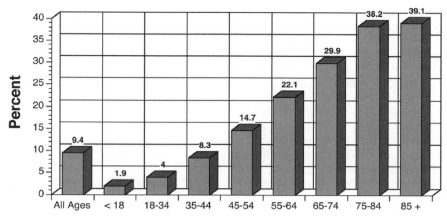

Figure 5-2 Best estimate of the prevalence of hearing impairment in the civilian, noninstitutionalized population of the United States. (Based on data from Adams, P., & Hardy, A. (1989). Current estimates from the National Health Interview Survey: United States (Vital and Health Statistics, Series 10, No. 173). Hyattsville, MD: National Center for Health Statistics; Gentile, A. (1975). Persons with impaired hearing, United States, 1971 (Vital and Health Statistics, Series 10, No. 101, DHEW Publication No. [HRA] 76–1528). Washington, DC: U.S. Government Printing Office; Glorig, A., & Nixon, J. (1960). Distribution of hearing loss in various populations. Annals of Otology, Rhinology and Laryngology, 69, 497–516; Goldstein, D. (1984). Hearing impairment, hearing aids, and audiology. ASHA, 27, 24–31, 34–35, 38; Hearing Industries Association. (1984). A market research study of the U.S. hearing-impaired population. Washington, DC: Author; Jatho, K. (1969). Population surveys and norms. International Audiology, 8, 231–239; Kochkin, S. (2005). MarkeTrak VII. Hearing Review, 12(7), 16–29; Moscicki, E. K., Elkins, E. F., Baum, H. M., & McNamara, P. M. (1985). Hearing loss in the elderly: An epidemiologic study of the Framingham Heart Study Cohort. Ear and Hearing, 6, 184–190; National Center for Health Statistics. (1980). Basic data on hearing levels of adults 25–74 years, United States, 1971–1975 (Vital and Health Statistics, Series 11, No. 215, DHEW Pub. No. [PHS] 80–1663). Hyattsville, MD: Author; National Center for Health Statistics. (1981). Prevalence of selected impairments, United States, 1977 (DHEW Pub. No. [PHS] 82–1562). Hyattsville, MD: Author; National Health Interview Survey. (1977). Hearing ability of persons by sociodemographic and health characteristics: United States (Vital and Health Statistics). Hyattsville, MD: National Center for Health Statistics; Ries, P. (1982). Hearing ability of persons by sociodemographic and health statistics (Vital and Health Statistics, Series 10, No. 140, DHHS Pub. No. [PHS] 82–1568). Washington, DC: U.S. Government Printing Office; Roberts, J. (1968). Hearing status in examination findings among adults, United States, 1960–1962 (Vital and Health Statistics, Series 11, No. 99, DHEW Publication No. 1000). Washington, DC: U.S. Government Printing Office; Staab, W. J. (2003). Hearing aids: A user's guide (3rd ed.). Phoenix, AZ: Wayne J. Staab Publisher; U.S. Census Bureau. (2004). U.S. interim projections by age, sex, race, and Hispanic origin. Retrieved March 18, 2004, from http://www.sba.gov/aboutsba/ sbastats.html; U.S. Department of Health and Human Services. (1988). Aging America: Trends and projections, 1987–88. Washington, DC: U.S. Government Printing Office; Wilder, C. (1975). Prevalence of selected impairments, U.S., 1971 (Vital and Health Statistics, Series 10, No. 99, DHEW Pub. No. [HRA] 75–1526). Washington, DC: U.S. Government Printing Office; and Williams, P. (1984). Hearing loss: Information for professionals in the aging network. Washington, DC: NICD/ASHA, Gallaudet College.)

more, you are gaining market share. There is no advantage in investing in a market that is shrinking in total population or total hearing aid sales volume (see part 3, Market Growth, Appendix 5–3). Some of the issues that influence population trends are the economic health of a community, taxes, the quality of life, rates of employment, business openings or closings, social conditions, crime, education, and pollution.

Market Conditions   What market conditions currently affect or are likely to affect your business within the next 3 to 5 years? Are these positive or negative influences? These may be somewhat difficult to quantify, but an attempt should be made to identify at least the economic, social, environmental, and governmental influences on your practice. If recognized, planning can be performed to minimize or take advantage of these as they occur. For example, plant closings often signal a reduction and distribution change in a population. The chamber of commerce in a community can provide information about employment opportunities and industries that draw certain groups of individuals. Data are also available on the Internet and from the public library

and often include incomes, demographics, growth, age comparisons, trends, and environmental conditions (see part 4, Market Conditions, Appendix 5–3).

Do market conditions have an impact on hearing aid sales? It is reasonable to expect they do, depending on the type and populations affected. For example, high employment might signal sales opportunities to populations who do not normally have large discretionary funds. Interest rates can have serious implications to retirees whose living standard is tied explicitly to savings. Higher interest rates, resulting in higher returns on certificates of deposit (CDs), money market funds, bonds, and so on, signal increased discretionary income and greater opportunities for hearing aid purchase. A bullish stock market and low national rates of inflation generally provide income increases not required for the necessities of life.

Industry trends and conditions can influence your market as well. New technologies supported in part by manufacturers can stimulate consumer interest and hearing aid sales purchases. Pricing policies, discount schedules, warranty plans, and return policies all affect the way dispensers operate their businesses (Jelonek, 1992b).

Consumer Analysis: Age and Income Demographics An analysis of age and income ordinarily includes both demographic and behavioral profiles. Demographic variables often list age, gender, income, occupation, race, marital status, housing, education, family size, and so on. Behavioral profiles include psychographics, purchase tendencies, risk concerns, interests, and driving forces.

Consumer analysis is an attempt to more specifically target your market. It is from much of these data that actual marketing programs will be developed. Collectively, consumer analysis data can be used to determine the age, retirement populations, disposable income, activity level, how geographically concentrated the market is, and potential purchasing

levels of the population in question. Purchasing decisions are influenced heavily, especially by seniors, on the basis of interest rates, CDs, and other investment incomes. They are more likely to purchase when investment income is high.

In the action plan example (part 5, Age and Income Demographics, Appendix 5–3), comparisons of age and income are made to national and state statistics, but they could be made to city, state, or county data, whichever are available or of interest. The following tables provide summary data for simple comparisons.

Tables 5–2 and **5–3** provide examples of the type of age and income data that are useful when comparing markets (Staab and Jelonek, 1995b). Both give information relative

Table 5–2 Use of Age Demographics in Market Analysis

	Population Median Age (y)	Population Age Distribution (%)				Population Age Distribution (n)			
	2002–2004	45–54	55–64	65–74	75+	45–54	55–64	65–74	75+
USA	36.2	14.4	10.1	6.4	5.6	41,219,069	16,227,169	30,782,295	16,041,551
California	34.2	13.5	9.0	5.4	5.2	4,859,899	3,225,197	1,950,085	1,872,872
Illinois	35.4	14.0	9.5	6.0	6.0	1,781,548	1,209,585	760,880	759,749
Indiana	35.7	14.2	9.9	6.2	6.2	885,589	613,524	387,698	384,312
New York	37.3	14.3	10.3	6.4	11.3	2,740,525	1,970,166	1,226,182	2,179,385
ZIP CODE									
NEW YORK	**37.3**								
10021 New York	39.6	14.0	12.1	8.3	7.6	14,482	12,367	8,530	8,001
10022 New York	45.6	15.2	14.9	11.4	9.2	4,601	4,566	3,522	2,835
10028 New York	38.2	14.8	11.3	7.2	6.1	6,674	5,262	3,303	2,610
INDIANA	**35.7**								
46342 Hobart	36.8	13.5	9.0	7.2	7.0	3,992	2,655	2,116	2,018
46368 Portage	35.6	14.5	8.8	6.2	5.4	5,131	3,167	1,573	2,051
46410 Gary	36.6	13.6	8.4	6.8	7.9	4,471	2,758	2,237	2,625
ILLINOIS	**35.4**								
60120 Elgin	29.7	11.3	5.9	3.3	3.2	5,497	2,910	1,615	1,556
60123 Elgin	33.6	13.4	7.7	5.1	5.3	7,557	4,303	2,863	2,960
60178 Sycamore	35.8	14.3	8.4	5.7	5.4	2,343	1,421	939	890
CALIFORNIA	**34.2**								
92025 Escondido	30.3	11.2	6.4	4.2	5.4	5,351	3,043	1,972	2,465
92056 Oceanside	36.6	11.8	7.1	8.4	9.2	6,392	3,793	4,391	4,807
92128 San Diego	41.2	13.1	8.4	9.2	13.0	5,619	3,665	4,080	5,828
95825 Sacramento	32.4	11.2	7.2	5.7	8.4	3,438	2,171	1,730	2,516
95608 Carmichael	40.7	15.3	9.9	8.5	9.3	8,892	5,663	4,941	5,719
95661 Roseville	38.4	16.0	8.7	5.8	8.9	4,308	2,188	1,445	2,234
94588 Pleasanton	35.6	15.9	8.6	3.7	2.0	4,571	2,387	1,012	549
94550 Livermore	36.4	14.8	9.5	5.1	4.1	10,740	6,292	3,364	2,468
94583 San Ramon	36.8	17.6	9.0	3.3	2.8	7,667	3,968	1,498	1,215
96002 Redding	35.8	12.6	9.4	7.4	7.5	3,836	2,857	2,280	2,264
96003 Redding	38.4	14.3	9.9	7.9	8.1	5,866	4,074	3,203	3,263
96007 Anderson	38.0	13.8	10.5	7.9	7.2	2,962	2,282	1,724	1,532
96067 Mt. Shasta	44.1	19.1	12.2	8.8	8.2	1,393	893	648	597
96080 Red Bluff	38.5	13.2	10.1	8.6	8.5	3,524	2,639	2,239	2,281
96097 Yreka	41.9	14.8	10.9	9.2	10.2	1,444	1,034	879	972

Data from U.S. Census Bureau. (2004). 2004 American community survey, American factfinder. Washington DC: U.S. Government Printing Office.

Table 5–3 Use of Income Demographics in Market Analysis

	HOUSEHOLD INCOME			HOUSEHOLD INCOME DISTRIBUTION - MEDIAN					
Zip Code	Median 2000–2004	Nat'l Rank 2004	Median 2000	Less Than $15,000	$15,000–$24,999	$25,000–$49,999	$50,000–$99,999	$100,000–$149,999	$150,000+
USA	$44,684		$42,257	15.2	12.3	27.5	30.1	9.4	5.6
California	$51,185	12	$47,493	14.0	11.5	26.6	30.6	13.7	6.9
Illinois	$48,953	17	$46,590	13.8	11.3	28.1	32.3	9.0	5.4
Indiana	$42,195	29	$41,567	13.8	13.0	31.0	31.7	7.4	3.2
New York	$47,349	22	$43,393	17.9	11.7	26.2	29.0	9.1	6.2
Zip Code	Adjusted Gross Income	Percentile							
New York	**$47,349**								
10021 New York	$56,263	99%	$75,472	8.5	5.5	16.9	19.5	13.3	26.5
10022 New York	$61,320	100%	$80,406	8.0	5.1	17.0	29.0	12.9	28.0
10028 New York	$57,849	99%	$77,565	7.6	5.5	18.2	28.7	13.8	26.1
Indiana	**$42,195**								
46342 Hobart	$36,263	65%	$46,212	11.0	11.2	32.6	37.3	6.0	1.8
46368 Portage	$41,064	69%	$48,021	12.0	11.7	28.4	39.6	6.2	2.1
46410 Gary	$41,123	68%	$48,191	9.8	10.1	32.2	39.6	6.5	2.0
Illinois	**$48,953**								
60120 Elgin	$44,723	71%	$52,067	8.2	8.7	30.4	39.6	9.8	3.3
60123 Elgin	$46,890	84%	$57,928	8.3	8.1	25.2	41.0	12.9	4.6
60178 Sycamore	$45,725	81%	$54,867	7.3	9.4	28.0	42.4	9.1	3.7
California	**$51,185**								
92025 Escondido	$32,411	78%	$38,828	14.4	15.7	31.2	26.7	7.8	4.2
92056 Oceanside	$34,022	80%	$33,676	8.6	9.1	28.2	39.9	10.1	4.2
92128 San Diego	$50,551	93%	$66,676	6.1	8.1	20.9	38.8	11.2	8.9
95825 Sacramento	$27,852	64%	$35,228	18.7	14.8	34.0	24.1	5.7	2.6
95608 Carmichael	$35,786	86%	$45,693	12.9	12.0	28.9	30.2	10.2	5.8
95661 Roseville	$47,454	89%	$58,606	9.4	7.7	25.0	36.8	13.6	7.6
94588 Pleasanton	$60,648	98%	$92,644	2.6	3.4	11.2	38.0	24.6	20.2
94550 Livermore	$51,984	93%	$75,026	5.4	5.0	17.9	41.3	19.0	11.4
94583 San Ramon	$62,821	96%	$95,588	3.0	2.7	12.6	25.6	26.6	21.9
96002 Redding	$25,927	56%	$34,507	18.5	17.1	33.5	25.0	4.1	1.9
96003 Redding	$24,550	61%	$35,917	18.8	16.8	31.0	26.1	5.3	2.2
96007 Anderson	$21,002	29%	$29,564	24.7	17.7	34.2	20.2	2.3	1.0
96067 Mt. Shasta	$23,407	65%	$32,933	22.8	8.9	29.2	32.5	12.2	3.3
96080 Red Bluff	$24,956	53%	$32,095	19.7	18.3	32.6	23.4	3.6	2.3
96097 Yreka	$19,760	55%	$29,392	24.7	19.1	31.2	18.9	3.2	2.7

Data from U.S. Census Bureau. (2004). 2004 American community survey; american factfinder. Washington, DC: U.S. Government Printing Office; and U.S. Census Bureau. (1999). Median household income in 1999. Retrieved May 9, 2007; from www.census.gov

to the United States and for select zip codes in four sample states: California, Illinois, Indiana, and New York. **Table 5–2** offers age statistics, and **Table 5–3** provides household income statistics. This kind of information is available from various sources. (These specific data can be obtained from www.freedomographics.com and from www.factfinder. census.gov.)

Keep in mind when using such statistics to direct marketing efforts toward the elderly population that older individuals either are well aware of loss of hearing function sufficient to create problems in understanding the speech of others or may be unaware of information-bearing signals in their acoustic environment. Regardless, marketing practices that stress the loss of hearing as a function of aging serve only to remind individuals of the inevitable changes in life that reduce one's participation in it. The elderly seem not to be as intimidated by the loss of sensory function as they are by the changes in interpersonal relations and the ability to actively participate in social activities—that should be the message of your marketing.

Information of Use when Comparing Markets

Market Served   When estimating the size of your market from population statistics, understand that there is an overall hearing-impaired market and a served market. Seldom, if ever, are they the same. What is the difference? The hearing-impaired market consists of the total number (percentage based on estimates) of individuals in the population considered to have a measurable hearing loss, regardless of how that marketing area is defined. The served market is a realistic expectation of those individuals within your marketing area that are accessible to hearing aid sales from your office.

Many audiologists use misguided information about their served market, using instead the entire population of hearing impaired within their area. However, allowances must be made for those populations not being served by your office and may exclude numbers associated with veterans; the deaf; the institutionalized; children; HMOs; age, income, and demographic populations within your area; companies that have insurance plans in which you or your patients do not participate; those having mild hearing impairments who do not believe that their hearing is severe enough to require hearing aids; and other exclusionary market segments. In reality, elimination of these untapped segments of the population could reduce the served market to much less than the 9.4% noninstitutionalized, national average. On the other hand, concentration of efforts within retirement communities could lead to a much higher percentage.

Whatever the served market, it should reflect the exceptions identified in the previous paragraph. This will require estimates on your part because every marketing area is expected to be different from all others. For example, if the population in your area is 35,000, based on the 9.4% estimate, you would expect 3290 hearing-impaired people in that area. However, when adjustments are made for age, type of employment, and so on, the number could be significantly different.

The Hearing-Impaired Population by Age, Degree of Loss, and Life Expectancy   The total population in the United States as of December 2005 was 297,800,900 (U.S. Census Bureau, 2005).

The total, civilian, noninstitutionalized hearing-impaired population is estimated at 9.4%, and of the total U.S. population at 11.2%. The incidence of hearing loss ranges from 4.4 to 27.8% and reflects variations in defining hearing loss, measurement procedures, intended use of the data, and so on. The percentage used in this chapter to describe the total hearing-impaired population is 9.4% because it appears to be based on the best and most extensive data analysis **(Fig. 5–2)**. This calculation provides the basis of the hearing-impaired totals shown in **Fig. 5–3**. Mild hearing

losses account for 47.3% (12.4 million) of the hearing-impaired total, moderate losses at 29.0% (7.6 million), severe losses at 16.6% (4.4 million), and the profound deaf category at 7.1% (1.9 million). World population percentages are expected to be similar; however, most other countries report much lower percentages, reflecting, perhaps, the lack of methods to adequately evaluate hearing. Data for **Figs. 5–2, 5–3**, and **Table 5–4** are derived from Adams and Hardy (1989), Gentile (1975), Glorig and Nixon (1960), Goldstein (1984), Hearing Industries Association (1984), Jatho (1969), Moscicki et al (1985), National Center for Health Statistics (1980, 1981), National Health Interview Survey (1977), Ries (1982), Roberts (1968), U.S. Census Bureau (2004), U.S. Department of Health and Human Services (1988), Wilder (1975), and Williams (1984).

Population projections show that a continuing and increasing incidence exists, especially in the over-65 category for hearing impairment **(Fig. 5–4)**. Life expectancy is projected to change from 75.8 years in 1995 (CDC, 2001) to 82.6 years in 2050 (U.S. Census Bureau, 2001). The percentage of individuals over 65 years of age is expected to grow from ~13% today to a little over 20% in 2050 ("Study: 2020 Begins Age of the Elderly," 1996). Individuals over age 85 comprised ~3 million in 1995; that number is expected to increase to ~20.8 million in 2050 (U.S. Census Bureau, 2004).

Trends in U.S. population figures are reflected in **Fig. 5–4**, as well as **Table 5–4**, which shows a population older than 65 increasing from 11.3% in 1980 to 20.6% in 2050. This reflects an increase in life expectancy from ~47.3 years in 1900 (U.S. Life Expectancy, 2007) to ~77.9 years today (National Center for Health Statistics, 2007), with a continued increase anticipated. This age group is of particular importance to audiology practices because it reflects the segment of the population that is most likely to seek hearing services, especially hearing aids. It is estimated that currently ~65% of all hearing aids are sold to individuals 65 years of age and older (Kochkin, 2005).

Some interesting statistics emerge from the U.S. Census Bureau in a study financed by the National Institute on Aging on the status of the elderly, considered to be those 65 years of age and older ("Study: 2020 Begins Age of the Elderly," 1996):

- The 65 and older population will grow from 1 in 8 today to 1 in 6 by 2020 and 1 in 5 by 2050.

- By 2020, the nation's elderly population will total 53.3 million—a 62% increase over the current elderly population of 33 million.

- Currently, Florida has the largest proportion of elderly, with 2.5 million, or 18.6% of the total population. It is expected that by 2020, nine other states will have a similar profile.

- In eight states, the number of people age 65 and over will more than double by 2020.

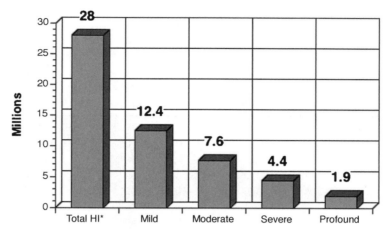

Figure 5–3 Best estimate of the prevalence of hearing impairment in the civilian, noninstitutionalized population in the United States by degree of loss. *9.4% of the civilian, non-institutionalized population. HI, hearing impaired. (Based on data from Adams, P., & Hardy, A. (1989). Current estimates from the National Health Interview Survey: United States (Vital and Health Statistics, Series 10, No. 173). Hyattsville, MD: National Center for Health Statistics; Gentile, A. (1975). Persons with impaired hearing, United States, 1971 (Vital and Health Statistics, Series 10, No. 101, DHEW Publication No. [HRA] 76–1528). Washington, DC: U.S. Government Printing Office; Glorig, A., & Nixon, J. (1960). Distribution of hearing loss in various populations. Annals of Otology, Rhinology and Laryngology, 69, 497–516; Goldstein, D. (1984). Hearing impairment, hearing aids, and audiology. ASHA, 27, 24–31, 34–35, 38; Hearing Industries Association. (1984). A market research study of the U.S. hearing-impaired population. Washington, DC: Author; Jatho, K. (1969). Population surveys and norms. International Audiology, 8, 231–239; Moscicki, E. K., Elkins, E. F., Baum, H. M., & McNamara, P. M. (1985). Hearing loss in the elderly: An epidemiologic study of the Framingham Heart Study Cohort. Ear and Hearing, 6, 184–190; National Center for Health Statistics. (1980). Basic data on hearing levels of adults 25–74 years, United States, 1971–1975 (Vital and Health Statistics, Series 11, No. 215, DHEW Pub. No. [PHS] 80–1663). Hyattsville, MD: Author; National Center for Health Statistics. (1981). Prevalence of selected impairments, United States, 1977 (DHEW Pub. No. [PHS] 82–1562). Hyattsville, MD: Author; National Health Interview Survey. (1977). Hearing ability of persons by sociodemographic and health characteristics: United States (Vital and Health Statistics). Hyattsville, MD: National Center for Health Statistics; Ries, P. (1982). Hearing ability of persons by sociodemographic and health statistics (Vital and Health Statistics, Series 10, No. 140, DHHS Pub. No. [PHS] 82–1568). Washington, DC: U.S. Government Printing Office; Roberts, J. (1968). Hearing status in examination findings among adults, United States, 1960–1962 (Vital and Health Statistics, Series 11, No. 99, DHEW Publication No. 1000). Washington, DC: U.S. Government Printing Office; Staab, W. J. (2003). Hearing aids: A user's guide (3rd ed). Phoenix, AZ: Wayne J. Staab Publisher; U.S. Census Bureau. (2004). U.S. interim projections by age, sex, race, and Hispanic origin. Retrieved March 18, 2004, from http://www.sba.gov/ aboutsba/sbastats.html; U.S. Department of Health and Human Services. (1988). Aging America: Trends and projections, 1987–88. Washington, DC: U.S. Government Printing Office; Wilder, C. (1975). Prevalence of selected impairments, U.S., 1971 (Vital and Health Statistics, Series 10, No. 99, DHEW Pub. No. [HRA] 75–1526). Washington, DC: U.S. Government Printing Office; Williams, P. (1984). Hearing loss: Information for professionals in the aging network. Washington, DC: NICD/ASHA, Gallaudet College.)

♦ The elderly population increased 11-fold from 1900 to 1994. The under-65 population increased just 3-fold.

♦ Of 80 million elderly projected for 2050, 8.4 million will be black, 6.7 million will be of races other than white or black, and 12.5 million will be Hispanic.

♦ The percentage of elderly living in poverty declined from 24.6% in 1970 to 12.9% in 1992.

♦ The ratio of elderly people to working-age people (ages 20–64) will nearly double between 1990 and 2050.

♦ In 2020, 25% of Floridians will be elderly. Arizona will have the largest percentage of seniors after Florida: 19.6%.

♦ The number of elderly will at least double in eight states between 1993 and 2020. The fastest growth will be in Nevada, where the over-65 group will surge 116%.

Other age group statistics and information that are of interest:

♦ The number of centenarians (those 100 years and older) more than doubled since 1980 to nearly 50,000. Four in five were women.

♦ Five states with the highest proportions of people age 85 and older in 1993 were in the Midwest: Iowa, North Dakota, South Dakota, Nebraska, and Kansas.

♦ From now until 2014, someone will turn 50 every 7.5 seconds.

♦ The old of 2020 will be healthier than their parents of 1920.

♦ Seniors 85 and older are the fastest-growing age group. Their numbers are expected to more than double, to 7 million in 2020.

Table 5–4 General and Hearing-Impaired Populations, 1980–2050

		DEMOGRAPHICS - 70 YEARS								
		General Population						**Hearing-Impaired Population**		
Year	**Total Population (thousands)**	**18–24**	**25–34**	**35–44**	**45–64**	**65+**	**% 65+**	**%***	**Total (thousands)**	**Total 65+** (thousands)**
1980	227,704	30,347	37,593	25,881	44,493	25,714	11.3	8.1	18,444	11,804
1985	238,631	28,739	41,788	32,004	44,652	28,608	12.0	8.6	20,522	13,134
1990	249,657	25,974	43,529	37,847	46,453	31,697	12.7	9.1	22,719	14,540
2000	282,125	24,601	36,415	43,743	62,440	34,921	12.4	10.1	27,063	17,320
2030	365,584	26,226	37,158	40,168	82,280	71,400	19.6	11.8	35,967	23,019
2050	419,854	25,296	37,237	38,222	73,748	86,600	20.6	13.0	40,399	25,855

* This % takes into consideration that the total percentage of the population with hearing impairment will increase as the population ages.
** This is based on 64.0% of those over 65 having a hearing impairment.
Source: U.S. Census Bureau (2005). Population statistics: Projections of the U.S. by age, sex, and race: 1983–2080 (Series P-25, No. 952). Hearing-impaired population data derived from Adams, P., & Hardy, A. (1989). Current estimates from the National Health Interview Survey: United States (Vital and Health Statistics, Series 10, No. 173). Hyattsville, MD: National Center for Health Statistics; Gentile, A. (1975). Persons with impaired hearing, United States, 1971 (Vital and Health Statistics, Series 10, No. 101, DHEW Publication No. [HRA] 76–1528). Washington, DC: U.S. Government Printing Office; Glorig, A., & Nixon, J. (1960). Distribution of hearing loss in various populations. Annals of Otology, Rhinology and Laryngology, 69, 497–516; Goldstein, D. (1984). Hearing impairment, hearing aids, and audiology. ASHA, 27, 24–31, 34–35, 38; Hearing Industries Association. (1984). A market research study of the U.S. hearing-impaired population. Washington, DC: Author; Jatho, K. (1969). Population surveys and norms. International Audiology, 8, 231–239; Moscicki, E. K., Elkins, E. F., Baum, H. M., & McNamara, P. M. (1985). Hearing loss in the elderly: An epidemiologic study of the Framingham Heart Study Cohort. Ear and Hearing, 6, 184–190; National Center for Health Statistics. (1980). Basic data on hearing levels of adults 25–74 years, United States, 1971–1975 (Vital and Health Statistics, Series 11, No. 215, DHEW Pub. No. [PHS] 80–1663). Hyattsville, MD: Author; National Center for Health Statistics. (1981). Prevalence of selected impairments, United States, 1977 (DHEW Pub. No. [PHS] 82–1562). Hyattsville, MD: Author; National Health Interview Survey. (1977). Hearing ability of persons by sociodemographic and health characteristics: United States (Vital and Health Statistics). Hyattsville, MD: National Center for Health Statistics; Ries, P. (1982). Hearing ability of persons by sociodemographic and health statistics (Vital and Health Statistics, Series 10, No. 140, DHHS Pub. No. [PHS] 82–1568). Washington, DC: U.S. Government Printing Office; Roberts, J. (1968). Hearing status in examination findings among adults, United States, 1960–1962 (Vital and Health Statistics, Series 11, No. 99, DHEW Publication No. 1000). Washington, DC: U.S. Government Printing Office; Staab, W. J. (2003). Hearing aids: A user's guide (3rd ed). Phoenix, AZ: Wayne J. Staab Publisher; U.S. Census Bureau. (2004). U.S. interim projections by age, sex, race, and Hispanic origin. Retrieved March 18, 2004, from http://www.sba.gov/aboutsba/sbastats. html; U.S. Department of Health and Human Services. (1988). Aging America: Trends and projections, 1987–88. Washington, DC: U.S. Government Printing Office; Wilder, C. (1975). Prevalence of selected impairments, U.S., 1971 (Vital and Health Statistics, Series 10, No. 99, DHEW Pub. No. [HRA] 75–1526). Washington, DC: U.S. Government Printing Office; Williams, P. (1984). Hearing loss: Information for professionals in the aging network. Washington, DC: NICD/ASHA, Gallaudet College.)

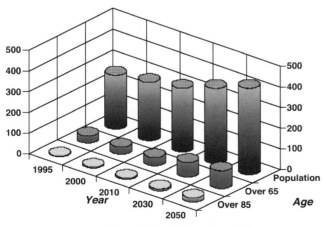

	1995	2000	2010	2030	2050
Total Population	261	282	309	364	420
Over 65	33.9	35	40.2	71.4	86.6
Over 85	3	4.2	6.1	9.6	20.8

All numbers are in millions

Figure 5–4 Projected total population in millions (1995–2050), with the over age 65 and over age 85 groups identified. (Data from U.S. Census Bureau. (2004). Current population reports. Population projections of the United States by age, sex, race, and hispanic origin: 1995 to 2050 (series p25–113). Washington, DC: U.S. Government Printing Office.)

Lifestyle Demographics Lifestyle demographics provide information about the types of goods and services that are important to people, and which help drive their activities and purchases. **Table 5–5** is a sampling of issues that were investigated for the cities and zip codes identified, and listed as a percentage of households that participate in that particular activity (Staab and Jelonek, 1995b). These can be compared with each other and also to the average in the United States. Other areas of interest that were represented in this comparison (but not shown) are real estate purchases; investments in such things as stocks and bonds, wine, electronics, home video games, and personal computers; cable TV use; interest in photography, crafts, crossword puzzles, coin and stamp collecting, gardening, and other leisure activities; participation in sports, including bicycling, boating, bowling, golf, physical fitness, jogging, snow skiing, tennis, walking, and camping; ownership of motorcycles and recreational vehicles; membership in wildlife and environmental organizations; church attendance; dieting; interest in current affairs and politics; grandchildren; home workshops; household pets; and membership in veterans' organizations.

The identification of populations that have higher than normal or lower than normal interests in certain areas provides significant information on how to market to that audience and with what kind of message. For example, under Dining Out, the information for zip code 10010 suggests a population that may be more affluent (35.70% participating) as opposed to zip code 15636 (13.90% participating). It also suggests that marketing hearing instruments that allow for speech understanding in noise might be better received by those who dine out often.

Lifestyle demographic information can tell you much about the population in your served market, and this should be taken into consideration when developing your marketing action plans. As an example, targeting advertising that features grandchildren to a group that does not rate grandparenting high is not a good use of marketing efforts and expenditures. This group might be more responsive to materials that illustrate travel destinations, for instance. Because of lifestyle interest differences, you may not be able to use a manufacturer's mass-produced advertising and promotional literature. Demographic differences can certainly explain why the same piece of literature pulls better in some places than in others. (The data in this discussion were obtained from services purchased from ESRI Business Information Solutions, www.esribis.com. ESRI is one of several companies that provide information on updated and projection demographics and consumer data and trends, including lifestyle demographics.)

Market Analysis (Competition)

Your business does not function in a vacuum. You have competition, and that competition is able to influence the success of your practice. It is, therefore, important to not only analyze the market potential of your own business but also that of the competition. This is key to the identification of market opportunities and the development of marketing strategies and promotions.

Profile and Evaluate the Distribution Structure of the Local Market Competition is anyone who, in the eyes of consumers, provides substitute products and/or services to yours, who promotes in your market, or who shares referral sources. **Table 5–6** provides a checklist of competitive analysis variables. If the competition is superior, their products and services will be chosen over yours. If they are inferior, they are vulnerable and represent a marketing opportunity for you.

Analyze the competition from the perspective of your patients. Who are your competitors? Why have patients chosen their services? Analyze their strengths and weaknesses (personally, educationally, and professionally). What would you say they do best? What do your patients and referral sources say about them? What is their facility, market share, growth rate and potential, equipment, accessibility, ambiance, length of time in business, image, and marketing message? How many offices and service centers do they have? What kinds of staff (type and number)? For what are they known? This analysis should be performed to determine if your competition has a marketing advantage that will make it difficult for your plans to succeed. This information can be obtained by reviewing telephone directories, reading competitive advertising, driving by the facility, or asking potential patients what they think about a given practice. Businesses that have a competitive advantage are rewarded in that they have performance that consistently is better than others, have continuous referrals, enjoy generous walk-in business, have a high incidence of word-of-mouth referrals, have a market share that is stable or growing, show close rates on advertising and promotion leads, and have high name recognition among hearing aid users and referral sources.

Competition can be analyzed from either a defensive or an offensive position. If defensive, attempt to determine if the competition seems to be satisfied with their current position. If they are, this can prove advantageous to you. If they present an offensive position (likely to move or shift what they are doing), what will these shifts be, and how dangerous are they to your practice? If analyzed from an offensive position, look to where the competition is vulnerable. What might you do to cause them to respond vigorously to your program(s), and how might you expect them to respond?

After you have finished analyzing your competition, analyze your practice in the same way. Determine if you have a competitive advantage, and if not, how you will motivate people to frequent your practice (objectives, strategies and tactics). It is important that you identify and develop your competitive advantage. Without this, a dispensing operation will not achieve and sustain superior market performance.

When do you have a competitive advantage? According to Jelonek (1992b), this occurs when you have a product or service that is

♦ *Unique* The product or service is not available from others.

♦ *Has value* Patients believe that they are receiving an exceptional value or deal. This value might be evidenced by the image of your practice, by your specialization, by the superiority of the product itself, by differentiation, or through exclusivity.

Table 5-5 Lifestyle Demographic Sample Data

City	Zip Code	1990 Population	CUL Good Life Cultural/Arts Events % Households Participating	CAR Good Life Career-Oriented Activities % Households Participating	FLY Good Life Frequent Flyer % Households Participating	FAS Good Life Fashion Clothing % Households Participating	ART Good Life Fine Arts/ Antiques % Households Participating	FOR Good Life Foreign Travel % Households Participating	GOU Good Life Dining Out % Households Participating	HFD Good Life Hshld Furn Decorating % Households Participating	MON Good Life Money Making Opportunities % Households Participating
UNITED STATES			15.10%	11.90%	11.50%	12.70%	10.30%	13.10%	20.20%	19.10%	9.20%
STRATFORD	06497	49,495	16.70%	11.70%	17.30%	14.40%	9.70%	16.90%	24.60%	19.90%	9.40%
BRIDGEPORT	06606	41,861	14.60%	12.00%	11.50%	19.90%	8.40%	17.10%	25.30%	19.60%	11.00%
TRUMBULL	06611	32,236	18.00%	12.90%	27.40%	15.50%	11.50%	21.10%	25.90%	21.80%	9.00%
DARIEN	06820	13,449	24.70%	13.10%	40.20%	16.10%	19.30%	34.50%	35.30%	25.90%	8.20%
NORWALK	06850	14,019	19.20%	16.10%	28.00%	18.20%	12.40%	23.40%	31.10%	19.90%	10.20%
WESTPORT	06880	21,737	32.00%	18.30%	45.20%	17.20%	21.20%	37.50%	35.20%	25.10%	10.20%
HACKENSACK	07601	36,932	19.40%	15.80%	22.30%	21.30%	11.20%	24.50%	27.80%	19.10%	12.00%
BOGOTA	07603	7,824	13.00%	15.10%	11.70%	12.60%	10.80%	17.50%	24.40%	17.50%	10.70%
HASBROUCK HTS	07604	11,489	12.40%	13.70%	17.30%	17.60%	8.40%	16.40%	25.60%	24.50%	7.60%
BERGENFIELD	07621	24,580	14.00%	8.70%	18.40%	15.50%	8.40%	20.10%	24.40%	18.10%	5.80%
PARAMUS	07652	25,059	17.00%	13.20%	24.40%	18.30%	10.00%	25.70%	26.60%	19.00%	12.90%
TEANECK	07666	37,815	27.60%	19.00%	24.80%	16.50%	13.00%	28.50%	25.40%	19.20%	10.50%
DENVILLE	07834	14,554	18.40%	15.80%	28.20%	13.90%	12.80%	21.60%	28.30%	24.70%	11.60%
MORRISTOWN	07960	38,515	27.10%	18.70%	38.00%	17.10%	16.50%	30.50%	29.80%	21.10%	8.90%
NEW YORK	10003	49,308	47.20%	25.10%	34.60%	24.10%	26.40%	43.90%	34.40%	18.30%	7.20%
NEW YORK	10010	24,606	43.00%	23.90%	33.80%	24.80%	21.70%	44.70%	35.70%	20.50%	9.00%
NEW YORK	10016	45,192	41.00%	25.90%	36.00%	30.30%	22.80%	44.30%	33.90%	21.20%	9.70%
NEW YORK	10021	93,571	42.60%	22.60%	40.30%	27.80%	25.90%	47.10%	34.60%	21.40%	9.30%
NEW YORK	10028	41,373	25.40%	21.20%	26.50%	21.60%	17.70%	56.00%	27.50%	23.80%	10.90%
NEW YORK	10128	48,417	41.80%	24.30%	40.30%	25.20%	22.30%	43.90%	34.50%	21.00%	8.40%
BRONX	10461	37,530	13.50%	12.10%	10.30%	19.00%	8.00%	18.50%	26.20%	19.00%	10.80%
BRONX	10465	27,638	11.00%	9.50%	10.70%	18.70%	7.20%	16.90%	26.80%	22.60%	11.60%
BRONX	10467	64,302	16.10%	13.90%	8.90%	21.50%	7.80%	19.60%	22.10%	19.20%	13.70%
MIDDLETOWN	10940	37,232	14.50%	13.00%	10.20%	15.20%	9.00%	14.00%	22.60%	18.20%	11.30%
BROOKLYN	11203	59,995	20.80%	17.30%	10.00%	25.50%	7.10%	28.60%	22.90%	20.10%	16.10%
BROOKLYN	11204	50,923	11.40%	9.90%	9.60%	20.70%	8.20%	19.80%	26.20%	17.00%	12.50%
BROOKLYN	11214	58,783	12.60%	10.40%	9.90%	19.60%	8.70%	19.00%	28.60%	18.30%	11.50%
BROOKLYN	11223	53,105	12.20%	9.10%	10.60%	21.60%	8.50%	20.00%	25.70%	20.00%	11.30%
BROOKLYN	11225	48,321	22.10%	15.60%	10.90%	27.60%	9.00%	28.30%	25.40%	20.10%	14.50%
BROOKLYN	11226	76,678	20.90%	17.50%	8.00%	28.40%	8.80%	26.90%	25.50%	20.30%	18.90%
NEWBURGH	12550	34,816	13.20%	12.50%	11.10%	14.80%	9.00%	14.60%	24.80%	18.50%	10.90%
NEWBURGH	12553		13.80%	13.30%	14.20%	15.60%	9.10%	15.40%	23.60%	24.50%	9.80%
GREENSBURG	15601	43,164	14.20%	9.80%	11.50%	44.10%	8.90%	8.00%	18.10%	20.90%	8.90%
HARRISON CITY	15636	3,313	7.70%	7.50%	9.70%	9.60%	7.60%	5.70%	13.90%	26.80%	10.80%
MURRYSVILLE	15668	8,860	19.70%	16.00%	29.60%	12.30%	11.10%	16.80%	19.50%	22.70%	7.50%
COATESVILLE	19320	29,226	10.70%	10.00%	9.50%	15.40%	10.70%	10.80%	21.60%	19.30%	7.70%
DOWNINGTOWN	19335	24,438	13.70%	14.30%	24.00%	13.30%	11.10%	15.40%	24.50%	23.30%	8.40%

Note: The percentages indicate the population within the zip codes identified that are likely to engage in the activity listed. This is a sampling only of the categories of lifestyle interests that can be evaluated and which are useful in directing marketing efforts.
Source: Staab, W. J., & Jelonek, S. (1995b). Building professional marketing skills. Presented at Towards 2000: Hearing Aid Marketing Workshop, Phoenix, AZ, with permission.

Table 5–6 Variables to Consider when Conducting a Competitive Analysis

Defensive Position
- Is your competitor satisfied with his or her current position?
- What likely future moves or shifts will your competitor make, and how dangerous are these shifts to you?

Offensive Position
- Where is the competitor vulnerable?
- What might you do to cause your competitor to respond vigorously?

Competitor Profile
1. What are your competitor's strengths and weaknesses?
2. What are your competitor's strategies?
3. Use the following categories to develop a profile of your competitor.

❏ Facility	❏ Market share
❏ Location	❏ Customer base
❏ Ownership	❏ Sales volume
❏ Decor	❏ Distribution area
❏ Type of facility	❏ Referral sources
❏ Financial	❏ People
❏ Profitability	❏ Credentials
❏ Cash flow	❏ Sales style
❏ Cash reserves	❏ Knowledge
❏ Prices	❏ Communication skills
❏ Discounts	❏ Staff size
❏ Staying power	❏ Advertising/promotion
❏ Product/services	❏ Media used
❏ Product or services mix	❏ Amount used
❏ Product brand	❏ Types used
❏ Test equipment	

Source: Adapted from Staab, W. J., & Jelonek, S. (1995b). Building professional marketing skills. Presented at Towards 2000: Hearing Aid Marketing Workshop, Phoenix, AZ, with permission.

- *Is defendable*   Your offering is difficult to copy or might include provisions that exclude others from providing something similar.

- *Is sustainable*   It has a momentum that can continue for a reasonable period of time without encroachment.

Pearl

You have a competitive advantage when your product or service (Jelonek, 1992a):

- Is unique

- Has value

- Is defendable

- Is sustainable

Develop a Competitive Advantage   The following approaches are suggested for developing a competitive advantage (Staab and Jelonek, 1994b):

Cost   Cost can be a competitive advantage only if everything associated with this offering can be obtained and provided at a lower cost than by the competition. This includes the entire management of the business. If a cost advantage exists, the focus should be on the cost, not on the price of the product. Selling a product or offering service at a low cost alone, or for a short period of time, does not provide a cost advantage. In reality, few practices are able to offer cost as a competitive advantage. Selling at a low price without a cost advantage is a certain route to failure.

Pitfall

- Selling a product or offering service at a low cost alone, or for a short period of time, does not provide a cost advantage. In reality, few practices are able to offer cost as a competitive advantage. Selling at a low price without a cost advantage is a certain route to failure.

Focus Specializing in a certain type of service or product, or on a specific segment of the market, might give you a competitive advantage. Examples of this include home service, cochlear implants, working with children, concentration on celebrities, service centers, the latest technology, and private label products. The specialty cannot be in name only. You must have associated with you all the skills, knowledge, and equipment to keep you ahead of the competition.

Timing This assumes that you can quickly and easily offer new products or services to the market, or it might mean that you are able to offer the products and services that others offer, but more quickly, with greater accessibility, and with greater quality.

Differentiation What do you do or have that is unique to the marketplace? Are you able to offer a value that others cannot and present it in a distinctive manner? Do you have credentials that others do not have, hospital or academic training program privileges, knowledge, quality, skills, offerings, a delivery system, managed care, cerumen management, or equipment? In what you do, is it the distinguishing characteristic or competitive strength of your practice?

However you differentiate your practice from others, make certain that you present your offering with added value, realizing that value is determined by the patient, not by you. Patients often consider cost, time, accessibility, and outcome as factors that determine value. It is this feature that the consumer will often refer to when asked about your business. If what you are offering is not perceived by the patient as having added value, it is considered a commodity, for which price is the only distinguishing competitive feature.

> **Pitfall**
>
> • If what you are offering is not perceived by the patient as having added value, it is considered a commodity, for which price is the only distinguishing competitive feature.

In a series of marketing seminars on hearing aids comanaged by me (Staab and Jelonek, 1994a,b), attendees were asked to identify what they thought their competitive advantage was. Almost without exception, each suggested that they were very caring and understanding of their patients, that they related to them extremely well, and that they considered them as people rather than as patients. They believed that their interaction with the patients was their primary competitive advantage. They considered this interaction with their patients to be very special, and perhaps it was. However, this relationship does not provide the basis for a competitive advantage because everyone in the room expressed the same "competitive advantage." How does this meet the requirements of uniqueness, value, defensibility, and sustainability? In other words, rather than being a competitive advantage, what seminar participants were expressing was a measure of standards of performance. This was expected of them to manage a business successfully.

> **Special Consideration**
>
> • The special care, understanding, and attention you give to your patients is not considered a competitive advantage; rather, it is a standard of performance.

Appendix 5–4 provides an action plan outline for determining your competitive advantage. It is important to have one so that you can be differentiated from the competition. It gives your office a focus, drives your marketing strategies and programs, helps to define your identity, and positions you relative to competition in the minds of your patients. Analysis of competition is a tool in establishing the uniqueness of your office. Your resourcefulness in using this information is the key to a successful practice.

How to Use Market Analysis Data Market data are used to help determine market sales potential, to assess the competitive intensity of the market, to develop market programs, to facilitate strategic planning, to determine service offerings and pricing levels, to target direct mail programs, to identify office locations and design, to determine what types of services and products should be offered, to develop promotional programs, and to select and direct market communications. The market potential is determined by several factors, including population size and growth rate, population mix, income and occupations, community economic health, and dispenser-to-population ratios.

Marketing Objectives

Goals or objectives? Goals are fine, but objectives may be better. Both are important. The difference between them is that goals are qualitative, and objectives are quantitative.

Goals should be considered for both personal and business reasons. Personal goals might consist of achieving income, preparing for retirement, or enjoying a particular lifestyle. Business goals might consist of increasing unit sales, increasing gross sales, increasing net income, improving productivity, expanding market position, increasing profitability, decreasing debt, repositioning the practice, expanding the practice with a new office, developing new patients, developing new markets or referral sources, increasing cash flow, lowering the return rate, decreasing the resale time period, increasing the lifetime value of current patients, increasing response rates to mailings, decreasing patient attrition, and providing better patient service. These are all examples of worthwhile goals on which marketing strategies are built.

It follows, naturally, that if goals are quantified, resulting objectives—if achieved—will provide a basis for measuring the value of the goal. For example, selected goals defined above could be restated as the following list of objectives:

• *Increase unit sales* by 10% from 20 units per month to 22 units per month without a decrease in gross profit margin.

• *Decrease debt* by 40% without absorbing more than a 10% loss from gross profits.

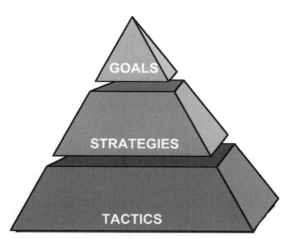

Figure 5–5 The arrangement of marketing features. Goals (objectives) define the overall direction of the business. Strategies are developed as general directions used to achieve the goals or objectives. The tactics consist of the day-to-day, detailed activities that allow the practice to survive and grow.

♦ *Increase the lifetime value of current patients* by 15% from an average of $8000 to $9200.

♦ *Increase response rates to prospect mailings* by 10% from 2.0 to 2.2%, while keeping the number of pieces mailed constant.

♦ *Decrease patient attrition by 20%* from 10 to 8%, without increasing marketing costs by more than $50 per first-time purchaser.

♦ *Reduce the average inbound call wait time* from 30 seconds to 20 seconds, without increasing total inbound telemarketing costs by more than 8%.

Regardless of how goals and/or objectives are stated, they should be (1) put in writing, (2) quantified, (3) considered realistic, and (4) limited in number.

In the hierarchy of events, goals or objectives are at the tip of a triangle, as illustrated in **Fig. 5–5**, with tactics, or the day-to-day activities, supporting strategies, which in turn support overall objectives.

Marketing Strategies

Marketing strategies are developed as general directions used to achieve the goals or objectives. They are the "how to" but not the detailed activity. The detailed activities are the tactics and are presented later in the marketing action plan under "Promotion."

Positioning is central to all marketing strategies. It is difficult to provide services and products if they are not proper for the market, if they are priced incorrectly, if the practice is not known to the market, or if the practice lacks a credible image (Hosford-Dunn et al, 1995a). Positioning is accomplished through strategies implementing the "marketing mix" categories of product, price, promotion, place, and people. How you position yourself relative to these categories defines the image of your practice. For small businesses like

audiology practices, categorization should be kept simple, with goals, strategies, and tactics kept to a manageable number.

Positioning Your Practice

To assist in understanding what these categories refer to, and how they help to build the image of the practice, the following brief explanations are provided.

Product *Product* refers to the overall nature of the goods and services you provide to your patients. Product strategies involve the selection of products, the brands managed (this includes the product skills, knowledge, and expertise needed for each brand), hearing analyses, outcome measurements, services, warranties, and return policies. Deciding which products to use is usually based on the image, profit margins, investment, technology, and reliability of each product, as well as the help (in the form of comarketing) offered by individual suppliers. This decision appears to be made on the basis of both product performance and business realities. For example, most dispensing audiologists have come to grips with the initial euphoria of the Americans With Disabilities Act (ADA) and recognize that persons with hearing impairment are not beating a path to their door to purchase assistive listening devices. Most find that their practices are sufficiently inventoried if they have alerting devices (especially for the doorbell or phone), something for television use, a telephone amplifier, and a hard-wired remote microphone-to-earphone communication device.

Suggestions for deciding how to position a product in the marketplace (modified from McKenna, 1986) are as follows:

Understand market trends If new technology is critical to your market, position your practice as the technology leader through your product offerings. For example, offer a variety of digital hearing aids, not just a single brand, to support that image.

Focus on intangible positioning factors having to do with quality A constant emphasis on new products (tangible items), while ignoring unrelated services, can have immediate adverse effects when the new product becomes obsolete. Obsolescence can occur rather quickly with some new products or technologies.

Focus on a specific audience and serve it better than anyone else You might choose to concentrate on home care service with the aged who have difficulty transporting to your office, or with children.

Experiment and pay attention to market reaction You may have preconceived ideas about products and services for a particular market, but they may not be consistent with consumer performance. For example, at one time many thought that in-the-canal and completely-in-the-canal hearing aids were not for the elderly because they might have difficulty managing the controls. The reality is that many elderly people can manage and prefer the smaller instruments. Failure to explore this with your elderly patients may result in their turning to a competitor.

Price   Price defines your pricing strategy and methodology and is integral to your marketing plan. Price strategies relate to pricing options, increased value, added services, multiple-tiered services, and products. Pricing must be consistent with the perceived value of your offerings and still allow your practice to survive, grow, and meet the overall financial goals as stated in your business plan. Because price plays such an important role in establishing the success and image of your practice, it is discussed in the section "Price as a Marketing Strategy."

Promotion   Promotion includes media advertising, publicity, brochures and literature, personal selling, sales promotion, direct marketing (including mail and telemarketing), patient education, and sales incentives. Although advertising is a part of promotion in the marketing mix, it is not the only way to promote. Advertising is a subset of promotion and is discussed later in this chapter; it is not just another word for marketing.

Place   Place refers to where your practice is located and by whom and when your offerings are made. It also defines your target geographical area: city, county, state, region, and so on. Place strategies include office location and design, relocation, the tracking of clientele, increasing outside service calls, remodeling/enlarging, the integration of new technologies, additional financing (long or short term), and functional uses of facilities. Suggestions for practice location are made in Chapters 6 and 14 in this volume.

People   People defines your staffing needs and division of labor relative to marketing and sales. People strategies are often patient based. These can involve existing patients, potential patients, or referral sources (from patients, the medical community, third parties, or managed care). They often involve knowledge of the lifestyle demographics and psychographics of the population in question. This category is not always identified separately in the "P's" of the marketing mix as is done here, but is listed under the "place" category.

Examples of Strategies

Having discussed in general the role of strategies in a marketing action plan, the following examples of strategies in support of a goal (to increase profitability) are presented. The specific strategies used would depend on how the goal was quantified.

1. Eliminate unprofitable activities

2. Increase prices

3. Sell premium priced products

4. Emphasize cost reductions

5. Sell more products or services

6. Add point-of-purchase products

7. Decrease spending

8. Improve effectiveness of patient service

9. Cross-train personnel

As can be seen in these examples, even though the goal is price related, the strategies cover a range of product mix elements: product, price, promotion, and people. (Place is not an element in these marketing strategies.) The critical element in strategic planning is to ensure that the strategies proposed help achieve the overall objective with which they are associated. There should be at least one or more strategies for each objective.

Price as a Marketing Strategy

Pricing is often considered the cornerstone of any marketing plan. It helps to determine not only current sales and earnings but, much more fundamentally, who your patients and competitors will be in the future. Whatever the price, it must reflect the business objectives, satisfy patients, and ensure a competitive status in the marketplace. The basic plan is to determine the pricing objective, to target the market, and then to provide appropriate pricing strategies. (An excellent overview of pricing, with detailed examples related to audiology practices, is presented by Hosford-Dunn et al, 1995b, particularly Chapter 14.)

Special Consideration

- The pricing decision must reflect management's objectives, satisfy customers, and ensure competitive status in the marketplace.

The price you charge for your products and services can determine the success or failure of your overall business. Some practices set prices based on simple criteria, such as recovery of costs, percentage markup over cost, competitors' prices, and the market price leader. The problem with such approaches is that they fail to take into account numerous other factors that affect the pricing decision. For example, would it not seem prudent to consider such issues as the patient base and mix, consumer demands, competitive forces, economic conditions, availability of money, and changes in interest rates? It is because of these issues, and others, that each practice should develop independently its own pricing policies and objectives. These decisions are essential because changing price levels affect cash flow and margins more rapidly than any other marketing decision.

Pricing Objectives

What are your pricing objectives? Do they include profit, return on investment (ROI), improved cash flow, liquidation of aging inventory, and increased sales volume or market share? In establishing pricing objectives, the ultimate sales and profit objectives must be determined. To accomplish this, the following issues must be resolved first:

1. Disagreements must be ironed out over objectives within your own organization.

2. The fundamental conflict between buyer and seller must be considered.

In terms of the buyer–seller relationship, the seller views prices as (1) expected revenue, (2) an accumulation of costs, and (3) a marketing feature (high prices indicate product quality; low prices provide a marketing advantage). The buyer views the purchasing decision on the basis of the perceived value of the product and on its price compared with the competition.

Pearl

- General pricing objectives include increasing profitability, increasing sales, gaining market share, eliminating competition, promoting an image of quality or service, discouraging any new competitors from entering your market, being accepted as a price leader in the market by competitors, and restoring order to a disorderly market.

What approach should be used when establishing sales and profit objectives? Three general pricing objective categories have been identified: (1) profit oriented, (2) sales oriented, and (3) the status quo (Hosford-Dunn et al, 1995b). These authors also review the target measures and pricing methods for each of these categories. The explanation of approaches that follows is intended to serve as a guideline for determining your general pricing objectives.

For Profit Price for profit is the most logical pricing objective, and most practices use the "cost plus" approach to obtain it. However, to achieve a predetermined profit, specific goals must be established; a specific percentage of sales as a rate of ROI, or as a rate of return on assets managed (ROAM).

To Maximize Profit When used as a short-term objective, maximizing profit may be incompatible with the almost certain long-term goal of profit maximization. For example, for some who have chosen to dispense primarily premium-priced hearing aids or charge high prices in an introductory product stage, high gross revenues may be realized, but the use of this approach may prevent the practice from gaining its ultimate market share because of the practice's increased dependence on a smaller number of consumers. Additionally, high gross revenues do not necessarily translate to high profits.

To Achieve a Certain Return on Investment Prices are set to generate the level of profit necessary to achieve a targeted ROI. This is a pricing approach based on net profit goals for an average sales volume, rather than on actual volume. A danger is that achieving this volume may take precedence over realizing adjustments that might allow an immediate high rate of cash return. Consider the following example:

Hearing aid sales of 8 per month = 96 per year

Fixed cost of product per year = $1000/aid or $96,000/year

Variable cost of product per year = $800/aid or $76,800/year

Desired profit margin = 20% ROI

With nontangible items, such as a hearing test, there is no cost associated with the product alone, but there are variable costs associated with giving the test. Tangible items, such as hearing aids, have both fixed and variable costs (in this example, a fixed cost of $1000 per unit and a variable cost of $800 per unit to dispense and maintain the instrument). The average cost per unit of products or services sold would be the sum of total fixed and variable costs, divided by the number of services or products sold. Using this information:

$$\text{Selling price} = \frac{\text{Net profit}}{\text{Sales}}$$

Selling price =

$$\frac{[(100 + \%\text{ROI})/100 \times (\text{Expenese} + \text{Cost of goods sold})}{\text{Sales (Number of products sold)}}$$

Selling price =

$$\frac{1.2 \times (\$96,00 + \$76,800)}{96 \text{ units}/\text{year}} = \$2160 \text{ per hearing aid}$$

A very simple method to determine how large the ROI must be to ensure an acceptable return after taxes and inflation is

$$\text{Break-even point} = \frac{\text{Rate of inflation (\%)}}{100 - \text{Rate of tax on gain}}$$

As a general point of information, and as an example, with inflation at 6%, a business in the 40% tax bracket must have net returns of more than 10% to come out ahead.

For Cash Flow At times you may have to adopt policies that conflict with profit objectives. For example, if you have committed large sums of money for a particular direct mail program on programmable hearing instruments, a pricing policy may have to be set in place, temporarily, which returns the maximum cash within a specific period.

To Increase Sales Pricing, either up or down, can impact sales volume faster than any other marketing technique. However, similar results can be achieved by improving product quality, service, or delivery. Understand fully the implications of price reductions on your gross profit margins (and the increase in product or service unit sales required) before instituting such programs (**Table 5–7**).

As shown in **Table 5–7**, the greater the discount, the greater the increase in units of product or service that are required to stay at the same profit margin. Shown also are the dollar volume increases required to continue to achieve the same profit margin (50% in this example), as well as the number of additional instruments that must be sold at each discount level. The figures change with different scenarios. For example, if a decision is made to offer a price discount (say, 30%), and an attempt is made to maintain the same gross profit (i.e., 50%, which is the sales minus the cost of goods sold), an increase in sales dollar volume of

Table 5–7 Impact of Price Discounts on Gross Profit

Sales dollars and unit increase required to maintain a 50% gross profit if discounts are offered. Modify numbers as required.						
			Selling price = $1000 – changes with discount offered, column (b)			
			Costs = $500 (assumes this is constant to offset volume purchasing lost)			
			Average sold = 20 units/month			
			Sales volume = $20,000/month (based on selling price of $1000)			
(a) Percent Discount per Hearing Aid	(b) Selling Price per Hearing Aid Minus Discount (Dollars)	(c) Monthly Sales Minus Discount (Dollars)	(d) Discounted Monthly Sales (Dollars)	(e) Profit Margin of Selling Price (%)	(f) Monthly Sales Volume Increase (%) Needed to Get Back to 50% Gross Margin	(g)* Monthly Unit Increase Needed to Get Back to 50% Gross Margin
0	1000	20,000 – 0	20,000	50.00	0	0
5	950	20,000 – 1000	19,000	47.37	5.26	1.05
10	900	20,000 – 2000	18,000	44.44	11.11	2.22
15	850	20,000 – 3000	17,000	41.18	17.65	3.53
20	800	20,000 – 4000	16,000	37.50	25.00	5.00
25	750	20,000 – 5000	15,000	33.33	33.35	6.67
30	700	20,000 – 6000	14,000	28.57	42.86	8.57

*$20,000 minus discounted monthly sales (d) divided by discounted selling price (b) (Staab, 1986).

42.86% would be required. This would amount to an increase in unit sales from 20.00 to 28.57 units (Staab, 1986). To determine the impact of a price increase, review the break-even analysis in **Fig. 5–6**.

To Maintain or Increase Market Share   Pricing to maintain or increase market share is a fairly common practice but is often misunderstood. The theory is that market share increase (new unit sales or patients) is a more meaningful

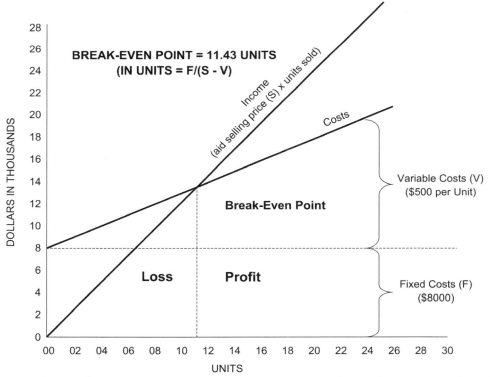

Figure 5–6 Break-even analysis chart based on a 1-month projection (although this could be displayed yearly as well). Fixed and variable costs are compared with projected units and revenues. In this example from the text, fixed costs, regardless of how many units are sold, are $8000. The variable cost per unit is $500. At a selling price of $1200, costs and revenue will equal each other ($13,715 each) at the 11.43 unit mark. (Put another way, when 11.43 units are sold, total cost is 11.43 × $500, or $5715, + $8000, or $13,715.) At the same price, the sale of each unit above 11.43 yields profit.

measure of success than growth in sales dollars, because expanding market share may permit a business to accomplish its long-term objectives more easily as a result of the broader patient base. It is for this reason that prices are sometimes set to ensure high sales volume, even at the expense of short-term profits.

To Stabilize Market Prices and Margins Pricing to stabilize market prices and margins is often done as a reaction to competition, especially during times of rising prices (but it can be done in times of falling prices as well). This approach should be used with caution because adjusting prices to competitors' often triggers price wars.

To Follow the Law of Demand (the Demand Curve) Pricing to follow the law of demand tailors the pricing strategy to selling less for a higher price, or more for a lower price.

A couple of pricing approaches that may not be directly related to increased profits or sales volume are (1) pricing to maintain image, in which a high price implies quality, value, or prestige; and (2) limiting the degree of price hikes. An example is if a 10% price increase is projected for next year; the increase can be tempered by initiating two 5% increases—one now or in another 6 months, and the other a year from now.

From Pricing Objectives to Pricing Strategies

It is not possible to anticipate every variable affecting the market, but be aware of certain general rules:

♦ With few exceptions, an increase in the price of a product will lead to a fall in the demand for that product. Conversely, a reduction in the product price will lead to an increase in demand for that item.

♦ No practice will be a product leader over its entire product line. In a competitive marketplace, even the strongest company will have weaknesses in some areas.

♦ Any pricing policy must be flexible enough to allow for minor price adjustments based on prevailing market conditions. To allow this flexibility, the pricing policy should have a basic reference point price. The price is then modified to take into account variations within a product line, market structure, geographic location, competition, terms, and quantity.

Not until all conflicts related to objectives are resolved can strategies be put into effect. To facilitate decisions regarding pricing strategies, do the following:

♦ Have a pricing policy that sets the basic philosophy for the entire marketing plan; price above, equal to, or below that of the competition. When setting this basic philosophy, remember that smaller practices may not be able to offer some products or services that are priced well above or well below the competition.

♦ Consider the relationship between pricing and the product's life cycle (see discussion later in this chapter). The price in a company's growth stage is usually different than in its mature stage.

♦ Establish and define your pricing objective.

Pricing Strategies

"Cost Plus" Pricing "Cost plus" pricing is the simplest approach, but it is also often the least rewarding. The reason is that, at the very least, operating expenses must be recovered. Total operating expenses are calculated, and a percentage markup is added for profit. What goes into total operating expenses? These generally include costs of all material, labor, and overhead. This approach fails to consider what the consumer is willing to pay and any differences in the product mix. It is best used for determining the minimum price to charge.

Markup Pricing Markup pricing has the advantage of simplicity. This approach adds a percent value to the cost of the products or services, including overhead. It is often a constant percentage added to each product or service (e.g., a doubling or tripling of the cost). The markup is usually a percentage of the selling price that is added to the cost, not the actual earnings. For example, using this approach, a hearing aid that has a wholesale cost of $1000 and is sold for $2000 has a 50%, not a 100% markup, as seen in the following equations:

$$\text{Markup} = \frac{\text{Selling price} - \text{Cost of product}}{\text{Selling price}} \times 100$$

$$\text{Markup} = \frac{\$2000 - \$1000}{\$2000} \times 100 = 50\%$$

$$\text{Selling price} = \frac{\text{Cost of product}}{100 - \text{Markup}} \times 100$$

$$\text{Selling price} = \frac{\$1000}{100 - 50\%} \times 100 = \$2000$$

This type of approach is also sometimes referred to as the gross profit, or gross margin, markup.

This approach does not attempt to determine what the product is actually worth to the patient. Be aware, however, that using a percentage markup can lead to underpriced labor-intensive products and overpriced material-intensive products. Its efficiency is undermined by the failure to reap the maximum profits (when patients are willing to pay a higher price for the product or service).

Consumer Pricing Consumer pricing determines that price must be based on consumers' perceived values, and not on your costs. This is often used by businesses that offer specialized products and services where each can be priced individually based on costs, expenses, and profit margins. Pricing strategies based on ROI often fall in this category. This type pricing often takes a multitiered approach where products and prices are offered at more than one level and the consumer selects based on what he or she is willing to pay.

Inflation Pricing Inflation pricing complicates pricing strategies because it drives costs up while the experience curve tends to go down (especially in the case of new products). If set too low, prices may not be able to keep up with inflation, or if too high, may not generate the volume needed to stay in business. This is not ordinarily used in audiology practices. Instead, other approaches are modified to compensate for inflation.

Competitive Pricing Competitive pricing is one of the simplest pricing approaches. Basically, fees are set at or below those of competitors, without regard to profitability. Because dispensing audiologists often use the same products or services, price is certainly a factor, and this is the approach used by many. In some highly competitive markets, this may be the most reasonable approach. Competitive pricing necessarily affects the price you can charge and what the competition can charge relative to your practice. But what should you do if your competitor raises or lowers prices? Before changing your price relative to theirs for the same or similar products, consider the following:

- What are the competitor's reasons for his or her prices? Do you have the same cost pressures? Is your competitor attempting to generate immediate cash, a liquidation of stock, or aggressively seeking market share?

- Consider responding with a non-price-related strategy, such as higher quality, better distribution, or an extended warranty.

- If the competitor offers a lower price, consider offering a lower priced product to compete with the offering.

- If the competitor offers a higher price, consider both your own costs and possible consumer reaction to the higher cost.

> **Controversial Point**
>
> - Many audiologists mimic market leaders when it comes to pricing. Unfortunately, this assumes that the leaders know what they are doing.

Price Skimming Price skimming deliberately sets a high price on products to maximize short-term contributions. This approach is often used with new products. A potential bonus is that the product or service may develop prestige, because high prices usually are associated high quality. However, make certain that the service and quality are commensurate with the price, or consumer resentment and loss of sales will develop.

Low-Ball Pricing Low-ball pricing is often used by extremely aggressive companies or those struggling to gain market share. In some cases, the products or services are sold at a loss. This is an attempt to buy market share in the short term, with an expectation that profits can be attained in the long term.

Penetration Pricing Penetration pricing revolves around the "experience curve" theory. The theory maintains that when prices are set deliberately low, a large market share can be captured quickly, resulting in economies of scale such that unit costs are low. The success or failure of this approach depends on the speed with which economies of scale can be achieved (and depends on the size of purchase discounts, low competition, no returns, and efficient use of overhead). This is often a high-risk strategy. This pricing approach is also used with low-cost, high-volume products, such as hearing aid batteries.

Opportunistic Pricing Opportunistic pricing can occur during severe supply shortages when patients are willing to pay more for products they value. This is seldom used in dispensing practices because substitute products seem to be readily available.

Price Bundling (or Unbundling) Price bundling (or unbundling) occurs when different products are sold together at a single price. This is very common with hearing aids, especially behind-the-ear (BTE) instruments where the earmold is sold as a part of the hearing aid. It occurs as well with the hearing aid evaluation cost being a part of the hearing aid sale, or when a service contract is sold as part of the instrument sale but not broken out with a separate fee. Unbundling occurs when each component of a product package or service is identified with a separate price. Audiologists bundle their goods and services 65% of the time (Strom, 2004).

Loss Leader Pricing Loss leader pricing is sometimes used to offer a full line of products and services or to attract new patients. The intent is to attract patients to products that are profitable (hearing aids) by offering something else at below or at no cost (free hearing aid batteries or free hearing testing), with the hope that patients will later purchase the higher priced, and profitable, product.

Defensive Pricing Defensive pricing is done when a loss of market share is anticipated. It is more common with established businesses as an attempt to discourage competitors from entering or remaining in the market. The discounted pricing is strategically timed to affect competitors when they are most vulnerable.

Price Milking Price milking is sometimes used by mature companies that wish to leave the market, or when a product life cycle has entered the mature stage. Maximum profits are sought by setting prices at levels higher than the market would normally justify. A certain percentage of patients who are loyal to a particular product will pay the higher price, even though marketing costs may have been significantly reduced.

Demand-Oriented Pricing Demand-oriented (or market-oriented) pricing is modified pricing according to the demand. Prices are raised when demand is high and lowered when demand is low. One type of demand-oriented pricing is margin analysis. Margin analysis is a method that searches for the best price and also identifies a range of profitability based on demand (Hosford-Dunn et al, 1995b). Readers are encouraged to read the referenced material for details.

Thoughts on Setting the Price: Average, Over-, or Underpricing?

This section will provide a philosophical explanation of the consequences when the price is not set appropriately. According to Miles (1986), "average pricing" should be avoided. Pricing should reflect the true competitive value of what is being provided, even as conditions change. When this is achieved, no money is left on the table unnecessarily, on the one hand, and no opportunities are opened for competitors through inadvertent overpricing, on the other hand. According to Miles (1986), average pricing is a major cause of gains and losses of market position. **Figure 5–7** illustrates average pricing in comparison to costs.

No average cost to an average patient exists. As a result, some are overcharged (overpriced), and others are undercharged (underpriced). In overpricing, "low-service" patients are forced to subsidize the "high-service" segments. This is likely to result in a loss of those patients being overcharged but a gain in market share among those being undercharged. The result may be a business that is apparently growing but has mysteriously decreasing profit margins. Worse, a focused competitor could capture this business

and still have ample margins. Progressive expansion by competitors could occur with the competitors moving to the next most overcharged segment. This would leave you with high-service segments at the "average" price.

In underpricing, there is a failure to charge up to the full value of what is being delivered to less price-sensitive patients (although focusing on this much smaller group can be quite rewarding financially). Underpricing overlooks the fact that price is frequently a key indicator of quality. More often, though, underpricing is the result of the seller's lack of understanding of consumers' needs, business economics, options available, and criteria for selection to gauge price sensitivity. If sufficient margins do not exist, your practice will cut back on what differentiates you from the others. Design, features, quality, innovations, and service will suffer. Additionally, opportunities will open for the insightful competitor.

A somewhat related issue to underpricing is the lower selling price on hearing aids and other services demanded by most managed health care programs as one of the conditions for dispenser participation. In many of these programs, the selling price of a hearing aid may fall below the established full-service cost **(Fig. 5–7)**. The price to nonmanaged care patients will have to be adjusted upward to subsidize the low gross profit business, or the audiology practice may find itself in a financially losing situation. Awarded discounts for volume purchases should not be passed on to these programs because this practice further exacerbates the problem.

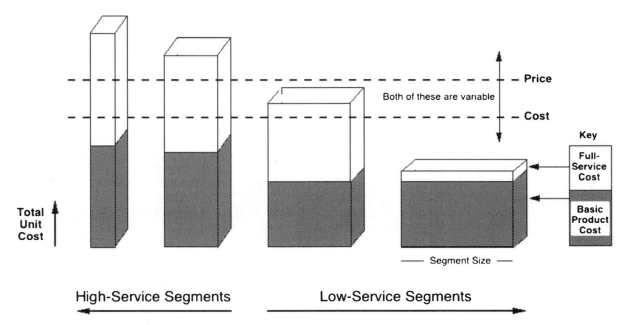

Figure 5–7 Simplified diagram of the dangers of average pricing. The shaded portion of each box represents the basic product cost for the segment size identified. The unshaded portion of each box indicates the total full-service cost of the product (everything other than the basic cost that goes into the delivery). The dotted "cost" line represents the average cost of the sale, including the full-service cost and the basic product cost. Using this average cost for setting price, if you charge too high a price (overpricing: dotted "price" line), the "low-service" patient segment is being forced to subsidize the "high-service" segment. If the price is set too low (underpricing), there is a failure to charge up to the full value of what is being delivered to less price-sensitive patients. (Adapted from Miles, A. W. (1986). Pricing. In Perspectives marketing series (pp. 1–5). Boston: Boston Consulting Group, with permission.)

What is needed to help set the price appropriately?

1. An understanding of the full costs of serving specific customer segments. Use a periodic in-depth review and analysis to obtain this information. Average costs often come from pooled data allocated such that they disguise the true cost of doing business with different service-level patients.

2. Up-to-date assessment of competitors' costs to serve the same segments. Try to determine these costs in detail.

3. Thorough understanding, from patients' perspectives, of their needs, decision criteria, and available alternatives.

4. An assessment of patients' likely responses, including price sensitivity, to potential offers that promise to provide new value.

Interestingly, three of the five deadly business sins identified by Drucker (reported in Hosford-Dunn et al, 1995b) have to do with pricing. These are (1) the worship of high profit margins and of "premium pricing," (2) the mispricing of a new product by charging "what the market will bear," and (3) cost-driven pricing.

When all is said and done, what are the basic marketing steps related to pricing?

1. Determine the minimum price you can offer your product for (cost-plus) and still remain in business.

2. Select the market segment you desire to satisfy with that pricing structure (target market).

3. Determine an image for the product/service that will satisfy that target market. Attach the price that is compatible with this image.

4. Test the price.

Testing the Price

Although several approaches could be used to test the price, multiple uses of the break-even point can provide you with much of the information you are seeking. It allows you to perform "what if" analyses rather quickly.

Break-even Analysis   A good approach to use when making pricing decisions is break-even analysis. The premise of this type of analysis is that certain fixed costs must be covered to break even. This approach considers the fixed versus variable costs, as well as the total costs of doing business, to determine the break-even point (in units and dollars). Once this point is exceeded, profits increase in direct proportion to the level achieved beyond this point. This method works best when products are rather homogeneous.

The following is an example of break-even analysis:

Total fixed costs   (costs unaffected by volume: lease, taxes, administration, insurance, etc.): $96,000/year

Variable costs   (costs that vary with volume: direct labor, telephone, power, hearing aids, supplies, commissions, etc.): $500/unit

Average selling price $1200/unit
Available for fixed costs $700/unit
The equation for calculating a break-even point volume in unit sales is

$$BEP = F/(S - V),$$

where BEP is break-even point, F is total fixed costs, S is selling price, and V is variable cost/unit.

$$BEP = \frac{\$96,000}{\$1,200 - \$500}$$
$$= 137.14 \text{ units per year or } 11.43 \text{ units per mc}$$

To recover the $96,000 in fixed costs in this example, 137.14 units would have to be sold in 1 year, or an average of 11.43 units/month at $1200 per unit.

Another way to show this is illustrated in **Fig. 5–6**, with costs given on a monthly basis ($8000/month fixed costs). The remaining assumptions are the same as in the previous example. **Figure 5–6** shows that 11.43 units and $13,716/month are required to break even. The profit increases substantially once the BEP has been exceeded. This break-even chart provides a method to monitor visually the impact of sales on profit, cost, and volume.

Using the same break-even formula, if the selling price of the product goes down to $1000 per unit, and all other costs remain constant, the break-even volume will now be 192 units/year, or 16 units per month. **Figure 5–6** shows only the BEP at a sales price of $1200 per unit. Other prices can be drawn on the chart or overlaid.

The BEP can be used to determine prices and necessary unit sales to achieve target ROIs before taxes. For example, if you wished to make $150,000 before taxes, had fixed overhead of $50,000, and variable costs per unit of $500, how many units would have to be sold at a price of $1200? The contribution margin in this case is $700 (suggested unit selling price minus the variable unit costs). Seven hundred divided into $150,000 is 214.29 units that would have to be sold at $1200 per unit. Scenarios can be projected by changing the number of units and selling price, assuming all other factors remain the same.

*Legal and Ethical Issues Related to Pricing
and Consumer Contacts*

Activities that inform, persuade, or communicate in some way with the market attract the attention of government regulatory agencies. As a result, regulations have been promulgated that are intended to protect the consumer.

The list of regulations that follows is adapted from the Federal Trade Commission (2007). It is not meant to be all inclusive, and a comprehensive discussion is not within the scope of this chapter. Readers are encouraged to check the laws and regulations in their own state. The actions discussed are unlawful only if they are taken by joint agreement with one or more competitors. However, it is a mistake to think that such an agreement must be either formal or conspiratorial. The federal government's position is that there is ordinarily no legitimate reason for competitors to be discussing such subjects and to do so may lead to investigation and possible indictment by the Justice Department.

Antitrust Regulations Promote Open Competition Antitrust regulations govern the acts of business. The basic purpose of these laws is to promote vigorous, free, and open competition in the marketplace. They are based on the belief that such competition provides the best guarantee that the American consumer will obtain the best product at the lowest price. The salient features of these regulations are the following.

Price fixing is illegal. Section 1 of the Sherman Antitrust Act of 1890 prohibits "every contract, combination . . . or conspiracy in restraint of trade of interstate commerce." Probably the clearest and most widely publicized violation of the act is price fixing between competitors—agreements between competitors to set prices, to establish minimum or maximum prices, to establish a common pricing system, or to otherwise affect competitive pricing in the industry. Several Supreme Court cases have dealt with a mere exchange of information among competitors concerning recent and specific price quotations to identified patients. Even when no express commitment was made by these competitors to adhere to any price schedule, and the prices charged by them were not uniform, the court found that the exchange of price information constituted sufficient "concerted action" with the expectation that reciprocal information would be given upon request, with the effect that prices were kept within a specified range.

For this reason it is important to avoid the exchange of sensitive business information with competitors. For example, even a seemingly innocuous activity such as the exchange of current price lists could conceivably constitute a violation of Section 1 of the Sherman Act because of its natural tendency to produce uniform prices, even in the absence of any agreement to fix prices. It is expected, of course, that as a vigorous competitor, the dispensing audiologist will obtain as much information as possible about the competition and the market for products, prices, or services. However, the point to remember is that such information should not be discussed openly with competitors to set prices or discounts, terms or conditions of sale, the creditworthiness of patients, profit margins or costs, for bids or intent to bid, and so on.

Interestingly, the proscription against price fixing does not apply only to the price, but to all terms and conditions of sale. Thus, agreements as to credit card charges, discounts, service charges, delivery terms, and the like are all per se illegal.

Pricing of products and services should be based on all relevant factors and not exclusively upon prices charged by competitors.

Formation of Monopolies Is Illegal The Clayton Act of 1914 was passed to strengthen Section 2 of the Sherman Antitrust Act by preventing the formation of monopolies.

Unfair Competition Is Illegal This was established with the Federal Trade Commission Act of 1914. This was passed to deal with unfair methods of competition not covered by the Clayton Act. The Federal Trade Commission (FTC) is empowered to take action against any business practices that are deemed harmful either to competing firms or to consumers.

Price Discrimination Can Be Illegal Price discrimination can be illegal (Robinson-Patman Act of 1936) if the same product is sold to different patients at different prices, unless it is performed as a justified approach to meet competition or is based on the costs of servicing the customers. This supplemented Section 2 of the Clayton Act.

Promotional Activities Are Regulated Promotional activities that are regulated by the Tax Reform Act of 1986 and the FTC are coupons and in-package promotions and other offers, including warranties. Unfair trade practice laws sometimes make it unlawful for retailers to sell products below cost.

Phony Price Lists Are Illegal The Wheeler Lea Amendment (1938) proscribed phony price lists.

Advertising and Sales Promotion Claims Must Be Supported by Documentation Be certain there is documented evidence in the files for claims made in advertising and sales literature. In general, statements made in advertising, sales literature, or orally will be held to violate Section 5 of the Federal Trade Commission Act if they have the capacity or tendency to deceive, considered in light of the entire advertisement, the entire sales brochure, or the entire sales presentation. The test for determining deception is the effect of the statement upon the ordinary or average person. Failure to qualify affirmative representations that are too broad also may constitute deception. In other words, a half truth may be just as false as a whole lie. The FTC, for example, holds that any claim that the average person would relate to safety of a product is a factual claim. Furthermore, absence of knowledge that a claim is false will not defeat an FTC proceeding.

◆ Risk Reduction

This topic most often elicits two types of thinking attributed to consumers: Will I get my money's worth? And will the hearing aids or products/services purchased live up to my expectations? In reality, hearing aid purchasers face at least five types of risk when making their buying decision. These are monetary, functional, social, psychological, and physical (Settle and Alreck, 1989; Staab and Jelonek, 1995a). The magnitude of each depends on the characteristics of the buyer and on the type of hearing aids or services being considered.

◆ Monitory risk is the fear that the purchased product/service will provide less value than the price leads the buyer to expect.

◆ Functional (performance) risk occurs when buyers have alternative brands, styles, services, and so on, to choose from.

◆ Social (occupational) risk relates to the affiliation or social status associated with the purchase of a good.

- ♦ Psychological risk
- ♦ Physical risk

Another type is buyer risk, which can be reduced by several methods. **Figure 5–8**, adapted from Settle and Alreck (1989), identifies 24 of these methods (some more significant than others) and rates them from best to of little help according to categories of risk outlined above.

Targeting promotions to fairly small, sharply defined audience segments means much more than just using highly selective media. It demands tailoring message content to the preferences and buyer risk profiles of each segment.

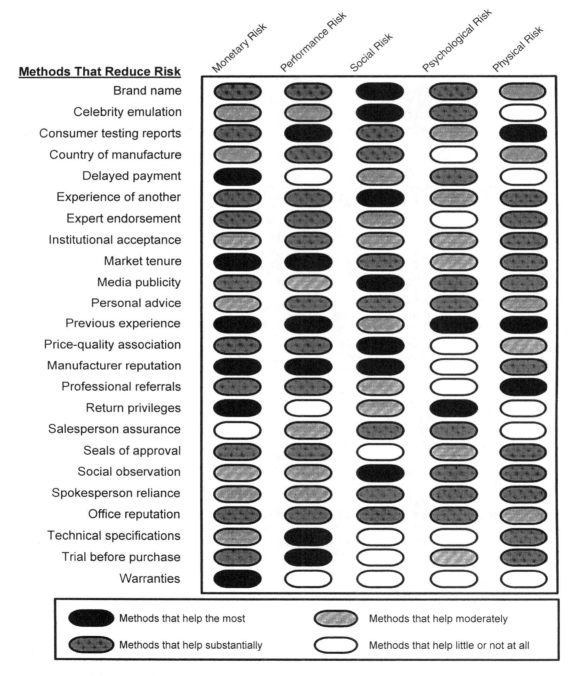

Figure 5–8 Overview of the types of risk a hearing aid purchaser may face, and a partial listing of methods used to help reduce that risk. The shadings indicate the extent to which the methods used actually help reduce the risk involved. (Adapted from Settle, R. B., & Alreck, P. L. (1989, January). Reducing buyers' sense of risk. Marketing Communications, pp. 34–39, with permission.)

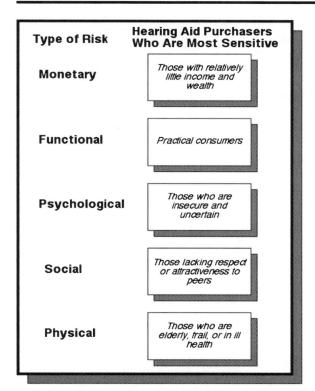

Figure 5–9 Forms of hearing products/services buyer risk.

What is required, as much as anything, is matching the hearing products and their promotional message (the language, social situation, and psychological state) to the social and internal realities of the target market segment. According to Staab and Jelonek (1995a, p. 25), "The best approach to reducing consumers' sense of risk is to provide successful performance and service with their current hearing aids. Nothing has more effect on hearing aid sales (either positive or negative) than previous experience." **Figure 5–9** identifies the type of risk and the hearing aid purchasers who are most sensitive to each of the risk categories.

♦ Marketing Programs (Tactics)

Marketing programs are the day-to-day sales promotional activities, or tactics, that generate the business to finance the practice. Programs direct how you interact with your patients. They emphasize the harsh realities of managing a business (set prices, formulate policies, and shape patient perceptions) and require detailed planning (objectives, strategies, programs, deadlines, schedules, budgets, and itemization). Marketing program efforts generally receive cursory, rather than the specific, attention they require. Often the programs offered consist of reactive marketing efforts to competitive programs. In this sense, much of what

we do is similar to the reactions of sheep—follow what someone else is doing.

A successful hearing aid marketing program requires targeting the market with the right blend of activities. If no marketing plan and programs support it, the practice may not reach the proper market or, even worse, may lose its existing market. To identify how marketing programs fit into the overall marketing plan, recall that the market analysis targets market segments, identifies marketing opportunities, and establishes the competitive advantage. Goals and objectives direct the marketing strategies, which, in turn, outline how the goals and objectives are to be obtained. Marketing programs (tactics) are developed to address a specific problem or take advantage of an immediate market opportunity. To this end, several marketing programs are generally required. These can be developed as individual programs or as part of a series of complementary synergistic programs serving different marketing strategies. The extent to which they are developed depends on the limited resources available (funds, labor, time, and personnel). Changes in dispenser uses of marketing media over the past several years dictate adjustments in the kinds of marketing tactics used. Interestingly, one expense that has not changed much over the years is that associated with the percent of sales dedicated to advertising and promotion (**Fig. 5–10**).

Many audiologists believe that if they follow what the competition does, that is, meet the average, they are doing as much as is required. Realize, however, that "average" is just as close to the bottom as it is to the top. To be successful rather than average, programs must result from the end product of detailed, systematic planning. This planning can be done using the same flow chart provided for the overall marketing program (**Fig. 5–1**). The discussion that follows identifies related issues to successful marketing programs.

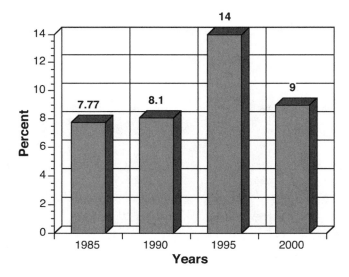

Figure 5–10 Percent of sales devoted to advertising and promotion. (Data from Strom, K. (2001). The HR 2001 Dispenser Survey. Hearing Review, 8(6), 20–22, 24–25, 28–32, 36–37, 40, 42.)

♦ The Promotional Mix

The tactics for presenting a promotional mix consist of a combination of personal selling (oral and face to face), advertising (paid presentation), public relations (your image with a public interest), and sales promotions. The offer might focus on just one element of the marketing mix (product, price, promotion, or place) or on linking multiple marketing elements.

When developing market plans, the dispensing office or clinic is rarely included as part of the marketing mix. This is unfortunate, because in hearing aid dispensing, the office should be considered as a dynamic marketing tool that can support sales, attract new patients, and help generate referrals. Jelonek and Staab (1994) suggest the use of a checklist as in **Table 5–8** to evaluate your office. Is it patient-oriented? Does it contribute to, or undermine, your marketing efforts?

Table 5–8 Evaluating Your Office as a Marketing Tool

Office Checklist

**How does your office measure up? Is it consumer-friendly?
Does it support sales, service efforts, and consumer expectations?**

Neighborhood
- ❑ Accessible by car
- ❑ Nearby parking
- ❑ Accessible by public transportation
- ❑ Safe (crime rate) during daylight hours
- ❑ Neighborhood ambience: retail
- ❑ Neighborhood ambience: professional
- ❑ Neighborhood ambience: medical
- ❑ Neighborhood ambience: residential

Building
- ❑ Visible, easy-to-read signage (business or building name, street address)
- ❑ Easy-to-find office location (on or near well-known streets, locations)
- ❑ Accessible office suite (stairs, elevators, ramps, hallway length, directions within building)
- ❑ Building ambience: retail
- ❑ Building ambience: professional
- ❑ Building ambience: medical
- ❑ Building ambience: residential
- ❑ Building condition (cleanliness, decor, smell, temperature, safety)

Office
- ❑ Decor: positive, professional or retail image
- ❑ Decor: consistency
- ❑ Lighting: easy to see, easy to read
- ❑ Furniture: easy to sit in and get up from
- ❑ Furniture: stable, secure
- ❑ Easy access and movement for clients with limited mobility, poor eyesight, using assistive devices (canes, walkers, wheelchairs, oxygen tanks)
- ❑ Test equipment looks professional, high tech, up-to-date
- ❑ Test equipment is visible
- ❑ Client can see computer screens and participate in the fitting or testing process (hearing aid fitting systems, hearing aid analyzers, real ear equipment)
- ❑ Individual offices/rooms: clean, uncluttered
- ❑ Dedicated offices for audiometric testing, fitting, service
- ❑ Accessibility of real ear test systems, hearing aid analyzers, hearing aid programming devices, computers
- ❑ Well-organized literature stands and tasteful point-of-purchase displays
- ❑ Magazines, books, etc., related to hearing

Evaluation
Rate each of the above areas using the following:
1. Excellent

Table 5–8 (Continued)

> 2. Above average
> 3. Average
> 4. Below average
> 5. Poor
>
> *If you rated any of the categories average or below, immediate action should be taken to improve your office as a marketing tool.*

Promotion Should Be Highly Focused on the Target Market

To whom should the message be directed? Decide if it should be for existing patients, prospective patients, referral sources, third-party payers, or some other group. Is the message to be targeted to a certain age group, sex, income, lifestyle, or purchase-decision style or group? Proper focus allows resources to be concentrated and increases the probability that the program will be successful.

Where to Present the Promotional Messages

Is this done better in the print media (telephone directories, newspapers, direct mail, printed materials, etc.), audiovisual media (television/cable, radio, television, or the Internet), outdoor media, personal contacts or advertising specialties. Regardless, use a story (headlines and content) and visuals to get attention, to direct the message, and to motivate potential purchasers to action.

Promotional Tasks

Promotional tasks for all the above are either to inform, persuade, or remind consumers about the products or services offered. Do you intend to provide awareness, value, life enhancement, education, or a call to action, or to position your practice competitively? If product related, the approach is closely tied to the stage of the product life cycle (see discussion later in this chapter). Regardless, the offer is important.

Promotional Tips in Message Presentation

Promotional tips should include a strategy of explaining the benefits, adding value, targeting as specifically as possible, cross-promoting if a program does well, using a theme identified to your office, focusing your message, and always asking the question the consumer will ask: What's in it for me?

Promotional Programs Have a Limited Life Span

A limited life span is characteristic of marketing programs. They are generally short term, lasting from a few days to perhaps a few weeks. Seasonal programs have their own built-in life span (Christmas, summer maintenance, May Is Better Hearing Month, year-end offer). It is possible that some programs will take on a life of their own after being initiated. Loss or damage, programmable hearing aids, and "essentially invisible" hearing aids are examples.

◆ Advertising and Promotion

Advertising

Advertising consists generally of media marketing (television, radio, newspapers, consumer/business publications, print media, Internet, etc.). It is purchased as a commodity, with the content controlled by the advertiser. It tends to use a shotgun approach in that it scatters its message of a broad objective toward the product or service. Immediate action is not expected. It should, however, eventually contribute to sales through its attempts to disseminate information, persuade purchasers, and influence attitudes. Advertising is used because products and services do not normally sell themselves. Therefore, advertising is employed as a predominant message as to how consumers form opinions about the products they buy, about the services they seek, and about the businesses they patronize. Its role is, purely and simply, to communicate, to a specified market, information and develop a frame of mind that stimulates action. If advertising is not intended to contribute to immediate sales, some have questioned its importance, but not advertising is like winking in the dark: you know what you're doing, but nobody else does. According to a survey by the American Association of Advertising Agencies (reported in Staab, 1992), the average person in the United States is exposed to over 16,000 different advertising messages every day. Of these, the average person remembers about six—meaning that something else may be required to complete the sale.

Pearl

- Not advertising is like winking in the dark: you know what you are doing, but nobody else does.

Advertising creates awareness, including long-term recognition. It helps to build your identity, to position yourself relative to the competition, and it builds and sustains momentum. Always make certain that the message is clear, that it tells the real "story." A famous example of a story gone wrong, albeit through translation, was John F. Kennedy's announcement to the people of Berlin: "Ich bin ein Berliner!" JFK thought he said, "I am a citizen of Berlin!" To some, what he "really" said was, "I am a jelly doughnut!" ("Berliner" is a German type of jelly doughnut.)

Public Relations (Publicity)

This marketing function relates the image of your practice with the public interest. Public relations (PR) is an effective marketing technique intended to (1) make your personal expertise known to the public, (2) promote respect for your services, and (3) provide a useful public service by imparting reliable information to a knowledge-hungry society. It is not always easy to get the attention of the press, but if you do, use it as follows:

♦ Identify the appropriate person to whom information should be sent.

♦ Try to send information on a periodic basis.

♦ Articles or interviews are perceived by the public as more objective than advertisements.

♦ Free publicity is generally better than paid-for advertising.

♦ The message should be informative and educational, rather than promotional.

♦ Use PR to help create your image.

Advertising objectives and strategies must be developed within the context of the marketing plan. They are generally divided into three basic categories: to inform, to persuade, or to remind (**Fig. 5–11**).

Basic Approaches to Advertising

How to Establish an Advertising Budget

Berkowitz (1992) identified the following approaches to establishing an advertising budget:

♦ What you can afford (what is left over after managing all other expenses)

♦ Competitive parity (based on what the competition does without regard to goal differences)

♦ Fixed percentage of sales (This does not allow for experimentation, countercyclical promotions, and opportunities. It is good to maintain a close relationship between expenses and sales per business cycle.)

♦ Percentage on future sales projections (This avoids using last year's figures for this year's budgeting.)

♦ Unit of sales/fixed dollar amount

♦ Task/objective approach based on the media selected, frequency, reach, continuity, repetition, ad size, length of commercial requirements, and so on

♦ Cooperative advertising with manufacturers to increase advertising budget (telephone directory ads under brand name listings, and also for direct mail inserts, newspaper ads, etc.)

How to Develop the Message

The message of the advertisement should emphasize awareness, interest, desire, credibility, or action. An acronym that can be used for this is SIMPLE: *s*top the reader, *i*nterest the reader in finding out more, *m*otivate the reader to want the product, *p*ersuade the reader that the product is right for him or her, *l*ogical reason for purchase, and *e*ase the path to purchase) (Berkowitz, 1992).

Pearl

• Keep it SIMPLE: *s*top the reader, *i*nterest the reader in finding out more, *m*otivate the reader to want the product, *p*ersuade the reader that the product is right for him or her, *l*ogical reason for purchase, and *e*ase the path to purchase.

Benefits, not features, should be sold in an advertisement. This approach determines the way patients perceive your business. A systematic approach to layout design follows the KISS principle (*k*eep *i*t *s*imple, *s*tupid) (Green Dot Advertising and Marketing, 2007).

♦ Use familiar serif face type.

♦ Use upper- and lowercase print.

♦ Reading (or scanning) is from top to bottom; if the layout follows this order, it can increase readership by 10%.

♦ Put the illustration on top (a picture is worth a thousand words).

♦ Place a headline under the illustration (headlines have 5 times the readership as body copy).

♦ Copy under the headline should emphasize the benefits. As few as 5% of readers may actually read the body copy, so use short sentences, short paragraphs, and the language of everyday conversation.

♦ Add a tracer so that the source of the ad can be determined when the patient makes an appointment.

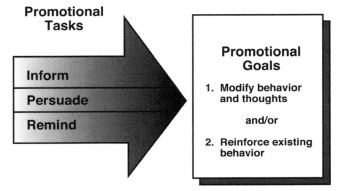

Figure 5–11 Promotional tasks are either to inform, persuade, or remind consumers about products and/or services. The choice of which to use depends largely on the product life cycle.

Types of Advertising Media

Newspapers provide good local coverage and depth penetration. Having a wide range of appeal and a broad acceptance, their highest readership is in the 45 to 64 age group (Matthouse and Calder, 2002). Newspapers allow for good timing and space flexibility and are an ideal medium for ads with clip-out inquiry forms. Limitations are their relatively short life (1 day), strong competition from all kinds of other ads, and the fact that the reader spends, on average, 30 minutes reading the paper with at most 50% involved in reading ads (Malthouse and Calder, 2002). It is important to note that newspapers are losing readership to the Internet and that currently 68% of newspaper readers are over age 55 (Sweep, 2002). The frequency with which ads should be placed varies. Berkowitz (1992) suggests that 13 exposures over 52 weeks is preferable to 13 in 13 weeks: the first 3 or 4 exposures get lost in the masking of other ads, the fifth and sixth exposures tend to be the ones that register with readers, and the seventh and eighth are those that register with the individual purchaser. Exposures 7 to 10 are important for their repetition and reminder value. These suggestions are consistent with the "rule of seven" (Moses, 2003), which states that the number of points in a presentation should be limited to seven or fewer.

Newspaper media kits (available from other media as well) allow for the determination of

- Which papers will reach the maximum number of your target audience
- Daily circulation figures to determine days with highest readership (for scheduling)
- Advertising rates (usually cost per thousand)
- Section in which to place the ad

Weekly papers and shopping papers are alternative approaches used to reach a localized circulation and keep costs low.

Television is often economically beyond the reach of small businesses. However, in small market areas, cable TV, public access channels, and paid programming have become more accessible and affordable.

The advantage of television is that it combines sight, sound, color, motion, and drama. It commands high attention and high exposure, along with the opportunity to project an image and deliver a message to people in their own homes with significant power and persuasiveness.

Weaknesses include its high absolute cost, the amount of clutter in fighting for the viewers' attention, brief exposure (generally 30 seconds), and less audience selectivity. It takes several exposures before a reaction is obtained and involves a higher cost, which is determined by the audience size, time of day, and commercial length.

Davis (2005) gives general pointers on TV advertising for small businesses, among them:

- As with newspapers, use the station representatives as a source of target market information. The message often involves a "slice of life" anecdote, testimonials, an offer for a demonstration, and problem solving.

- Name identification and repetition are very important for recall.
- An attention grabber in the first frame can offer visual surprise; other attention grabbers are close-ups, sound effects, and showing the product in use.
- TV ads can run more frequently than radio ads because TV offers both visual and auditory stimulation and therefore does not have the same fatigue factor.

Web sites are emerging as popular sources of advertising. There is no single magic formula to a successful site. It is possible, however, to design a Web site using a mix of marketing programs that are right for you, based on your overall goals and strategies. By aligning online marketing with other efforts, you can better achieve overall company objectives. Additionally, you will present a consistent style and message across all points of contact with your target audience. The tactics that will help you reach your goals may be completely different from the tactics that are right for a competitor's Web site. Unless you are proficient in Web site management and have the time, however, it will be necessary to employ the services of someone to serve as a Web master.

A few tactics that might be implemented on a Web site are

- Write and distribute articles available for free republication.
- Rewrite sales pages provided by the suppliers of the hearing aids you offer, but observe copyrights.
- Send postcards or notes to Web site customers/visitors.
- Spend 1 hour per day on prospecting new customers.
- Survey visitors to the site as part of market research.
- Provide a discount coupon, available only online, and advertise it in other, more traditional, media (this is intended to pull new and repeat visitors to your Web site).
- Include a weekly, or monthly, interactive discourse with site visitors (to provide reasons for repeat visits).
- Implement a customer loyalty program (to increase repeat purchases and build a more loyal customer base).
- Partner with other online businesses by mentioning each other's products/services in your Web site links.
- Have a limited time offer.
- Add testimonials (helps establish credibility and shows experience).
- Put a "refer-a-friend" link on every page (reminds people to tell others about your site).
- Develop a mailing list of "hot prospects" and send them a brochure about your Web site.
- Communicate your Web site address at every point of contact with patients and prospects.
- Install a "bookmark this page" script on each page (encourages repeat visits).

Implement the Web site to your greatest ability, then persist. Improve upon and tweak the implementation of each marketing program until it works for you.

Radio formatting is highly selective and fragmented (all news, talk shows, music, ethnic programs, etc.). Commercials are 15, 30, and 60 seconds, and sold in time grids (morning and evening drive times: 6:00 to 10:00 AM and 3:00 to 7:00 PM; daytime, evening overnight; and weekend). Radio offers a variety of advertising packages, including combinations of day and evening commercials. Benefits include mass use, high geographic and demographic selectivity, and low cost. Advantages are that the listener tunes to stations, not programs, as compared with TV, where viewers watch programs, not channels. Limitations of advertising on radio are that the message is presented in audio only and therefore requires numerous repetitions. Also, radio tends to attract a lower attention level than TV. Additionally, rate structures are not standardized.

The task is to get people to listen. To accomplish this, the following elements are used: surprise, arousal of curiosity, repeated promise of the benefit, and repeat identity. A radio account executive can help you determine which stations are appropriate for you. They will provide current market research to allow you to make an informed decision and match your prospects to the appropriate stations. Account executives can also assist you in writing and producing the commercial. Except for rare conditions, there should be no additional cost for development of the advertisement (as opposed to TV).

Outdoor advertising is more limited in scope and is used much less frequently by audiologists than any of the other media approaches. Advertising includes billboards, benches, bus signs, and taxi advertising. These outlets offer little flexibility because their size (and often their content) is highly standardized, regulated, and disciplined. The message view time is extremely short (2–3 seconds). Outdoor advertising is considered supplementary to other major media.

Promotion

Promotion is often associated with all activities other than personal selling, advertising, or public relations. As compared with advertising, promotional activities have specific objectives and are intended to stimulate immediate action. They are more precise than advertising. The goals of promotional programs are to modify behavior and thoughts and to reinforce existing behavior. Promotional activities are relatively short term, usually no longer than 2 weeks. They should be directed toward the consumer and should stimulate a specific action.

Promotion was originally referred to as sales promotion and was used largely as a defensive or retaliatory price weapon. Today it is used to build long-term business and to convert consumers to full-fledged clients. As such, it is considered a strategic tool and not just an opportunistic tactic. Promotion by audiology practices is used to (1) combat the intensification of competition due to increasing numbers of audiologists, without comparable increases in hearing aid sales or profits; (2) satisfy patient

wants, rather than needs,; (3) promote sales during economic decline, with the purpose of retrenching and surviving; (4) increase market share during good business times; (5) create new patients; (6) build a list of qualified prospects; and (7) build the dispensing practice image (Staab, 1992).

Promotion should continue in times of heavy demand because the market is dynamic, and patient loyalty is not a given. Heavy demand also draws more competition, requiring promotional activities to maintain market share. In the face of a declining demand for products or services, promotional activities may discourage competitors from entering the marketplace.

Salient Characteristics of the Promotional Mix

Purpose of Promotion

The purpose of promotion is to change the image and shape of the demand curve for the products and services offered.

Primary Objectives

The primary objectives are generally short-term activities above and beyond the normal advertising or routine selling activities.

Definition of Promotion

- A short-term activity
- Directed toward the consumer
- Intended to stimulate some specific action by means of informing, persuading, reminding

Factors that Influence the Promotional Mix

Amount of Funds Available for the Promotion

The amount of funds available for the promotion is the true determinant of what the promotional mix will be.

Nature of the Market

The influence of the nature of the market is felt in at least three ways: geographic scope of the market, market concentration, and type of patients.

Nature of the Product

Are hearing aids considered a shopping, specialty, or unsought good (Staab, 1990)? The promotional approach will be different, depending on the consumers' perception. Equally important is whether the audiologist is using a "push" or "pull" strategy. Pushing strategies are more likely to use advertising, point-of-purchase (POP) displays, or personal selling to convince consumers to purchase products/services. Pulling strategies are in reaction to consumer demands for certain products/services.

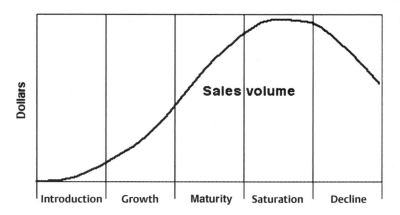

Stages of the Product Life Cycle

Advertising and promotional strategies relate closely to the market situation and should vary depending on the life cycle stage of a product **(Fig. 5–12)**. If not product related, strategies can be used to correct misinformation (e.g., all hearing aids are the same), to reduce consumer risk and/or fears, to create an image, and to suggest new uses of a product.

In the introductory stage of the product life cycle, consumers do not realize that the product is wanted, or even how it will help. Personalized attention is required, and the interest is in features and functions. Consumers considered early innovators and adopters are most readily reached in this stage. The promotional strategies are to inform and educate, to let consumers know of the existence of the product, what it is, its satisfying benefits, and how it is to be used.

In the growth stage, consumers are now aware of the benefits of the product, it has good acceptance, and promotion requires much less personal selling. Consumers are interested in the use of a particular product (primary demand), as contrasted with the demand for a particular product (selective demand). The promotional strategies

here are to stimulate selective demand—to show why this particular product is desirable. Promotion and advertising should be increased during this stage.

In the maturity and saturation stages, competition has intensified, and sales have leveled off. Consumers considered late adopters are somewhat immune to promotion, depending primarily on word-of-mouth referrals. The strategy at these stages is to use promotions and advertising techniques to persuade these late adopters to purchase the product. Promotional activities at these stages are costly and often contribute to profit decline.

In the decline stage, sales and profits are declining. New and better products are being produced. The strategy is to cut back on all promotional efforts, unless something has occurred that can revitalize the offering such as behind-the-ear hearing aids with open fittings.

How to Present the Promotional Program

As has been mentioned previously, the presentation of the promotion program **(Fig. 5–13)** mirrors the general marketing program (**Fig. 5–1**). The primary difference is that the

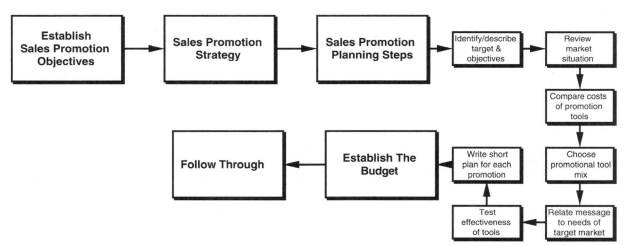

Figure 5–13   Diagram of the marketing programs (promotional, tactical) phase of the overall marketing process action plan. Detailed steps of the sales promotion plan are included.

activities of the promotion program are specific rather than related to the general marketing program. Basic elements in the promotional presentation (adapted from Staab, 1992) follow.

Identify the Market Opportunity or Threat You Wish to Pursue (Situational Analysis)

Although the overall marketing objectives set the stage in establishing the promotional objectives, this phase should not repeat those same objectives, but should add new dimensions.

In this phase, the opportunity or competitive threat is described. The market and market conditions are then analyzed to determine if the opportunity or threat is worth pursuing in your served market. Data from the overall market analysis (described earlier in this chapter) are reviewed. A course of action is then identified.

Marketing programs are often set for smaller market segments, where the message can be directed specifically. This often results in less complicated programs, making them more personal and easier to develop and evaluate. How you choose to segment the market depends on what your program is intended to do. In general, the closer your program meets the needs of the target, the better the results.

Examples of opportunities for an audiology practice include unserved or poorly served patient needs, products or services not being provided, competitor financial or management problems, discontinued or resold offices, competitor inactivity, changes in personnel, new uses of hearing aids, basic industry marketing changes, or population adjustments. Threats exist when new technology is introduced in a timely fashion by competitors, additional offices are added in your marketing area, negative FDA or consumer announcements are made, highly financed and visible competition is present, the stock market drops dramatically, the economy changes for the worse, heavy advertising and promotions to your market segment are made by others, exclusivity of a product or service takes business from you, or a price discount offering that could have an immediate impact on your sales is introduced.

Some situations do not lend themselves well to promotion. For example, promotion is not recommended when the product is inadequate or overpriced, when overnight success is expected, when the cost of the promotion is so costly that the investment might be better spent on improving service, when used with an established product with declining market share, or when the promotion is used alone.

Set Strategies that Will Provide Means to Resolve the Market Opportunity or Threat

Think of strategies at this level that are extensions of the general marketing strategy:

- Sample consumers' interests in a given hearing aid or related services.
- Convert patients from other dispensers, rather than merely borrowing patients.

- Deplete inventories of existing hearing aids, batteries, or other supplies to make room for new products.
- Encourage the sales force (if one exists) to focus on a particular product or service.
- Introduce the trial of hearing aids, a specific test, or some other service available.
- Create excitement about a product, or call attention to the new uses of products or services.
- Increase consumer demand for hearing aids or other service or product supplied by your practice.

Sales Promotion Planning Steps

Define Who and Where the Target Market Is

This is perhaps the most important ingredient in the success of a promotional campaign. According to the Direct Mail Marketing Association ("The Competitive Advantage," 1986), the success of the marketing campaign is attributed as follows: 15% on the promotional copy, 25% on the offer, and 60% on how well the target market is defined. Include information about the target's habits, characteristics, wants, and needs. What appeals to this market segment?

Special Consideration

- The success of the marketing campaign depends on the promotional copy, on the offer itself, and on how well the target market is defined.

Review the Market Situation (Product, Sales History, Product Life Cycle, Competitive Strategies)

These factors, along with the sales trends, pricing, and budget constraints, determine the optimum promotion mix.

Know the Capabilities of Different Promotional Approaches and Comparative Costs

Keep files on the competition as reference material.

Choose the Promotional Tools that Are Best Suited to Reach the Target with Maximum Results

You usually will not know what these are before the promotional campaign. However, measure performance so that future promotions can use information based on (1) past experience, (2) results of other promotional programs that have been run, and (3) the product's place in its own life cycle.

Relate the Theme and Message of the Promotion to the Real or Imagined Needs of the Target Market

The promotional offer is the heart of the marketing program. To motivate the target audience, the offer should have a premium or added value that will encourage consumers to purchase the product now, not later. As a tangible item, the offer could be a product, service, or saving. It can also be intangible, such as enhanced performance or patient support. The offer can be price, product, promotion, delivery (place), or people driven, or a combination of these.

- Price-driven examples include battery club programs, a backup set of hearing instruments at a reduced price, and a percent off on cleaning.
- Product-driven examples are digital technology, completely-in-the-canal aids, noise cancellation, and array microphone systems.
- Place (delivery) examples include rapid turnaround, expanded office hours, service centers, and on-site repairs.
- A people example is the use of specific staff members within the office to manage particular patients.

Is there a cost or savings associated with the offer (direct or indirect), and what will its effect be on the marketing program? Does it add value and demand a premium price, or is it an offer of savings? What will the result be to the bottom line?

Time limitations specify the start and end of a program. By definition, marketing programs are short in duration, but they can be repeated if they are cyclical or seasonal. Materials that are media promoted or mailed to the consumer directly have relatively short response interest.

Test the Effectiveness of the Promotional Tools Used

A simple way to test the effectiveness of a particular promotional tool is to use a return on promotion (ROP) approach.

$$ROP = \frac{Sales - Cost\ of\ sale}{Cost\ of\ sale}$$

In this example, assume that sales for one month are \$9000, and the cost of sales is \$2000. Using this equation,

$$ROP = \frac{\$9000 - \$2000}{\$2000} = \$3500$$

Write a Short Plan for Each Promotion

The plan should include the following:

- Statement of objectives
- Target market(s)
- Message and marketing tools to be used, and why
- The time line for the promotion (when it will occur, with dates for start and end)
- How to measure the promotion's effectiveness

Establish the Budget

This includes all resource requirements (the investment in time, labor, funds, personnel, and equipment required to make the program function). Have these been allocated properly? What is the mechanism for financing the program (budgeted funds, existing funds, debt)? Create a budget that itemizes all costs, direct and indirect, and set up a schedule. Calculate a BEP and project an ROI. Compare the cost and returns of alternate programs. Develop the schedule to allocate personnel, time, duration of the program, and expected results. Consider contingency plans if the program does not progress as expected. The plan should be in written form to prevent omissions and errors.

How much should you budget? Some marketing texts place this figure between 2 and 35% of the total marketing/advertising budget. In a personal communication, Strom (2005) said that the average dispensing audiologist in 2004 designated 10% of the budget for marketing, down from 13.5% the previous year.

Ideally, funds should be allocated to specific promotions based on market potentials or past history. Other approaches to establishing a budget include the following:

- *Relation to income* The budget is based on a percentage of past or anticipated sales. It is sometimes based on per unit sales. If the budget is based on past experiences, however, the promotional program is a result of sales, when in fact it should cause sales.
- *Task or objective* Determine what the promotion is intended to accomplish, then determine what the cost of the promotional activity must be (or what is acceptable). This is a fairly sound approach to establishing a budget that is not too complicated.
- *All funds available* This requires deep pockets and puts all the company's financial eggs into one basket.
- *Follow the competition* This assumes that what the competition is doing is right. However, a competitor's program may not have the same goals, targets, and so on, that you have.

Program Execution and Follow-through

Program execution and follow-through require that the promotion's schedule and plans have been set and are followed. Results should be monitored to track the progress and success (or failure) of the promotional program. Use some unit of measure that is easy to quantify (e.g., new unit sales, new patients, resales, leads generated, or inquiries), and be prepared to modify the program to increase its effectiveness or to terminate the program if it becomes a drain on your practice. Results can be used to direct additional marketing programs.

◆ Promotional Program Tactics

Some tips for promotional programs (Staab, 1992):

- Try to add value, rather than discounting products.
- Put your imprint on the promotions. Make them exclusive and identifiable to your office.

- Focus on the future. Look for repeat business, not just new business.

- Give your promotions a theme to help reinforce your other promotional efforts.

- Target your promotions as specifically as you can, and make the results measurable.

- Try to find ways to reward your best patients, the lifeblood of your business.

- If the promotion does well, look for cross-promotional opportunities.

- Find ways to make your patients feel good about you and your office.

- Promotions should be presented in a quality manner but within your affordability range.

- If you have a sales staff, the promotion should be exciting and rewarding for them, or they will not perform well.

- Make the promotion fun and easy to execute.

- Keep testing different promotions, even if specific promotions are working well.

- When designing the promotion, ask, "What do hearing aid consumers want us to do for them?"

A myriad of sales promotional activities exist but only general categories and examples will be identified and/or discussed here. More complete descriptions can be found in Staab (1992) or in observing what the competition offers. Keep in mind that sales promotion activities are supplementary to advertising. Sales promotions work better on products where advertising has *already* generated recognition and acceptance. Advertising creates value, promotion induces trial, and the product provides the satisfaction. The type and number offered are limited only by your imagination and budget. Promotions that have been successful in the past continue to be reintroduced and modified, reinforcing the belief by many that no promotion device is actually new.

Although most promotion approaches are directed primarily at attracting new patients, few will pay for themselves on this basis alone. They are just as important in retaining existing patients, creating excitement about you and your products, stimulating the sales force (even if it is only you), and in combating competitive promotions.

Pearl

- Advertising creates value, promotion induces trial, and the product provides the satisfaction.

Types of Tactics

Word of Mouth

Experience indicates that word of mouth, that is, messages conveyed from one consumer to another, strongly influences a company's reputation and consumers' plans to buy that company's products. The opinion of a company is generally formed by the experience of the individual consumers with the products and services provided. Although it is difficult to quantify word-of-mouth marketing for audiology practices, the Technical Assistance Research Programs Institute (reported in Hosford-Dunn et al, 1995a) developed some statistics (see also Word of Mouth Marketing Association's Web site: http://www.//ads.womma.org):

- Consumers were 5 times more likely to stop doing business with a company because of poor service than because of poor product quality or high cost.

- Ninety-six percent of dissatisfied patients never complained to the practice, but 90% stopped doing business with that practice.

- The average dissatisfied patient complains to 9 other people; 13% complain to at least 20 people.

- The cost of losing a patient is 5 times the annual value of the patient's account.

- An undifferentiated product accompanied by outstanding service may command up to a 10% price premium.

- A patient who is pleased with a practice will tell five other people.

- Almost all patients (95%) with a complaint will stay with a practice if their complaint is resolved quickly.

- Improving quality of service is much more cost-effective than other promotional efforts: it costs 5 times as much to get a new patient than to keep one.

In-Office or In-Home Demonstrations

In-office demonstration are more economical, but the home offers an environment freer from obligation (it is less threatening and, in some cases, essential because of limited mobility on the part of the patient).

Special Offers

These are essentially price discounts (e.g., free batteries and a percent off on cleaning). Care should be exercised with such promotions because, although they may generate short-term sales, they can erode profits and dilute the image of your practice. In reality, they are often used as an easy-out solution, to resolve a panic situation, or to generate a database. Their use to reduce inventory, however, can work to your advantage. Cash with order and senior citizen discounts fall under this category as well.

Premiums/Incentives

Premiums/incentives are combination orders, for example, offering one pack of batteries with another free or at a reduced price. Other examples are a year's supply of free batteries with the purchase of a hearing aid, coupons that can be redeemed for cash or product, mail-in offers of free books or other literature, direct premiums to the first 50 individuals who attend an opening, and "finder's fees" for references to other customers.

Coupons

Coupons are less expensive than other promotional programs, have low up-front costs, and have no cost until they are redeemed. They can be used, for example, to encourage trial of a product or service; to clean, recheck, adjust, test, or repair instruments; as an in-pack insert to battery club members for the purchase of additional products; as a dollar off the next purchase to competitive product users; as a Welcome Wagon introduction to new members of a community; or to generate additional purchases by current users. A potential drawback with coupons, however, is that customers may feel that the original price of the product or service that is being discounted was too high.

Direct Mail

Direct mail allows promotional campaigns to be directed to specific markets, and it is the easiest way to reach large numbers of prospects. The message comes to the prospect without competition from other advertising or from editorial matter. Direct mail permits great flexibility in materials and production, is statistically projectable, is cost-effective, can be produced and distributed quickly, and can make use of professionally prepared materials supplied by manufacturers. Prospects come from lists (compiled, response, or consumer) that can be purchased or self-developed.

Direct mail does not come without drawbacks, however. Rising postage and production costs can limit its usefulness, an error in conception or execution can make the marketing effort worthless, mailing lists deteriorate, and some recipients consider it all "junk mail." Objectives of direct mail may be to arouse or renew interest in an audiology practice, its products, or its services; to familiarize prospects with products and services available at the practice; to encourage continued patronage by current patients and to resell old patients; and to favorably predispose prospects to a personal demonstration of the product or service.

Direct marketing, direct mail, direct response: These terms are used interchangeably, but there are differences. Direct marketing refers to marketing efforts by the manufacturer that are directed at the end-user. Direct mail advertising uses the mail service to deliver promotional materials directly to prospects. Direct response advertising is any advertising (print ads, broadcast commercials, or direct mail materials) that invites the recipient to contact you directly through a toll-free number, a mailing address, or a business reply card.

Point of Purchase

POP displays are devices (e.g., materials placed in the waiting room of your office) by which a product is displayed in such a way as to stimulate immediate sales. They are intended to capitalize on the impulsive nature of buyers. The POP becomes a last-minute inducement to purchase a product. POP promotional programs are low cost and can be easily evaluated. They allow a distinct consumer focus, precise target marketing, communication of new ideas or performance, and reinforcement of brand awareness. POP displays help sell even when no salesperson is present by allowing patients to help themselves. Examples are hearing aid battery displays, ear wax removal kits, hearing aid listening demonstration comparisons, and hearing aid user's guides.

Posters/Displays

Posters and displays help to hold patients' interest and educate them about issues and products. Examples include pamphlets about a new product's specific uses, testimonial letters on a bulletin board, and issues-oriented fact sheets.

House Organs (Newsletters)

Newsletters help develop personal rapport with patients. Quick and easy to read, they present information directly and personally and at relatively little expense. Newsletters can be a forum for patient education, promote new products and services, offer special battery sales, familiarize readers with staff members, announce changes in office hours, duplicate media content from trade and the consumer press, explain why a given hearing aid might be best for a given population, summarize articles of consumer interest, present legislative matters, provide maintenance reminders, and present testimonials from satisfied users, among other things. They can be distributed at no charge to both existing and potential patients, as well as to referral sources. Publication should be at least twice a year, but quarterly is better.

Telemarketing

The use of the telephone to promote products or services is construed by most audiologists as something anathema. Because telephone contact is part of every practice, to some degree, telemarketing is a readily available promotional program. Some practices use telemarketing as a follow-up to a direct mail promotion, in recognition that a 35% chance exists that the mailing was discarded without having been read. The call provides a second opportunity to introduce the hearing aid or service and provide a detailed promotional message. It is often used to qualify or activate a potential patient or to follow up on leads. Telemarketing should be used to set and confirm appointments, provide postorder or postdelivery support, follow up on service contracts (e.g., cleaning, evaluation, accessories, or batteries), confirm that instruments are working well, and answer patients' questions.

Telephone Directory

Telephone directories are almost a necessity for any business. Whether you believe they are effective or not, when a consumer has opened a telephone directory to a particular section, the decision has already been made to purchase. The only question that remains is, from whom? It is your responsibility to develop a directory listing or ad that will direct consumers to your practice. Directory salespeople suggest that you use multiple listings, advertise prominently, make your listing stand out (e.g., by using a boxed ad or color), and advertise in directories of nearby communities. In developing a directory ad, consider highlighting all the major brands or services that you offer; note the length of time you have been in business, if you are established; include a map or description of your location, if it is difficult to find, and perhaps a photo of your building. For many users who consult telephone directories, the size of the ad implies reliability and success, the length of time you have been in business implies trustworthiness, and a photo of your building implies a solid status.

Open House (Consultation)

The general purpose of an open house is to provide for high traffic flow and sales in a short period of time (say, 3–5 days). An outside consultant is often employed to provide technical information about the product in question, to review patients' hearing loss and fit them with appropriate instruments, and to set appointments. A combined media promotional approach is used to contact potential attendees, with the mailing list coming from the audiologist or from a purchased mailing list that targets the market. The open house has a theme: a new product, solutions to special problems, instrument cleaning, a research study, demonstrations, free hearing testing, a new or remodeled office, or some special event. Discount coupons are often included to help entice attendees. Open house programs can generate substantial cash flow in a short time (but they may also entail substantial upfront costs). A potential drawback is the possibility of a substantial drop-off in sales following the event, unless some other promotional activity is planned to continue patient participation. Another drawback is that the consultant may be more interested in generating sales that are less likely to be successful, leaving the practice with unanticipated problems following the conclusion of the open house.

Public Relations

PR involves the generation of positive publicity for your practice, generally for little or no cost. Publicity can be generated, for example, by staging an event at your facility, with an invitation to the press to attend. Variations of this include school field trips, special recognition ceremonies, hosted seminars, individual and office tours for local media. Maintain an updated, single-page media handout that provides information about you, your qualifications, what your practice does, and your staff. Press releases to local media can often provide hundreds of dollars in free advertising (remember that the best advertising is often that which you do not pay for). It is important to ensure that the information released is newsworthy. Human interest stories are good (e.g., hearing aid donations, special fittings).

Special Events

Some marketing programs are intended to improve recognition of your practice by mass exposure during a short period of time. Special event sponsorship seems to work well for products or services that are difficult to differentiate from the competition (think of automobiles or hearing aids). Although not used often by audiologists, they can be good on a local level and seem to provide the greatest impact when the dispensing practice is the sole sponsor of a small event.

Tie-in Promotions

Tie-in promotions consist of joint, cooperative, or umbrella programs that allow participating businesses to share the costs and reap the benefits. They work best when the businesses are noncompetitive (e.g., hearing aid and eyewear manufacturers). Advantages include enhanced product image, shared media costs, a widened market penetration, expanded product usage, and added visibility in nontraditional locations. Some of the promotions are cross-branded, meaning that products are drawn from the same business environment (e.g., hearing aids and batteries); some feature "common-thread" products (e.g., hearing aids and ear wax removers); and some highlight complementary use relationships (e.g., hearing aids and assistive listening devices). Some tie-in promotions are event-oriented, that is, associated with some major event or celebration. Many are identified with lifestyles (e.g., hearing aids in nursing homes) or with special events (e.g., May Is Better Hearing Month). Tie-in promotions are not without their problems, especially when associated with another business or group. Difficulties arise in partner selection, longer lead times for coordination, creative and promotional differences, and logistical and legal difficulties.

Printed Material

Printed material promotions take many forms. As the name implies, they include almost everything that is printed: brochures, booklets, bulletins, circulars, pricing schedules, business cards, letterheads, manuals, correspondence, and other promotional materials. When developing printed material for the elderly, experts advise using relatively short words and sentences (less than 20 word/sentence on average) and large type size (12 points or larger).

Hearing Screening Programs

Screening programs, whether conducted with audiometers or by telephone, are often performed in pharmacies, clinics, retirement homes, senior centers, or at health fairs. If conducted by telephone, they have a much greater impact if not performed on a daily basis, but rather during limited time periods (about 2 weeks) at select times of the year, not too closely related in time.

Community Events

Certain events within the community provide important opportunities for your name to come before the people. You can use these to your advantage as a member of any of local committee, as a sponsor of the event, or as a participant.

Personal Contacts

The term *networking* may be a holdover from the 1990s, but the practice of meeting with other professionals is not new. Avenues for developing personal contacts include service groups (e.g., Rotary, Kiwanis, and Lions Clubs), professional organizations, local chambers of commerce, country clubs, and churches.

Advertising Specialties

These provide your message on useful, give-away items (pens, rulers, flyswatters, caps, key rings, calendars, mugs, etc.). These items should have a fairly long use life, offer repeated exposure to your name, and be practical. If cheap or not useful, they reflect on your practice.

Alternative Print Media

Not used often by audiology practices, these consist of package inserts (the message is carried with another's purchased item as often seen in the computer industry), ride-along/co-ops (your message with several other advertisers using non-standard formats), statement stuffers (including a mailing piece in another's or your own statements), or card decks (along with several other unrelated advertisers with the message on similar 3x5 inch cards). Another form, free-standing inserts (most often recognized as loose inserts in newspapers), is more commonly used by audiologists.

Information Lunches

Information lunches bring groups of potential patients together for the purpose of presenting useful information, with the intent that attendees will be influenced to consider your practice when a product or service is desired. These are also used to introduce new products.

Personal Selling

Personal selling is the primary method by which marketing promotion occurs, and it is an essential part of a dispensing audiologist's daily activities.

♦ Summary

The hearing health care world is changing dramatically, and those who change to meet its needs will succeed. As we move ahead, the ability to target specific markets, monitor costs, and change tactics will be critical to maximizing profits. Successful audiologists will be those who are flexible, who rethink their products and services, as well as their marketing strategies, and who adjust to changing market needs.

What marketing challenges will you accept in your next marketing plan? What marketing mountains will you climb? The year ahead is filled with opportunity, and those years that follow, even more so. What is required on your part is a destination, a marketing action plan, basic marketing skills, and a willingness to succeed and persevere.

Appendix 5–1

Glossary

advertising Any paid form of nonpersonal sales or promotional effort made on behalf of goods, services, or ideas by an identified sponsor.

advertising agency A firm that specializes in providing promotional services to other businesses for a fee. Services offered include development of advertising copy, selection of advertising media, and placement of the advertisement.

advertising copy The communication that a prospective buyer actually sees or hears.

advertising media The broadcast or print vehicles through which an advertisement is communicated—such as radio, television, magazines, newspapers, and billboards.

assets The resources that a business uses in attempting to earn a profit.

average markup A single percentage used to determine the selling price of each item in a given product line.

brand A name, term, symbol, or design (or a combination of these) used by a business to identify its goods or services and to distinguish them from those of competitors.

budget A planning statement that shows the projected revenues and expenses of an organization.

business Any privately owned and operated organization primarily devoted to securing profits or other benefits desired by its owners or managers.

capital A factor of production, including machines, tools, and buildings used to produce goods and services.

cash An asset that includes currency, checking and savings deposits in commercial banks, cashier's checks, bank and postal money orders, and bank drafts.

cash discounts Discount prices offered in return for prompt payment for goods or services.

channels of distribution The various ways that goods flow from manufacturers to industrial customers or ultimate consumers.

compensation The total wages, salaries, and fringe benefits received by employees.

competition The process of determining the price, quality, and available quantity of an item through the impersonal interactions of numerous businesses.

consumer behavior How people make buying decisions.

consumer market Individuals or households that purchase goods and services for personal use.

cooperative advertising An arrangement whereby national advertisers and local merchants share the cost of local advertising.

cost of goods sold The direct material costs incurred by a business in producing its products.

couponing A technique for spurring sales by offering a discount through redeemable coupons.

demand The ability and willingness of consumers to buy specific quantities of a good in a given time period.

direct mail A method of promotion in which the business uses mailing lists to reach its most likely customers.

discount A reduction in the price offered to a customer for prompt payment or for buying in large quantities.

entrepreneur Person who starts a business and takes the financial and personal risks involved in keeping it going.

expense A cost of doing business.

gross profit The difference between a business's net sales and its cost of goods sold. Also called *gross margin*.

gross sales The total dollar amount of goods sold.

inflation An increase in price levels, often measured by the annual change in consumer or wholesale prices.

interest A sum paid or charged for the use of money or for borrowing money.

inventories In retailing, goods available for sale to the consumer.

inventory control The processes whereby managers determine the right quantity of various items to have on hand and keep track of these items' movement and use within the organization.

labor A factor of production, consisting of the human resources used to produce goods and services.

management The process of coordinating resources to meet an objective.

market A group of people who have needs to satisfy, money to spend, and the ability to buy.

market research Research that attempts to find out what products or services the consumer wants; what forms, colors, packaging, price ranges, and retail outlets the consumer prefers; and what types of advertising, public relations, and selling practices are most likely to appeal to the consumer.

market segmentation An approach to marketing in which the marketer splits the total market into smaller, more homogeneous groups, and aims production and selling strategies at these target markets.

markdown A reduction in the original retail selling price of an item.

market value The price of a good, service, or security as determined by demand and supply.

marketing That area of business that directs the flow of goods and services from producer to consumer to satisfy buyers and to achieve company objectives.

marketing concept The principle that stresses shaping products to meet consumer needs rather than attempting to mold those needs to the products.

marketing mix The blend of the five basic marketing activities (product, place, promotion, people, and price) that a business employs to reach its target market effectively.

markup The difference between the cost of an item and its selling price.

markup percentage The difference between an item's cost and its selling price, expressed as a percentage.

media All of the different means, including broadcasting and publications, by which information, or advertising, reaches its audience.

money Anything that is generally accepted as a means of paying for goods and services.

net income The actual profit or loss of a company, obtained by subtracting expenses from revenues.

net operating income Gross profit minus operating expenses.

net sales The figure obtained after discounts to customers are deducted from gross sales.

objectives Broad, long-term goals that provide direction for an organization.

operating expenses All the costs of business operations that are not included in costs of goods sold.

operating income The income left for a business after operating expenses are deducted from gross income.

organization A group of people with a common objective.

outdoor advertising Any public information about a company's products or services placed out of doors; includes skywriting and neon signs, but consists mainly of billboards and posters.

penetration pricing An approach to pricing in which the manufacturer introduces the product at a low price, planning to get back the initial investment through big sales.

personal income Total income from wages, salaries, receipts, dividends, rent, interest, and government payments to individuals.

personal selling Any personal communication between seller and buyer that is performed by salespeople operating inside or outside the company.

place The element of the marketing mix that involves finding appropriate channels of distribution, including retailing and wholesaling institutions, to get the product to the target market at the right time and in the right place.

planning Establishing objectives for an organization and determining the best way to accomplish these objectives.

plans The means by which an organization's objectives are achieved.

point-of-purchase (POP) display A device by which a product is displayed in such a way as to stimulate immediate sales.

policy A guideline established by management for a specific type of activity in an organization.

price The element of the marketing mix that involves establishing a monetary value for the product that gives value to the customer and adequate revenue to the producer; also, the money and goods exchanged for the ownership or use of some assortment of goods and services.

price discrimination The practice of charging customers different prices for products of like grade and quality.

price leader The producer who tends to set prices in an industry.

price fixing An arrangement among competitors to set prices at designated levels.

price stability An economic pattern in which prices change very little, on the average, overall.

pricing above the market An approach to pricing in which the marketer charges prices that are higher than those of competitors.

pricing below the market An approach to pricing in which the marketer charges prices that are below those of competitors.

pricing with the market An approach to pricing in which the marketer charges prices that match those of competitors.

product The element of the marketing mix that involves developing the right good (or service) for the target market; also, a physical item or service that satisfies certain customer needs.

product life cycle The stages of growth and decline in sales and earnings, through which most products go after they have been introduced in the marketplace.

product line The array of products offered for sale by a business.

product mix The list of all products offered by a seller.

profit The money left over from all sums a business has received from sales, after expenses have been deducted.

promotion Persuasive communication designed to sell products, services, or ideas to potential customers.

promotional mix A combination of advertising, personal selling, publicity, and sales promotion designed to communicate persuasively with the target market.

psychographics The study of the behavior or consumers of an individual level.

publicity Any information relating to a business, product, or services, that appears in any medium on a nonpaid basis.

receivables Money owed to a business.

recession A decline in the real gross national product (GNP) for two consecutive quarters.

retail selling Direct, face-to-face selling that takes place mostly in department and specialty stores.

retailer An establishment that purchases only consumer goods from manufacturers or wholesalers and sells them to ultimate consumers.

return on investment (ROI) The total return, or profit, obtained from a project divided by the amount of money invested in it.

revenue The financial receipts of a business.

risk management The process of reducing the threat of loss due to uncontrollable events.

rules Procedures covering a specific situation.

salary A method of compensation based on the amount of time the employee works, where the unit of time is a week, a month, or a year instead of merely an hour.

sales promotion Those marketing activities other than personal selling, advertising, and publicity that stimulate consumer purchasing and dealer effectiveness.

selling expenses The expenses a business incurs through marketing and distribution of the products it buys or makes for sale.

skimming A pricing method in which a manufacturer charges a high price during the introductory stage of a product and later reduces it when the product is no longer a novelty.

small business One that is independently owned and operated and is not dominant in its field.

target market The specific group or groups of customers to whom a company wishes to sell its products or services.

theory of supply and demand The theory that the supply of a product will rise when demand is great and fall when demand is low; also, that prices will be higher when supply is low, and lower when supply is great.

trading area The geographic region from which a business draws most of its customers and obtains most of its sales and revenues.

Appendix 5–2

Ballpark Estimate of Retirement Needs (Single Earner)

Planning for retirement is not a one-size-fits-all exercise. What follows is a simple, rough estimate to provide a basic idea of the savings you will need to make today for when you plan to retire. This simplifies some issues, such as projected Social Security benefits and earnings assumptions on savings. It reflects today's dollars; therefore, you will need to recalculate retirement needs annually and as your salary and circumstances change. It assumes also that your wages will increase in the future at the same rate as inflation.

Worksheet assumes you will realize a constant real rate of return of 3% and that wages will grow at the same rate as inflation.

1. How much annual income will you want in retirement? $_____

♦ Estimate 70 to 80% if most of your medical bills will be paid for, you don't plan to travel much, or are older and/or in your prime earning years, to maintain current standard of living.

♦ Estimate 80 to 90% if you must pay for medical costs above Medicare, plan to take some small trips, and know that you will need to continue to save some money.

♦ Estimate 100 to 120% if you need to cover all Medicare and other health costs, are younger and/or have prime earning years ahead of you, want a retirement lifestyle that is more than comfortable, and/or need to save for the possibility of long-term care.

2. Subtract the income you expect to receive annually from

Social Security (if you make $40,000+, enter $14,500)	– $_____
Traditional employer pension (in today's dollars)	– $_____
Part-time income	– $_____
Other (reverse annuity mortgage payments, earnings on assets, etc.)	– $_____
This is how much is needed to make up for each retirement year	= $_____

3. To determine the amount you will need to save, multiply the amount you need to make up (2) by the factor below.
   Estimate of how much you will need in the bank the day you retire.

Age You Expect to Retire	Choose Your Factor Based on Life Expectancy (at age 65)					
	Male, 50th Percentile (age 82)	Female, 50th Percentile (age 86)	Male, 75th Percentile (age 89)	Female, 75th Percentile (age 92)	Male, 90th Percentile (age 94)	Female, 90th Percentile (age 97)
55	18.79	20.53	21.71	22.79	23.46	24.40
60	16.31	18.32	19.68	20.93	21.71	22.79
65	13.45	15.77	17.35	18.79	19.68	20.93
70	10.15	12.83	14.65	16.31	17.35	18.79

$_____

4. If you expect to retire before age 65, multiple your Social Security benefit in (2) by the following factor.

Age you expect to retire:	55 years	Your factor is:	8.8
	60 years		4.7

+ $_____

5. Multiply your savings to date by the factor below (include money accumulated in a 401(k), individual retirement account (IRA), or similar retirement plan).

If you want to retire in:	10 years	Your factor is:	1.3
	15 years		1.6
	20 years		1.8
	25 years		2.1
	30 years		2.4
	35 years		2.8
	40 years		3.3

– $_____

Total additional savings needed at retirement: = $_____

Don't panic. Another formula to show you how much to save each year to reach your goal amount is below. This factors in compounding interest.

6. To determine the annual amount you will need to save, multiply the total amount by the factor below.

If you want to retire in:		Your factor is:	
10 years			.085
15 years			.052
20 years			.036
25 years			.027
30 years			.020
35 years			.016
40 years			.013
			= $_____

Appendix 5–3

Marketing Action Plan: Market Analysis

1. Market Definition

Define the geographical market you serve.

Use zip codes, cities, counties, or multiple counties if in a sparsely populated area. Include only those places that account for at least 5 to 10% of your current client base or those places from which you draw at least 10% of your new clients. An example is shown.

Market	Zip Code	City	County	Multiple Counties
Example 1.	85351			
Example 2.		Fountain Hills		
Example 3.			Yavapai	
Example 4.				Cochise/Havasu (AZ)
5.				
6.				
7.				
8.				

2. Market Size

What is the size of your market?

a. Population

Use zip code, city, or county(ies).
(samples)

	Sample	Population
Example 1.	85351	31,737
Example 2.	Fountain Hills	11,999
3.		
4.		
5.		
6.		
7.		
8.		
Example TOTAL		43,736

b. Hearing aid sales

List all competitors in your geographical market. Guesstimate their average monthly unit sales of hearing aids. Total these averages to estimate the monthly unit sales. Multiply this number by 12, to estimate total annual unit sales. An example is shown.

	Your Office		Traditional Dispensers	Dispensing Audiologists	Medical Facilities
Example 1	20	a.	15	20	12
Example 2		b.	25		
		c.			

	d. _____	_____	_____
	e. _____	_____	_____
	f. _____	_____	_____
	g. _____	_____	_____
Total (example)	240	480	240	144
				120

This process can be repeated to determine the total market volume for audiological procedures, surgeries, etc., if this information is important to your practice and planning.

Total	1224

Example

3. Market Growth

a. Is your market's population:

    Growing? ❏   Shrinking? ❏   By what %? _____

Why? _____

_____

What are the long-term growth prospects for your market? _____

_____

b. Is your market's total hearing aid sales volume:

    Growing? ❏   Shrinking? ❏   By what %? _____

Why? _____

_____

c. What are the long-term growth prospects for your market?

_____

4.   Market Conditions

a. What market conditions are currently affecting your business (population, economic cycles, socioeconomic conditions)? (Check those that apply.)

Economic
- ❏ Unemployment
- ❏ Plant openings, closings
- ❏ Cost of living
- ❏ Interest rates
- ❏ Inflation

Social
- ❏ Crime
- ❏ Senior services
- ❏ Health care services: availability, accessibility
- ❏ Transportation
- ❏ Accessibility of cultural, social, sports activities

Environmental
- ❏ Pollution
- ❏ Weather extremes
- ❏ Natural disasters
- ❏ Probability of future natural disasters
- ❏ Environmental ambience
- ❏ Proximity of parks, open space, vacation sites

Government
- ❏ Senior services
- ❏ Taxation
- ❏ Licensing laws

b. What market conditions are likely to affect your business in the next 3 to 5 years (population, economic cycles, socioeconomic conditions)? (Check those that apply.)

Economic
- ❏ Unemployment
- ❏ Plant openings, closings
- ❏ Cost of living
- ❏ Interest rates
- ❏ Inflation

Social
- ❏ Crime
- ❏ Senior services
- ❏ Taxation

Environmental
- ❏ Pollution
- ❏ Weather extremes
- ❏ Natural disasters
- ❏ Probability of future natural disasters
- ❏ Environmental ambience
- ❏ Proximity of parks, open space, vacation sites

Government
- ❏ Senior services
- ❏ Health care services: availability, accessibility
- ❏ Licensing laws
- ❏ Transportation
- ❏ Accessibility of cultural, social, sports activities

c. What can you do to minimize the ill effects of negative events or conditions? How can you take advantage of positive events or conditions?

5. Age and Income Demographics for Your Market

What are the age and income demographics for your market (from available demographics data)? Examples are shown.

Zip Code, City, or County	45–64 (%)	65–84 (%)	45+ (%)	65+ (%)	85+ (%)	Median Age	Median Income	Nat'l/Stat Centile
USA	19.3	11.4	32.0	12.7	1.3	33.7	$33,900	
Arizona	18.0	12.2	31.4	13.4	1.2	32.9	$29,833	
85351	11.0	68.0	68.0	83.0	15.0	76.1	$27,151	45 / 51
Fountain Hills	24.2	17.7	17.7	18.2	0.5	40.2	$44,946	89 / 91
Yavapai	23.5	25.0	25.0	27.0	2.0	45.4	$21,493	18 / 9
Cochise/Havasu	20.2	22.4	22.4	83.0	2.3	41.1	$20,725	15 / 26

Appendix 5–4

Marketing Action Plan: Determining Your Competitive Advantage

1. Competitive Profile

a. List all competitors in your market (within a certain distance, area, or market profile).

b. Place an asterisk next to the names of your key competitors (those who are a substitute for you in your served market).

c. Note the ownership, type of business, and professional credentials of your key competitors (*Ownership* = sole proprietor, MD, investor, corporation, hospital, multisite chain, major company, government, etc. *Type of business* = MD, clinic, health maintenance organization (HMO), hospital, private practice, hearing aid dispensary, franchise, retail store. *Professional credentials* = audiologist, hearing aid specialist, MD, etc.).

	Name	Location	Ownership/Type	Credentials
Example 1.	*Audiology Associates	5 miles	Private practice	Audiologist
2.				
3.				
4.				
5.				
6.				
7.				
8.				

2. Competitive Intensity

Total number of competitors _____

Market size (population) _____

Population per office _____

> **Example:**
> Total number of competitors = 8
> Market size = 250,000
> Population per office = 31,250

3. Competitive Performance Analysis

Estimate all competitors' unit sales per month, market share, growth (compared with overall market), and client base. Add revenue if you are able to estimate it.

	Name	Unit Sales (Hearing Aids)	Market Share (%)	Growth (+ or −)	Client Base (Active Users)
Example 1.	Audiology Associates	30	25	+	1000
2.					
3.					
4.					
5.					
6.					
7.					
8.					
9.					
10.					
11.					
12.					
13.					
TOTALS					
	# Competitors	Aids per Month	100%	+ or −	# Customers

4. Market Potential

Market size (population) _____

Hard-of-hearing (HOH) population (9.4% of total) _____

40% of HOH population _____

60% of HOH population _____

Example:
Market size = 250,000
HOH (9.4% of total) = 23,500
Of the HOH total, what percentage do you believe are potential purchasers?

20% = 4700
40% = 9400
50% = 11,750
60% = 14,100

5. Market Penetration

Cumulative total of client bases _____

Market size (population) _____

Hard-of-hearing (HOH) _____

population (9.4% of total)

Population per office _____

Example:
Client base = total customers from #2
Market size = 250,000
HOH (9.4%) = 23,500
Population per office = 31,250

6. Competitive Strengths and Weaknesses

Assess key competitors' strengths and weaknesses. Use + for strength and − for weakness.

Competitor A
❏ Client Base
  ❏ Size
  ❏ Location
  ❏ Income
❏ Finances
  ❏ Assets
  ❏ Creditworthiness
  ❏ Cash

Competitor B
❏ Client Base
  ❏ Size
  ❏ Location
  ❏ Income
❏ Finances
  ❏ Assets
  ❏ Creditworthiness
  ❏ Cash

Competitor C
❏ Client Base
  ❏ Size
  ❏ Location
  ❏ Income
❏ Finances
  ❏ Assets
  ❏ Creditworthiness
  ❏ Cash

<table>
<tr><td>

❑ Technology
  ❑ Test Equipment
  ❑ Programmable Hearing Aids
  ❑ Computerized Office
❑ Knowledge, Skills
  ❑ Hearing Aids
  ❑ Audiology
  ❑ Counseling
  ❑ Sales
  ❑ Service
❑ Communication Skills
❑ Credentials
❑ Reputation
❑ Visibility, Name Recognition
❑ Marketing Communications
❑ Office
  ❑ Location
  ❑ Decor

</td><td>

❑ Technology
  ❑ Test Equipment
  ❑ Programmable Hearing Aids
  ❑ Computerized Office
❑ Knowledge, Skills
  ❑ Hearing Aids
  ❑ Audiology
  ❑ Counseling
  ❑ Sales
  ❑ Service
❑ Communication Skills
❑ Credentials
❑ Reputation
❑ Visibility, Name Recognition
❑ Marketing Communications
❑ Office
  ❑ Location
  ❑ Decor

</td><td>

❑ Technology
  ❑ Test Equipment
  ❑ Programmable Hearing Aids
  ❑ Computerized Office
❑ Knowledge, Skills
  ❑ Hearing Aids
  ❑ Audiology
  ❑ Counseling
  ❑ Sales
  ❑ Service
❑ Communication Skills
❑ Credentials
❑ Reputation
❑ Visibility, Name Recognition
❑ Marketing Communications
❑ Office
  ❑ Location
  ❑ Decor

</td></tr>
</table>

COMPETITIVE ADVANTAGE   **COMPETITIVE ADVANTAGE**   **COMPETITIVE ADVANTAGE**

| ❑ Cost Structure ❑ Timing ❑ Focus ❑ Differentiation — Ⓐ | ❑ Cost Structure ❑ Timing ❑ Focus ❑ Differentiation — Ⓑ | ❑ Cost Structure ❑ Timing ❑ Focus ❑ Differentiation — Ⓒ |

7. Your Strengths and Weaknesses

Business Assessment. Assess your strengths and weaknesses. Use + for strength and − for weakness.

+   −

_____ _____   ❑ Client Base
_____ _____   ❑ Size
_____ _____   ❑ Location
_____ _____   ❑ Income
_____ _____   ❑ Finances
_____ _____   ❑ Assets
_____ _____   ❑ Creditworthiness
_____ _____   ❑ Cash
_____ _____   ❑ Technology
_____ _____   ❑ Test Equipment
_____ _____   ❑ Programmable Hearing Aids
_____ _____   ❑ Computerized Office
_____ _____   ❑ Knowledge, Skills
_____ _____   ❑ Hearing Aids
_____ _____   ❑ Audiology
_____ _____   ❑ Counseling
_____ _____   ❑ Sales
_____ _____   ❑ Service
_____ _____   ❑ Communication Skills
_____ _____   ❑ Credentials
_____ _____   ❑ Reputation
_____ _____   ❑ Visibility, Name Recognition
_____ _____   ❑ Marketing Communications
_____ _____   ❑ Office
_____ _____   ❑ Location
_____ _____   ❑ Decor

```
_____  _____
_____  _____
_____  _____
_____  _____
_____  _____
```

Competitive Advantage
❏ Cost Structure
❏ Timing
❏ Focus
❏ Differentiation

Total ════════ ════════

How do you rank your competitive situation? Are you positive or negative on these? Add these up to obtain your totals.

8. Competitive Advantage

Describe your current and planned competitive advantage using the following categories.

❏ Cost
❏ Focus
❏ Timing
❏ Differentiation

Based on these, how is your competitive advantage relative to:

Value? _____

_____

_____

Uniqueness? _____

_____

_____

Sustainability? _____

_____

_____

Defensibility? _____

_____

_____

Competitive Analysis					
	Competitor A	**Competitor B**	**Competitor C**	**Competitor D**	**Competitor E**
Competitive Environment					
a. Estimated unit sales, hearing aids					
b. Estimated $ custom-molded aids					
c. Estimated % noncustom aids					
d. Market share trends					
Success Factors					
a. Product quality					
b. Product reliability					
c. Product price					
d. Product recognition					
e. Company image					
f. Product breadth of line					
g. Market coverage sales					
h. Effectiveness					
i. Location					
j. Buyer–seller relationship					
k.					

l.					
m.					
Major Strength					
Major Weakness					
Strategy					

9. Marketing Strategies of Competitors

1. Describe the current *product strategies* employed by primary competitors.
   Competitor A _____

   _____

   Competitor B _____

   _____

   Competitor C _____

   _____

2. Describe the current *pricing strategies* employed by primary competitors.
   Competitor A _____

   _____

   Competitor B _____

   _____

   Competitor C _____

   _____

3. Describe the current *distribution strategies* employed by primary competitors.
   Competitor A _____

   _____

   Competitor B _____

   _____

   Competitor C _____

   _____

4. Describe the current *advertising strategies* employed by primary competitors.
   Competitor A _____

   _____

   Competitor B _____

   _____

   Competitor C _____

   _____

5. Describe the current *sales promotion strategies* employed by primary competitors.
   Competitor A _____

   _____

   Competitor B _____

   _____

   Competitor C _____

   _____

References

Adams, P., & Hardy, A. (1989). Current estimates from the National Health Interview Survey: United States (Vital and Health Statistics, series 10, No. 173). Hyattsville, MD: National Center for Health Statistics.

American Savings Education Council. (2005). Fact sheet. Retrieved December 12, 2005, from http://www.asec.org

Antitrust laws policy guide. (1988). Santa Monica, CA: Lear Siegler.

Berkowitz, A. (1992). Advertising to fulfill the marketing plan. In W. Staab (Ed.), Applied hearing instrument marketing (pp. 165–185). Livonia, MI: National Institute for Hearing Instruments Studies.

Centers for Disease Control and Prevention. (2001). Retrieved May 7, 2007, from http://www.cdc.gov/nchs/data/hus/tables/2003/03hus027.pdf.

Davis, G. (2005). Television advertising for small business and professionals. Retrieved May 3, 2007, from http://www.television advertising. com

Epromotional Products and Gifts. Statistics show the following why customers leave. Retrieved May 15, 2007, from http://www.epromotionalproductsandgifts.com/loyalty.aspx

ESRI Business Information Solutions. (2005). Retrieved May 3, 2007, from http:// www.esribis.com

Federal Trade Commission, Retrieved May 13, 2007. Promoting Competition, Protecting Consumers: A plain English guide to antitrust laws. http://www.ftc.gov/bc/compguide.

Gentile, A. (1975). Persons with impaired hearing, United States, 1971 (Vital and Health Statistics, series 10, No. 101, DHEW Publication No. [HRA] 76–1528). Washington, DC: U.S. Government Printing Office.

Glorig, A., & Nixon, J. (1960). Distribution of hearing loss in various populations. Annals of Otology, Rhinology and Laryngology, 69, 497–516.

Goldstein, D. (1984). Hearing impairment, hearing aids, and audiology. ASHA, 27, 24–31, 34–35, 38.

Green Dot Advertising and Marketing. (2007). Newspaper advertising. Retrieved May 2, 2007, from http://www.greendotonline.net/newspaperads.html

Hearing Industries Association. (1984). A market research study of the U.S. hearing-impaired population. Washington, DC: Author.

Hosford-Dunn, H., Dunn, D. R., & Harford, E. R. (1995a). Marketing. In Audiology business and practice management (pp. 295–319). San Diego, CA: Singular Publishing Group.

Hosford-Dunn, H., Dunn, D. R., & Harford, E. R. (1995b). Pricing. In Audiology business and practice management (pp. 295–319). San Diego, CA: Singular Publishing Group.

Jatho, K. (1969). Population surveys and norms. International Audiology, 8, 231–239.

Jelonek, S. (1992a). Conducting a market analysis. In W. Staab (Ed), Applied hearing instrument marketing (pp. 35–58). Livonia, MI: National Institute for Hearing Instruments Studies.

Jelonek, S. (1992b). The importance of good marketing programs. In W. Staab (Ed.), Applied hearing instrument marketing (pp. 59–88). Livonia, MI: National Institute for Hearing Instruments Studies.

Jelonek, S., & Staab, W. J. (1994). The hearing aid office as a marketing tool. Hearing Instruments, 45(4), 27–28, 30.

Kochkin, S. (2005). MarkeTrak VII. Hearing Review, 12(7), 16–29.

Malthouse, E., & Calder, B. (2002). Measuring newspaper readership: A qualitative variable approach. International Journal on Media Management, 4(4), 248–260.

McKenna, R. (1986). The Regis touch. In New marketing strategies for uncertain times (pp. 7–15). New York: Addison-Wesley.

Miles, A. W. (1986). Pricing. In Perspectives marketing series (pp. 1–5). Boston: Boston Consulting Group.

Moscicki, E. K., Elkins, E. F., Baum, H. M., & McNamara, P. M. (1985). Hearing loss in the elderly: An epidemiologic study of the Framingham Heart Study Cohort. Ear and Hearing, 6, 184–190.

Moses, J. (2003). Frequency is the key to advertising success. National Federation of Independent Business. Retrieved May 3, 2007, from http://www.nfib. com/object/3985727.html

National Center for Health Statistics. (1980). Basic data on hearing levels of adults 25–74 years, United States, 1971–1975 (Vital and Health Statistics, series 11, No. 215, DHEW Pub. No. [PHS] 80–1663). Hyattsville, MD: Author.

National Center for Health Statistics. (1981). Prevalence of selected impairments, United States, 1977 (DHEW Pub. No. [PHS] 82–1562). Hyattsville, MD: Author.

National Center for Health Statistics. (2007). Retrieved May 5, 2007, from http://www.cdc/nchs/fastats/lifexpec.html

National Federation of Independent Business (NFIB). (2002). Education Foundation survey. Retrieved May 7, 2007, from http://www.nfibonline.com

National Health Interview Survey. (1977). Hearing ability of persons by sociodemographic and health characteristics: United States (Vital and Health Statistics series 10, No. 140 (8/82)). Hyattsville, MD: National Center for Health Statistics.

108th Congress. (2004, October). Report by the House Small Business Committee. In Small business record. Washington, DC: U.S. Government Printing Office.

Ries, P. (1982). Hearing ability of persons by sociodemographic and health statistics (Vital and Health Statistics, series 10, No. 140, DHHS Pub. No. [PHS] 82–1568). Washington, DC: U.S. Government Printing Office.

Roberts, J. (1968). Hearing status in examination findings among adults, United States, 1960–1962 (Vital and Health Statistics, series 11, No. 99, DHEW Publication No. 1000). Washington, DC: U.S. Government Printing Office.

Settle, R. B., & Alreck, P. L. (1989, January). Reducing buyers' sense of risk. Marketing Communications, pp. 34–39.

Small Business Notes. (2007). About small business. Retrieved May 15, 2007, from http://www.smallbusinessnotes.com/aboutsb.html

Staab, W. J. (1986). Hearing aid dispensing. In W. Hodgson (Ed.), Hearing aid assessment and use in audiologic habilitation (3rd ed., pp. 266–300). Baltimore: Williams & Wilkins.

Staab, W. J. (1990). Marketing hearing aids—an overview. In C. Killingsworth (Ed.), Directions in marketing audiology: Turning up the volume. Chicago: Academy of Dispensing Audiologists.

Staab, W. J. (1992). Sales promotion for office traffic control. In W. Staab (Ed.), Applied hearing instrument marketing (pp. 201–254). Livonia, MI: National Institute for Hearing Instruments Studies.

Staab, W. J. (2003). Hearing aids: A user's guide (3rd ed). Phoenix, AZ: Wayne J. Staab Publisher.

Staab, W. J., & Jelonek, S. (1994a). Are you finding your competitive advantage? Hearing Instruments, 45(7), 20–21.

Staab, W. J., & Jelonek, S. (1994b). Building professional marketing skills. Presented at Towards 2000: Hearing Aid Marketing Workshop, Phoenix, AZ.

Staab, W. J., & Jelonek, S. (1995a, January–March). Reducing hearing aid purchasers' sense of risk. Audecibel, pp. 19–25.

Staab, W. J., & Jelonek, S. (1995b). Building professional marketing skills. Presented at Towards 2000: Hearing Aid Marketing Workshop, Phoenix, AZ.

Strom, K. (2001). The HR 2001 Dispenser Survey. Hearing Review, 8(6), 20–22, 24–25, 28–32, 36–37, 40, 42.

Strom K. (2004). The HR 2004 Dispenser Survey. Hearing Review, 6(11), pp. 14–35.

Strom, K. (2005). Personal communication, December 6, 2005.

Study: 2020 begins age of the elderly. (1996, May 21). USA Today, p. 4A.

Sweep, D. (2002). MORI online survey of 11,000 adults. Retrieved May 5, 2007, from http://www.mori.com

The Marketing Edge, Hearing Industries Association, Washington, D.C.

U.S. Census Bureau (2001). Population projections of the United States, by age, sex, race, and hispanic origin: 1993 to 2050 (Series P25–1104). Washington, DC: U.S. Government Printing Office.

U.S. Census Bureau. (2004). Current population reports. Population projections of the United States by age, sex, race, and hispanic origin: 1995 to 2050 (Series P 25–1130). Washington, DC: U.S. Government Printing Office.

U.S. Census Bureau. (2004). U.S. interim projections by age, sex, race, and Hispanic origin. Retrieved May 5, 2007, from http://www.sba.gov/aboutsba/sbastats.html

U.S. Census Bureau. (2005). Population statistics: Projections of the United States by age, sex, and race: 1983–2080 (Series P-25, No. 952). Washington, DC: U.S. Government Printing Office.

U.S. Department of Health and Human Services. (1988). Aging America: Trends and projections, 1987–88. Washington, DC: U.S. Government Printing Office.

U.S. Life Expectancy 1900–1960. Retrieved May 5, 2007, from http://www.nsf.gov/news/speeches/colwell/rc02_asm_keynote

Wilder, C. (1975). Prevalence of selected impairments, U.S., 1971 (Vital and Health Statistics, series 10, No. 99, DHEW Pub. No. [HRA] 75–1526). Washington, DC: U.S. Government Printing Office.

Williams, P. (1984). Hearing loss: Information for professionals in the aging network. Washington, DC: NICD/ASHA, Gallaudet College.

Chapter 6

Private Practice Issues

Teresa M. Clark and Darcy Benson

Practicing audiology in the private sector is akin to parenting: until we actually do it, it is difficult to understand how broad the task is. And like parenting, we seldom feel we have been adequately trained. A general guide, whether for developing parenting skills or for starting a private practice in audiology, can give some idea of what to anticipate. That is the goal of this chapter. And just like children with their own identities, visions, and desires, so too are private practices. The building and running of a private practice often sends one into regions far from the familiar clinical experience. It is a frustrating, exhilarating, and incredibly rewarding experience. Though each practice is different in terms of personality, context, and style, there are several issues that are common to all of them.

This chapter is directed to audiologists who are considering starting up private practices and need general information on what that entails. Those clinicians already engaged in private practice know these issues all too well. The other chapters in this volume deal with specific areas of practice management. It is hoped that this chapter will provide a broader view of private practice issues and serve as a springboard to an understanding of the information found elsewhere in this volume.

This chapter explores the defining aspects of a private practice and briefly touches on a multitude of issues that are important to running an efficient, successful practice. It begins with a definition of private practice and a discussion of the development of the underlying values and goals. Different ways of acquiring practices and the necessary resources required to purchase and run a practice are addressed. A section on how to create an image and develop and maintain a good reputation follows. More specific topics are then explored: equipment needs, staffing, and organizational systems necessary for running a private practice. Business issues are tackled next, including marketing, establishing relationships with vendors, managing the practice's cash flow, and introducing new sources of revenue. The chapter concludes with a review of trends in private practice.

◆ Defining Private Practice

A private practice is a professional organization that functions independently of any larger institution. The organization accomplishes objectives, seeks knowledge, and provides vocations and avocations (see Chapter 1). In a private audiology practice, one or more clinicians come together to form a professional organization and take responsibility for defining all aspects of how the organization will function with regard to patient care, fiscal management, marketing management, human resources, and ethical standards. Under these primary categories are more specific issues that must be defined, to put in motion the practice of audiology in such an organization.

The roots of audiology private practice are in the medical model of private practice. Audiology private practice is often a unique melding of diagnostic and rehabilitative services, together with a retail establishment that sells products. The audiologist works as the health care provider, rendering services to the patients of the practice and in many cases fitting products that improve and/or protect hearing. Front office personnel take phone calls, schedule appointments, accept payments for services and products, and manage a myriad of other details.

There are some defining parameters to private practice, common to all. A private practice is an entity, an independent institution that allows the health care practitioner (i.e., the audiologist) to provide services for his or her population (i.e., persons with hearing and/or balance disorders) and receive direct payment for these services. It is a combination of both a professional enterprise and a business endeavor. The owner of a private practice invests his or her own time and money, carries the power of decision making without outside intervention, and has ultimate responsibility for the outcome. The enterprise shows that the owner is not only an autonomous professional but also an autonomous businessperson. No one else shoulders the burden; the owner controls the bottom line.

The most common type of audiology practice is the hearing center, which provides diagnostic hearing evaluations aimed primarily at individuals with hearing impairment who need or are interested in amplification systems and/or rehabilitative services. Many offices also provide a range of diagnostic services to support medical doctors in the area and perhaps even specialized diagnostic services for the evaluation of the central auditory system. A smaller number of practices provide diagnostic services only. Balance centers, which offer diagnostic and rehabilitation services, have been experiencing rapid growth at the time of this writing. The 2005 Compensation and Benefits Study by the American Academy of Audiology (AAA, 2005) shows the breakdown of audiologists by setting, with 19% of the survey respondents being in a private audiology practice (**Fig. 6–1**).

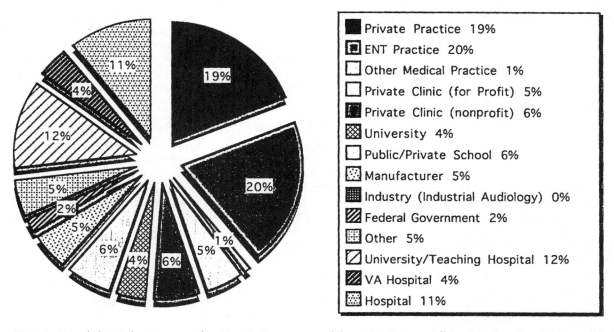

Figure 6–1 Audiologists by primary work setting. ENT, ear, nose, and throat; VA, Veterans Affairs. From American Academy of Audiology. (2005). Compensation and benefits survey.)

Many private practice audiologists look outside the traditional core of hearing and balance services for ways to expand their practice and market their services to the nonimpaired population at large. Some audiologists have explored the world of occupational and nonoccupational audiology, providing services to the music industry (e.g., in-ear monitors and musicians' earplugs) and/or to individuals whose leisure activities put them at risk for hearing impairment (e.g., skeet shooters and hunters). Other professionals might provide services to individuals who use communication devices on the job (e.g., monitors for security personnel and anchorpersons) or to the general public looking to customize their personal devices (e.g., cell phones, MP3 players, and personal digital assistants [PDAs]). The area of hearing conservation for industry provides an avenue for audiologists to expand into the world of occupational audiology.

Other audiologists augment their practice by engaging in clinical research projects with manufacturers in the hearing health care industry. Additionally, these audiologists may act as educational trainers, introducing new concepts and products to other audiologists. Some also are sales consultants for the hearing health care industry on a part-time basis.

The private practice model is helping to further define the audiologist as an autonomous health care practitioner. To gain autonomy, the profession "must have a large viable independent private practice component. This is mandatory in order to gain and maintain autonomy and equality in the health care system" (Harford, 1993, p. 11). Increasing the autonomy of audiology and having a greater number of audiologists with doctor of audiology (Au.D.) degrees are stepping-stones in the quest to become limited license practitioners in the coming years.

The world of private practice offers the audiologist a variety of avenues to provide services and products to different populations. In fact, there are probably as many different private practice settings as there are audiologists in private practice.

♦ Developing a Vision of the Private Practice

Core Ideology

There are certain principles that are basic to a successful private practice, and to other hearing health organizations. These principles in turn define the vision, mission, and values of the practice (mission statement and practice philosophy). The organizational values set the tone for the practice and influence every aspect of it, from patient care to human resources to marketing. These organizational values have been described as the "core ideology" of an organization (Collins and Porras, 1996). The core ideology is key to success, as it "defines the enduring character of an organization," and it "is the glue that holds an organization together through time" (Collins and Porras, 1996, p. 66). The core ideology of the practice should not change over time, as it is

Table 6–1 Core Ideology, Goals, and Vision

Core Values
Honesty
Integrity
Patients' needs come first

Core Purpose
To improve the quality of life for the patients served
To provide excellence in the delivery of hearing and balance care

Goals
To have gross receipts of $500,000 in 5 years
To add balance remediation services
To develop a strong referral base from primary care physicians

Long-Term Vision
To have three locations throughout the county
To be known as the authority in hearing and balance care in the local area

a reflection of the values of the owner. The owner must ensure that the employees who work in the practice know and understand the practice's core ideology and agree to uphold the practice's philosophy in the course of working in the practice.

Fundamental to the core ideology is the practice's core values and purpose. The core values are the practice's "small set of timeless guiding principles" and the "essential and enduring tenets" of the practice (Collins and Porras, 1996, p. 66). The core purpose is the practice's reason for being. No matter how large or small, the practice's core values and purpose must be outlined and upheld, ideally by all persons who are involved with the practice (**Table 6–1**).

The practice's core ideology must exist before the actual creation of the practice. Ideally, these values are given in the practice's written mission statement and are incorporated into the business plan. The mission statement outlines the practice's mission, its fundamental purpose, and its sole reason for being. It affirms what the organization is, what it does, what it stands for, and why it exists. The practice, like any business, is built around its mission statement.

Goals and Long-Term Vision

From the core values, purpose, and mission, the envisioned future of the practice is outlined. This includes the long-term vision and the goals of the practice. The long-term vision may initially be difficult to define, but it should include the "dreams, hopes, and aspirations" (Collins and Porras, 1996, p. 73) of the owner. The goals should succinctly articulate what the private practice owner hopes to accomplish and should be "clear and compelling . . . the focal point of effort . . . a catalyst for team spirit" (Collins and Porras, 1996, p. 73). The goals may also include the mechanisms that will be used to reach them. They should be clear so that the practice owner can determine when the organization has achieved these goals. The goals of the practice may be influenced by many internal and external factors and, in contrast to core ideology, may change over time as goals are reached.

The professional expertise and preferences of the owner, and in some cases, the employees, will influence the goals. Questions such as the following should be answered: Is the owner's interest primarily in diagnostics, hearing conservation, hearing rehabilitation via amplification, or in balance remediation? Will diagnostics be limited to a battery of basic tests or include more specialized testing, such as auditory brainstem response (ABR) and videonystagmography (VNG)? Does the owner prefer to serve a broad range of ages or focus on children or on adults?

The constraints of the practice, such as financial reserves, location, space, and equipment, will affect its goals. Diagnostic services are influenced by how much room is available for specialized diagnostic equipment. The number of patients that can be seen is determined by how many treatment rooms are available. The ability to serve multiply handicapped patients is affected by the accessibility of wheelchair ramps, elevators and other accommodations required by the Americans with Disabilities Act.

The population the owner wishes to serve and how it is served affect where the private practice is located. A practice whose mission is to provide diagnostic services should be established in a location that has a large physician base for referrals. A practice whose goal is to serve children should be located in a community of young families, or near a children's hospital. Offices that wish to dispense hearing devices to older adults should be located near retirement communities.

It is the core ideology and goals of a private practice that establish its uniqueness. The practice takes on a persona of its own, reflecting the personality and values of the owner. The core ideology is transferred to the support and professional staff, and is reflected in their interaction with the patients and in the day-to-day operation of the office. It is this individuality that establishes the identity of a practice and separates competitive practices from each other. The services provided by various offices may be similar, but the personae of the offices may be very different from one to the other. These factors related to core ideology can determine the success of a private practice, as the people in the community ultimately will decide which practices are most suited to their needs.

The goals of a successful practice also may change over time. As the practitioners broaden their skill levels and as more capital is available for equipment purchases, other services may be added. Changes in the managed care arena alter the kinds of services and products provided and thus influence the practice's goals. In a field so closely tied to advances in technology, rapid technological changes provide new ways to address problems and find solutions, thereby influencing the practice's goals.

A shift in interest areas may also contribute to a change in goals. Private practice owners may develop an interest in related areas, such as business solutions and marketing techniques. The methods that have proved to be profitable for them are repackaged and marketed to their colleagues (e.g., patient newsletters and aural rehabilitation materials). Practice owners may become cogent negotiators in the managed care arena and contract their time in assisting other colleagues in obtaining managed care contracts. These ancillary business activities are performed within the boundaries of the private practice, providing new sources of revenue for the business.

Practice Goals and the Community

Each community has its own blend of people and needs. The community in which the practice is established affects the goals of the practice by influencing what the practice does and does not offer. Practices located in poor urban neighborhoods, for example, must consider taking third-party reimbursement, such as Medicaid, to serve the community better. As another example, providing a hearing conservation program might be considered in areas with a lot of factories.

Not only does the community shape the private practice goals, but the practice also becomes a part of the community that it serves. The owner, as an audiologist, becomes a part of the medical and nonmedical health care community by providing audiology services at physicians' offices, medical clinics, and hospitals and in nursing home facilities. The owner, as a professional colleague, becomes part of the local audiology community by belonging to regional and state audiology organizations, and, as an audiology advocate, can influence local and state regulations and legislation that affect the profession. The owner, as a businessperson, becomes part of the business community by joining the local chamber of commerce, for instance, and provides support to other businesses. Joining volunteer civic organizations such as Rotary International and Sertoma International allows the owner to become part of the service community. Being active in business and civic groups serves more than one purpose. For a young practice, it helps in establishing relationships with other businesses (banking institutions, insurance agencies, local media, etc.) and can be a valuable source of referrals to the practice. Also, by establishing a solid relationship with these groups, the owner demonstrates support for the community and as a professional sends a message that he or she believes in public service. The patients of the practice will have a high level of confidence that the owner is not only an audiology professional but also a responsible member of the community.

The Business Plan

Once the core ideology, goals, and long-term vision of the practice are defined, they are incorporated into the practice's business plan. The business plan is a written document that clearly articulates how the practice's business activities are envisioned and how they are to be performed. It is a concise description that begins with the practice's mission and then spells out in detail the services and products that will be provided. The plan includes a description of the target market and the population to be served, the marketing plan, an outline of operations, a description of the short-term goals and long-term vision, a financial analysis with financial projections, a risk assessment, and an overall schedule. The mission and activities described in the business plan should be consistent with the owner's core ideology as originally defined. (For more information on writing a business plan, see Chapter 13.)

Ethics in Private Practice

Any private practice is a blend of providing professional services and making a living by operating a business. Both endeavors must be considered high priorities. An audiologist may provide high-quality professional care, but if equal attention is not paid to the business aspect of the practice, the success of the practice could be jeopardized. A private practice audiologist who dispenses hearing devices engages in retail sales within the framework of a professional practice. The practice owner must understand the difficulty in striking a balance between the need to "serve the hearing impaired public in the highest ethical manner and still make good business decisions" (Metz, 2000, p. 73). Sound business practices, patient needs, and professional goals can at times be in conflict. When conflicts do occur, the private practice owner may find that models of ethical decision making provide much needed assistance in resolving them (Bernstein, 2000). A clear understanding of the practice's core ideology, goals, and vision is also imperative in bringing the various components into harmony. (For a further discussion of ethics, see Chapter 2.)

◆ Considerations in Opening a Private Practice

There are many ways to start up private practice. Many audiologists do this by assembling all of the necessary tools of the trade (or at least the bare minimum) and developing a patient base over time. Unfortunately, this approach can leave the owner without sufficient revenue in the first few years to cover overhead costs and earn a small profit. In the United States, one estimate is that 90% of small businesses fail within the first 5 years (Kiyosaki, 2005).

Other audiologists looking to start a private practice find that buying an existing practice is easier, providing an instant patient base and an immediate influx of revenue (a so-called turnkey business, or one that is ready for immediate use). Many of the practices that audiologists purchase are not audiology practices per se, but hearing aid retail stores founded by hearing aid dealers who are trained to fit and sell hearing aids. When hearing aid dealers retire, many of them sell their practices to audiologists. Diagnostic testing and rehabilitative services are then added to the dispensing services the offices provide.

A less common way for an audiologist to go into private practice is to inherit a practice from a family member. Perhaps a parent who was an audiologist or hearing aid dealer encouraged his or her children to pursue the field of audiology as preparation for taking over the family business. Another avenue for getting into private practice is to become a junior partner in an established practice, with a partnership buy-in over time. Senior audiologists in private practice who are ready to retire look for potential partners to buy into their businesses or to buy them out completely. Still others initiate partnerships with audiologists or other medical or health care professionals, sharing the cost of space and equipment. When looking to partner with medical or other professionals, audiologists need to be mindful of the federal and state laws that govern such arrangements. These include federal antikickback statutes, which govern the exchange of patient referrals; the Stark laws, which restrict the referral of patients to a designated health service with which the physician has a financial relationship; so-called safe harbor regulations, which clarify business practices that are and are not acceptable under law; and HIPAA regulation for handling patient information.

Thus, the primary ways to get into private practice are to start out on one's own, to purchase one, to inherit one, to partner with other professionals, and to buy into an existing practice. The approach chosen often is related to financial resources and constraints, either real or perceived.

When starting up in private practice, the audiologist will need to enlist the services of outside professionals. Many audiologists who embark on private practice realize quickly how ill-prepared they are for running a small business. Master's level audiology training programs typically did not prepare students for the critical responsibilities that are necessary for being a small business owner. Historically, audiologists received little or no business training, and what they did receive barely touched on the broad scope of knowledge needed to run a solid practice. The little that many audiologists know about business and practice management often comes from what they observe from working in other private practices, clinics, and hospitals. What they learn through these experiences may or may not be sound business practices. Residential Au.D. and distance–learning Au.D. programs have curricula that address some of these shortcomings.

Whether purchasing an existing practice or starting from scratch, it is imperative to enlist the services of an attorney and accountant. These professionals will assist in formulating the purchase price of the business, in negotiating the terms and conditions of the purchase, and in writing the purchase agreement. After the sale is complete, the attorney and accountant will also advise the new owner (or owners) on setting up the business structure of the practice, such as sole proprietorship, partnership, or corporation. These decisions will affect the legal, tax, and liability implications of the business. The attorney and accountant can also be instrumental in reviewing and revising the business plan. The business plan is not only essential for any business to have in place, but it will be needed if the business is to secure loans from lending institutions. (For a discussion of purchasing a private practice, see Hosford-Dunn et al, 1995.)

Regardless of the purchase approach, many resources are required to start a practice, particularly financial resources. If an audiologist starts his or her own business, some capital must be available to purchase furniture and office and diagnostic equipment, to pay rent, to buy products for retail sale, and to have enough cash on hand to operate the business. Additionally, it may take a relatively long time before the business is profitable enough to support the owner and any other ancillary or professional staff. Some outside funding is often needed while the business is growing.

Purchasing an existing business obviously requires a larger capital investment. In the best scenario, the owner has sufficient personal assets to fund the initial deposit on the business purchase and to provide a minimum amount of operating capital. If the owner does not have adequate personal assets to start and run the business, or if he or she chooses not to fund the business personally, then the owner must obtain private loans from individuals or secure business loans from lending institutions. With an existing business, the cash flow may be positive enough to pay overhead expenses and to draw off a modest amount to survive during the initial years. With a new business, however, this is rarely the case. Having a sound financial practice plan is essential to the practice's long-term survival. (For a detailed discussion of the financial aspects of private practice, see Hosford-Dunn et al, 1995.)

In addition to the financial outlay in purchasing or starting a small business, there are high demands on the owner's physical and emotional resources. If a turnkey business is purchased, the owner not only starts seeing patients the first day the practice opens, but s/he suddenly assumes all of the additional responsibilities that come with owning the practice. Seeing patients in a new work environment and at the same time hiring support personnel, setting up new accounts, and sorting through belongings left behind by the previous owner can be overwhelming. The new owner is suddenly in charge of many different areas. Regardless of whether one is starting or purchasing a practice, tasks that are not in the traditional job description of an "audiologist" will fall to the audiologist, because s/he is the owner. Being the director of audiology may be a familiar role, but the owner is now also the director of finance, human resources, information systems, sales and marketing, operations, organizational systems, professional services, and facility maintenance. The different roles the audiologist, as private practice owner, must assume are shown in **Fig. 6–2**.

The challenges of private practice require energy, determination, a willingness to acquire new information, and an openness to developing new talents. Good "people" skills are essential. Certain personality characteristics help the new owner to succeed in private practice. One is a positive, can-do attitude manifested by someone who makes things happen rather than lets things happen (Winslow, 1995). This includes the ability to see life as a series of opportunities and possibilities and the desire to explore them. It also helps to be a risk taker, or to have the ability to tolerate risk. Those with organizational skills and tenacity in getting things done will find these traits helpful when running a practice. Another valuable characteristic is the ability to appreciate different points of view: from patients, employees, referral sources, and vendors. Perhaps most important is the ability to be creative at problem-solving, as owning a private practice continually presents challenges with no clear-cut solutions. Those who have strong risk aversion, a limited ability to cope with uncertainty and change, and a generally negative attitude about the possibilities of life should think twice about entering private practice.

Work hours for new private practice owners may be longer than those of salaried professionals. Private practice owners often feel that there are never enough hours in the day to keep up with the demands of the business, seldom feeling that headway is being made on the tasks required to keep the business running. Most new private practitioners eat, sleep, and breathe their business, often at the expense of their health and personal relationships. Trying to manage stress can become a major issue. The stress that the private practitioner shoulders is not different from the stresses for any small business. Starting a practice from scratch can provide some relief, as the first several years can be slow, and there is time to learn how to manage the business before the patient load gets heavy. However, the lack of financial rewards during the early years can cause unease for the new practice owner as he or she tries to make ends meet, both personally and in the business. The stress from trying to nurture a new business and the inherent financial burdens can create an ever-present anxiety. Stress is often cited anecdotally as a major reason for the selling of practices. The owner's core ideology, goals, and long-term vision are all-important as touchstones for holding the business together in the critical early years.

◆ Creating an Image and Reputation in Private Practice

The core ideology, goals, and long-term vision of a private practice define that practice, but their implementation imparts the image of the practice to the community. Image is multifaceted, but the core image should reflect the philosophy of the practitioner. Image must be a true projection of who the owner is, who he or she feels comfortable serving, and in what capacities he or she provides these services. Professionalism should be the foundation for any audiology practice. However, individual practices will want to present

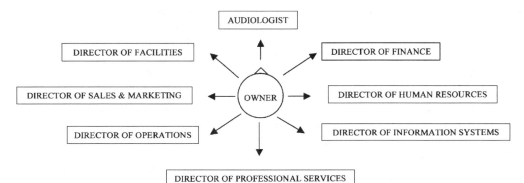

Figure 6–2 The different roles the audiologist, as private practice owner, must assume.

themselves in different professional contexts to their patients, colleagues, and referring professionals. These contexts should be unified, and the unified presentation will result in the overall image of the practice.

It is important to remember that image is perception. Perception creates a picture in the mind that arises when something interests a person. It is subject to a multitude of internal forces. When something interests a person, there is an internal judgment about the image and a feeling of pleasure or displeasure toward it. Constructing a perceived image for a private practice requires the careful manipulation of a variety of factors that contribute to the total image of the practice and produce the desired result. This includes both tangible and intangible aspects of the practice. All of these must support and interconnect with one another seamlessly to produce the desired result.

It is critical that the owner identify early in the development of the practice how he or she wishes the practice to be perceived by the community. In order for the owner to attract a certain clientele, the corresponding image needs to be created in the minds of both the lay and professional community. The image is created by the practice's physical layout and surroundings, its personnel and personal attitudes, the competency of its audiologic services, and the quality of the products it provides. It is formed by the appearance of the marketing and multimedia materials, the telephone directory ad, the newspaper ads, and the office newsletter. All of the practice's printed materials, the stationery, business cards, appointment cards and office brochure should have similarities that identify them with the practice. **Figure 6–3** illustrates ways of presenting a unified image through the use of a consistent logo and logotype on printed materials. In addition, the location of the office, the sign on the building, the physical layout, and the office furnishings contribute to the perception of the practice. All of these should be consistent with the image and "branding" the owner wants to convey to the community.

Perhaps of greater importance are the intangible items that imprint the practice's image in the minds of patients and referral sources. Support staff must have a clear understanding of the image the practice is trying to portray, as they have the greatest direct contact with the community. It is imperative that these individuals comport themselves in a manner consistent with the office image and good manners. A training workbook and videotape published by the AAA points out common faux pas and scenarios that support good imaging (AAA, *Best Practices Initiative,* n.d.). Professional staff must also have a clear idea of the community's perception of the office. If the conduct of just one employee is out of sync with the desired image, the carefully crafted image the owner has created is undermined.

Equally important is the practice of good etiquette, which generates the perception of warmth, respect, and compassion for the patients who are served. The office personnel can solidify a perception of confidence by being accessible to patients, by being flexible with appointment times, and by seeing patients on time.

Central to the idea of creating an image in any private practice is the perception of competence. Competence is reflected not only in high levels of patient satisfaction and in

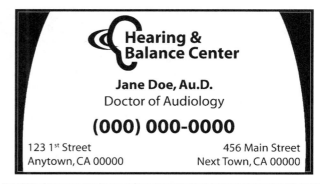

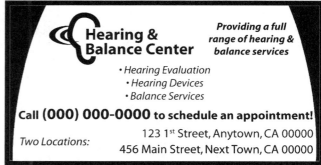

Figure 6–3 Sample office card and newspaper ad showing a consistent use of the practice's logo.

the professional delivery of services, but also in the efficient operation of the entire office. This perception runs from front office scheduling to the back office bookkeeping functions. An aura of competence translates into patient confidence and trust in the services of the practice in general. For the professional community, being prompt in the return of phone calls, sending reports in a timely manner, and sending thank you letters help to create confidence in the practice. Creating a perception of competence generally develops over time with repeated contact with patients and referral sources. However, it is wise to remember that first impressions can be lasting impressions.

Creating a competent professional image in the marketing climate requires incorporating a variety of interactive equipment in the practice environment. The public often expects a dazzling demonstration of technology in action, from hearing device fitting using probe microphone measurements to programming changes shown on a flat-panel computer monitor. Although, as clinicians, we know the merits of sophisticated instrumentation in testing protocols as well as in rehabilitation, inviting patients to observe technology in action allows them to participate in a more "patient–driven" process. In theory, this approach provides enhanced care while simultaneously educating patients and creating greater confidence in the practice and the clinician.

Fundamental to creating a positive image is the concept of quality and continuous quality improvement (CQI). CQI requires the practice and clinician go beyond the expected and strive for higher levels of patient care (see Chapter 3). Every few years the private practice owner should step back and review the tangible and intangible items that make up the practice to ensure that the right image is being created. Office questionnaires sent to the patients of the practice and to referral sources can be a good "reality check" as to how the practice is being perceived by the community. Revising printed materials periodically can give the practice a fresh look and instill a sense of confidence that the practice is continually seeking ways to improve in its effort to provide quality service. (See Chapter 3 for a discussion of quality.)

♦ Equipment Needs for a Private Practice

Technology is revolutionizing most industries and professions today, and the field of audiology is no exception. Microprocessors are incorporated into almost every piece of instrumentation in use in an audiology practice. Audiometers and immittance meters/bridges are all microprocessor controlled and can be programmed with automated test sequences to facilitate testing. At the time of this writing, personal computer (PC)–based audiometers are becoming available, using special software applications and customized hardware. Other diagnostic equipment that previously used dedicated computer systems, such as equipment for evoked potential testing, now runs on standard PCs. Hearing aids, once adjusted to the patient's hearing loss using analog potentiometers, are fitted to the patient using proprietary software programs developed by hearing aid manufacturers and run on a standard software platform, such as the NOAH system, developed by the Hearing Instrument Manufacturers' Software Association (HIMSA).

Personal Computers: Hardware and Software

The core office equipment of a private practice is the PC. Patient scheduling, database maintenance, hearing device tracking, record keeping, accounts management, office correspondence, intraoffice forms, marketing, and financial functions are all done on the PC. A practice may use stand-alone PCs for different functions, each with its own individual software application programs. As the practice grows, it may become advantageous to group PCs in a network so that information can be accessed and shared between computers. PCs can be networked to each other or can connect to a common PC, the server. Any user on the network can store and retrieve files on the server. One advantage to using a server is that data backup, an important and often overlooked function, can be automated.

> **Pitfall**
>
> - In a small practice, a single computer could be used for all office tasks, whether patient-related or business functions. Although the use of a single PC can be appealing from a cost point of view, it does have its limitations. Using multiple computers, on separate dedicated systems, prevents a digital "traffic jam" and allows diagnostic and business tasks to be done at the same time.

Most business, audiology, and hearing aid software applications are run under the Microsoft Windows operating system using IBM-compatible PCs. Many are used in combination with the Microsoft Office software suite. The software suite can be useful to import/export data between the different software applications that are used in the practice.

In addition to networking the practice's PCs, using an integrated practice management program may be more efficient for processing large amounts of information. These software programs combine many different functions into one software application. Patient scheduling, hearing aid tracking, bookkeeping, and marketing are common functions that are combined. Other programs allow interface with the NOAH hearing aid fitting platform and financial programs such as Intuit's QuickBooks. Data are transferred more seamlessly between these integrated software applications than with separate programs requiring the import/export of data.

Some practice management application programs are purchased, whereas others are available via monthly subscription. For purchased software, the practice must buy individual licenses for each PC onto which the software will be installed. For subscription software, the applications are Internet-based, residing on mainframe computers external to the business. The office's data are held in large data centers, password protected, and accessed by the office when needed. In the latter case, a broadband Internet connection is required. An Internet-based system relieves the practice of the responsibility of backing up office data and allows access to office information from any location that has an Internet connection.

For the most part, software programs for audiology practices are run on IBM-compatible PCs, not on Apple Macintosh computers. Unless the private practice owner wants to take on a considerable challenge in modifying a Macintosh to run these programs, it is best to stay with the IBM-compatible PC. Laptop or desktop PCs should meet or exceed the current minimum requirements for memory for the programs that will be run. Because computer technology evolves rapidly, the practice owner will want to make sure the equipment configuration will meet the needs of software upgrades in the near future.

Broadband Connections for Internet and E-Mail

Broadband connections are now integral to the running of any business, allowing access to the Internet and e-mail services. The most common Internet connections are via digital subscriber line (DSL) or cable modems. Wireless routers can also be used should the practice want to be free from hard-wire connections. Another necessary Internet-related piece of equipment a practice should consider is a firewall for guarding against Internet hackers, an unfortunate reality in today's world of cyberspace. (See Chapter 18 for a discussion of computer hardware and software.)

General Office Equipment

A private practice also needs general office equipment. The office's telephone system should meet current office needs and be capable of hardware and/or software expansion as the business grows. Telephones should be telecoil compatible, especially for practices that dispense hearing aids. If the practice serves the deaf population, a telecommunications device for the deaf (TDD) is recommended for contacting patients and scheduling appointments. The practice will also need other standard office equipment: a copy machine, a fax machine, and calculators or adding machines. A label printer or label maker is a handy investment for creating labels for patient charts, labeling hanging folders, and organizing a practice's hearing aid repair laboratory, with its multitude of small hearing aid components.

Clinical Equipment

When choosing equipment for a private practice, the owner must keep in mind the services the practice provides, as outlined in the initial business plan. The specific services that are provided determine which equipment is needed. For example, a practice that focuses primarily on hearing aid dispensing requires an electroacoustic analyzer and a probe microphone system. A practice that focuses primarily on differential diagnosis should consider evoked potential equipment. Practices that serve the needs of persons with balance disorders would invest in diagnostic and remediation equipment. A practice that contracts with industry for hearing conservation should consider a sound-level meter and a portable audiometer.

The most basic equipment that is needed for an audiology private practice is the equipment for performing a diagnostic hearing evaluation: the audiometer and the sound room. In addition to generating pure-tone and live-voice speech stimuli, the audiometer should be capable of delivering calibrated speech materials via built-in digitized speech recordings or via external compact disc (CD) player. A variety of recorded speech materials for assessing speech recognition in quiet and/or noise are available commercially in CD format. Additionally, the audiometer should be equipped with a set of insert earphones and a sound-field system. Other diagnostic equipment that should be considered for the basic diagnostic evaluation includes an immittance bridge/meter and otoacoustic emissions (OAE) equipment.

For otoscopy and cerumen management, a practice needs a good-quality halogen otoscope and specula in a variety of sizes. Cerumen management equipment and supplies will depend on whether cerumen will be removed via instrument, suction, irrigation, or a combination of several methods. For instrument removal, a curet and forceps will be needed. For suction, a high-quality suction pump and related accessories will be needed. With irrigation, the practice owner may wish to invest in the Welch Allyn Ear Wash system (Welch Allyn Inc., Skaneateles Falls, NY) or use the standard ear syringe and basin. For greater visualization and illumination of the ear canal and tympanic membrane, a headlamp or magnifying headlight such as the Welch Allyn LumiView could be added to the practice's equipment. Lastly, a video-otoscope can provide excellent visualization of the canal and eardrum and can allow for a permanent record of a patient's ear.

For infection control, the practice will need to decide what supplies will be needed according to its infection control plan. These may include one-time-use disposable supplies (e.g., otoscope specula, immittance tips, OAE tips, wax curettes) or investing in reusable equipment that require cleaning, disinfecting and sterilization. Regardless of which approach is taken, infection control supplies will be needed.

Pearl

- Although the AAA and the Academy of Doctors of Audiology (formerly the Academy of Dispensing Audiologists) have recognized that cerumen management is clearly within an audiologist's scope of practice, audiologists are legally allowed to remove cerumen only when removal is included under state licensure. Audiologists should check with their state licensing board to make sure that cerumen removal is within the audiologist's scope of practice, as regulations vary from state to state.

For practices that dispense hearing aids, the appropriate equipment must be obtained. This will include, at the minimum, an electroacoustic analyzer and universal programming interface equipment, for example, the GN Otometrics (Taastrup, Denmark) HI-PRO hard-wired box or HIMSA's Bluetooth wireless interface NOAHlink. Other equipment that should be considered are a probe microphone system for speech mapping, a small but well-equipped repair laboratory, and a stock of new and loaner hearing aids.

As practices become more specialized, the instrumentation needs become apparent to the practitioner. Some diagnostic equipment is costly and may not be practical to include in a small practice. Conversely, a large practice that sees many patients and provides a range of services will be able to justify owning a wide variety of equipment. Practices that provide a broad range of diagnostic hearing services may own an evoked potential system for measuring evoked cochlear, brainstem, and cortical responses. Practices that focus on balance evaluation and/or remediation require electronystagmography (ENG) or VNG instrumentation. These practices may also need equipment for posturography and perhaps a rotary chair. If a practice offers intraoperative monitoring, a portable evoked potential system may need to be purchased or made available through the operating theater where the audiologist provides such services.

It can be overwhelming for the private practice owner to itemize the equipment necessary for an audiology private practice and to compute the cost of such equipment. Clearly, there are certain pieces of equipment that are necessary to any audiology practice. Other pieces may be optional and may be purchased at a later date. How, what, and when equipment is acquired depend greatly on available capital and cash flow.

Pearl

- An owner of a private practice that provides primarily hearing aid services notices there is only one facility in the area doing evoked potential testing, and that facility has a several-week backup for scheduled testing. The owner concludes that he or she should purchase an evoked potentials unit and add this service to the practice. Even though this looks inviting, underlying stumbling blocks, such as billing and physician referral, must be considered. Unlike hearing instrument purchases, patients will not pay for these diagnostic services out of pocket. Managed care constraints may dictate that the patient cannot be seen at the owner's practice. In addition, the referring physicians may have loyalties to the hospital clinics and refer all special testing to them. The purchase of the equipment cannot be supported.

Methods for Purchasing Equipment

There are different ways to purchase equipment, and some can help to decrease the equipment costs up front. Buying used equipment can be more cost-effective and can reduce the start-up costs of the business. Leasing equipment can be attractive; however, the long-term costs of leasing must be compared with the actual purchase price of the equipment. When diagnostic equipment is costly, as in the case of VNG and balance equipment, leasing may be the only option. Almost all office equipment is available for lease, including telephone systems, copiers, and fax machines. Leasing may also be attractive because the practice owner is not required to keep the equipment at the end of the lease. During the period of the lease, there may have been substantial upgrades in technology and changes in test protocols that warrant obtaining different equipment than that which was leased.

Controversial Point

- Some hearing aid manufacturers provide equipment purchase programs known as "co-ops." With these programs, equipment is purchased at a reduced cost in exchange for a commitment from the audiologist to purchase a specified quantity of hearing aids from that manufacturer at a preset price over a specified period of time. Although these co-op arrangements may seem attractive to the new private practice owner, the long-term costs of such contracts and their ethical ramifications must be considered. For example, hearing aids bought through such arrangements are often not subject to volume discounts, and the audiologist may end up paying more for the equipment, through the loss of volume discounts, than if the equipment were purchased outright. The contract also ties the audiologist to a particular product or family of products over a long period of time. Under such arrangements, the professional objectivity of the audiologist's advice could be compromised, or appear to be compromised, from patients' point of view. (Refer to AAA, *Ethical Practice Guidelines*, n.d.)

There are many other books and journal articles that provide a detailed list of the instrumentation needed for a private practice. One source is Hosford-Dunn et al (1995), which discusses whether to purchase new or used equipment and provides a summary of general equipment that may be needed. A further discussion regarding computer software and its relationship to the organizational systems of the office will follow later in this chapter. (See Chapter 14 for additional information on equipment. Refer to Chapter 18 for a more detailed discussion of information systems.)

◆ Task Allocation and Human Resources Management

Even before the first patient walks through the door, the private practitioner will quickly see that a number of tasks must be performed to produce a smoothly running practice. When practices are young, the owner usually does much of the work; seeing patients and running the practice with minimal support personnel. Because the owner is the primary revenue generator, the time spent running the practice takes away from his or her opportunity to see patients. As practices grow, more staff is added to assume some of the owner's responsibilities. Therefore, the owner must weigh the costs of additional staff to run the office versus the cost of lost revenues if he or she continues trying to run the office alone.

Generally, in private practice there are front office and back office staff. The front office staff interfaces with the public and patients directly, whereas the back office staff works behind the scenes on bookkeeping and billing. Unless a practice is very large, it is likely that the front and back office tasks are performed by the same staff members, who take on a variety of roles.

Front Office Staff

The front office is one of the most important entities in any private practice organization. In small, single-audiologist practices, there may be only one person who performs the front office tasks; however, as clinicians are added, the number of front office personnel need to grow as well. In most established private practices, the front office performs the daily functions of running the office. These are the responsibilities traditionally associated with a receptionist and include handling the telephone, scheduling patient appointments, greeting patients, having patients complete necessary paperwork, and assembling patient charts. Front office personnel also maintain patient records by filing pertinent information in the patient charts and storing charts appropriately. They typically input patient information into the office computer database and keep the database updated with changes in patient information. In addition, front office staff frequently handle over-the-counter sales of small items, such as hearing aid batteries.

One of the most important and detail-oriented responsibilities of the front office job is shipping and receiving. During the course of each day, products will arrive and leave the office via the mail, small parcel service, or overnight air express service.

This duty includes tracking the inflow and outflow of all resale items and supplies in the office, including new earmolds, hearing aids, accessories, batteries, and hearing assistive technology (e.g., assistive listening devices). This is an especially important task in offices that dispense hearing aids. New orders and repair orders need to be placed, tracked, received, and logged in; patients need to be contacted; and devices must be delivered. It is critical that all earmold and hearing aid orders get to and from the manufacturer expeditiously and that their whereabouts are carefully tracked.

Pitfall

- Valuable time is lost if the tracking system is not efficient. When new hearing instruments are ordered, patients should be given a realistic expectation of when the aids will be ready. In some offices, return appointments are scheduled in advance with an estimate of when the devices will arrive. If the instruments are not received on time, valuable office and patient time is wasted, as the appointment must be canceled. An inconvenienced patient may be disappointed, frustrated, or angry if the appointment must be rescheduled. This reflects poorly on the office and shows a lack of professionalism.

In practices that are driven by diagnostic evaluations, it is imperative that the materials needed for testing be on hand, clean, and ready to use when the patient comes in for the appointment. A staff member must take periodic inventory of supplies to ensure that appropriate materials are available. This includes items such as insert earphone tips, electrodes, specula, and test forms.

Front office personnel are often responsible for tracking saleable inventory, as they are continually handling the products that come in and out of the office. They may be in charge of maintaining general office supplies, such as copy paper, pens and pencils, and forms.

Because many prospective patients are unfamiliar with audiologists, the front office staff serves in a de facto patient relations capacity, providing information to the public about audiology and the nature of different audiologic test procedures. They may give patients basic information about different styles and types of hearing aids and encourage hearing aid "shoppers" to schedule appointments. Front office staff can be instrumental in quieting nerves, calming down disgruntled customers, and providing a friendly smile to timid newcomers.

Pearl

- A receptionist may be highly skilled but is shy or has difficulty in engaging patients in light conversation. This characteristic may be perceived as unfriendliness and indifference by patients who are new to the office. The patients' perceptions of the office are created by their initial interaction with the front office staff. The receptionist should create a sense of comfort and confidence by showing an interest in the patients, by showing understanding, and by being compassionate. A friendly smile goes a long way.

In some offices, front office staff members are trained as hearing aid technicians for troubleshooting basic hearing aid problems, checking batteries, cleaning earmolds, changing tubing, and performing simple in-house repairs, such as replacing broken battery doors. The front office staff may collect payments from patients when the appointments are completed and carry out some of the billing functions.

Additional Support Staff and Services

As the practice grows, additional support staff and services may be added. An office manager can be a valuable addition to a private practice, covering a variety of services, such as managing patient accounts, handling third-party billing, supervising front office staff, and serving as administrative assistant to the owner. The office manager can provide invaluable support with the marketing activities of the practice. He or she can help the practice owner implement the office's marketing plan by interfacing with the design and print companies that produce the individual marketing pieces, working with the mailing houses, and acting as liaison with newspaper advertising and other marketing representatives.

A private practice may also have an in-house bookkeeper to carry out the bookkeeping functions of the practice or may use the services of an outside bookkeeping service. Often, several people in the office share some of the bookkeeping tasks. For example, the front office staff may collect patient payments, the office manager may do the third-party billing and send out patient statements, the bookkeeper may keep track of accounts payable and receivable, and the owner may pay the bills and take care of banking transactions. In very small or young practices, the audiologist and front office staff may perform all of these activities themselves.

A private practice also needs clerical services. Most small offices have the front office staff or office manager provide the clerical services needed for general office correspondence. Hiring a part–time high school or college student for basic filing, confirming appointments, and special projects may help the office run smoothly while keeping personnel costs down. With office computerization, many professionals handle other word processing work themselves.

Outside Consultants

Most small business owners use the services of an accountant to prepare quarterly and annual financial statements and tax returns. Professional accounting services can be especially helpful in providing an understanding of potential tax liabilities and consequences of business decisions and events. Practices will also need services of legal counsel from time to time.

Private practices may hire outside consultants for a variety of needs, such as information technology support for computer maintenance and upkeep, mailing–house services for marketing materials, and printing services for designing and printing of office stationery, forms, and other documents.

Professional Staff

Larger private practices have a staff of audiologists to provide the services of the practice, in addition to the owner. Some supervise students in residential Au.D. programs who are in their fourth year of study, master's level graduates who may be required to complete a clinical fellowship year for the American Speech-Language-Hearing Association, and audiology students interested in on-site practical experience. Some offices have a certified and/or licensed audiology assistant to help with basic hearing testing, test assisting for diagnostic evaluations, and hearing aid support services.

Human Resources Management

In most practices, hiring both professional and nonprofessional staff is required to complete all of the functions needed in private practice. Hiring and managing people are some of the most baffling activities many private practice owners will encounter. Audiologists typically have little training in the area of human resources. For many audiologists, human resources management is a skill learned gradually over time.

The broad issues and nuances of hiring and managing staff for a private practice are well beyond the scope of this section. It is always important to be aware of legal issues surrounding employment. If the practice owner is unsure of the legality of a particular hiring practice, it is a good idea to pose questions to an attorney familiar with human resources management.

Hiring competent personnel is not an easy task, even for a seasoned manager. It is important to find a potential employee who not only has the skills required for the job, but who can connect with the core ideology and goals of the practice. It is of equal importance to find an individual with the personality type that suits the position for which he or she will be hired. Most employers want to hire good team players and people who will stay with them for a reasonable period of time. Finding the right person requires patience and takes time. It generally involves reviewing a large number of résumés and conducting numerous, in-depth interviews to find the person who most closely fits the owner's criteria. The up-front effort may be worth it, however, because hasty hiring can result in choosing an individual who is not a good fit for the organization. The owner may be faced, often for the first time, with the unfortunate task of terminating people soon after they are hired. It is an uncomfortable responsibility, at best.

Depending upon the position, employee searches often start with newspaper advertisements, on-line employment Web sites, announcements at local professional meetings, or professional newsletters. Frequently, personal networking provides the best candidates for open positions. Family members and friends are sources that can yield good candidates. (A detailed discussion of human resources can be found in Chapter 4.)

Of equal importance is the task of retaining good employees. It is often hard for small practices to offer expansive benefit packages, but this is one of the keys to retaining staff. The more benefits offered, the more reluctant an employee might be to leave. As evidenced by the above litany of tasks that one employee may perform in a private practice, the cost of replacing a good employee far outweighs simple wage issues. Benefits in a small office may not always be in the form of monetary remuneration. Private practices can sometimes offer more flexibility in work schedules. Allowing

children to come into the office on sick days, for instance, can be extremely important for working parents of young children. Small offices can offer a level of familiarity and conviviality that a large office or corporation cannot match. There is a feeling of camaraderie that develops in a staff when everyone rolls up their sleeves to accomplish the tasks at hand and works toward a common goal. Expressing thanks to the staff many times a week makes employees understand that their worth is recognized and valued.

For small practices with one or two staff members, policies and procedures are usually unwritten and decided on an as-needed basis. As practices grow, it is necessary and highly desirable to write down office policies in an employee handbook. Each employee should receive, read, and review the policies with the practice owner or manager. A comprehensive employee handbook makes the policies of the office clear, thereby resolving questions early and thwarting problems that would arise if policies varied between employees. Office policies should be consistent with state and federal laws and local labor codes. The practice owner may wish to bring in an outside human resources consultant when writing the employee handbook.

Performance reviews should be performed regularly and at least annually. This gives the practice owner the opportunity to discuss with the employees their progress in their job performance and to reward employees for a job well done by increasing their compensation.

Motivated employees often attend outside classes, seminars, or conferences where they can hone their skills and can come in contact with their peers in similar positions. In our experience, it is gratifying to see how much most individuals value these benefits, especially those in nonprofessional positions. Asking employees to attend outside classes sends a clear signal that the practice owner is making an investment in them. In most cases, such investments benefit everyone involved: the employees usually recognize the investment and are flattered by the owner's commitment to them; the owner gains happier and more highly skilled employees. This type of investment also engenders employee loyalty, a highly prized commodity in the world of small business.

◆ Organizational Systems for Private Practice

Few offices run efficiently or effectively without proper organizational systems. An office's organizational system is the framework of the practice, the foundation upon which the practice is built. The way an office is structured ultimately affects every aspect of it, from its internal efficiency to the external image of the practice. From the patients to the referral sources and the other companies with which the office does business, a well-run office contributes positively to the practice's image of professionalism.

Familiarity with organizational systems and an understanding of their impact on the operation of a business are important to running a private practice. Inappropriate organizational systems hinder practice growth, whereas appropriate systems can facilitate growth. Implementation of proper organizational systems is one of the most important components of an efficiently run and successful business.

Audiologists who are new to private practice may overlook the importance of being organized, but they quickly will gain appreciation of good organizational systems as their practices grow. It is helpful to have prior experience with organizational systems in previous employment settings or from experiences working in well-run clinics as part of audiology training programs. Systems that work well for a small, single office, sole proprietorship with one or two support personnel are quite different from those that are required for multiple-location practices with numerous professional and nonprofessional employees.

Some of the most important organizational systems are those involving scheduling, patient databases (i.e., patient recall, patient records, and hearing aid tracking), billing/finance, purchasing, and shipping/receiving. In constructing these systems, the practice owner must answer questions such as: How are patients to be scheduled? For how long should each appointment be scheduled? How will walk–ins be handled? When should recall letters be sent out? How will the office track hearing aid repairs? How will ABR test results be reported? When will physician report letters be sent out? Who orders supplies? Who orders equipment? How will collections be handled?

Organizational systems are generally interdependent. In a well-run practice, these systems are conjoined to ensure that patients, goods, and payments flow through the practice with the greatest of efficiency.

In creating the practice's organizational framework, the private practice owner must decide whether these systems will be performed with computer software programs, with a manual system, or with a combination of both. In the past, a schedule book was used for patient appointments, a log sheet for tracking hearing aid orders and repairs, a day sheet for accounts receivables, and a manual ledger for bookkeeping. These manual systems, however, become less efficient and unwieldy as the number of patients increases, the audiology staff grows, the sale of hearing aids increases, and the number of services performed expands. It is surprising that, at the time of this writing, many small offices continue to use manual systems to run their practices.

The use of computer software programs allows greater efficiency and flexibility over manual systems. The practice owner may decide to use readily available software programs for some office tasks. Quicken and QuickBooks are popular software programs for finance. FileMaker Pro is a comprehensive database application that can be customized to the practice's own patient database requirements. Numerous scheduling programs are also available for keeping track of meetings and patient appointments. Software tools for implementing customer relationship marketing (CRM) can facilitate the management of all aspects of patient interactions. "Office automation with the right architecture provides a strategic framework for focusing on patients, minimizing administrative costs, and maximizing long-term transactions with those patients" (Hosford-Dunn, 2006, p. 2).

An alternative to these off-the-shelf programs is integrated office management software. This special-purpose program is designed specifically for audiology and hearing aid private practices and combine many, if not all, of the necessary organizational systems. Independent software companies design some of them; others are available through hearing aid manufacturers that offer proprietary programs for private practices. Offices that fit hearing aids with the NOAH software-based system can use that database system for other office functions. Offices that specialize in industrial audiology can use software specifically designed for industrial audiology. Regardless of the type of practice, using an integrated office management system is the most efficient way to manage organizational systems.

In a busy practice, the task of data entry required to keep current the office's software programs falls to the support personnel. This data upkeep typically requires good communication between the audiologist and the staff. The use of an internal tracking sheet can facilitate communication between office personnel for data entry, scheduling, and other purposes as well. **Figure 6–4** shows an example of an intraoffice form, created for our practice, that ties together many of the office systems (scheduling, ordering, computer data entry, etc.).

The intraoffice form serves as an instruction sheet from the audiologist to the support personnel. The form accompanies the patient chart when the patient is seen in the office. Each box on the form represents one or two information systems. The audiologist checks the appropriate boxes for the patient on any given visit, and the support staff follows the audiologist's instructions as shown on the form.

Using this type of flow sheet can serve many purposes. It links office systems together, ensures that important information is transmitted among the staff and that appropriate action is taken, and facilitates the tracking of hearing aids. All office personnel are trained in the use of the form. Therefore, little or no verbal exchange is needed when the form is handed off from person to person. Obviously, this system works only if everyone completes the form correctly and carries out the requests appropriately. When errors do occur, the cause of the problem can be tracked more easily.

Patient records usually form the core of clinical care and information. It is of great importance that patient charts have a standardized organizational format for easy access to information. Likewise, it is mandatory that a handling system be implemented and followed by all staff members to enable quick access to all patient records.

Much of the office's organizational system comprises patients' private health information. All employees must be given training in the handling of this information as required by the Health Insurance Portability and Accountability Act (HIPAA) of 1996 (Public Law 104–191). The act includes detailed provisions for ensuring confidentiality of protected health information. (For more information on HIPAA, see Chapter 7.)

♦ Audiology Protocols in Private Practice

Much of this chapter is related to business aspects of private practice. But how does the owner manage the way audiology is practiced within the context of private practice? Not

___ DB ___TMC ___ AW ___ MO'M

Name: _____

Last Office Visit: _____
Last Hearing Test: _____

SCHEDULING

Type of Visit:

___ BAB
___ HDC

___ F2
___ F2/AT

___ OV1
___ OV2

___ EMI
___ EMF or SMF

___ OVC
___ OVB

___ HDR

When:

___ 1 week
___ 2 weeks
___ 3 weeks
___ 4 weeks
___ 6 months
___ 1 year (Recall)

Audiologist/Dispenser:

___ DB   ___ AW

___ TMC   ___ MO'M

___ HDF : Regular ___
          Remake ___
          Exchange ___
          Loss ___

___   & F2/AT   date: _____

___ HEF : Regular ___   date: _____
          Remake ___
          Exchange ___
          Loss ___

___   & F2/AT   date: _____

date: _____

RECALL

date: _____

___ OVC   ___ OVB   ___ BAB

FDA MD CLEARANCE

___ *Medical Clearance* from:

_____ M.D.

PAYMENTS

HDC Visit: ___ Deposit
            ___ Copy Purchase Agreement (for Patient)

HDF Visit: ___ Payment on account
            ___ Copy Purchase Agreement (for Patient)

BTE ORDERS

___ Right: Make & Model _____

            Color _____

___ Left: Make & Model _____

            Color _____

___ Remote Control _____

Order taken by: _____ on _____

REPAIRS

___ HDR Appointment _____

___ Pick up ok _____

___ Appt or pick up (patient's choice)

___ Send to patient via: _____

___ REMINDER: Get loaner back

LETTERS & QUESTIONNAIRES

___ TYRF Letter & Batteries to:

_____

___ Office Questionnaire in ___ weeks
___ IOI Questionnaire in   ___ weeks

___ Thinking letter in   ___ weeks

Figure 6–4 An example of an intraoffice form that ties together several office systems.

only should the basic tenets of audiology be kept clearly in mind as professional tasks are performed, but systems must be put in place to ensure that the way they are performed is consistent, regardless of who does the job. This topic is about not only quality assurance but also continuity of care. Establishing practice protocols resolves many of the issues associated with the practice of one's profession in the context of private practice. (For a discussion of quality assurance, refer to Hosford-Dunn et al, 2000.)

Protocols should be developed with several goals in mind. They should be consistent with the core ideology, goals, and vision of the practice. They establish continuity of care by specifying what information needs to be obtained during each procedure and by outlining the minimum data requirements necessary to indicate the procedure has been performed correctly and accurately. Protocols establish a level of efficiency by assigning a time frame for each procedure and using the correct diagnosis and billing codes for each. They can give support in preparing clinical reports. This is especially true if templates or checklists are used to create the reports. A further discussion of the use of templates or checklists can be found in Gardner and Stone (1998).

Protocols should give the clinician guidance in providing care. They can be thought of as a framework for achieving the goals basic to each patient consultation, evaluation, and rehabilitation plan. The goals are tied to the immediate patient problems and the proposed short- and long-term solutions. They should be aimed at guaranteeing that each patient receives consultation, evaluation, and/or rehabilitation procedures that provide results that can be tracked over time and that stand the test of validity and reliability. For example measurement of treatment outcomes should be included in the protocols to determine if the solutions applied have true validity. Protocols should also ensure high test–retest reliability.

Protocols help the clinician evaluate data quickly. They also provide guidance to the clinician when questions arise or problems occur. Protocols and their attendant forms can also serve as a ready-made paper trail for the owner or managing audiologist to document patient encounters.

The educational and clinical background of the owner (or managing audiologist) and the clinicians on staff will be reflected in the protocols. The protocols should also be in line with the current standards of care. Although protocols are in place to ensure continuity, they should be flexible enough to allow for variations in patient populations (e.g., non-English-speaking patients). Clinicians will also add and subtract from protocols based on their own experiences and biases. In some instances, alternate protocols may exist for the same procedures, as long as each protocol is consistent with current professional practices. Although slight variations may be allowed, the protocols must be clearly defined (i.e., written) and followed by all clinicians.

The use of evidence-based practice (EBP) will guide the owner in developing the protocols for the practice. EBP integrates clinical expertise with the best available clinical evidence derived from systematic research. AAA has incorporated evidence-based decision making into the academy's clinical practice guidelines (Valente et al, 2005). The practice owner may find these guidelines useful, as they can help the clinician translate research into evidence-based patient care. Using EBP helps to distinguish the practice from other hearing health care providers in terms of public confidence and respect from other medical specialties, state and federal health care agencies, and third-party payers. (See Chapter 8 for discussion of EBP.)

In this age of managed care, test protocols and measurements of treatment outcomes are beginning to take on greater importance. Savvy managed care companies are more likely to award contracts to practices that have clearly defined protocols and that have outcome measures in place. Many outcome measures assess benefit, generally

by employing some type of pre- and postevaluation assessment, and are viewed as indicators of patient satisfaction.

Pitfall

- Many testing protocols in private practice are trimmed to save time, contain costs, and guarantee payment from third-party payers. When trying to provide the best patient care in the most abbreviated manner possible, private practice audiologists find themselves in a battle similar to that faced by physicians. It is not always possible to win the battle without casualties, however.

An important topic in a discussion of protocols in audiology practice is the issue of infection control. The initiative for developing infection control protocol came from heightened awareness in the 1980s of bloodborne pathogens, including human immunodeficiency virus (HIV) and hepatitis; this became the "catalyst for global change in infectious disease control across all health care professions" (Bankaitis and Kemp, 2003, p. 38). The scope of practice in audiology has changed substantially since its inception in the middle of the last century. Audiologists are now involved with procedures that expose them to bodily fluids, such as blood and mucus, that are potentially infectious. Audiology practice requires patient contact, and many objects used in practice come in contact with multiple patients. Many persons seeking audiologic care may be immunocompromised. As a result, infection control has become an important issue in audiologic practice. (For further discussions of infection control, see Chapter 10 and Bankaitis and Kemp, 2003.)

The development and implementation of protocols are closely tied to quality assurance, continuity of care, billing, office efficiency, professional development, and patient satisfaction. Determining what procedures should have established protocols and the specific content of those protocols affects how professional work is performed along many dimensions.

In addition to protocols, there are other information-based mechanisms that ensure appropriate patient care throughout the consultation, evaluation, and rehabilitative processes. Many private practices provide new patients with information packets that describe the nature of the evaluation and/or rehabilitative processes. Diagnostic procedures are sometimes daunting to patients. Knowing ahead of time about the procedures can allay their fears and make patients relax during testing, allowing for better test results. It is essential that patients and families embarking on habilitative or rehabilitative paths have a basic understanding of hearing loss and how it affects communication. Providing such information makes it easier for patients to comply with directives during diagnostic and therapeutic procedures. It also facilitates the development of a trust relationship, increasing the likelihood of a positive outcome for patients.

Some private practices send out questionnaires to patients asking them a variety of questions about the office and about their satisfaction levels. This type of inquiry provides insight regarding the kind of care that patients feel they have received, the office's physical setting, and other observations about the practice and staff. Solicited constructive criticism allows for growth of any private practice and ultimately results in providing better patient care.

◆ Marketing Issues in Private Practice

Marketing is much more than just advertising. It comprises a constellation of different activities designed to ensure adequate patient flow for the purpose of generating the necessary revenues for the business. Marketing efforts in medical communities have long been grounded in cultivating relationships with other medical practitioners to win referrals. Formal advertising, which was seldom used until recently, has become ubiquitous in all forms of media. Over the last several years, there has been a substantial increase in advertising by insurance companies, drug companies, and independent physician associations (IPAs) contracted with community hospitals. Communities are constantly being courted to obtain the best policies, drugs, and health care available. Consumers are accustomed to physicians and dentists advertising their skills on the radio, television, and in newspapers with special offers. For example, "lunch and learn" seminars are offered, and mass mailings for seminars or open houses are common. If an audiology practice does not participate in some forms of marketing in today's health care environment, it will surely languish.

Marketing, in any business, is an ongoing process. For the private practice owner, it is a mind-set about how the practice carries out its services and approaches each patient. It is an understanding that every patient that is seen by the practice has the opportunity to share, with anyone who cares to listen, his or her positive or negative experience with the practice.

Patients will be referred from a variety of sources, depending on the type of practice. One of the most common referral sources for new and established private practices is local ear, nose, and throat (ENT) physicians. Audiologists specializing in balance assessment and remediation may find physical therapists in the area an especially valuable resource and referral source. Contracting with IPAs, health maintenance organizations (HMOs) or other insurance companies, unions, and related organizations increases patient referrals. Practices that have been in business for many years, even if under different ownership, also have a built-in referral system from their existing patient base. Word-of-mouth marketing, that is, opinions expressed between patients, is one of the most powerful methods of promoting the practice. This type of personal referral not only brings in new patients but also ensures that those who recommend your business return themselves.

The patient database is perhaps the most valuable asset for hearing aid practices. The average hearing instrument user requires follow-up care over many years. Using newsletters, annual recall notices, and other direct mail pieces keeps patients abreast of new developments, therapies, and advances in hearing aid technologies. The practice's patient base, through word-of-mouth referrals and repeat business, may constitute the bulk of the revenues of the practice.

Pearl

- If an existing patient refers a friend or family member to the practice, he or she should be thanked personally. A handwritten note or a personal phone call gives the patient a positive feeling about the office. The patient will be inclined to refer others to the practice.

Private practice owners must always look for ways to increase their patient base. Actively marketing to the existing referral sources and recruiting new referral sources provides for an ever-growing practice. Marketing to a broader segment of the medical community beyond the otolaryngologist can expand the practice's patient base. Increasingly, pediatricians, family practice doctors, internists, cardiologists, neurologists, and gerontologists refer patients to an audiology practice. In managed care environments, these primary care and specialty providers gain special importance as direct referral sources. Physician referrals are especially important for a diagnostic practice. Over the past several years, a variety of marketing programs through the Better Hearing Institute (BHI) have focused on connecting with primary care physicians and alerting them to services that audiologists can provide their patients (Kochkin, 2004). These connections may be initiated by personal contact followed by quarterly newsletters written specifically for physicians about hearing and balance-related topics.

Pearl

- In any professional community, it is considered proper professional protocol to refer a patient back to the original referral source if the patient needs the care of that specific health care provider again. Working in a professional community demands that the protocols of that community be learned and followed to garner respect not only from other professionals but also from one's patients and peers. (For a further discussion of this and the problem of "stealing" patients, see Stach, 1998.)

Outside contracts with residential communities and nursing homes is another avenue for patient referrals. Providing in-services in the community increases name recognition of the practice and establishes the owner as the expert within the community. Being perceived as the expert in one's specialty typically ensures more referrals. Business contacts in the community through local business meetings, civic service clubs like Rotary International, or organizations such as the Better Business Bureau and chamber of commerce can also provide the occasional referral.

Office employees may also generate referrals to the practice, as they generally are part of the local community and have ties to organizations that the owner may not. Knowledgeable and enthusiastic employees are often eager to refer patients to the office and can be a valuable source of word-of-mouth referrals.

Regular weekly or monthly advertising in small town local and larger city newspapers will put the practice in the public eye. Advertising serves as a constant reminder that the practice is a viable, community-based business. Print ads are especially useful for hearing aid dispensaries, as these ads are often product-driven. Telephone directory listings are another good way to reach local consumers. Some practices also advertise on local radio and cable TV stations. Regardless of the media, it is important that advertising be consistent with the practice's image and that the content conforms to state advertising laws for health care–related businesses.

Additionally, the practice's personnel can visit community senior centers or residential communities in an effort to promote business. Making contact with the administrators or health liaisons at these institutions may result in referrals. Some facilities will allow the posting of office brochures or business cards on a community bulletin board or the distribution of copies of the practice's newsletter in residents' mailboxes. Still other sources of referrals are music stores, which may welcome information about noise exposure, musicians' earplugs, and sound monitors; and manufacturers, which may need assistance with implementing hearing conservation programs at their plants.

It is a good custom to acknowledge all referrals, as a note of appreciation often encourages more referrals. In the case of direct referrals from health care professionals, it is customary to thank the professional for the referral in a letter or report referencing the patient. With patient referrals, phone calls or thank-you letters are appropriate. Giving small thank-you gifts is another way of expressing appreciation for a referral. However, when giving thank-you gifts for referrals, the practice owner should make sure they are of nominal value and are not in violation of federal antikickback statutes. (For additional information on marketing, see Chapter 5.)

Pearl

- In today's world, it is advisable that practices have a Web site so that consumers are able to find out about the practice and "browse" who you are. The presence of a good Web site inspires confidence in the business.

♦ Business Issues in Private Practice

Audiologists who venture into private practice generally have little preparation for managing the business aspects of the practice. They receive formal education in audiology and have professional experience in clinical services or research, but little training or experience in business and practice management. Typically, they do not take business classes as part of their bachelor's or master's programs, and most clinical positions in audiology do not expose them to the business aspects of the clinic. It has been only with the advent of residential and distance-learning Au.D. programs that audiology students are exposed to the business side of audiology. How, then, does the new private practice owner learn the many aspects of running a small business?

Once the business has been started (or, ideally, before it has been purchased), the audiologist must learn how to manage the financial aspects of the practice. For some, it is with on-the-job training; for others, via classes at local learning centers or community colleges, or a combination of both hands-on learning and classes. At a minimum, hiring a competent bookkeeper is essential if the audiologist does not have any prior experience in business.

Pitfall

- Although some audiologists do their practice's bookkeeping themselves, they should weigh the cost of hiring a bookkeeper against the cost of doing their own books. This cost may include the potential errors resulting from a lack of expertise, the potential loss of revenue if the bookkeeping is done during business hours, and the personal time constraints if the bookkeeping is done after work.

Regardless of who does the actual bookkeeping, the audiologist, as owner, must have an understanding of basic bookkeeping and accounting. Managing the assets and liabilities of the business requires an understanding of cash flow (receipts and disbursements), accounts receivable, accounts payable, cost of goods, inventory, depreciation, and collections. Understanding state and federal tax filings and knowing how to budget for taxes are fundamental to running a small business. Sound business practices must be established from the beginning. For example, collecting for services at the time of the patient's visit helps maintain a positive cash flow, as does the timely billing of third-party payers. Positive cash flow allows for on-time payments to vendors and other payable accounts and maintains the practice's good credit.

Besides a bookkeeper, the owner will need to hire a professional accountant to look after the broader financial well-being of the practice. An accountant will do a periodic financial analysis of the business and prepare state and federal income tax returns. He or she can assist the practice owner in understanding and interpreting the two main business financial reports: the income statement (a summary of income and expenses over a specified period of time) and the balance sheet (a summary of the assets and liabilities of the business at a specified point in time). Ideally, the accountant assists in interpreting these reports, gives advice regarding the overall financial status of the business, and helps the owner understand the tax implications of various business decisions (equipment purchases, leases, employee retirement plans, etc.).

It is important for a private practice owner to find an accountant whose expertise he or she trusts and with whom the owner can have a good working relationship. A problem exists when the owner and accountant do not have a good line of communication, what Fleury (1992) describes as an accountant–client gap: "the perceptual difference between what the small business owners think they are buying in accounting services and what the accountant is trained to provide." (p. 21) A clear understanding of what the client expects from the accountant and what the accountant expects of the client is imperative.

Pearl

- A good owner–accountant relationship can be a key ingredient to the success of a young business. The owner may put a lot of faith in the accountant, as the owner is not yet business savvy. The accountant's job, however, is dependent on the owner's providing business documents that are accurate, complete, and timely. The accountant's financial statements and advice are only as good as the data from which they are generated. A good accountant will provide document templates to guide the business novice.

Taxation issues are often confusing to the new small business owner. They also can cause the demise of a practice that is bringing in revenue and is otherwise profitable. Many small business owners learn about business and personal taxation through a baptism of fire, if they are lucky enough to survive it. It is imperative that bookkeeping information be forwarded to the accountant in a timely manner in order for the owner to ascertain the tax liabilities of the business, to meet the dates taxes are due, and to budget appropriately.

Without a rudimentary knowledge of basic accounting and bookkeeping principles, the private practice owner is not in a position to make critical decisions regarding the finances of the practice. Questions such as the following must be answered: Is the business profitable? What is the break-even point? Should expenses be reduced? Should prices be increased? Is the ratio of cost of goods to gross revenue acceptable? Is there a cash flow problem? Should equipment be purchased this year or next? These decisions will have a direct impact on the financial health of the practice and will affect its tax liability. Although it is the bookkeeper who prepares the books and the accountant who does the financial analysis and gives advice, it is the owner who must make the final decisions. The owner may also want to enlist the services of a professional financial planner or licensed investment adviser who can assist him or her in managing the investments of the business. This may include establishing and managing pension/profit-sharing plans, money market and mutual funds, and stock accounts, along with personal financial planning. A financial planner can be of great assistance in helping the practice achieve its goals. (A detailed discussion of practice accounting can be found in Chapter 15.)

Relationships with Vendors

For most small businesses, it is necessary to establish relationships with wholesalers and retailers. In an audiology practice, office supplies and accessories are needed for conducting diagnostic evaluations (e.g., otoscope supplies, insert earphone tips, and electrodes). If hearing aids are dispensed, it is necessary to establish relationships with a variety of hearing aid manufacturers, companies that carry hearing aid accessories, battery suppliers, and companies that specialize in hearing assistive technology.

Most vendors require a credit application before entering into a business relationship with the practice. The credit application asks for banking information and credit references from other vendors. For a newly established business, it is prudent to establish a few initial relationships to prove that the practice is solvent enough to pay its bills in a timely manner. These vendors can serve as references to increase the practice's credit pool. Typically, it is easier to establish accounts with larger hearing aid companies than with smaller businesses, whose cash flow is at the mercy of small practices.

For audiologists who dispense, it is wise to limit the number of manufacturers that will provide products for the practice. This is advantageous for several reasons. From a business perspective, it is important to manage effectively the profit margin on products sold. Profit margins naturally increase when higher numbers of products are purchased from a single vendor, because of quantity discounts. Buying with quantity discounts applies to all types of products, from hearing aids to tubes of electrode paste. Additionally, it is easier for the audiologist to attain a high level of expertise with products if the number of product lines used is limited. Because of this, many dispensing audiologists try to purchase hearing aids from a few companies that have a full line of instruments (e.g., economy, essential, advanced, and premium digital hearing devices). The practice can then offer patients the highest quality instruments at the best price point for all concerned. Lastly, special considerations are often needed for certain patients, and having a close working relationship with a few manufacturers helps to secure special attention when needed.

A vendor's customer service can be as important as quantity discounts. Companies that provide good products at reasonable prices but have very poor turnaround time for new orders and repairs may not be worth the money saved in product pricing. Equally important is the manufacturer's quality control. Although patients may acknowledge that the audiologist is the liaison between the manufacturer and the patient, when products are faulty, the finger of blame is pointed at the audiologist. High customer satisfaction will be realized if the practice uses vendors with fast turnaround time and reliable products, even if they cost a few dollars more. The adage "You get what you pay for" holds true in this case.

In working with hearing aid manufacturers, the practice is doing more than just ordering products from vendors. Many manufacturers are interested in helping businesses increase hearing aid sales by providing marketing support. This support often comes in the form of advertising dollars and human resources (i.e., regional sales representatives). For example, as new hearing aid technologies come onto the market, the manufacturer and private practice owner will want to make the products known to the public at large. This is done through direct mail, seminars, open houses, newspaper ads, and television and radio commercials. Sometimes vendors will offset the costs of such marketing (where their products are promoted), by paying part or all of a newspaper ad or announcement. At other times, manufacturers may help the practice host an informational seminar or open house by advertising the activity and by sending a company representative to the practice to provide first-hand information about the new products. Because the manufacturer and practice are promoting the same products together, they are forming a strategic alliance to help each other. Such an alliance may come at an unacceptable cost to the owner, however, if it creates an ethical conflict of interest or if there is a financial burden in the long run (e.g., the forfeiting of volume discounts).

Controversial Point

- Although marketing support from hearing aid manufacturers can be helpful to a practice, the type of support varies from company to company. It is important for the owner to have a full understanding of manufacturers' terms and conditions before entering into any marketing arrangement. The particular product line being promoted may not be appropriate for every patient, and it is incumbent on the owner to make sure patient care is not compromised during any marketing event. The audiologist must put patients' needs first without any real or perceived conflict of interest (see AAA, *Ethical Practice Guidelines*, n.d., on Financial Incentives from Hearing Instrument Manufacturers).

◆ Introducing New Sources of Revenue

Revenues from Patient Services and Sales

As a practice grows, more and more individuals in the community become aware of the expertise the practice offers, and greater opportunities for expansion arise. For many practices, this means establishing outside contracts with other facilities. A common outside contract involves providing audiology support for local otolaryngology offices. This type of arrangement will bring in more revenue dollars from diagnostic testing done at the physicians' offices. Diagnostic services may be billed directly to the patient in such a situation, or remuneration may come in the form of an hourly rate paid by the physician. However, the primary increase in revenue is often in the form of physicians' referrals to the audiology private practice for hearing aid services. Such arrangements require monitoring to ensure the

arrangement is profitable and does not create any conflicts of interest. For example, if too much time is spent servicing contract arrangements away from the practice, the revenue that is brought in may be less than the revenue that would be generated by focusing on the practice's own patients.

Other common sources of outside revenue are from nursing home and senior residential communities, which contract for the provision of services provided at the facility using the practice's portable equipment. These types of arrangements require tight organization on the part of the facility and clear guidelines from the managing audiologist regarding the practice's requirements for providing services on-site. In order for these visits to be profitable, it is important that several patients be seen on the same day and that the schedule is as efficiently organized as possible. For instance, patients should receive otoscopic examinations prior to the audiologist's visit and have excessive cerumen removed so that hearing evaluations can be performed and ear impressions can be made, if needed. If rehabilitative services and products are provided, it is mandatory to arrange in-service training to the nursing home staff, in addition to counseling and support to the patients, thus ensuring successful rehabilitative outcomes. Reimbursement for some services may be difficult to obtain. Billing issues must be ironed out prior to administering services and/or selling products.

Public health agencies and government programs such as Medicare, Medicaid, state children's services, and vocational rehabilitation services may contract with audiologists to provide hearing health care for their recipients. Service may include hearing screening and evaluation, hearing aid consultation and fitting, and follow-up, as well as counseling and training. Typically, this type of contract will bring in revenue, but at a rate far below what is billed to private-pay patients. Billing and collecting can be time-consuming and expensive. Therefore, resources that are expended for services and products that bring in limited revenue must be weighed against seeing fewer patients, but at a standard rate of reimbursement.

Providing occupational hearing conservation services, including establishing or maintaining programs for industry or school systems, can increase revenue. Nonoccupational services, such as for recreational activities, lend themselves to this type of outside consultation. Related to this are specialized subcategories of patients. Trapshooters and musicians, for example, need hearing protection; commercial and recreational pilots need earmolds for communications, as do news commentators and security personnel. Indeed, there are audiologists who have structured their private practices almost exclusively on recreational or occupational audiology.

Obviously, marketing efforts will provide a mechanism for increasing revenue in a private practice. Hearing aid practices, for example, routinely market to patients by sending fliers and informational newsletters. Advertising to the general hearing-impaired population via the local newspaper and television and radio stations can bring in new patients. Lectures at service organizations and professional or civic groups can increase confidence in the practice, resulting in more referrals (see Chapter 5).

Revenues from Outside Consulting and Contracting

For many audiologists in private practice, outside contracting with hearing aid and other equipment manufacturers can bring in additional revenue. Some audiologists are hired to train other clinicians to fit and use a particular manufacturers' products. Other audiologists act as part-time regional sales managers for these companies, providing equipment information and support to fellow audiologists using the products. Acting as a consultant to a hearing aid company or equipment manufacturer may entail doing clinical research on new products, assisting in new product development, interacting with engineers, and providing general audiologic support. These types of relationships can be very advantageous to the audiology field at large. Clinicians who handle products or use equipment have a mechanism, through their consulting contracts, to provide direct input to companies that design their products. It also brings them in direct contact with other audiologists who use the products.

Special Consideration

- Some outside contractual arrangements may bring up ethical considerations. Professional and personal ethics should govern the audiologist's decision-making process and guide him or her in the provision of audiology services and products. Disclosing to patients the nature of outside contracts will avert potential questions and concerns.

Because the private practice venue allows for more autonomy than many other clinical positions, audiologists in private practice may discover an interest in a related area and find a way to segue this interest into the practice, adding a new source of revenue. For example, some private practitioners bring in additional revenue by developing marketing materials or practice management products for other private practices to purchase and use. Others develop accessories that they manufacture and sell to other audiologists. Still others have gone on to develop an altogether different business, based on the needs of their own private practice and on the practices of others (e.g., sponsoring or arranging continuing education events and products).

Private practice challenges an audiologist not only as a professional but also as an individual. It serves as an important mechanism for professional and personal growth. The audiologist, as business owner, comes in contact with other business owners in different fields and disciplines and establishes new relationships with them. In this way, his or her frame of reference is broadened. A private practice can be a very dynamic entity. It allows the managing audiologist to touch on tasks, disciplines, and fields in which he or she has little or no experience. This can be overwhelming at times, but it is also an exciting and exhilarating touchstone for exploring the world anew.

♦ Future Trends in Private Practice

In the first edition of this volume, our speculation on the future focused heavily on managed health care and the effects it may have on audiology private practice. Our speculation has not been borne out. There has not been a broad consolidation of practices into IPAs to gain contracts with large managed care groups. The threat of hostile takeover from practice management companies has passed, and the independent private practice has survived intact. Today there continue to be different types of private practice, whether small, single-location practices focusing on hearing aid dispensing or large, multilocation hearing and balance centers.

As of this writing, there is no clear financial advantage for a hearing-impaired person to seek out one hearing health care delivery system over another. Most health care insurance companies do not provide hearing aid benefit, and there is little assistance from the state or federal government (with the exception of Veterans Affairs). Thus, the patient is not tied financially to a particular delivery system, as the burden of costs still resides with individual patients.

Question remain: What can the private practice model offer that other delivery models cannot? With technology becoming more sophisticated, will there come a time when the audiologist has very little role in the fine-tuning and maintenance of the hearing aids? How will this change the audiologist's role in the care of hearing-impaired patients?

This is where private practice audiologists may have an edge. Even with changes in technology, having a hearing loss, and subsequently being fitted with amplification, is a life-changing event for patients. Private practice audiologists will continue to have a role in counseling patients and providing postfitting support. They will continue to implement powerful psychological interventions in the context of diagnosing and treating hearing loss. Perhaps with less emphasis on the technological aspect of hearing aids, audiologists will be able to focus more on the important components that comprise audiologic rehabilitation. At this writing, there is a renewed interest in focusing less on devices and more on nourishing the neural plasticity of the auditory system. This potentially could maximize patients' benefit from amplification. These listening "retraining" programs, such as the Listening and Communication Enhancement System (Sweetow and Henderson-Sabes, 2004), may help audiologists to redefine their role in the fitting process.

Private practice audiologists may be in a better position to provide this type of personal care than those in retail or medically based practices. In the fast-paced world in which we live, more and more people may be looking for the extra care that a private practice can offer. Having a hearing loss is a very personal issue, and private practice audiologists are well positioned to give the type of individualized care that the new generations of the hearing-impaired may want. It will be incumbent on private practice audiologists not only to offer this extra value but also to make sure that potential patients are aware of this difference. They need to separate themselves from corporate retail chains and medical/audiology practices by marketing the level of service that sets them apart. The public must know what the private practice audiologist has to offer, and they must know it before they walk in the door.

In this chapter, the core issues common to private practice audiology have been reviewed. Private practice can have a significant role in the future of hearing health care as it offers a flexible, adaptive model that can respond effectively to changing technologies and market conditions. Those of you considering going into private practice should have a clear vision of what audiology is and can be in this context. You should understand how unique private practice is in its ability to offer personalized, individual, private care, compared with other delivery models. We hope we have given you a foundation for a better understanding of the private practice model, one that we believe has a strong future and can provide one of the most enriching and rewarding experiences in the profession.

References

American Academy of Audiology. (n.d.). AAA best practices initiative: Phase 1, Frontline office training kit–initiating the journey. McLean, VA: Author.

American Academy of Audiology. (n.d.). Ethical practice guidelines on financial incentives from hearing instrument manufacturers. Retrieved May 4, 2007, from http://www.audiology.org/NR/rdonlyres/12EE4F66-1F1B-461F-B736-7531318D9D69/0/financialincentives.pdf.

American Academy of Audiology. (2005). Compensation and benefits survey. Retrieved May 4, 2007, from http://www.audiology.org/-aboutacademy/newsroom/pressreleases/compsurveyintro.htm?PF=1.

Audiologists by current practice setting. (1998, June). Audiology Express, p. 4.

Bankaitis, A. U., & Kemp, R. J. (2003). Infection control in the audiology clinic. Chesterfield, MO: Oaktree Products.

Bernstein, M. (2000, October). The method to arrive at an ethical decision. Paper presented at the Third Annual Meeting of the American Society for Bioethics and Humanities, Salt Lake City, UT.

Collins, J. C., & Porras, J. I. (1996). Building your company's vision. Harvard Business Review, September-October 1996, 65–77.

Fleury, R. E. (1992). The small business survival guide (pp. 21–23). Naperville, IL: Sourcebooks Trade.

Gardner, H. J., & Stone, M. T. (1998). To save time and labor, consider these audiological report checklists. Hearing Journal, 51, 86–89.

Harford, E. (1993). Impact of the hearing aid on the evolution of audiology: American Auditory Society Carhart Memorial Lecture. AAS Bulletin, 18(2), 7–12, 103, 108.

Hosford-Dunn, H. (2006). Integrated marketing communications (IMC), Part I – CRM: The Ginsu Knife for Marketing. Retrieved May 4, 2007, from http://www.audiologyonline.com/articles/pf_article_detail.asp?article_id=1630.

Hosford-Dunn, H., Dunn, D. R., & Harford, E. R. (1995). Creating the office. In Audiology business and practice management (pp. 147–170). San Diego, CA: Singular Publishing.

Kiyosaki, RT. (2005). Rich dad's before you quit your job: 10 real-life lessons every entrepreneur should know about building a multimillion-dollar business. New York: Warner Business Books.

Kochkin, S. (2004). BHI physician referral development program. Hearing Journal, 8, 27–29.

Metz, M. J. (2000). Some ethical issues related to hearing instrument dispensing. Seminars in Hearing, 21, p. 73.

Stach, B. (1998). Clinical audiology: An introduction. In J. L. Danhauer (Ed.), Reporting and referring (pp. 401–437). San Diego, CA: Singular Publishing.

Sweetow, R. W., & Henderson-Sabes, J. H. (2004). The case for LACE: Listening and auditory communication enhancement training. Hearing Journal, 57, 32–40.

Valente, N., Abrams, H., Benson, D., et al. (2005). Guidelines for the audiological management of adult hearing impairment. Audiology Today, 18(5), 32–36.

Winslow, W. (1995). The making of Silicon Valley. Palo Alto, CA: Santa Clara Valley Historical Society.

Section II

Practice Management Applications

Chapter 7

Health Insurance Portability and Accountability Act (HIPAA) Fundamentals

Kadyn Williams, Helena Stern Solodar, and H. Carol Saul

This chapter discusses the Health Insurance Portability and Accountability Act (HIPAA) and its impact on health care providers and their patients. An overview of this broad legislation is followed by more in-depth insight into the basics of the privacy and security rules.

♦ Background

Think of HIPAA as a new way of conducting business that alters the way in which all health care providers, including audiologists, create, share, use, and disclose health information. Prior to 1996, when the act was passed, the order of the day was one of relative openness; today it is one of increased privacy and security. Besides the issue of quality of care, today the issues of privacy, confidentiality, and security of health information must be daily concerns for audiologists. This chapter provides an overview of the fundamentals of HIPAA compliance, with numerous references that will lead the reader to more detailed guidance on this complex body of law.[1]

The Health Insurance Portability and Accountability Act, also known as the Kennedy-Kassebaum bill, is an expansive federal law that affects Americans' health care in several ways. First, it allows persons to qualify immediately for comparable health insurance coverage when they change jobs. Second, it strengthens the enforcement weaponry in the government's arsenal aimed at detecting and punishing fraud and abuse in the health care industry. Third, it contains provisions addressing medical savings accounts and access to long-term care and

---

[1]This material does not constitute legal advice, which can only be given by legal counsel in response to specific questions and facts. This material is believed to be accurate as of the date of its printing; however, because HIPAA is an evolving body of law, the reader should check for changes in law before relying on any statements.

coverage. As focused on in this chapter, HIPAA also governs the privacy and security of health information.

Once the HIPAA statute was passed by Congress, the Department of Health and Human Services (DHHS) was charged with developing regulations to implement its broad provisions. This was done over several years, and for certain portions of the regulations, is still under way at the time of this writing. As a result, there are different effective dates and compliance deadlines for different parts of administrative simplification. Provisions generally are aimed at promoting the transmission of health care information electronically and lessening the paperwork burdens on the health care sector, while strengthening patients' rights of privacy of their health records. An authoritative source on HIPAA compliance deadlines may be found at http://www.cms.hhs.gov/HIPAAGenInfo/Downloads/HIPAACompliance Deadlines.asp.

◆ Administrative Simplification Rules

Ironically, the "administrative simplification" provisions of HIPAA are anything but simple. They address five broad areas, including standard transactions and code sets, unique health identifiers, electronic signatures, privacy rules, and security rules, of which the latter two are the focus of this chapter.

1. *Standard transactions and code sets*   These identify types of transactions that must be communicated using standard formats and codes. They include (1) health care claims or equivalent encounter information, (2) health care payment and remittance advice, (3) coordination of benefits, (4) health care claim status, (5) enrollment or disenrollment in a health plan, (6) eligibility for a health plan, (7) health plan premium payment, and (8) referral certification and authorization. Other standard transactions, such as claims attachments, are likely to be added in the future. The compliance deadline for the standard transactions and code set rules was October 16, 2002, unless a 1-year extension was granted, in which case compliance was required by October 16, 2003. For a period after the deadline, the Centers for Medicare and Medicaid Services (CMS) continued to accept claims in nonstandard format; however, as of October 1, 2005, CMS announced that noncompliant claims would not be processed. For additional information on HIPAA's standard transactions and code set rules, go to http://www.cms.hhs.gov/hipaa/hipaa2/regulations/transactions/default.asp.

2. *Unique health identifiers*   HIPAA directs DHHS to develop standards for the adoption of unique health identifiers for employers, health plans, and health care providers. The provider identifier is referred to as the national provider identifier (NPI). The final rule adopting the HIPAA standard unique health identifier for providers was published February 23, 2004, and as of May 23, 2005, all providers may apply for their NPI. The compliance deadline for all covered entities was May 23, 2007, except that small health plans do not need to comply until May 23, 2008.

After these dates, covered entities must use the assigned 10-digit NPIs in all standard transactions. Therefore, providers will no longer have to keep track of different numbers to identify themselves in standard transactions with multiple health plans. To apply online, go to http://nppes.cms.hhs.gov. Additional information regarding the NPI is available at http://new.cms.hhs.gov/NationalProvidentStand/01_overview.asp. Rules implementing a national employer identifier became effective on July 30, 2004. The final rule adopted the Internal Revenue Service's employer identification number (EIN) as the standard for employers. Rules for a national health plan identifier remain under development.

3. *Electronic signatures*   HIPAA mandates the adoption of an electronic signature standard whereby an electronic signature is used in the transmission of a standard transaction. A rule on electronic signatures has not yet been finalized.

4. *Privacy rules*   Establish who may have access to protected health information.

5. *Security rules*   Set the standards for ensuring that only those who should have access to electronic health records will actually have access.

Who Must Comply with HIPAA's Administrative Simplification Rules?

Covered Entities

HIPAA directly governs the actions of individuals or entities that come within HIPAA's definition of covered entities (CEs). CEs are (1) health plans or payers (including self-insured health plans and government payers, such as Medicare and Medicaid programs); (2) health care clearinghouses, such as billing services that process health information into or out of standard format; and (3) certain health care providers, such as audiologists, physicians, hospitals, and pharmacies.

Health care providers, such as audiologists, are CEs only if they transmit health information electronically in connection with a standard transaction covered by the HIPAA transaction rule. Thus, a health care provider who does nothing electronically, if such exists today, is not a CE for purposes of the privacy rule.

> **Pitfall**
>
> - It is a common misconception that small companies are exempt from HIPAA compliance. All health care providers that are covered entities must comply regardless of the size of the organization.

Business Associates

Although they are not required to comply with HIPAA as a CE (and are not subject to government fines for noncompliance), another category of entity—the business associate—will be indirectly affected. HIPAA's business associate provisions stem from Congress's concern that the safeguards afforded by HIPAA could be avoided, whether intentionally or unintentionally, by a CE's use of the services of third parties, such as consultants, collection agencies, information technology providers, or others who are not themselves directly subject to HIPAA. HIPAA therefore provides that a CE may disclose protected health information to a business associate, and may allow a business associate to create or receive protected health information on its behalf, only if the CE obtains "satisfactory assurances" that the business associate will appropriately safeguard the information. HIPAA requires that those satisfactory assurances be in the form of very specific provisions contained in a written agreement (commonly referred to as a business associate agreement) between the CE and its business associate.

A CE may be liable for its business associate's breach of the agreement if it knows that the associate is breaching the

terms of the agreement and if it fails to cure the breach or terminate the contract (or report the breach to DHHS if termination is not feasible).

So, how does a CE determine who its business associates are? A business associate is an entity who (1) on behalf of the CE, performs or assists in the performance of a function or service that involves the use or disclosure of individually identifiable health information (IIHI); or (2) provides legal, actuarial, accounting, consulting, data aggregation, management, accreditation, administrative, or financial services to the CE if the service involves the disclosure of IIHI from the CE or from another business associate of the CE. A flow chart to assist in analyzing business associate relationships is given in **Fig. 7–1**.

In an audiologic practice setting, business associates may include billing and collection agencies, information

Who Is a Business Associate?

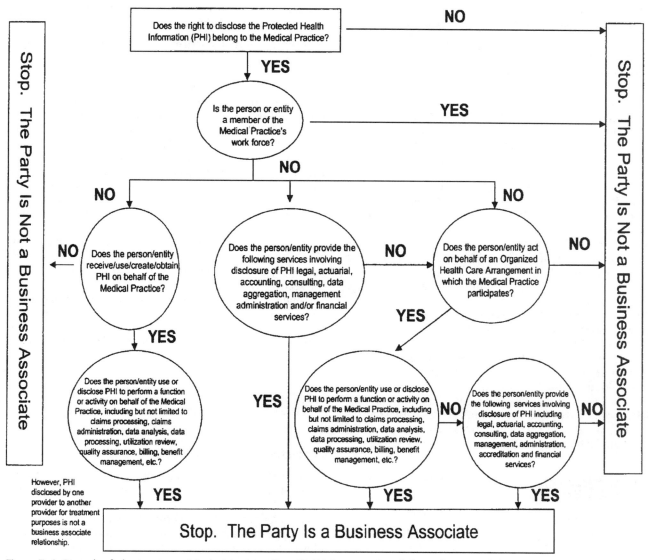

Figure 7–1 Example of a business associate decision tree. (From Health Insurance Portability and Accountability Act (HIPAA) privacy manual: A how-to guide for your medical practice. (2003). Gates Moore & Company, Epstein Becker & Green, P.C., with permission.)

technology services, marketing consultants, and legal and accounting services. Who is considered a business associate will vary from practice to practice. The question is whether or not this outside source uses or discloses patients' protected health information (PHI) to carry out functions for the practice. For example, the relationship between an attorney and a practice does not always involve the attorney's use or disclosure of PHI. If, however, the practice is sued by a patient, the practice's attorney likely will need access to the patient's PHI, and a business associate agreement will be required. Similarly, a hearing aid manufacturer that accesses PHI for treatment purposes is not a business associate. However, a hearing aid manufacturer whose representative assists the office with a software application and has access to PHI is a business associate.

Pearl

- Business associate agreements are not necessary if the sharing of PHI with the manufacturer is for the purpose of treatment.

Entities that merely act as conduits for IIHI (e.g., the U.S. Postal Service) are not business associates because no disclosure is intended, and the probability of disclosure is small. Also, financial institutions that process consumer payments for health care services are not business associates, provided that the CE complies with HIPAA's minimum necessary disclosure requirements, discussed below. Finally, keep in mind that a CE itself may be a business associate if it provides services for or on behalf of another CE.

HIPAA's definition of *business associate* includes a specific exception for members of a CE's workforce. *Workforce* is defined as employees, volunteers, trainees, and others whose work for a CE is under the direct control of the CE, regardless of whether they are paid by the CE.

There remains a great deal of confusion throughout the health care industry as to when a business associate agreement is required to be put in place, and if put in place, which entity is the CE and which is the business associate. It will be helpful to keep in mind that the business associate provisions do not apply to disclosures by a CE to a health care provider concerning the treatment of the patient. In fact, HIPAA generally allows communications between or among CEs that are directly related to treatment, payment, or health care operations (TPO).

Special Consideration

- Protected health information may be shared without patient authorization if there is reason to believe that the patient is being (or will be) treated by the other health care provider.

What terms are required to be in the business associate agreement? HIPAA is very specific as to those terms. As noted, a CE must enter into a written agreement with each of its business associates that provides "satisfactory assurances" that the business associate will safeguard the PHI as required by HIPAA. The business associate agreement must provide that the business associate shall

- Use or disclose PHI only as permitted pursuant to the business associate agreement and not in a manner that would violate the privacy rules if such actions were taken by the CE

- Use appropriate safeguards to prevent use or disclosure of PHI except as permitted by the agreement

- Report any known misuse of PHI to the CE

- Impose the same requirements on the business associate's subcontractors and agents

- Make PHI and an accounting of disclosures available to patients as required by the privacy rules

- Make its internal practices, books, and records relating to use and disclosure of PHI available to DHHS

In addition, the business associate agreement must allow a CE to terminate the agreement if the CE determines that the business associate has breached a material term of the agreement. Upon termination, the business associate must be required, if feasible, to return or destroy all PHI and retain no copies. If return or destruction is not feasible, then the obligations in the business associate agreement must continue. A sample business associate agreement form may be accessed at http://www.hhs.gov/ocr/hipaa/contractprov.html. However, the form has not been updated for compliance with the security rule.

Additional provisions required to be included in business associate agreements were established in the security rule and apply to electronic PHI (EPHI). These are discussed in the security rule section of this chapter.

If one is willing to sign another party's business associate agreement, it should be reviewed carefully by competent legal counsel. This ensures that additional terms, not required by HIPAA and perhaps detrimental to the signer, have not been added.

◆ The HIPAA Privacy Rule

Protected Health Information

The privacy rule addresses confidentiality of PHI. With certain exceptions, PHI is all IIHI that is transmitted or maintained in any form, including oral, written, or electronic information. Health information is any information created or received by a health care provider, health plan, public health authority, employer, life insurer, school or university, or health care clearinghouse *and* relates to the past, present, or future provision of health care to an individual, or the past, present, or future payment for the provision of those services. Note that both educational records and student medical records are specifically excluded from HIPAA's definition of PHI.

Deidentified Protected Health Information

If there is a reasonable expectation that health information does not identify an individual, then the information is not protected by the privacy rule. There are two ways in which information may be deidentified by a CE: either by removing all 18 identifiers, or by having a statistician determine and document that there is a very small risk of linking the information with an individual. The 18 designated identifiers listed within the privacy rule may be found in **Table 7–1**.

When PHI is used for the purpose of research, public health, or health care operations, uses and disclosures of a limited data set are permitted. A limited data set removes 16 of the 18 identifiable items, with the only remaining items being either references to dates, such as dates of admission, discharge, or service, date of death, age, and any geographic subdivision, including a town, city, state, or zip code; however, specific street addresses cannot be included in a limited data set.

To use a limited data set, a CE must obtain a data use agreement from the entities that are using the information. The data use agreement may be customized, as there are no specific requirements regarding the format of this agreement; however, the following must be included: the permitted uses and disclosures of the data by the recipient, a limitation on who can use or receive the data, and a statement that the recipient agrees not to reidentify the data or contact the patient.

Limitations on Use and Disclosure of Protected Health Information

Understanding the terms *use* and *disclosure* is essential to understanding what information may or may not be divulged by a CE. *Use* is defined as the sharing, employment, application, utilization, examination, or analysis of PHI within a CE. *Disclosure* is the release, transfer, or giving access to or divulging in any other manner PHI to anyone outside the CE. HIPAA permits CEs to use and disclose PHI for limited purposes. To use or disclose PHI, one of the following four conditions must exist: (1) written authorization is obtained from the patient; (2) the information falls within the privacy rule permitted uses of TPO, as defined in the glossary in Appendix 7–1; (3) the information falls within a more stringent state regulation; or (4) the disclosure is required by law (e.g., disclosures related to law enforcement, national security, or other similar purposes; disclosures related to public health oversight or similar activities; disclosures regarding victims of abuse or crime; and disclosures related to workers' compensation).

Pearl

- Common office practices are permissible, such as the use of sign-in sheets and calling patients back for treatment, as long as care is taken to protect the privacy of patients.

Additionally, HIPAA requires CEs to limit the use and disclosure of PHI to the minimum necessary to accomplish the purpose of the disclosure or request, unless that information is shared with the patient, between health care providers for treatment purposes, the disclosure is required by a state law, or is requested by a government agency. Thus, CEs frequently must make reasonable efforts to use or disclose only the minimum necessary amount of PHI required to achieve the purpose of the particular use or disclosure. Every CE should implement policies to identify the persons or classes of persons in its workforce who need access to PHI to carry out their duties, and should limit access only to those identified persons and only to necessary PHI.

Special Consideration

- Under the privacy rule, health care providers are permitted to leave messages unless the patient requests otherwise. The rule permits the disclosure of limited information to family members or others regarding patient care even when the patient is not present.

Table 7–1 Eighteen Identifiers Designated in the Privacy Rule

1. Name
2. Social Security number
3. Any address specification, such as street, city, county, precinct, and zip code (entire zip code must be removed if the geographic unit formed by combining all zip codes with the same three initial digits has a population of ≤ 20,000 people; otherwise, only the last two digits must be removed)
4. Electronic mail address
5. Web site address
6. Certificate or license number, such as driver's license number
7. Health plan beneficiary number
8. Account number maintained by the health care provider
9. Medical device identifier and serial number, such as hearing aid serial number
10. Telephone number
11. Fax number
12. All dates except for the year, including birth date, admission date, discharge date, date of death, and all ages > 89
13. Internet protocol address number
14. Full-face photographic images and any comparable image
15. Vehicle identifier and serial number, including license plate number
16. Medical record number
17. Biometric identifier, including finger and voice prints
18. Any other unique identifying number, characteristic, or code

To prevent violations of the privacy rule, there are several commonsense steps that should be taken:

- No one should be given access to information that they do not need.

- Employees and other third parties should be informed and educated about the CE's HIPAA policies. A confidentiality agreement should be signed by non–business associate third parties, such as a cleaning service or security personnel, who might accidentally access PHI. (A sample confidentiality agreement for this purpose is in Appendix 7–2.) In effect, this confidentiality agreement should state that the party will not access PHI and that, in the event that it is either accidentally or incidentally seen, it will not be used or disclosed by that party.

Pearl

- A family member can pick up hearing aids or products from the practice on the patient's behalf unless the patient directs otherwise.

HIPAA also contains very specific requirements governing a CE's response to a third-party request for medical records, such as a subpoena or attorney's discovery request for documents. Before providing documents in response to such a request, consult with competent advisers to ensure compliance.

◆ What Rights Does HIPAA Give to Patients?

HIPAA gives patients the right to:

- Receive a copy of the CE's notice of privacy practices (NPP)

- Authorize use and disclosure of PHI for certain non-TPO purposes

- Request restrictions on certain uses and disclosures of PHI

- Receive PHI via alternative means

- Inspect and copy PHI

- Request an amendment of PHI

- Request an accounting of disclosures of PHI made by the CE for non-TPO purposes

- Complain to the CE and the DHHS about alleged violations

Notice of Privacy Practices

Although the privacy rule clearly gives patients certain rights to their own health care records and addresses their control of the use and disclosure of this information, it also allows CEs the ability to use and disclose information as long as it is in connection with TPO activities. To exercise this right, the CE must

- Provide the patient with a copy of the NPP, which outlines in plain language the patient's rights with regard to PHI, as well as the CE's common practices for PHI use (e.g., the use of reminder cards)

- Obtain, or make a concerted effort to obtain, patient signature acknowledging receipt of the NPP

The NPP is the key HIPAA document that informs patients of their rights regarding their PHI and how it is protected. The NPP must be in "plain English," reflect true practice policy, and be conspicuously displayed. A copy of the NPP should be posted on the CE's Web site if the Web site describes the services and benefits of the practice. Except in emergent circumstances, discussed below, patients must receive the NPP on the date that the first service is rendered, and the CE is required to make a good faith effort to document that the NPP was received by the patient. Subsequent revisions to the NPP also must be posted conspicuously and, upon request, must be given to patients. An abbreviated version is unacceptable. For useful guidance on drafting an NPP, go to http://www.hrsa.gov/language.htm.

There is no specific format to use for acknowledgment of receipt of the NPP. For example, a practice may choose to have the patient initial a copy of the NPP or sign on a separate sheet of paper, as long as the acknowledgment is retained by the practice. **Figure 7–2** contains a sample NPP acknowledgment form.

If an emergency visit is required, the NPP can be given to the patient in a reasonable amount of time after the visit. Additionally, if a patient refuses to acknowledge receipt of the NPP, the practice should document this refusal but provide treatment nevertheless. Only in a research setting may treatment be withheld based on the patient's refusal to sign the NPP.

Pitfall

- Audiologists cannot withhold treatment even when the patient refuses to sign a written acknowledgment of receipt of the NPP. Remember to document the effort and refusal.

Authorizations

A CE must obtain a written authorization to use PHI when the use or disclosure of PHI is being made for purposes other than TPO. There may be variations in the content of the patient authorization depending on the purpose of the use or disclosure. Minimally, an authorization must

- Contain a specific expiration date that relates to the patient or the purpose of the use or disclosure (except for those authorizations related to research, which must post either an expiration date/event or a statement that no such expiration date/event exists)

____
Practice Name

ACKNOWLEDGMENT OF RECEIPT
OF NOTICE OF PRIVACY PRACTICES

I, ______________________ , have received a copy of ______________________'s
Patient Name — Practice Name

Notice of Privacy Practices.

______________________ ______________
Signature of Patient or Legal Guardian — Date

Figure 7–2 Example of a notice of privacy practices (NPP) acknowledgment. (From Health Insurance Portability and Accountability Act (HIPAA) privacy manual: A how-to guide for your medical practice. (2003). Gates Moore & Company, Epstein Becker & Green, P.C., with permission.)

- Name the person/entity authorized to make the requested use or disclosure (e.g., the CE)
- Name the person/entity authorized to receive the PHI from the CE
- Describe the PHI to be used or disclosed
- Include a description of each purpose of the use or disclosure
- Inform the patient of his or her right to revoke the authorization, including exceptions to this right and a description of how to revoke the authorization
- Warn the patient that additional disclosures may occur and that the PHI may no longer be protected by the privacy rule
- Include a statement that treatment may not be conditioned on receipt of the authorization, or under the circumstances where it can be conditioned, such as for research purposes, a statement about the consequences of refusing to sign the authorization
- Be signed by the patient or his or her personal representative
- If signed by a personal representative, contain a description of his or her authority to act for the individual

There are three basic forms of authorization that a CE may need:

- Authorizations upon which treatment may not be conditioned
- Authorizations upon which treatment may be conditioned, such as for research purposes
- Authorizations for marketing purposes, unless exceptions apply

A copy of the signed authorization must be provided to the patient, and a CE must retain authorizations for a minimum of 6 years; however, if a state law is more stringent, then the state law retention requirement prevails. See Appendix 7–3 for a sample form of authorization.

Marketing to Patients

HIPAA defines *marketing* as any communication about a product or service, a purpose of which is to encourage recipients of the communication to purchase or use the product or service. Although most audiologic practices engage in a variety of marketing activities, many of these fall within the exceptions to HIPAA's marketing rule. It is imperative that a practice understand the applicability of this rule to its various marketing activities. Therefore, as a general rule under HIPAA, a patient's authorization is required before using or disclosing PHI for marketing purposes. Several exceptions may apply to the marketing definition and to the authorization requirement.

The HIPAA marketing definition does not include activities that constitute TPO. Thus, CEs may use and disclose PHI for TPO without securing an authorization. Communications made by a CE for the purpose of describing its network, the scope of its services, and the services for which it pays do not constitute marketing. Additionally, communications tailored by the CE to the circumstances of a particular individual for treatment purposes or for furthering the individual's care are not within the definition of marketing. This permits activities such as recall/reminder cards, referrals, prescriptions, recommendations, and other communications that address how a product or service may relate to the individual's health. Moreover, communications made by the CE to an individual in the course of managing the treatment of that individual or for recommending alternative treatment, therapies, providers, or settings of care are not marketing communications. This exception permits CEs to discuss products or services in the course of managing an individual's care or providing treatment.

Other exceptions fall within the definition of marketing but involve specific situations where an authorization is not required. First, face-to-face, verbal communications with an individual do not require an authorization: an audiologist who simply tells a patient about a new product or service during an office visit is not conducting a marketing activity. Additionally, communications involving products or services of nominal value do not require an authorization. Thus, giving patients private-labeled batteries, birthday cards, or similar promotional products is permissible. Third, communications involving health-related products or services of the CE or of a third party are permitted, but only if the communication (1) identifies the CE as the marketer; (2) reveals whether the CE receives any payment from a third party for making the communication; (3) tells the individual how to opt out of future communications; and (4) if PHI was used to target an individual about a particular product or service, discloses why the individual was chosen and how the product or service could benefit the individual. Additionally, to market health-related products or services, the CE must have determined, prior to making the communication, that the product or service may be beneficial to the health of the type or class of individual targeted.

Unless one of the above exceptions is met, marketing using patients' PHI should not be conducted. In fact, the selling or giving away of the patient list to anyone, including a business associate or another vendor, without a signed authorization from each patient contacted, could be a criminal violation of HIPAA.

Pearl

- Giveaways of nominal value are permitted, as are most of the provider's own marketing activities, such as annual reminders and newsletters.

Personal Representatives

A personal representative is someone who has the authority under existing law (e.g., state law) to make decisions related to health care and act on behalf of an individual, such as guardians or persons with a power of attorney. The privacy rule refers to decisions related to health care as those pertaining to treatment and payment decisions on behalf of the patient. For example, in an emergency situation, a spouse may make decisions relating to immediate health care but may not be provided with PHI received many years ago. Note also that, in the case of a deceased patient, PHI remains protected, and the patient's rights of privacy belong to the patient's estate.

Minors

State laws may be more or less stringent than HIPAA, but in either case, HIPAA defers to all state laws regarding the disclosure of a minor's health information to a parent as the minor's personal representative. Thus, each audiologist must be cognizant of the laws governing the PHI of minors in the state in which he or she practices.

Other Administrative Steps Required by the Privacy Rule

In order for CEs to be compliant with HIPAA, additional administrative requirements must be met. A privacy officer, who is held responsible for developing and implementing the policies and procedures of the privacy rule, must be designated by the CE. The privacy officer may be either someone who is currently employed or someone specifically hired to take on the role. This individual should also be in charge of tracking and documenting wrongful disclosure incidents, as shown in **Fig. 7–3**, as well as more routine, permitted disclosures (see sample log to track disclosures of PHI in **Fig. 7–4**), and implementing changes or modifications identified during a risk assessment. The CE also must provide and document training regarding PHI policies and

---

Practice Name

PRIVACY OFFICER'S INCIDENT EVENT LOG

Date Received	Date Investigation Complete	Nature of Complaint	Results of Investigation	Sanctions

Figure 7–3 Example of a privacy officer's incident log. (From Health Insurance Portability and Accountability Act (HIPAA) privacy manual: A how-to guide for your medical practice. (2003). Gates Moore & Company, Epstein Becker & Green, P.C., with permission.)

Practice Name

LOG TO TRACK DISCLOSURES OF PHI

Patient Name_____

For each patient, you are required to keep a log of all disclosures of PHI for non-TPO reasons for which you did not receive a signed authorization from the patient. For each disclosure, fill in the date it occurred along with a description of the type of disclosure. In addition, you need to provide a description of the PHI disclosed along with the names and titles to whom it was disclosed.

DATE	DESCRIPTION OF DISCLOSURE	DESCRIPTION OF PHI	Who Requested	To Whom PHI Was Disclosed	Approve/Deny (+ initials)	REASON FOR DENIAL, COMMENTS

Figure 7–4 Example of a protected health information (PHI) disclosure log. TPO, treatment, payment, and operations. (From Health Insurance Portability and Accountability Act (HIPAA) privacy manual: A how-to guide for your medical practice. (2003). Gates Moore & Company, Epstein Becker & Green, P.C., with permission.)

procedures for all workforce (a sample training checklist is given in Appendix 7–4); provide a complaint process for individuals regarding the policies, procedures, and compliance with such policies and procedures of the privacy rule; and develop and apply appropriate sanction policies against the workforce members who fail to comply with HIPAA policies and procedures.

♦ The HIPAA Security Rule

Overview of the Security Rule

The security rule requires that the audiologic practice implement safeguards to protect the confidentiality, integrity, and availability of certain PHI. The compliance deadline for the security rule, for all CEs except small health plans, was April 20, 2005. Currently, the security rule applies only to EPHI. (The privacy rule, in contrast, applies to PHI in any format, including paper, electronic, or oral.) DHHS has reserved the right to propose standards for the security of PHI in nonelectronic form at a later date.

The security rule is designed to be technology neutral, adaptable to organizations of different sizes, and not to mandate specific technology solutions to security problems. It is not meant to reflect "best practices" in the information technology security area, but instead to mandate a "floor of protection" for EPHI. As with the privacy rule, if PHI is "deidentified" so that the data cannot be linked to a particular individual, the security rule does not apply.

Whereas the privacy rule sets standards for how PHI may be used and disclosed, the security rule sets standards for how to protect EPHI from unauthorized access, alteration, deletion, and transmission. The security rule requires CEs to assess their own unique security needs and risks to devise, implement, and maintain appropriate security. This mandated risk analysis should be documented and should consider "all relevant losses" that could result if the security measures were not in place (e.g., losses caused by unauthorized uses or disclosures and loss of data integrity).

As shown in **Table 7–2**, the security rule sets out security standards that must be implemented, including "required" and "addressable" implementation specifications. As the name suggests, required implementation specifications must be implemented. Addressable implementation specifications, in contrast, oblige the CE to assess how reasonable and appropriate the specification is, in light of the CE's operations. If reasonable and appropriate, the CE should implement the addressable specifications; if not reasonable and appropriate, the CE must document why it is not implementing the specification and use instead some alternative measure to achieve the desired security goal.

In deciding which addressable security measures to use, a CE must take into account (1) its size, complexity, and capabilities; (2) its technical infrastructure, hardware, and software security capabilities; (3) the costs of the security measures; and (4) the probability and severity of potential risks to EPHI. DHHS advises, however, that cost is only one factor to be taken into consideration and is not meant to free CEs from the responsibility of implementing adequate security measures.

Table 7–2 Security Standards

Security Standards	Required Specifications	Addressable Specifications
Administrative Safeguards		
1. Security management processes	Risk analysis Risk management Sanction policy Information system activity Review	
2. Assigned security responsibility	Identify security officer	
3. Workforce security		Authorization and/or supervision Workforce clearance procedure Termination procedures
4. Information access management	Isolating health care clearinghouse functions	Access authorization Access establishment and modification
5. Security awareness and training		Security reminders Protection from malicious software Log-in monitoring Password management
6. Security incident procedures	Response and reporting	Testing and revising procedures
7. Contingency plan	Data backup plan Disaster recovery plan Emergency mode operation plan	Applications and data criticality analysis
8. Evaluation	Evaluation	
9. Business associate agreement and other arrangements	Business associate agreement	
Physical Safeguards		
10. Facility access controls		Contingency operations Facility security plan Access control and validation procedures Maintenance records
11. Workstation use	Required	
12. Workstation security	Required	
13. Device and media controls	Disposal Media reuse	Accountability Data backup and storage
Technical Safeguards		
14. Access control	Unique user identification Emergency access procedures	Automatic log-off Encryption and decryption
15. Audit controls	Required	
16. Integrity		Addressable
17. Person or entity identification	Required	
18. Transmission security		Integrity controls Encryption
Organizational Requirements		
19. Business associate agreements and other arrangements	Required	
Policies, Procedures, and Documentation Requirements		
20. Policies and procedures	Required	
21. Documentation	Time limit Availability	

The security safeguards are further divided among administrative, physical, and technical safeguards. Two additional categories of requirements are prescribed: (1) organizational requirements and (2) policies and procedures and documentation requirements.

In general, the security rule provides that CEs must

- Ensure the confidentiality, integrity, and availability of all EPHI the CE creates, receives, maintains, or transmits

- Protect against any reasonably anticipated threats or hazards to the security or integrity of such information

- Protect against any reasonably anticipated uses or disclosures of such EPHI that are not permitted or required under the privacy rule

- Ensure compliance with the security rule by their workforce

With apologies for the necessarily technical nature of the material, the following provides a concise summary of the security rule's requirements, organized by the three categories of administrative, physical, and technical safeguards. Each safeguard is labeled as either required or addressable.

This may require obtaining the assistance of someone who is able to fully understand and implement security rule compliance.

Administrative Safeguards

Administrative safeguards are implemented through nine security standards:

1. *Security management process (required)*   Requires policies and procedures to prevent, detect, contain, and correct security violations. The security management process is the "foundation" of security and is implemented by four required specifications:

   a. *Risk analysis (required)*   Conduct an accurate and thorough assessment of the potential risks and vulnerabilities to the confidentiality, integrity, and availability of EPHI held by the CE.

   b. *Risk management (required)*   Implement security measures sufficient to reduce risks and vulnerabilities to a reasonable and appropriate level.

   c. *Sanction policy (required)*   Apply appropriate sanctions against workforce members who fail to comply with the CE's security policies and procedures.

   d. *Information system activity review (required)*   Implement procedures to regularly review records of information system activity, such as audit logs, access reports, and security incident tracking reports.

2. *Assigned security responsibility (required)*   Involves identifying the security officer who is responsible for the development and implementation of the required security policies and procedures. Given the technical nature of compliance, a CE's security officer should be someone who has a sufficient level of understanding of information technology.

3. *Workforce security*   Involves implementing policies and procedures to permit or deny access by the CE's workforce to EPHI, as appropriate. Workforce security is implemented by three addressable specifications:

   a. *Authorization and/or supervision (addressable)*   Implement procedures for the authorization and/or supervision of workforce members who work with EPHI or in locations where it might be accessed.

   b. *Workforce clearance procedure (addressable)*   Implement procedures to determine that the access of a workforce member to EPHI is appropriate. (Note: DHHS indicated that there is no absolute requirement for background checks, but that some personnel screening process is required, ranging in stringency based on the CE's risk analysis.)

   c. *Termination procedures (addressable)*   Implement procedures for terminating access to EPHI when the employment of a workforce member ends or as required by workforce clearance procedures.

4. *Information access management*   Involves the implementation of policies and procedures for authorizing access to EPHI in conformity with the privacy rule. Information access management is implemented by one required implementation specification and two addressable implementation specifications:

   a. *Isolating health care clearinghouse functions (required)*   If a health care clearinghouse is part of a larger organization, the clearinghouse must implement policies and procedures that protect the EPHI from unauthorized access by the larger organization.

   b. *Access authorization (addressable)*   Implement policies and procedures for granting access to EPHI.

   c. *Access establishment and modification (addressable)*   Implement policies and procedures based on the CE's access authorization policies that establish, document, review, and modify a user's right of access to a workstation, transaction, program, or process.

5. *Security awareness and training (required)*   Involves implementing security awareness and training for all members of the workforce, including management. (Note: DHHS states that security training is a "critical activity, regardless of an organization's size." Business associates also must be made aware of security policies and procedures, e.g., through contract language, but CEs have no obligation to provide security training to their business associates.) Security awareness and training is implemented by four addressable implementation specifications:

   a. *Security reminders (addressable)*   Periodic security updates.

   b. *Protection from malicious software (addressable)*   Procedures for guarding against, detecting, and reporting malicious software.

   c. *Log-in monitoring (addressable)*   Procedures for monitoring log-in attempts and reporting discrepancies.

   d. *Password management (addressable)*   Procedures for creating, changing, and safeguarding passwords.

6. *Security incident procedures*   Involve the implementation of policies and procedures for addressing security incidents. The security incident procedures standard is implemented by one required specification:

   a. *Response and reporting (required)*   Identify and respond to suspected or known security incidents; mitigate, to the extent practicable, harmful effects of security incidents that are known to the entity; and document security incidents and their outcomes.

7. *Contingency plan*   The establishment and implementation of emergency response policies and procedures to protect systems that contain EPHI from emergencies and other occurrences, such as fire, vandalism, system failure, and natural disaster. A contingency plan is implemented by three required implementation specifications and two addressable specifications:

a. *Data backup plan (required)* Establish and implement procedures to create and maintain retrievable exact copies of EPHI.

b. *Disaster recovery plan (required)* Establish (and implement as needed) procedures to restore any loss of data.

c. *Emergency mode operation plan (required)* Establish (and implement as needed) procedures to enable continuation of critical business processes for protection of the security of EPHI while operating in emergency mode.

d. *Testing and revision procedures (addressable)* Implement procedures for periodic testing and revision of contingency plans.

e. *Applications and data criticality analysis (addressable)* Assess the relative criticality of specific applications and data in support of other contingency plan components.

8. *Evaluation (required)* The performance of a periodic technical and nontechnical evaluation, based initially upon the standards of the security rule and thereafter in response to changes in the CE's environment or operations affecting the security of EPHI, that establishes the extent to which the CE's security policies and procedures meet the requirements of the security rule.

9. *Business associate agreements and other arrangements* Permitting a business associate to create, receive, maintain, or transmit EPHI on the CE's behalf only if the business associate gives assurances to appropriately safeguard the EPHI. This standard has one required specification:

a. *Business associate agreement (required)* The CE must enter into an agreement that documents the business associate's assurances to appropriately safeguard the EPHI.

Physical Safeguards

Physical safeguards are implemented through four security standards:

1. *Facility access controls* Implement policies and procedures to limit physical access to its electronic information systems and the facility (or facilities) in which they are housed, while ensuring that properly authorized access is allowed. The term *facility* refers to the physical premises and the interior and exterior of a building. This standard is implemented through four addressable specifications:

a. *Contingency operations (addressable)* Establish (and implement as needed) procedures that allow facility access in support of restoration of lost data under the disaster recovery plan and emergency mode operations plan in the event of an emergency.

b. *Facility security plan (addressable)* Implement policies and procedures to safeguard the facility and its equipment where EPHI is stored or accessed from

unauthorized physical access, tampering, and theft. (Note: A CE retains responsibility for considering facility security even if it shares space within a building with other organizations.)

c. *Access control and validation procedures (addressable)* Implement procedures to control and validate a person's access to facilities based on his or her role or function, including visitor control, and control of access to software programs for testing and revision.

d. *Maintenance records (addressable)* Implement policies and procedures to document repairs and modifications to the physical components of a facility that are related to security.

2. *Workstation use (required)* Implement policies and procedures that specify the proper functions, manner of functioning, and physical attributes of the surroundings of the CE's workstations that can access EPHI. (Note: The definition of *workstation* includes portable devices, such as laptop computers.)

3. *Workstation security (required)* Implement physical safeguards for all workstations that access EPHI, to restrict access to authorized users.

4. *Device and media controls* Implement policies and procedures that govern the receipt and removal of hardware and electronic media that contain EPHI into and out of the facility and within the facility. This standard is implemented through two required implementation specifications and two addressable specifications:

a. *Disposal (required)* Implement policies and procedures to address the disposal of EPHI, and/or the hardware or electronic media on which it is stored.

b. *Media reuse (required)* Implement policies and procedures for removal of EPHI from electronic media before the media are made available for reuse.

c. *Accountability (addressable)* Maintain a record of the movements of hardware and electronic media and any person responsible for such movements.

d. *Data backup and storage (addressable)* Create a retrievable, exact copy of EPHI, when needed, before movement of equipment.

Technical Safeguards

Technical safeguards are implemented through five security standards:

1. *Access control* Implement technical policies and procedures for electronic information systems that maintain EPHI to allow access only to authorized persons and programs. This security standard is implemented through two required implementation specifications and two addressable specifications:

a. *Unique user identification (required)* Assign a unique name and/or number for identifying and tracking user identity.

b. *Emergency access procedure (required)*   Establish (and implement as needed) procedures for obtaining necessary EPHI during an emergency.

c. *Automatic logoff (addressable)*   Implement electronic procedures that terminate an electronic session after a predetermined time of inactivity.

d. *Encryption and decryption (addressable)*   Implement a mechanism to encrypt and decrypt EPHI.

2. *Audit controls (required)*   Implement hardware, software, and/or procedural mechanisms that record and examine activity in information systems that contain or use EPHI. (Note: Although DHHS supports the use of a risk assessment and risk analysis to determine how intensive any audit control should be, it stresses that audit controls are mandatory. Furthermore, DHHS cautions that the audit controls under the security rule do not satisfy the privacy rule's requirement regarding accounting for disclosures of PHI, because audit trails record uses within an information system, whereas disclosure accounting applies to disclosures outside of the entity.)

3. *Integrity (addressable)*   Implement policies and procedures to protect EPHI from improper alteration or destruction. This security standard is implemented through a mechanism to authenticate EPHI. (Note: DHHS states that error-correcting memory and magnetic disk storage are examples of built-in data authentication mechanisms and that processes that employ digital signatures or check sum technology can also accomplish data authentication.)

4. *Person or entity authentication (required)*   Implement procedures to verify that a person or entity seeking access to EPHI is the one claimed. (Note: Although DHHS advises that digital signatures and tokens, among other technologies, may be used to implement this standard, smaller entities may decide simply to check picture identification.)

5. *Transmission security*   Implement technical security measures to guard against unauthorized access to EPHI that is being transmitted over an electronic communications network. This security standard is implemented through two addressable specifications:

a. *Integrity controls (addressable)*   Implement security measures to ensure that electronically transmitted EPHI is not improperly modified without detection until disposed of.

b. *Encryption (addressable)*   Implement a mechanism to encrypt EPHI whenever deemed appropriate.

Organizational Requirements

Organizational requirements are implemented through two standards. (The second, applicable only to group health plans, is omitted here.)

1. *Business associate agreements or other arrangements (required)*   A CE must take reasonable steps to cure a business associate's violation of the business associate agreement once the CE knows of a violation. If the reasonable steps are unsuccessful, the CE must either terminate the business associate agreement or report the problem to DHHS, if termination is not practical. The business associate agreement must provide that the business associate will (a) implement safeguards that reasonably and appropriately protect the confidentiality, integrity, and availability of the EPHI; (b) ensure that any agent, including a subcontractor, to whom it provides this information likewise agrees to implement reasonable and appropriate safeguards; (c) report to the CE any security incident of which it becomes aware; and (d) authorize termination of the business associate agreement by the CE if the CE determines that the business associate has violated the business associate agreement. CEs may need to amend their existing business associate agreements to add these terms, particularly (a) and (c), as these provisions were added by the security rule. In addition, the business associate agreement must provide that the business associate will make its policies and procedures, and required documentation relating to the safeguards, available to the secretary of DHHS for purposes of determining the CE's compliance with the security rule.

Policies, Procedures, and Documentation Requirements

Policies, procedures, and documentation requirements are implemented through two standards:

1. *Policies and procedures (required)*   CEs must implement reasonable and appropriate written policies and procedures to comply with the standards, implementation specifications, and other requirements of the security rule.

2. *Documentation (required)*   CEs must maintain written documentation (which may be electronic) of the implemented policies and procedures and of any action, activity, or assessment that is required to be documented. Two required specifications relate to this standard:

a. *Time limit (required)*   Retain the documentation required under the above standard for 6 years from the date of its creation or the date when it last was in effect, whichever is later.

b. *Availability (required)*   Make documentation available to those persons responsible for implementing the procedures to which the documentation pertains.

◆ Risks of Noncompliance

The maximum civil penalty for a HIPAA violation is $100 per violation, up to $25,000 for all violations of an identical requirement during a calendar year. HIPAA also imposes criminal liability for knowingly obtaining or disclosing IIHI, including a fine of up to $50,000 and/or imprisonment for not more than 5 years. However, if a violation is done with the intent to sell, transfer, or use IIHI for commercial advantage, personal gain, or malicious harm, the fine may be up to $250,000, and imprisonment may be as much as 10 years. The enforcement responsibility under the privacy rule is delegated to a director of DHHS's Office for Civil Rights (OCR). The agency's Web site (http://www.hhs.gov/ocr/hipaa/) includes some helpful, frequently asked questions about HIPAA. OCR may consider such things as the nature of the violation, the circumstances under which it occurred, the degree of culpability by the CE, any history of prior violations, and the financial condition of the CE in determining the amount of a penalty. DHHS has also announced its intent to make publicly available information regarding any CE who is found to have violated the privacy rule.

Patients (or their personal representatives) may file a complaint with OCR if they believe that their rights under the privacy rule have been violated, without notifying the CE in advance. When OCR receives a complaint, its investigation may include a review of a CE's written HIPAA policies, as well as the circumstances regarding the alleged violation.

In addition to complaint investigations, OCR is empowered to conduct compliance reviews to determine whether a CE is complying with the HIPAA privacy rule. Currently, due to a lack of enforcement resources, OCR is not conducting compliance reviews and has limited its enforcement activity to complaint investigations.

Whereas OCR is charged with enforcement of the privacy rule, CMS is charged with enforcement of the HIPAA security rule. Final rules addressing the imposition of penalties for CEs who violate HIPAA's privacy or security rules went into effect March 16, 2006. These enforcement rules detail the investigation process, bases of liability, determination of penalty amounts, grounds for waiver of penalties, and the hearing and appeal process that will be followed. To access detailed information or the final rule itself, go to http://www.hipaadvisory. com/regs/regs_in_PDF/finalenfor.pdf.

CEs also must factor in the likely negative publicity and damage to customer relationships that may accompany wrongful disclosures of PHI. Although HIPAA does not give an individual patient the right to sue a CE for violation of the act, failure to comply may expose the CE to private lawsuits under other theories of recovery, such as the constitutional right of privacy and applicable state laws.

Special Consideration

- Patients cannot sue health care providers for violations of their rights under HIPAA. However, patients can file complaints with government agencies, which can lead to government investigations and penalties. Furthermore, a CE may be liable under state law for violations of patient privacy.

◆ Relationship between State Laws and HIPAA

Prior to enactment of HIPAA, legal protections for the confidentiality of health information largely were left to a patchwork of state laws. Although it might be a neat result if one uniform federal law simply replaced the many different state laws, HIPAA does not lead to this result. Under HIPAA's preemption rules, state laws still must be followed if the state law is more protective of patient rights than HIPAA; or if the state law provides for the reporting of disease or injury, child abuse, birth, or death, or for public health surveillance, investigation, or intervention; or where the state law requires health plans to report or provide access to information on management and financial audits, program monitoring, or licensure or certification of facilities or individuals. As a result of HIPAA's preemption doctrine, CEs must continue to consider not only HIPAA but also whether there are any state laws that govern their actions.

◆ Summary

HIPAA represents a fundamental change in the way audiologists must conduct business and is a force we must all reckon with. It is neither a one-time nor a one-size-fits-all event; rather, HIPAA is a process that evolves over time as a practice develops and grows. Although it permits a degree of flexibility and latitude within its framework, there is one absolute: compliance for CEs is not optional; it must be obeyed.

There is a wealth of information readily available to help guide compliance, including the easily accessible Internet materials noted in the References. Use only current materials from reputable sites, such as national trade associations or the government agencies responsible for HIPAA implementation.

Appendix 7–1

Glossary

addressable A security standard that, though not required to be implemented, does require that the covered entity assess whether it is reasonable and appropriate, and either implement it or document why it is not reasonable or appropriate and implement an alternative measure.

authorization   A form that a health care provider must have executed by the individual patient or personal representative to use or disclose the protected health information for purposes other than for treatment, payment, and operations or for specific purposes listed in the privacy rule, such as public health or law enforcement.

business associate (BA)   A person or entity that is not a member of a practice's workforce who uses or discloses protected health information to carry out certain functions or activities on the practice's behalf.

covered entity (CE)   Under the Health Insurance Portability and Accountability Act (HIPAA), this means health plans, health care clearinghouses, and any health care providers (audiologists, physicians, hospitals, nursing homes, etc.) who transmit any health information in electronic form in connection with a HIPAA transaction.

data use agreement   An agreement that sets forth the permitted uses and disclosures of limited data sets, including who may use or receive the data and limitations on the receiving party's ability to reidentify or contact the individuals who are subjects of the limited data sets.

Department of Health and Human Services (DHHS)   A department of the executive branch of the federal government that has overall responsibility for implementing HIPAA.

designated record set   A group of records maintained by or for a covered entity, that is, (1) the medical records and billing records about individuals maintained by or for a covered health care provider; (2) the enrollment, payment, claims adjudication, and case or medical management record systems maintained by or for a health plan; or (3) used, in whole or in part, by or for the covered entity to make decisions about individuals.

disclosure   The release, transfer, provision of, access to, or divulging in any other manner of information outside the entity holding the information.

disclosure history   A list of any persons or entities that have received protected health information for uses unrelated to treatment, payment, and operations.

electronic protected health information (EPHI)   Protected health information that is created, maintained, or transmitted in electronic form. *See* Protected health information (PHI).

health information   Any information created or received by a provider that relates to the past, present, or future physical or mental health condition of a patient, or the past, present, or future payment for the provision of health care to a patient, or the provision of health care to a patient.

Health Insurance Portability and Accountability Act of 1996 (HIPAA)   A federal law that allows persons to qualify immediately for comparable health insurance coverage when they change their employment relationships. Title II, Subtitle F of HIPAA gives the Department of Health and Human Services the authority to mandate the use of standards for the electronic exchange of health care data; to specify what medical and administrative code sets should be used within those standards; to require the use of national identification systems for health care patients, providers, payers (or plans), and employers (or sponsors); and to specify the types of measures required to protect the security and privacy of personally identifiable health care information. Also known as the *Kennedy-Kassebaum bill.*

health care   Includes, but is not limited to, the following: preventive, diagnostic, therapeutic, rehabilitative, maintenance, or palliative care, and counseling service, assessment, or procedure with respect to the physical or mental condition, or functional status, of an individual or that affects the structure or function of the body; and sale or dispensing of a drug, device, equipment, or other item in accordance with a prescription.

health care clearinghouse   An entity that processes or facilitates the processing of information received from another entity in a nonstandard format, or nonstandard data content into standard data elements or a standard transaction, or that receives a standard transaction from another entity and processes or facilitates the processing of that information into nonstandard format or nonstandard data content for a receiving entity.

health care operations   Activities related to a practice's business, clinical management, and administrative duties. Some examples of these activities are use of protected health information to obtain a referral, quality assurance, quality improvement, case management, training programs, licensing, credentialing, certification, accreditation, compliance programs, business management, and general administrative activities of the practice. Includes all activities associated with the selling, merging, transferring, or consolidation of medical practices and other covered entities.

health care provider   A person or organization that provides, bills, and is paid for health care services.

health plan   An individual or group plan that provides, or pays the cost of, medical care.

incidental use or disclosure   A secondary use or disclosure that cannot reasonably be prevented, is limited in nature, and that occurs as a by-product of an otherwise permitted use or disclosure.

individually identifiable health information (IIHI)   Any health information (including demographic information) that is collected from the patient and (1) is created or received by a health care provider or other covered entity or employer and (2) that relates to the past, present, or future physical or mental health or condition of an individual, or the past, present, or future payment for or the provision of health care at the practice *and* that could potentially identify an individual.

limited data set   Protected health information that excludes specific, readily identifiable information about individual patients as well as their relatives, employers, and members of their households. It may include admission, discharge and service dates, date of death, age (including ages 90 and over), and any geographic subdivision (including town or city, state, and 5-digit zip code, but excluding postal addresses).

marketing   To make a communication about a product or service that encourages the recipients of the communication to purchase or use the product or service.

minimum necessary   The principle that, to the extent practical, individually identifiable health information should be disclosed only to the extent needed to support the intended purpose of the disclosure of the information.

notice of privacy practices (NPP)   A document that health care providers and other covered entities must use to inform patients about their rights surrounding the protection of their protected health information.

Office for Civil Rights (OCR)   A subdepartment of the Department of Health and Human Services responsible for the enforcement of the HIPAA privacy rules.

operations   *See* Health care operations.

payer   In health care, an entity that assumes the risk of paying for medical treatments. This can be an uninsured patient, a self-insured employer, a health plan, or a health maintenance organization (also spelled *payor*).

payment   The activities by the practice to obtain reimbursement for health care services. This includes billing, claims management, collection activities, and verification of insurance coverage and precertification of services.

personal representative   A person who, under applicable law, has the authority to act on behalf of an individual in making decisions related to health care.

protected health information (PHI)   With few exceptions, this includes individually identified health information held or disclosed by a practice regardless of how it is communicated (electronically, verbally, or written).

required   A security standard that is required to be implemented.

security incident   A security incident means the attempted or successful unauthorized access, use, disclosure, modification, or destruction of information or interference with system operations in an information system.

treatment   The provision, coordination, or management of health care and related services by one or more health care providers; the referral of a patient for health care from one provider to another.

treatment, payment, and operations (TPO)   *See* Treatment; Payment; Health care operations.

use   With respect to individually identified health information, the sharing, employment, application, utilization, examination, or analysis of such information within an entity that maintains such information.

workforce   Employees, volunteers, trainees, and other persons under the direct control of a covered entity, whether or not they are paid by that entity.

Appendix 7–2

Sample Workforce Confidentiality Agreement

_____

Practice Name

I understand that _____ has a legal and ethical responsibility to maintain patient privacy, including obligations to
                        Practice Name

protect the confidentiality of patient information and to safeguard the privacy of patient information.

In addition, I understand that during the course of my employment/assignment/affiliation at _____, I may see or hear
                                                                      Practice Name

other Confidential Information such as financial data and operational information pertaining to the practice that _____
                                                                                     Practice Name

is obligated to maintain as confidential.

As a condition of my employment/assignment/affiliation with _____, I understand that I must sign and comply with this
                                                                 Practice Name

agreement. By signing this document, I understand and agree that:

I will disclose Patient Information and/or Confidential Information only if such disclosure complies with _____ 's policies, and
                                                                        Practice Name

is required for the performance of my job.

My personal access code(s), user ID(s), access key(s), and password(s) used to access computer systems or other equipment are to be kept confidential at all times.

I will not access or view any information other than what is required to do my job. If I have any question about whether access to certain information is required for me to do my job, I will immediately ask my supervisor for clarification.

I will not discuss any information pertaining to the practice in an area where unauthorized individuals may hear such information (for example, in hallways, on elevators, in the cafeteria, on public transportation, at restaurants, and at social events). I understand that it is not acceptable to discuss any practice information in public areas even if specifics such as a patient's name are not used.

I will not make inquiries about any practice information for any individual or party who does not have proper authorization to access such information.

I will not make any unauthorized transmissions, copies, disclosures, inquiries, modifications, or purgings of Patient Information or Confidential Information. Such unauthorized transmissions include, but are not limited to, removing and/or transferring Patient Information or Confidential Information from _____'s computer system to unauthorized locations (for instance, home).

      Practice Name

Upon termination of my employment/assignment/affiliation with _____

           Practice Name

I will immediately return all property (e.g., keys, documents, ID badges, etc.) to _____.

              Practice Name

I agree that my obligations under this agreement regarding Patient Information will continue after the termination of my employment/assignment/affiliation with _____.

     Practice Name

I understand that violation of this Agreement may result in disciplinary action, up to and including termination of my employment/assignment/affiliation with _____ and/or suspension, restriction or loss of privileges, in accordance with _____'s

    Practice Name   Practice Name

policies, as well as potential personal civil and criminal legal penalties.

I understand that any Confidential Information or Patient Information that I access or view at _____ does not belong to me.

             Practice Name

I have read the above agreement and agree to comply with all its terms as a condition of continuing employment.

_____   _____

Signature of Employee/Physician/Student/Volunteer   Date

_____

Print Your Name

Source: Health Insurance Portability and Accountability Act (HIPAA) privacy manual: A how-to guide for your medical practice. (2003).Gates, Moore, & Co., Epstein Becker & Green, P.C., with permission.

Appendix 7–3

Sample Patient Authorization for Use and Disclosure of Protected Health Information

_____

Practice Name

By signing this authorization, I authorize _____ to use and/or disclose certain Protected Health Information (PHI)

        Practice Name

about me to _____.

    Name of Entity to Receive This Information

This authorization permits _____ to use and/or disclose the following individually identifiable health information

      Practice Name

about me (specifically describe the information to be used or disclosed, such as date(s) of services, type of services, level of detail to be released, origin of information, etc.):

_____

_____

The information will be used or disclosed for the following purpose:

_____

If requested by the patient, purpose may be listed as "at the request of the individual."

The purpose(s) is/are provided so that I can make an informed decision whether to allow release of the information. This authorization will expire on _____

     Expiration Date or Defined Event

The practice will _____ will not _____ receive payment or other remuneration from a third party in exchange for using or disclosing the PHI.

I do not have to sign this authorization to receive treatment from _____

                                            Practice Name

In fact, I have the right to refuse to sign this authorization. When my information is used or disclosed pursuant to this authorization, it may be subject to redisclosure by the recipient and may no longer be protected by the federal HIPAA Privacy Rule. I have the right to revoke this authorization in writing except to the extent that the practice has acted in reliance upon this authorization. My written revocation must be submitted to the

Privacy Officer at:

_____

Address

_____   _____   _____

City   State   ZIP Code

Signed by: _____   _____

       Signature of Patient or Legal Guardian   Relationship to Patient

_____   _____

Patient's Name   Date

_____

Print Name of Patient or Legal Guardian

Patient/Guardian to Be Provided with a Signed Copy of Authorization

Source: Health Insurance Portability and Accountability Act (HIPAA) privacy manual: A how-to guide for your medical practice. (2003).Gates, Moore, & Co., Epstein Becker & Green, P.C., with permission.

Appendix 7–4

Privacy Policy Training Checklist

_____

Practice Name

Training conducted on _____ by _____

                        Date   Name of instructor

Attendees included those persons on the Training Documentation Form.

Training included: (Please check next to action item to indicate training completion.)

_____ Introduction to HIPAA and the Privacy Rule

_____ Introduction to Privacy Officer and Overview of Privacy Officer Responsibilities

_____ Explanation of Workforce Confidentiality Agreements

_____ Overview of Practice's Privacy Policies and Procedures

_____ Overview of Practice's Notice of Privacy Practices

_____ Explanation of Privacy Forms

_____ Patient Authorization Form

_____ Form Requesting Restriction on Uses and Disclosures of PHI

_____ Form to Inspect and Copy PHI and to Implement Access Denial

_____ Form to Amend PHI

_____ Form to Receive Accounting of Disclosures of PHI

_____ Patient Complaint Form

_____ Explanation of Who Can Disclose PHI

_____ Discussion of Job Responsibilities as They Relate to PHI

_____ Explanation of Minimum Necessary Standard

References

Health Insurance Portability and Accountability Act (HIPAA) privacy manual: A how-to guide for your medical practice. (2003). Gates Moore & Company, Epstein Becker & Green, P.C.

Ingrao, B. (2005, May–June). HIPAA security. Advance for Audiologists, pp. 22–31.

Jacob, D. (2002). How to comply with HIPAA: A practical guide for hearing healthcare providers. Hearing Journal, 55(9), 36–39.

Jacob, D. (2003). Ten steps to HIPAA compliance. Hearing Journal, 56(2), 24–26.

National Institute of Standards and Technology. Computer Security Resource Center (CSRC). Retrieved February 21, 2006, from http://csrc.nist.gov/

National Plan and Provider Enumeration System. Retrieved October 1, 2005, from http://nppes.cms.hhs.gov/NPPES/Welcome.do

Pallarito, K. (2004). A year after privacy rules take effect, hearing professionals seem to be adapting. Hearing Journal, 57(6), 19–24.

Sullivan, J. M. (2004). HIPAA: A practical guide to the privacy and security of health data. Chicago: ABA Publishing.

U.S. Department of Health and Human Services, Centers for Medicare and Medicaid Services. (1996). Health Insurance Portability and Accountability Act of 1996: Public law 104–191.

U.S. Department of Health and Human Services, Centers for Medicare and Medicaid Services. HIPAA compliance deadlines. Retrieved October 1, 2006, from http://www.cms.hhs.gov/hipaa/hipaa2/general/deadlines.asp

U.S. Department of Health and Human Services, Centers for Medicare and Medicaid Services. National provider identifier. Retrieved February 21, 2006, from http://new.cms.hhs.gov/NationalProvIdentStand/01_overview.asp

U.S. Department of Health and Human Services, Centers for Medicare and Medicaid Services. Transactions and code sets standards overview. Retrieved October 1, 2005, from http://www.cms.hhs.gov/hipaa/ hipaa2/regulations/transactions/default.asp

U.S. Department of Health and Human Services, Health Resources and Services Administration. Plain language principals and thesaurus for making HIPAA privacy notices more readable. Retrieved October 1, 2005, from http://www.hrsa.gov/language.htm

U.S. Department of Health and Human Services, Office for Civil Rights. (2000). Standards for electronic transactions (Part III, 45 CFR, parts 160, 162, and 164). Federal Register. Retrieved October 1, 2005, from http://www.cms.hhs.gov/TransactionCodeSetsStands/Downloads/txfinal.pdf

U.S. Department of Health and Human Services, Office for Civil Rights. (2002). Standards for privacy and identifiable health information: Final rule (Part V, 45 CFR, parts 160 and 164). Federal Register. Retrieved October 1, 2005, from http://www.hhs.gov/ocr/hipaa/privacyrule.pdf

U.S. Department of Health and Human Services, Office for Civil Rights. (2003). Health insurance reform: Security standard, final rule (Part II, 45 CFR, parts 160, 162, and 164). Federal Register. Retrieved October 1, 2005, from http://www.hhs.gov/ocr/hipaa/SecurityStandard/Downloads/securityfinalrule.pdf

U.S. Department of Health and Human Resources, Office for Civil Rights. Medical privacy—national standards to protect the privacy of personal health information. Retrieved October 1, 2005, from http://www.hhs.gov/ocr/hipaa

U.S. Department of Health and Human Services, Office for Civil Rights. Medical privacy national standards to protect the privacy of personal health information—sample business associate contract provisions. Retrieved October 1, 2005, from http://www.hhs.gov/ocr/hipaa/-contractprov.html

Workshop for Electronic Data Interchange. Retrieved October 1, 2005, from http://www.wedi.org

Chapter 8

Outcome Measures and Evidence-Based Practice

Theresa Hnath Chisolm and Harvey B. Abrams

"You got to be very careful if you don't know where you're going, because you might not get there."

– Yogi Berra

The general goal of outcomes measurement is to provide objective information to patients and to promote data-driven decision making by managers. In the context of this chapter, the term *outcome measures* refers to those methods and tools that can be used to evaluate a patient's status as a result of audiologic intervention. Although the use of outcome measures is critical for all audiologic services, the focus of this chapter will be on hearing aid selection and fitting. It is the hearing aid that will ultimately define the profession and discipline of audiology. Turner (1998) argues that by virtue of their education, research productivity, knowledge transfer, and clinical services, audiologists should be the recognized hearing aid experts. To truly claim the right to declare themselves as the hearing aid providers of choice, however, it is imperative that audiologists objectively document the benefits achieved as a result of their expertise.[1] These collective measures of treatment effectiveness coupled with carefully conducted clinical trials create a foundation of evidence upon which the clinician can draw to maximize the opportunity for positive patient outcome—a process known as evidence-based practice (EBP). EBP is defined as the "conscientious, explicit, and judicious use of current best evidence in making decisions about the care of individual patients. The practice . . . means integrating individual clinical expertise with the best available external clinical evidence from systematic research" (Sackett et al, 1996, p. 71).

---

[1] The interested reader is referred to the 1993 Carhart Memorial Lecture delivered by Dr. Earl Harford (Harford, 1993) to the annual meeting of the American Auditory Society. Dr. Harford offered an eloquent and convincing case for the indispensable role of the hearing aid in the past, present, and future of audiology.

> **Pearl**
>
> • Use outcome measures to modify the fitting as well as to determine the success of the fitting.

The move to EBP requires data-driven decision making and underscores the need for performance measures that provide quantitative information on the outcomes of care. As the evidence base grows, the profession of audiology will be in a position to develop clinical practice guidelines that will lead to:

♦ Reduced variability

♦ Increased reproducibility

♦ Consistent outcomes

♦ High-quality patient care

♦ Minimized risks

♦ An increased relationship between knowledge and clinical practice

♦ Rationale for Hearing Aid Outcomes Assessment

We are firmly entrenched in an era of increasing accountability and shrinking health care resources. As a result, administrators, third-party payers, and patients themselves are seeking evidence that medical treatments make meaningful differences in the patients' lives. An impressive array of outcome measures is available for documenting the effectiveness of intervention with hearing aids. One application of outcome measures is the performance of an economic analysis of hearing aid options. For example, to economically justify the selection of a high-end digital instrument compared with a less expensive digital or nondigital alternative, the measured benefits with the more expensive option would need to increase in proportion to the additional costs to demonstrate cost-effectiveness. Beck (2000) posits that, although cost will always remain a concern in health care decision making, the question will be reframed to determine if the most expensive treatment necessarily leads to the best outcome. In addition to their use in measuring treatment effectiveness and in conducting economic evaluations of treatment options, outcome measures can be used for purposes such as adjusting the hearing aid parameters, counseling patients regarding expectations of benefit, and documenting patient satisfaction.

> **Special Consideration**
>
> • Outcomes are for all "stakeholders"—patients, employers, families, insurers, coworkers, and accrediting organizations.

♦ Conceptual Framework for Establishing Goals of Hearing Aid Intervention

The choice of an appropriate outcome measure depends on the establishment of clear goals for hearing aid intervention. This process can be facilitated by application of the World Health Organization (WHO) classification scheme for describing the consequences of health conditions (i.e., disorders and diseases). Initially, WHO (1980) used the terms *impairment, disability,* and *handicap* to describe the multidimensional impact of a health condition. Recently, however, as a result of changes in health care practices and a new social understanding of disability, the classification system was revised and is now referred to as the International Classification of Functioning, Disability, and Health (ICF; WHO, 2001). The WHO-ICF is a biopsychosocial model of functioning and disability that provides a framework for evaluating success in all areas of intervention and treatment, including hearing aid rehabilitation (Kiessling et al, 2003). The WHO-ICF systematically organizes and codifies the consequences of an individual's health condition, such as a hearing loss, into the broad dimensions of body structure and function, activity, and participation.

> **Special Consideration**
>
> • WHO dropped the domains *disability* and *handicap* from its revised classification document because of the negative connotations associated with this terminology.

As illustrated in **Fig. 8–1**, these three dimensions interact and are influenced by contextual factors related to the environment and the person. Environmental factors include social attitudes, architectural characteristics, legal and social structures; personal factors allow for consideration of a person's gender, age, coping style, socioeconomic background, education, and other demographic variables. The WHO-ICF can be accessed at http://www3.who.int/icf/.

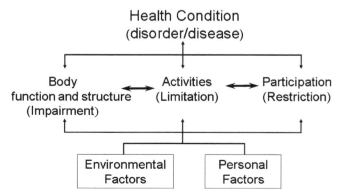

Figure 8–1 Interactions between the components of the World Health Organization International Classification of Functioning, Disability, and Health.

The WHO-ICF is important, not only because it provides a conceptual framework, but also because it allows for a detailed classification of human functioning. In theory, any function or disability can be assigned an ICF alphanumeric code that identifies a functional category and a level of functioning. To clarify the classification principles, consider the code for "hearing functions," which is b230. This code refers to "sensory functions relating to sensing the presence of sounds and discriminating the location, pitch, loudness, and quality of sounds" (WHO, 2001). The *b* refers to body functioning. The 2 refers to Chapter 2 in the ICF, titled "Sensory Functions and Pain." The 30 refers to the section of that chapter on hearing functions. Most domain codes at this level have statements about "inclusions" and sometimes "exclusions" that help coders to avoid some common errors. In the case of b230, inclusions are specified as "functions of hearing, auditory discrimination, localization of sound source, lateralization of sound, speech discrimination," and "impairments such as deafness, hearing impairment and hearing loss" (WHO, 2001).

ICF coding for body structures and function, activity, and participation are applicable to all aspects of audiology. For example, body structures are the anatomical parts of the body, including the external (s240; WHO, 2001), middle (s250; WHO, 2001), and inner (s260; WHO, 2001) parts of the ear. Body functions are the physiological and psychological functions of body systems and include the aforementioned hearing functions (b230; WHO, 2001). An anatomical deviation, such as occurs in otosclerosis, results in an impairment in body structure. A deviation in function, such as occurs when middle ear pathology or cochlear damage results in elevated auditory thresholds, causes a person to exhibit an impairment in body function. Surgical treatment for otosclerosis would be aimed at alleviating an impairment of body structure, and the use of a hearing aid by an individual with elevated auditory thresholds would be aimed at alleviating an impairment of body function.

The full range of life areas is encompassed in the dimensions of activity and participation. The broad domains assessed under activity and participation include learning and applying knowledge; general tasks and demands; communication; mobility; self-care; domestic life; interpersonal interactions and relationships; major life areas (e.g., employment, education, and economic life); and community, social, and civic life. *Activity* is defined as a person's ability to perform or execute an action or task in a uniform environment, or, more simply, what a person "can" do. *Participation* is what a person "does" do in his or her everyday environment. For example, "can" a person with sensorineural hearing loss, who has difficulty with sound detection, "communicate with—receive—spoken messages" (d310; WHO, 2001) or engage effectively in a "conversation" (d350; WHO, 2001)? Even if a person "can" do these activities, he or she may not participate in communication and conversational activities for a variety of reasons, such as the effort involved, embarrassment from potentially misunderstanding a message, and lack of readily available communication partners. The process of audiologic rehabilitation, the cornerstone of which is the use of hearing aids, is aimed not only in assuring that a person "can" engage in activities dependent on hearing, but also in helping a person to participate fully in hearing-related communication and conversational activities. Indeed, addressing the whole of a person's functioning through audiologic rehabilitation is necessary to minimize the potential impact of a hearing impairment on an individual's health-related quality of life (HRQoL, National Institutes of Health [NIH], 1993). Although HRQoL[2] is not a specific dimension within the WHO-ICF classification system, it is understood that it represents the sum of the effects of each of the dimensions shown in **Fig. 8–1**.

It is generally accepted that activity limitations, participation restrictions, and consequent reductions in HRQoL are related to the magnitude and type of hearing loss. However, there is widespread clinical recognition that it is not possible to accurately predict the nature and extent of an individual's limitations and restrictions solely on the basis of audiometric data alone. Two persons with the same degree of impairment may have very different perceptions regarding their HRQoL. Similarly, we cannot measure the effects of audiologic intervention solely in terms of a reduction of impairment. If this were the case, the provision of reasonably good audibility across a broad frequency range, without making average and loud speech uncomfortable, would be the only determinant of a successful hearing aid fitting. Because activity limitations and participation restrictions are significantly influenced by the individual's personality, communication needs, and the environment, as well as the degree of impairment, assurance of audibility at comfortable listening levels, unfortunately, does not guarantee an improvement in HRQoL.

Pitfall

- Assuring audibility at comfortable listening levels does not guarantee an improvement in quality of life.

◆ Goals of Hearing Aid Intervention

Alleviate Impairment

Based on the WHO-ICF, hearing aid intervention can be conceived of as having several general goals. The first goal is to alleviate, as much as possible, the impairment resulting from health conditions affecting the auditory system's structure and/or function. As is well known, the primary impairment resulting from a conductive disorder is a decrease in the ability to detect sounds. When there is damage

---

[2] The term *health-related quality of life* is used here, but in the health care literature, this term is often used interchangeably with health status, functional status, and quality of life to refer to the same concept of health.

to the sensorineural mechanism, however, impairments in loudness perception, temporal resolution, and frequency resolution often accompany the impairment in detection. Although future technology may allow us to address frequency and temporal resolution impairments, current hearing aid technology provides the audiologist with the ability to address impairments of detection and loudness perception through the preselection of electroacoustic characteristics, while also considering the style of the instrument (e.g., behind the ear, in the ear, in the canal, or completely in the canal), the hearing aid arrangement (e.g., monaural, binaural, or contralateral routing of signals), circuitry options (e.g., linear, output compression, and wide dynamic range compression), and user options (e.g., T-coil, directional/omnidirectional switching, and multiple programs).

In current practice, the selection of hearing aid parameters begins with obtaining data from a complete audiologic evaluation. Standard audiometric data are often supplemented with information from additional perceptual measures, such as speech recognition performance in quiet and in noise, and loudness comfort and growth. In addition, relevant information may be obtained through informal discussions or formal assessment of an individual's self-perceived listening difficulties, needs, and concerns. To select an initial set of electroacoustic characteristics, these data are often applied to one of several available prescriptive approaches. The prescription defines several parameters, including the frequency/gain response at one or more input levels, the output sound pressure level for 90 dB input level (OSPL-90), and additional characteristics such as crossover frequency between channels and dynamic/static characteristics of compression circuitry.[3]

Electroacoustic and other hearing aid parameters are typically selected to meet three specific goals: to make soft sounds audible, to make normal conversational speech comfortably loud and understandable, and to make loud sounds loud but tolerable. Outcome measures selected to demonstrate that these specific goals are achieved involve verifying that the electroacoustic and other hearing aid characteristics meet the objective criteria used in their preselection. Once it is determined that the electroacoustic and other characteristics of the hearing aid(s) are optimal for meeting the impairment level goals, we need to determine that general and specific goals set at the levels of activity and participation are also met. At these levels, the outcome measures selected will be used to validate that the use of hearing aid(s) makes meaningful differences, that is, that the treatment is efficacious.

Pearl

- Use outcome measures to modify the fitting as well as to determine the success of the fitting.

---

[3] Although not common in current clinical practice, technological advances may result in the incorporation of techniques such as paired comparisons of sound quality and/or perceived intelligibility for selection and/or adjustment of electroacoustic characteristics.

Reduce Activity Limitations

The general goal of hearing aid fitting in the activity dimension is to improve a person's ability to understand speech, thus leading to improvement in communication functioning. Currently, outcome measures used to validate the effectiveness of hearing aid intervention in these dimensions include objective performance measures and subjective self-report measures of speech understanding and communication performance. It is important to keep in mind that as more sophisticated and nonlinear signal-processing technologies are introduced in amplification systems, other types of outcome measures aimed at validating the effectiveness of hearing aid intervention at the activity level may be seen in the audiology clinic. For example, it would not be unreasonable to include a measure of sound localization ability when evaluating multiple-microphone versus single-microphone technology. Indeed, techniques for addressing localization performance in the clinic are currently available (Besing and Koehnke, 1995). In addition, a recently developed questionnaire, the Speech Hearing, Spatial Hearing, and Qualities of Hearing Questionnaire (SSQ; Gatehouse and Noble, 2004), which is administered through interview, includes several specific questions regarding perceptions of distance and movement and sound-source segregation.

Reduce Participation Restrictions

The measurement of restrictions in participation resulting from a hearing impairment and its consequent activity limitations is not a common focus in standard audiologic testing protocols. We often infer this data, however, through the case histories we obtain from patients. For example, patients may report seeking our services because they can no longer enjoy attending social gatherings or are having difficulty with communication at work. Post–hearing aid fitting, we may informally ask patients if they experience less difficulty in these or similar situations. Although this informal approach may help to determine if the goal of reducing participation restrictions has been met, more formal assessments allow for the quantification of successful outcomes. There are a variety of self-report measures that can be used for this purpose. Because the level of participation is highly influenced by the environmental factors described earlier, the audiologist may need to take a more active role in evaluating the social, occupational, and living environments in which the patient exists. As a result, the audiologist may become involved in the development of hearing accessibility programs for communities or groups of listeners with hearing impairments (see, e.g., Pichora-Fuller and Robertson, 1994). Such programs are designed to address the needs, wishes, and abilities of the listener within specific communication situations with specific communication partners in specific communication environments.

Improve Health-Related Quality of Life

We are also concerned that meeting clinical objectives in terms of reductions of impairment, activity limitations, and participation restrictions will result in measurable changes in self-perceived HRQoL. Although HRQoL measurement has received little clinical application among audiologists, it is a construct that is receiving increased attention in the research literature, including those studies aimed at demonstrating the efficacy of hearing aid intervention (e.g., McArdle et al, 2005; Saunders and Jutai, 2004). Review of this literature provides information regarding available tools and approaches that can be adopted for use in clinical protocols.

Increase Patient Satisfaction

Finally, no hearing aid fitting could be considered fully successful without demonstrating that the patient was satisfied with the device and services received. Satisfaction does not always correspond to significant or quantifiable reductions in impairment, activity limitations, participation, or HRQoL. In addition to improvements in communication and real-world functioning, the domain of satisfaction involves the patient's relationship with service providers, the ease of access to services, as well as the influence of factors such as cosmetics, comfort, expectations, and perceived value. It is a construct that needs independent assessment.

♦ Clinically Useful Outcome Measures for Hearing Aid Effectiveness

The remainder of this chapter provides a detailed discussion of clinically useful outcome measures that provide a means for demonstrating that in the clinical processes of selection, fitting, and counseling in the appropriate use of hearing aid(s), we have met the goals selected at the levels of impairment, activity limitation, participation restriction, HRQoL, and satisfaction. These data can be used to demonstrate treatment effectiveness for individual patients and as part of program evaluation. The discussion focuses on measures appropriate for use in the adult population. It is important to note that outcome assessment for children requires age-appropriate tests, tasks, and approaches.

Measuring Outcomes for Impairment-Level Goals

As discussed, the general goal at the level of impairment is to improve audibility of speech, while maintaining listening comfort. This goal is accomplished through the selection of appropriate electroacoustic parameters and other hearing aid characteristics (i.e., style, arrangement, and circuitry). While 2 cm^3 coupler measurements may be used to ensure that the hearing aid satisfies manufacturer quality control standards and to make initial adjustments on the hearing aid, it is now standard practice to use real ear measurements (probe microphone measurements of real ear insertion gain [REIG] and real ear aided response [REAR], or functional gain for severe to profound losses) to adjust the parameters of the hearing aid and verify results. The primary goals of this verification process are to ensure that the measured electroacoustic characteristics are as close as possible to those prescribed for the patient, and that the hearing aid provides adequate audibility of the important speech energy without feedback or loudness

discomfort. Recently, manufactured probe microphone systems have incorporated "live speech mapping" capabilities. Although using actual speech (recorded or live) may intuitively seem preferable to speech-shaped stimuli (e.g., composite noise), there is no evidence that patient outcome is any better with live speech mapping. This should come as no surprise, as composite or speechlike noise used in most systems closely resembles the long-term average speech spectrum (LTASS). There are those who argue that "mapping" the response to a particular voice (e.g., spouse) will lead to better hearing and understanding of that person. Unfortunately, the acoustic properties of the particular voice in the real world will vary as a function of distance, reverberation, direction, and presence of background noise and will likely bear very little resemblance to those properties in the clinical environment.

Root Mean Square Difference

Documentation that the impairment-related goals have been met can be accomplished in several ways. For example, one approach would be to specify the root-mean-square (rms) difference between the REIG and the target frequency response. Byrne (1992) has described such a procedure using the formula

$$\text{rms difference} = d_1{}^2 + d_2{}^2 + d_3{}^2 + d_4{}^2$$

where $d_1{}^2 \ldots d_4{}^2$ equals the difference between the target gain and measured gain at 500, 1000, 2000, and 4000 Hz. Byrne discovered that his subjects were able to detect a difference in the sound quality of the hearing aid with an rms difference of as little as 3 dB.

Articulation (Speech Intelligibility) Index

Another approach to verifying hearing aid selection uses the articulation index (AI), sometimes referred to as the speech intelligibility index (SII). The AI provides a numerical value between 0 and 1. Higher AI scores are achieved by placing more of the acoustic speech signal in the audible range. Theoretically, the higher the AI score, the greater the ability to understand speech at comfortable levels. Several calculation methods are available, each with benefits and limitations (e.g., American National Standards Institute [ANSI], 1997; Fletcher, 1950; Pavlovic, 1984). The ANSI (1997) and Fletcher (1950) methods require complex calculations and are not appropriate for routine clinical use. The Pavlovic (1984) methods involve simpler calculations and are easy to use but lack precision. Unfortunately, existing AI approaches that best predict performance are not presently available for clinical implementation (Rankovic, 1997).

Patient Acceptability Factors

In addition to documenting improvements in speech audibility, it is important to achieve a good physical fit, acceptable cosmetics, adequate volume wheel range, and satisfactory sound quality. The assessment of these important outcomes is typically determined at follow-up visits, through telephone interviews, or by mailed questionnaires.

Acclimatization

Following the fitting process and a complete orientation to the use and care of the hearing aid(s), patients wear their instruments for a period of time (at least a few weeks) prior to obtaining measures which provide validation of the efficacy of hearing aid selection and fitting at a follow-up appointment. During the period between fitting and the follow-up appointment, it is expected that "acclimatization" to amplification may occur, at least for some new hearing aid users (Gatehouse, 1992), and that the patient will have experienced a variety of listening environments. Acclimatization may result in improved speech recognition ability over time, particularly for those patients who have more severe losses, but also may refer to the fact that the patient becomes accustomed to wearing the hearing aid(s) at a higher volume setting or becomes less bothered by such aspects of amplification as the occlusion effect, common background sounds, and the physical presence of the instrument(s) in the ear.

Measuring Outcomes for Activity Limitation and Participation Restriction Goals

Outcome measures used to validate the efficacy of hearing aid intervention at the activity and participation levels include objective performance measures of speech recognition and self-report measures assessing activity limitations and/or participation restrictions. Each of these categories is discussed.

Objective Performance Measures of Speech Recognition

The use of speech recognition testing as an outcome assessment tool in hearing aid fitting is controversial. Such testing has generally fallen out of favor since the Carhart (1946) comparative speech approach to hearing aid fitting was determined to be too time consuming and the phonetically balanced (PB) word lists were found to be insensitive to small differences among hearing aids (Walden et al,

1983). In addition, it has not been adequately demonstrated that performance on these clinical tests accurately predicts performance in everyday listening environments. There are those who argue, however, that the use of phoneme scoring, rather than whole-word scoring of PB words, allows for an increase in the reliability of test scores without increasing test time, such that their use as a hearing aid outcome measure warrants further consideration (Boothroyd, 1998). However, the use of phoneme scoring does not appear to be gaining widespread acceptance among clinicians.

In recent years, new speech-in-noise testing materials have been developed, ranging from phoneme-level identification tasks to whole-sentence recognition. Recently, multiple target words concatenated into syntactically correct sentences or whole-sentence recognition tests, both administered in noise, have begun to gain popularity among clinicians, on the assumption that speech that includes contextual cues and is presented in a background of noise will have greater predictive validity as an outcomes measure for amplification. Two tests that have seen increasing use both clinically and in hearing aid research are the Hearing in Noise Test (HINT; Nilsson et al, 1994) and the speech-in-noise evaluator known as QuickSIN (Killion et al, 2004). In HINT, the speech spectrum noise level is fixed at a moderate intensity. The signal-to-noise ratio (SNR) is varied adaptively to determine the ratio at which a 50% correct sentence performance is obtained. The patient is required to repeat the entire sentence correctly.

QuickSIN uses a descending paradigm with administration of one sentence, composed of five target words, at each of six SNRs that start at 25 dB signal-to-noise (S/N) and decrease in 5 dB decrements. The level of the sentences is fixed, and the level of the multitalker babble, which is continuous throughout the list of sentences, is varied in 5 dB increments from 25 to 0 dB S/N. QuickSIN is scored by quantifying the 50% point in terms of dB S/N and subtracting 2 dB, which is the mean score for young normal-hearing listeners, to identify the SNR loss of an individual. The QuickSIN guide (QuickSIN Speech-in-Noise Test, 2001) provides the number of pairs of sentences required for comparison between two conditions, such as two different hearing aids or two different hearing aid adjustments.

A similar approach to measuring SNR as described above was created using Northwestern University Auditory Test No. 6 (NU No. 6) words in multitalker babble. The Words-in-Noise (WIN) protocol (Wilson, 2003) consists of (1) 35 monosyllabic words from NU No. 6 spoken by the female speaker on the VA compact disc, which enables the evaluation of recognition performance in quiet and in babble with the same materials spoken by the same speaker; and (2) 5 unique words presented at each of 7 signal-to-babble (S/B) ratios from 24 dB S/B to 0 dB S/B in 4 dB decrements. In WIN, the level of the babble is presented continuously and is fixed, with the level of the words varying; the 50% point is quantifiable with the Spearman-Kärber equation (Finney, 1952). Both QuickSIN and WIN provide ~8 dB separation in terms of SNR between performance by listeners with normal hearing and performance by listeners with hearing loss.

Two benefits of SNR testing that quantifies the 50% point are that, for the majority of patients, there is no ceiling or floor effect, and the test can be administered quickly. In addition, a speech-in-noise task can be administered in sound field pre- and postamplification to estimate the performance of a hearing aid user in the most difficult of situations, such as when the signal and the noise are both presented from the same location. Caution is advised when using speech-in-noise testing procedures to compare performance between hearing aids that have nonlinear signal-processing functions, because the presentation level of the test materials may vary differently with each hearing aid and adversely affect performance as a function of level more so than SNR.

There remain several outstanding issues in speech recognition testing. Some of the speech materials available do not have normative data, are not available in recorded form, or the recordings are not standardized. One issue that has been noted by some is that the recording or playback process may seriously limit the dynamic range of the test materials relative to everyday listening environments, which may be an issue in predictive validity, particularly with nonlinear signal-processing hearing aids. Another issue is that most of the speech materials are male voices, which may not tap into the perception of important high-frequency phonemes that are so difficult for many patients who have sloping hearing losses. Finally, there are questions about what levels the speech and noise should be set at to represent the "real world," what type of noise should be used, and what loudspeaker array should be used to simulate everyday environments. (For a further discussion, see Chapter 14 in Volume 1 of this series.)

Pitfall

- Most of the recorded speech materials use a male voice, which may not tap into the perception of important high-frequency phonemes that are so difficult for many patients who have sloping hearing losses.

Subjective Self-Report Measures Examining Activity Limitations and/or Participation Restrictions

In real-world rather than clinical or laboratory conditions, the activity of speech understanding and the participation in events that require speech understanding are heavily influenced by contextual factors related to both the environment and the individual. As a result, many inventories have been developed to assess the impact of a hearing impairment on the individual in the areas of communication functioning, activity limitation, and participation restrictions. **Table 8–1** provides references to some of the more common self-report hearing aid outcome measures for use in the general adult population. This list is by no means exhaustive. Numerous additional inventories are available for use in assessing the outcomes of hearing aid intervention in

other populations (e.g., children and prelingually deafened adults) and for assessing outcomes in other areas of audiologic intervention (e.g., tinnitus management, dizziness). The interested reader is referred to Bentler and Kramer (2000) for a review of other outcome measures applicable to the general adult population and to Johnson and Danhauer (2002) for outcome measures used in all aspects of audiology.

The inventories reviewed in detail here are those reported to be either most commonly used by audiologists who dispense hearing aids and other instruments (Strom, 2005) or less commonly used, but which meet criteria that are considered important for clinical utility: (1) they are valid (i.e., the inventories measure what they claim to measure, (2) they are easy to administer in a short period of time (i.e., they are practical), (3) they are sensitive (i.e., the measure is able to detect change if change occurs), (4) they have test–retest reliability and/or critical difference data available, and (5) they are comprehensible (i.e., they are understandable to the end users of the information) (Hyde, 2000). The exclusion of any instrument here is not intended as a commentary on its psychometric properties or utility in research endeavors. Rather, we have chosen to focus our discussion on inventories that we believe are likely to be the most useful in clinical practice.

Pearl

- A clinically practical outcome measure should be easy to administer in a short period of time, provide easily quantifiable scores, and have established test–retest reliability data.

Three well-documented questionnaires warrant special mention, although they are not discussed in detail. The first is the Communication Profile for the Hearing Impaired (CPHI; Demorest and Erdman, 1986), which is an excellent research tool and useful for in-depth clinical assessment. With 145 items, however, the CPHI is time-consuming to administer. Another useful instrument is the Hearing Aid Performance Inventory (HAPI; Walden et al, 1984), which at 64 items is also quite long to administer. Although shortened versions of HAPI (SHAPI/SHAPI-E) have been introduced, these inventories provide aided scores only. Because they do not allow for difference scores, their value, for individual patients, is likely to be most applicable to examining differences between hearing aids. The final measure of note is the SSQ (Gatehouse and Noble, 2004). This instrument assesses auditory attention, perceptions of distance and movement, sound-source segregation, listening effort, prosody, and sound quality. Although the SSQ takes a more ecological approach to examining self-perceived hearing difficulties than does any other available self-report instrument, with 80 questions, the SSQ, like the CPHI and HAPI, is a time-consuming instrument to administer.

Table 8–1 Comparison of Self-Report Outcome Measures

Instrument/Authors	Purpose	Domain	Number of Items	Scoring and Interpretation
Abbreviated Profile of Hearing Aid Benefit (APHAB) Cox & Alexander, 1995	Quantify hearing loss disability and reduction of disability after using a hearing aid	Activity	24	Four subscale scores provided: ease of communication (EC); background noise (BN); reverberation (RV); aversiveness (AV). EC, BN, and RV combine to provide global score. Equal percentile profiles determined for aided, unaided, benefit scores. Lower scores are indicative of fewer problems for EC, BN, and RV, while higher scores indicate fewer problems for AV.
Client Oriented Scale of Improvement (COSI) Dillon, James, & Ginnis, 1997	Subjective identification of situations of listening difficulty and benefit from hearing aid intervention	Activity Participation	1–5	Patient judges degree of change attributable to intervention and final ability as a result of intervention. Higher scores indicate better outcomes. Proportion of patients obtaining degree of change and final ability scores is available.
Communication Profile Hearing Inventory (CPHI) Demorest & Erdman, 1987	Provides systematic and comprehensive assessment of a wide range of communication difficulties and reactions to those difficulties	Activity Participation	145	Results plotted as a profile of 3 importance ratings and 22 scale scores grouped into four categories: Communication performance, communication environment, communication strategies, and personal adjustment. Higher scores indicate lesser difficulty or involvement. Data can also be examined as z-scores for five factors: communication importance, communication performance, adjustment, reaction, and interaction.
Glasgow Hearing Aid Benefit Profile (GHABP) Gatehouse, 1999	Assess hearing aid benefit and satisfaction over time	Activity Participation HRQoL	4–8 items; up to 7 questions per item	5-point scale; can convert to 100-point scale; higher score indicates greater problems.
Hearing Aid Users Questionnaire (HAUQ) Dillon, Birtles, & Lovegrove, 1999	Quantify hearing aid use, difficulty, and benefit	Satisfaction	11	Different scale for each question. In all cases a higher score indicates greater hearing aid satisfaction.
Health Utilities Index (HUI) Furlong, Feeney, Torrance & Barr, 2001	Measure comprehensive health status and HRQoL for a broad range of subjects	HRQoL	15	Scoring algorithm based on 8 attributes: vision, hearing, speech, ambulation, dexterity, emotion, cognition (including memory and thinking ability), and pain or discomfort, with 5 or 6 levels each, ranging from severely impaired to normal, describing 972,000 unique health states. The single-attribute utility functions provide utility scores for each level with scores ranging between 0, dead, and 1, full health. Scores provide a measure of attribute-specific morbidity and a single summary measure of HRQoL.
Hearing Aid Performance Inventory (HAPI) Walden, Demorest & Helper, 1984	Assesses effectiveness of hearing aids in a variety of listening situations	Activity	64	5-point scale where 1 is very helpful and 5 hinders performance, based on four listening situations: noisy, quiet, reduced signal, and nonspeech stimuli. Numbers are added for individual items and the sum divided by total number items answered. The closer the score is to 1, the greater the hearing aid benefit.

Table 8–1 (*Continued*)

Instrument/Authors	Purpose	Domain	Number of Items	Scoring and Interpretation
Hearing Handicap Inventory for Adults (HHIA)/the Elderly (HHIE) Ventry & Weinstein, 1982	Measure perceived handicap from hearing loss	Participation	25	Three scores can be generated: 0–52 for emotional score; 0–48 for social/situational score; 0–100 for total score. Higher scores indicate greater difficulty.
International Outcome Inventory for Hearing Aids (IOI-HA) Cox, Hyde, Gatehouse et al, 2000	Assess a broad range of outcome domains in a short, practical mini-profile	Use Benefit Activity Participation Satisfaction HRQoL	7	5 point scale, where 1 is most negative and 5 is most positive. Norms for each item are available.
Medical Outcomes Study-Short Form 36 (MOS-SF 36) Ware & Sherbourne, 1992	Assess limitations in daily life and general health	HRQoL	36	8 subscale scores, 2 to 10 items each: physical function, role-physical, bodily pain, general health, vitality, social function, role-emotional, and mental health. Subscale aggregate scores: physical component summary (PCS) and mental component summary (MCS), reported as standardized scores with mean of 50 (SD = 10) in general healthy U.S. population.
Satisfaction with Amplification in Daily Life (SADL) Cox & Alexander, 1999	Quantify satisfaction in social daily life from hearing aid intervention	Satisfaction	15	Four subscale scores provided: positive effects, service and costs, negative features, and personal image, and a global score. Higher scores indicate greater satisfaction.
Sickness Impact Profile (SIP) Bergner, Bobbitt, Carter & Gilson, 1981	Measure changes in behavior based on the impact of sickness	Participation	136	Overall score, 2 domain scores, and 12 category scores; items are weighted according to a standardized weighting scheme. Subscales: ambulation, mobility, body/care movement, social interaction, communication, alertness, emotional, sleep/rest, eating, work, home management, and recreation/pastimes. A high score suggests greater functional difficulty. Based on three scales of health (physical, psychosocial, and overall function).
Speech Hearing, Spatial Hearing and Qualities of Hearing Questionnaire (SSQ) Gatehouse & Noble, 2004	Measures disability and handicap in a realistic range of contexts	Activity	80	0–10 scale, where 0 is not at all and 10 is perfectly. Higher score indicates greater ability. In addition to traditional speech intelligibility items, addresses issues of sustaining and switching attention, monitoring multiple input streams, analysis of spatial hearing (location, distance, and movement) and qualities of hearing such as listening effort, sound segregation, and prosody.
World Health Organization Disability Assessment Schedule II (WHO-DAS II) WHO, 1999	Examine consequences of a disease or disorder in three dimensions: body function and structure, activities, and participation.	HRQoL	36	5-point scale: 1 (none) to 5 (extreme/cannot do). Six domain scores: communication, mobility, self-care, interpersonal, life activities at home and work, and participation. Can convert to a 100-point scale; lower score indicates greater difficulty.

HRQoL, health-related quality of life; SD, standard deviation.

Abbreviated Profile of Hearing Aid Benefit A commonly used tool for quantifying the changes in the WHO-ICF activity dimension as a result of hearing aid use is the Abbreviated Profile of Hearing Aid Benefit (APHAB), developed by Cox and Alexander (1995). The APHAB, a 24-item questionnaire, is composed of situational-specific questions that assess speech understanding and hearing in a variety of situations. Scores are provided for four categories: ease of communication (EC), which examines the communication effort under favorable conditions; reverberation (RV), which examines communication in reverberant environments such as classrooms; background noise (BN), which examines communication in high levels of background noise; and aversiveness of sound (AV), which examines the unpleasantness of environmental sounds.

Cox (1997) describes the administration and application of APHAB. Patients are asked to indicate the percentage of time they experience problems hearing under these situations. There are seven response alternatives, ranging from "always" to "never." The patient uses these response alternatives to indicate answers to the 24 situational-specific items both "without my hearing aid" and "with my hearing aid." Responses can be recorded in a paper-and-pencil format or keyed directly on a computer. A software program available from Cox is used for scoring. The scores generated are displayed graphically and numerically. A subscale score can then be produced for unaided and aided listening. *Benefit* is defined as the difference between the aided and unaided scores. For individual subscale scores for EC, RV, or BN, a difference of 22 percentage points is needed between aided and unaided scores for the clinician to be reasonably certain that the scores represent a real difference between conditions. When pattern performance across these three subscales is examined, the clinician can be confident that real benefit has been achieved (at least for linear hearing aids) when the aided scores exceed the unaided ones by at least 10 percentage points. A downloadable version of APHAB as well as normative data and other information can be found at http://www.ausp.memphis.edu/harl/aphab.html.

Clinical experience with APHAB suggests several factors to consider in its use. One of these is the administration format. In one approach, the unaided responses are provided prior to hearing aid fitting, and aided responses are obtained following an appropriate period (~30 days) of hearing aid use. During the second administration, Cox (1997) suggests that reliability and validity are increased if the patients are allowed to see their unaided responses. If they no longer agree with their assessment of their unaided difficulties, they are permitted to change the response. Although this is acceptable, this format differs from that used when the APHAB was normed, when subjects were asked to provide unaided and aided responses in the same sitting. In addition, recent work by Joore and colleagues (2002) demonstrated a response shift through administration of a second pretest completed at the time of posttest on hearing-specific measures in adults being fitted with hearing aids for the first time. A response shift may occur for a variety of reasons, including the individual undergoing changes in internal standards of measurement, values, or conceptualization of a target construct (Schwartz and Sprangers, 1999).

Another problem associated with APHAB is that not all of the situational-specific items are relevant to individual patients. Because patients are discouraged from leaving items blank, they need instruction about how to respond to situations that they do not or are not likely to experience. Finally, there is some concern regarding the reading level associated with the scale. It is recommended that questionnaires and other documents designed for patient use and education (e.g., informed consents and drug information pamphlets) be written at the 7th or 8th grade reading level. The readability level of the APHAB exceeds the 11th grade, according to the Flesch-Kincaid grade-level scale (Flesch, 1948).

Pitfall

- The validity of some self-report questionnaires is limited because they require the patient to respond to situations that he or she has not encountered or may never encounter.

Hearing Handicap Inventory for the Elderly One of the most commonly used, and studied, outcome measures for audiologic intervention is the Hearing Handicap Inventory for the Elderly (HHIE; Ventry and Weinstein, 1982). This measure focuses on how a hearing loss might affect participation. The original version, with 25 questions, contains 13 items that are classified as eliciting information from an "emotional" domain and 12 from a "social" domain. The inventory is scored on the basis of the total number of "yes" (4 points), "sometimes" (2 points), and "no" (0 point) responses. The total score (range 0–100) provided the clinician with a relative indication of how handicapping the patient perceives the hearing impairment to be. That is, the higher the value, the greater the self-perception of hearing handicap. The questionnaire is repeated after audiologic intervention, which may include hearing aids and/or aural rehabilitation. The change in the HHIE score provides the outcome measure. When administered in a face-to-face format, a reduction in score of 18.7 points is needed for the clinician to conclude that real benefit has been attained. If a paper-and-pencil format is used, however, test–retest reliability diminishes, and the 95% confidence interval for a true change in score becomes 36 points (Weinstein et al, 1986). An example of an emotional domain item from the HHIE is "Does a hearing problem cause you to feel embarrassed when meeting new people?" "Does a hearing problem cause you difficulty when listening to radio or TV?" would fall into the social domain group of questions.

Variations of the HHIE include the HHIE-S, a 10-item short form version (Ventry and Weinstein, 1982); the HHIA, which is a 25-item version, including occupationally related questions (and its shortened version, HHIA-S; Newman et al, 1990); a full-length Spanish version (Lopez-Vazquez et al, 2002); and a shortened Spanish version (Lichtenstein and Hazuda, 1998). Clinical experience suggests that the HHIE is most effective with inexperienced hearing aid users, because experienced users may not accurately recall their "pre–hearing aid" self-perception of hearing handicap after a significant period of hearing aid use.

Client-Oriented Scale of Improvement Of concern with inventories such as APHAB and HHIE is that some items may not be relevant to some individuals. Thus, in contrast to scales that list specific questions or situations, the Client-Oriented Scale of Improvement (COSI; Dillon et al, 1997) requires the patient, with guidance from the clinician, to identify up to five situations that cause the most communication difficulties. At the completion of treatment, the patient assesses the degree to which the identified problems have resolved. Degree of change is ranked on a 5-point scale, from "worse" (1) to "much better" (5). Patients rate their final ability from "hardly ever" (1) to "almost always" (5). Test–retest correlation coefficients for COSI degree of change ($r = .73$) and COSI final ability ($r = .84$) were found to be higher than that obtained for the HHIE total score ($r = .54$) in 98 adults fitted with hearing aids for the first time, leading Dillon et al (1997) to conclude that COSI was particularly suitable for clinical use. An individual patient's score can be compared with the proportion of patients with mild to moderate hearing loss who obtained different COSI change and final ability scores (Dillon, 2001). Depending on the specific situations identified, the COSI goals can be focused on WHO-ICF dimensions of activity and/or participation. In a recent survey, COSI was used by more respondents than any other standardized outcome measure (Strom, 2005). One reason for COSI's popularity may be the assumption that by focusing on and measuring the treatment effect of problems that are most relevant to the patient, the outcomes measured will most accurately reflect the true functional impact of intervention as perceived by the patient.

The concern about COSI is that its application to program evaluation may be limited because each patient identifies problem situations that are unique to him or her. Dillon et al (1999), however, reported their use of COSI and the Hearing Aid Users Questionnaire (HAUQ) as outcome measures for monitoring the National Australian Hearing Services Program. The authors determined that many individual needs identified by the subjects could be grouped into 16 categories that can be analyzed for program effectiveness. For example, communication needs associated with hearing or understanding speech in restaurants, at parties, or in unique social situations can be categorized as "conversation with 1 or 2 in noise" or "conversation with group in noise." Approximately 75% of the subjects reported wanting to be able to hear television or radio at normal levels. In addition, Zelski (2000) found that inter-rater agreement was quite high (0.887).

Controversial Point

- Although COSI may be an effective outcome measure for individual patients, there is concern that it may be inappropriate for analyzing programs.

Glasgow Hearing Aid Benefit Profile Another instrument that allows for the assessment changes in both activity limitations and participation restrictions as a function of hearing aid use through identification of individualized listening needs is the Glasgow Hearing Aid Benefit Profile (GHABP;

Gatehouse, 1999). In addition to allowing for the identification of four patient-specific goals, the GHABP includes four prespecified questions: listening to television with other people, conversing with one other person in quiet, conversing on a busy street or in a shop, and conversing with several people in a group. For the preset items, patients are first asked whether or not the situation occurs in their lives. If it does, they are then asked how much difficulty they have in the situation and how much if any difficulty in the situation caused them to feel worried, annoyed, or upset. For each question, patients can report that the item is not applicable or select on a scale of 1 to 4 the amount of difficulty and degree of emotional response, with 1 equivalent to "no difficulty"/"not at all" and 4 indicating "great difficulty"/"quite a lot." Patients are also asked to answer the same two questions for individually identified situations. Gatehouse (2000) refers to the first of these questions as assessing initial disability, which in current WHO-ICF (2001) terminology would be equivalent to initial activity limitations, and the second as assessing hearing handicap, or in current WHO-ICF (2001) terminology, initial participation restrictions. After a period of hearing aid use, patients are asked, for each situation, how often they use their hearing aid, how much the hearing aid helps (i.e., hearing aid benefit), how much difficulty they still have (i.e., residual disability or activity limitations), and how satisfied they are with their hearing aid (i.e., satisfaction). Response scales for each question range from 1 to 4, with 1 indicating the least favorable response and 4 the most favorable. Test–retest correlations are reported to be a minimum of .86, indicating excellent stability across time (Gatehouse, 1999). Gatehouse (2000) reports that each of these scales can be manipulated on a scale varying from 0 to 100, with higher scores indicating more positive responses. Although quite comprehensive, the fact that up to six questions can be addressed for up to eight items (four preset and four individualized) means that GHABP can become time-consuming in a clinical situation. To assist in administration, a downloadable version of GHABP can be found at http://www.ihr.gla. ac.uk/products/ghabp.php.

Pearl

- A comprehensive outcome assessment is best achieved by using a combination of instruments or a single instrument that is designed to measure the treatment effect on impairment, activity, participation, satisfaction, and HRQoL.

International Outcomes Inventory—Hearing Aids In 1999, an international workshop, "Measuring Outcomes in Audiological Rehabilitation Using Hearing Aids," took place in Eriksholm, Denmark. The workshop focused on issues related to the use and promotion of outcome measures, as well as the design and selection of appropriate tools (Cox et al, 2000). As a result of the workshop, a new instrument, the International Outcomes Inventory—Hearing Aids (IOI-HA), was developed. The instrument, which contains seven questions, was designed to be practically oriented and was viewed as more of a mini-profile than a scale. The IOI-HA was not intended to be used as a substitute outcome measure but rather as a supplement. If used as a supplement in studies, the IOI-HA has the potential to generate a core of data that can be compared across the investigations (Cox and Alexander, 2002), and thus increase the evidence to direct practitioners in the use of the most efficacious approaches to hearing aid intervention. Each of the IOI-HA items is designed to target a different outcome domain: number of hours per day of hearing aid use, benefit in terms of improvement in hearing-related activities, residual activity limitations, satisfaction, residual participation restrictions, impact on others, and quality of life. Each item has five response choices and is scored on a scale from 1 to 5, with 1 indicating the most negative response and 5 the most positive. Psychometric data for the IOI-HA have been developed (Cox and Alexander, 2002). Initially designed to be appended to research protocols without significant cost in time or other resources, the brevity and inclusiveness of the IOI-HA has made it attractive to practitioners as well as researchers. Cox and colleagues (2003) provided normative data that can be used by clinicians to determine the relative success of a hearing aid fitting for an individual patient. Information about the IOI-HA is available at http://www.ausp.memphis.edu/harl/ioiha.html.

The outcome measures reviewed here as well as others that assess activity limitations and/or participation restrictions are useful for documenting hearing aid treatment efficacy (Cox et al, 2000). Currently, however, less than half of individuals (46%) dispensing hearing aids report using a standardized self-report outcome measure in the hearing aid fitting process (Strom, 2005). As we move forward in this era of EBP, it will be increasingly more important that the routine use of clinically applied standardized outcome measures becomes usual and ordinary practice for all practitioners. Only by routinely obtaining outcome measures can audiologists be assured that their interventions make a difference and that their patients have benefited from their care.

Measuring Outcomes for Health-Related Quality of Life

There is increased interest in examining the impact of hearing impairment in terms of HRQoL. An assessment of an individual's HRQoL involves more global considerations than those normally associated with impairment, activity limitations, or participation restrictions, although each of these necessarily affects an individual's perceived HRQoL. An HRQoL assessment commonly involves consideration of four separate factors, or domains: physical and occupational function, psychological function, social interaction, and somatic sensation. HRQoL assessments are multifactorial; that is, they encompass more than one domain of human experience, they are self-administered, they are time-variable (i.e., HRQoL may change from day to day depending on changes to any one of the four domains), and they are subjective. Although specific clinical disciplines such as psychiatry, rehabilitation, cardiology, and oncology use HRQoL measurements to assess outcome, little is

known about how audiologic disorders and interventions affect HRQoL, particularly when compared with other health-related disorders and treatments.

HRQoL measures can be categorized as disease-specific or generic. Disease-specific measures are useful for comparing different treatment options for the same health condition. Generic HRQoL measures are designed for use across health conditions. For example, generic HRQoL measures have been used to demonstrate the cost-effectiveness of cochlear implantation relative to other health disorders (e.g., Palmer et al, 1999). In choosing a specific or a generic instrument, the benefits and limitations of both approaches should be considered. Disease-specific instruments are clinically sensible; that is, the questions are similar to those used when talking to a patient. As a result, these instruments tend to be sensitive to the effects of treatments that are directed toward alleviating the specific problems identified. Using disease-specific instruments creates problems, however, when comparing treatment benefits across populations or conditions. Conversely, generic instruments allow comparisons across populations or conditions, but they may be insensitive to a particular condition or treatment. As a result of these benefits and limitations, the NIH consensus statement on HRQoL (NIH, 1993) currently recommends both types of measures.

Pearl

- The NIH consensus statement on HRQoL currently recommends the use of both disease-specific and generic measures when assessing patient outcome.

Disease-Specific Measures

The HRQoL disease-specific instruments were created to measure a specific portion of an individual's health. The questions associated with this type of measure are customized to the HRQoL burden of a specific disorder and its treatment options. The IOI-HA, GHABP, and other measures summarized in **Table 8–1** may be considered disease-specific HRQoL measures. For example, Mulrow and colleagues (1990) used the HHIE, a disease-specific measure of hearing aid benefit, in a randomized trial of the effect of hearing aid use on HRQoL.

Generic Measures

There are two styles of generic measures: health profiles and utilities. Health profiles are self-report instruments that attempt to measure all important aspects of HRQoL. These aspects often include mobility, self-care, depression, anxiety, and well-being. Utility measures are derived from economic and decision theory. They represent the preferences of patients for treatment process and outcomes. With utilities, HRQoL is summarized as a single number on a continuum from 0 (usually representing death) to 1 (usually representing full health), although there can be scores less than 0 that represent states worse than death. Thus, with utilities, an individual can express positive and negative effects

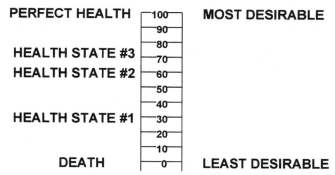

Figure 8–2 An example of a generic utility measure known as a "feeling thermometer." The patient is asked to rate his or her overall quality of life on the thermometer before and after treatment. The difference may indicate the degree to which intervention has improved the patient's overall quality of life. (From Feeny, D., Torrance, G., & Labele, R. (1996). Integrating economic evaluations and quality of life assessments. In B. Spilker (Ed.), Quality of life and pharmacoeconomics in clinical trials (2nd ed., p. 259). Philadelphia: Lippincott Williams & Wilkins, with permission.)

of a health disorder or treatment protocol within one score. One utility measuring device uses a scale known as a "feeling thermometer" (**Fig. 8–2**). A patient may be asked to rank his or her present health state on this thermometer before and after audiologic intervention to determine the extent to which treatment has improved the patient's perceived quality of life.

Standard Gamble Another utility measure technique is known as the "standard gamble" (**Fig. 8–3**). In this approach, the patient is offered a choice between two alternatives: living with health state B with certainty (which is presumably their present health state) or gambling on treatment A. Treatment A can lead to either perfect health or immediate death. The interviewer manipulates the probabilities of perfect health and death in choice A until the patient is indifferent between his or her present health state (B) and choice A. Obviously, the higher the probability of death the patient is willing to consider, the lower the health state (or quality of life) inherent in remaining with choice B.

Although the standard gamble is most commonly used for theoretical purposes to elicit "utility values" associated with serious life-threatening diseases such as cancer and heart disease, this technique may be useful in determining the impact of an individual's hearing impairment on his or her overall perceived quality of life. It might be useful, for example, to apply the standard gamble approach to potential cochlear implant recipients, particularly if candidacy continues to become less stringent. Instead of choosing between "perfect health" and "immediate death," the choice for the cochlear implant candidate might be "normal hearing" and "total deafness." If the patient is reluctant to gamble on a small risk of total deafness, the clinician may assume that the patient perceives his or her quality of life to be relatively good and not likely to significantly improve with an implant, even if hearing is substantially improved.

Time Trade-off An alternative approach to the standard gamble is the time trade-off (**Fig. 8–4**). In this technique, the patient is offered a choice between living a normal life span in his or her present health state or a shortened life span in perfect health. The interviewer reduces the life span spent in perfect health until the patient is indifferent between the shorter period of perfect health and the longer period in the less desirable state. An individual who is willing to "trade off" a significant part of his or her life for a shorter life in perfect health is revealing a great deal about his or her perceived quality of life.

Several computer-assisted programs have been developed to measure utilities, including the U-Titer (Sumner et al, 1991) and the Utility Measures for Audiology Application (UMAA) software (Roberts and Lister, 2005), currently being evaluated at the Veterans Affairs (VA) Medical Center in Bay Pines, Florida; the University of South Florida; and the American Institute for Balance. The U-Titer was used by Yueh and colleagues (2001) in a comparative evaluation of the effect of different amplification strategies on HRQoL and by Abrams, Chisolm, and Kenworthy (2002), who demonstrated the sensitivity of utilities to hearing aid intervention.

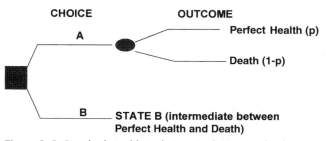

Figure 8–3 Standard gamble technique to determine the degree to which a patient's health impacts on his or her perceived quality of life. p, probability of perfect health; $1-p$, probability of death. p and $1-p$ are manipulated until the patient is indifferent between choice A with its associated risk and choice B, the patient's present health state. (From Feeny D., Torrance, G., & Labele, R. (1996). Integrating economic evaluations and quality of life assessments. In B. Spilker (Ed.), Quality of life and pharmacoeconomics in clinical trials (2nd ed., p. 260). Philadelphia: Lippincott Williams & Wilkins, with permission.)

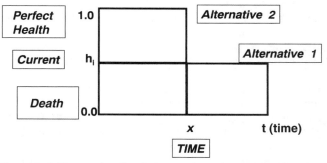

Figure 8–4 Time trade-off technique to determine perceived quality of life associated with hearing loss. h_i, perceived quality of life; x, total time with perfect health. x and t are manipulated until the patient is indifferent between a normal life span with existing health and shorter life expectancy with perfect health. (From Feeny, D., Torrance, G., & Labele, R. (1996). Integrating economic evaluations and quality of life assessments. In B. Spilker (Ed.), Quality of life and pharmacoeconomics in clinical trials (2nd ed., p. 260). Philadelphia: Lippincott Williams & Wilkins, with permission.)

Health Profiles   As noted earlier, health profiles are designed in the form of a questionnaire and provide individual scores for each category of health separate from a general health score. Examples of generic profiles referenced in the audiologic literature are Sickness Impact Profile (SIP; Bergner et al, 1981), MOS SF-36 Health Survey (SF-36; Ware and Sherbourne, 1992), Health Utilities Index (Furlong et al, 2001), and the WHO's Disability Assessment Schedule II (WHO-DAS II; WHO, 2001). Information about these measures is included in **Table 8–1**. The SIP measures sickness-related behavior by either direct report from the individual or from observations by another respondent referring to the individual. The MOS SF-36 measures eight subscales of general health that can be categorized into physical and mental components of health status. The Health Utilities Index (HUI) is a generic, preference-scored, comprehensive system for measuring health status, HRQoL, and producing utility scores. Individuals are required to select their level of functioning for several attributes. For example, in the Health Utilities Index Mark 3 (HUI3), a person is asked to select one of six descriptors that best represents his or her hearing. Each descriptor (1–6) is associated with a different utility value, such that $1 = 1.0$, $2 = 0.95$, $3 = 0.89$, $4 = 0.80$, $5 = 0.74$, and $6 = 0.61$. In the HUI3, utilities are measured for the multiple domains of vision, hearing, speech, dexterity, ambulation, emotion, cognition, and pain, and a summary measure is calculated to provide an overall utility value. The HUI has not been used in hearing aid research. The WHO-DAS II consists of 36 items organized into 6 domains: communication, mobility, self-care, interpersonal, life activities, and participation in society. It assesses difficulties with functioning and disability in each of these six domains over the past 30 days. For each question, an individual is asked, "In the last 30 days, how much difficulty did you have in. . . ." Responses are given on a 5-point Likert-type scale from 1 ("none") to 5 ("extreme"/"cannot do"). Six domain scores are generated along with a total score. Raw scores are transformed into standardized scores that range from 0, indicating the highest level of functioning, to 100, indicating the lowest level of functioning. The domains of communication, mobility, and self-care reflect the WHO-ICF dimension of activity, and the interpersonal, life activities, and participation domains reflect the WHO-ICF dimension of participation.

The SIP and the SF-36 were designed to measure the impact of illness and disease on an individual's HRQoL. The SIP is devised of multiple subscales with a grand total of 136 items. It is time consuming and not easy to administer, which limits its clinical utility. The SF-36 is much shorter, easy to administer, and is gaining popularity within quality of life research. Unfortunately, in reviewing the use of the SIP and the SF-36 as outcome measures for hearing aid intervention, Bess (2000) concluded that, although currently available generic health status instruments were successful in determining the impact of hearing loss on functional status and HRQoL, the instruments were not particularly responsive to hearing aid intervention. Since Bess's review, the responsiveness of the WHO-DAS II to hearing aid intervention was demonstrated in a large clinical trial (McArdle et al, 2005).

One reason that HRQoL assessment is receiving increased attention throughout health care is that the outcomes data obtained can be combined with economic data to examine the cost-effectiveness of particular treatments. In one approach, the relationships among cost, benefit, and time are examined and reported in terms of dollars spent for each quality-adjusted life year (QALY) gained. For example, Mulrow and colleagues (1990), using the HHIE, determined that hearing aids were a very cost-effective treatment for veterans with sensorineural hearing loss, costing only $200 per hearing QALY gained. In a study comparing hearing aid use alone with hearing aid use in conjunction with short-term group postfitting audiologic rehabilitation (AR), Abrams, Chisolm, and McArdle (2002) determined that hearing aid alone treatment cost $60.00 per QALY gained, whereas hearing aids plus AR cost only $31.91 per QALY gained, making hearing aids plus AR the more cost-effective treatment. The concept of QALY and other economic assessments of outcome will be discussed in greater detail later in this chapter.

Pearl

- QALY analyses demonstrate that maximum benefit is achieved per dollar spent when intervention is begun as early as possible.

Measuring Outcomes for Satisfaction

The measurement of satisfaction as a clinical outcome presents unique problems. Whereas measures of impairment, activity, participation, and HQoL can be referenced to a specific treatment intervention, a patient's perception (judgment) of satisfaction involves a constellation of factors that are peripheral to the treatment. These may include but are not limited to expectations of success, perceived value, cosmetic appeal, comfort, ease of use, and competent, efficient service delivery.

The concept of value warrants elaboration. For paying patients, the issue is fairly clear: they can return the hearing aid if they do not feel they are getting their money's worth. For VA patients, the issue of determining the influence of value on satisfaction can be problematic. Individuals in the VA system might keep the instruments even if they are dissatisfied, as there is no economic incentive to return the aids. However, for these individuals, the concept of value is often related to such noneconomic factors as their perception of service-related entitlement. Interestingly, an investigation of the impact of cost on perceived benefit (Newman et al, 1993) revealed that HHIE scores were no different between groups of insured and uninsured hearing aid recipients.

The most common way of documenting satisfaction is through questionnaires. Numerous surveys are available; however, only a few have been subjected to psychometric evaluation. The most extensive instrument is the Marke-Trak, developed by Kochkin (1990) for the hearing aid industry. It allows for the evaluation of satisfaction for device and service delivery. Other questionnaires are HAUQ (Dillon et al, 1997), an 11-item clinical instrument developed and evaluated on an Australian adult population, that assesses both device and service delivery satisfaction; and Satisfaction with Amplification in Daily Life (SADL; Cox and Alexander, 1999), a 15-item instrument that assesses the patient's level of satisfaction among several hearing aid–related dimensions, including perceived positive and negative effects of amplification, service and cost, and perceived effect on personal image. Many clinics have developed their own measures to assess patient satisfaction.

◆ The Economics of Outcomes

The emphasis on the bottom line in health care has refocused discussion of outcomes to the costs as well as the results of treatment. It is no longer sufficient to demonstrate that an intervention has made a difference in the impairment, participation, activity, satisfaction, or quality of life domains. Sufficiency now demands that the outcome has been achieved at "reasonable" costs. The definition of *reasonable* is often left up to the entity paying the bills—the insurer, health maintenance organization (HMO), government agency, or patient. It is becoming increasingly important for audiologists to understand the concepts of health care economics to analyze their costs, compare the costs of different treatment options, operate efficient and competitive practices, and determine costs as a function of benefit achieved for audiologic intervention. An understanding of health care economics is essential for analyzing costs and benefits of present services as well as for planning future programs. The discussion below is designed to introduce the reader to the basic concepts of health-care economics. **Table 8–2** illustrates the differences among several commonly used health economic measures. For a comprehensive treatment of the subject, the interested reader is referred to Drummond et al (1997).

Pitfall
• Just whose outcomes are you measuring, the patient's or yours?

Cost Analysis

Cost analysis is the simplest and most straightforward of health care economic analyses. It answers the question What does it cost to deliver the service? To answer this question, the clinician needs to identify the resources required to deliver the particular service. These resources can be separated into direct and indirect costs. **Figure 8–5** illustrates a spreadsheet that can be used to calculate the cost of an audiologic assessment. Labor costs include not only the time spent by the audiologist with the patient but also the time spent by the receptionist, who checks the patient in and schedules the patient for a return appointment, and the file clerk, who is responsible for locating the file, transporting it to the clinic, and reshelving the records. Fringe benefits must also be included in the calculation of labor costs. These include vacation and sick time, employer-paid health and disability insurance, employer contributions to retirement and Social Security programs, and workers' compensation. Fringe benefits can add 25 to 30% to the labor costs. Supplies and materials used for the procedure are also considered direct costs. The indirect costs are primarily associated with equipment and space. If these are leased, the costs can be easily calculated. If the equipment and space (building) is owned, the costs are depreciated over the life expectancy of the equipment and building.

A spreadsheet can be a very powerful tool for cost analysis purposes. The clinician can easily manipulate components of the analysis (salary, equipment, and time) to examine various alternatives and the resultant costs. For example, the clinician or manager can answer the following questions: How will the audiologic evaluation costs change if I buy a new audiometer? What will happen if I reduce evaluation time by 10 minutes? and How will costs be affected by the 10% increase in the lease for office space?

Although a cost analysis is critical for determining the dollars spent to deliver services, it reveals nothing about the value of those services, that is, the benefits achieved for the dollars spent. In economic evaluation of health care services, the costs of treatment, both direct and indirect, are compared with the measured outcomes resulting from the treatment. Three methods are used to evaluate the relationship between costs and outcomes. Cost/benefit analyses measure outcome by assigning monetary values to morbidity and suffering incurred from treatment. Cost-effectiveness evaluations measure outcomes as specific increments of clinical effects, such

Table 8–2 Comparison of Cost Analysis Procedures

This Economic Measure	Answers This Question	As Measured By
Cost analysis	How much does it cost me to deliver my service?	Dollars
Cost-benefit analysis	Will the generated revenue or cost avoidance associated with delivering my service exceed my expenditures?	Dollars versus dollars
Cost-effectiveness analysis	Which service option, among several, offers the best clinical results for each dollar spent?	Clinical improvement (%, dB, etc) per dollars spent
Cost-utility analysis	Which service option, among several, offers the largest improvement in quality life, as determined by the patient, for each dollar spent?	Dollars per quality-adjusted life years

PROCEDURE: AUDIOLOGICAL ASSESSMENT (AA)

NUMBER OF PROCEDURES: [ ]

I. DIRECT COSTS:

A. LABOR COSTS:

POSITION	SALARY/ HOUR[1]	PROCEDURE TIME (MIN)	COST/ PROCEDURE
Audiologist			$ -
Receptionist			$ -
File Clerk			$ -
			$ -
			$ -

[1] Divide yearly salary by 2080 to determine SALARY/HOUR and multiply this value by .26 (or other %) to account for fringe benefits.

Total Labor Costs Per Procedure $ -

B. SUPPLIES & MATERIALS:

ITEM	COST PER ITEM	NO. PER PROCEDURE	COST/ PROCEDURE
Specula			$ -
Boxes			$ -
Glue			$ -
Impression Material			$ -
Earphone Covers			$ -
Impedance Tips			$ -
Insert Phones			$ -
Miscellaneous			$ -

Total Supplies & Materials Costs Per Procedure: $ -

Figure 8–5 An example of a spreadsheet for analyzing costs associated with a comprehensive audiologic assessment.

(Continued)

186

TOTAL DIRECT COSTS PER PROCEDURE: _____ $ ___

II. INDIRECT COSTS:

A. EQUIPMENT COSTS:

ITEM	PURCHASE COST	LIFE EXPECTANCY	DEPRECIATED VALUE	COST/ PROCEDURE
Computer				
Audiometer				
Immittance				
Otoscope				
Sound Booth				
Real Ear				

Total Equipment Costs Per Procedure: _____ $ -

B. BUILDING DEPRECIATION

BLDG COST/YR	# SQ FT	COST/ SQ FT	CONTRACT	AUDIO SQ FT	TTL M&R	COST/ PROCEDURE

BLDG COST/YR is calculated by dividing the cost of the building by 40 (life expectancy)

Total Building Depreciation Costs Per Procedure: _____ $ -

C. ADMINISTRATIVE SUPPORT:

TTL DIRECT COSTS/PROC	% ADMIN SUPPORT(DEFAULT IS 15%)	TOTAL COST
$ -	0.15	$ -

Total Administrative Support Costs Per Procedure: $ -

TOTAL INDIRECT COSTS PER PROCEDURE: $ -

TOTAL COST PER AUDIOLOGICAL ASSESSMENT: $ -

Figure 8–5 (Continued)

as percent correct for word recognition tasks when comparing various hearing aids. Cost-utility analyses measure outcomes in terms of quality of life produced by the clinical effects. Cost-utility analyses are widely used in the medical field because they allow for comparison of the cost-effectiveness between different treatment interventions.

Cost-Benefit Analysis

A cost/benefit analysis answers the question If I apply this intervention strategy, will the dollars earned or saved exceed the dollars spent? This type of analysis requires assigning monetary units to both the costs of treatment and the benefits achieved. For example, the costs of a balance rehabilitation program, including evaluation and therapy (as calculated through a cost analysis process), is compared against the dollars saved by reducing the need for office visits and medication or the dollars gained by allowing the individual to return to work. If the money gained and/or avoided exceeds the money spent, the service can be considered cost-beneficial. However, health care is not a manufacturing business, where the price of a widget must exceed the cost of manufacturing the widget for the outcome to be considered successful. As a society, we do not treat cancer or kidney disease with the expectation that the monetary benefits associated with treatment will exceed the costs spent on that treatment. There is an expectation that properly delivered health care will improve outcomes in domains that are not necessarily economic. Nonetheless, a cost/benefit analysis may be a useful exercise when comparing treatment alternatives that have the potential to reduce personal or societal costs.

Willingness to Pay

A special subset of cost/benefit analysis is the willingness to pay (WTP) concept, that is, determining how much the individual is willing to pay for the increased benefits associated with the intervention. There are several examples in the audiologic literature that have examined this issue. Palmer et al (1995) asked subjects to make sound quality judgments while listening to class A and class D amplifiers. The subjects were then asked how much they would pay for a hearing aid with the associated sound quality. The results indicated that the subjects would be willing to pay up to $200 more for a

hearing aid with better sound quality. Newman and Sandridge (1998) compared objective and subjective outcome measures among subjects who were fitted with three levels of hearing aid technology. Whereas more than 75% of the subjects preferred the fully digital technology, one third of those switched their preference to a lower level of technology after being informed of the cost. Chisolm and Abrams (2001) used a WTP approach to examine the value associated with self-perceived hearing aid benefit as measured by the APHAB global score. Results suggested that the participants were willing to pay $22.06 more for a hearing aid for each 1-point increase in APHAB global benefit. In a study of how much individuals were willing to pay above the base price of a hearing aid for specific signal-processing features, Abrams and colleagues (2004) asked 100 participants to view several computer-simulated vignettes. Experienced hearing aid users were willing to pay the most for feedback cancellation, followed by directional technology, expansion, and noise management, in that order.

There are some problems associated with WTP assumptions. The same amount of money may be perceived as having inherently greater or lesser value depending on one's income. An individual who earns the minimum wage is likely to assign a much greater value to hearing aids for which he or she is willing to pay $500 than an individual earning a six-figure salary.

Cost-Effectiveness Analysis

A cost-effectiveness analysis compares the costs of treatment alternatives with a specific outcome measure that is a result of that treatment. For example, we accept the fact that improved intelligibility in noise is a highly desirable outcome of hearing aids. We may want to examine the cost-effectiveness of several hearing aid alternatives—a single-microphone, analog instrument; a single-microphone, fully digital hearing aid; and a dual-microphone, digitally programmable hearing aid—by determining the relative cost per intelligibility point gained (**Table 8–3**). Until recently, there has been little research examining the relative cost-effectiveness of hearing aid intervention. Newman and Sandridge (1998), however, conducted a comprehensive benefit, satisfaction, and cost-effectiveness analysis comparing three hearing aids representing different levels of technology: a

Table 8–3 Example of a Hearing Aid Cost-Effectiveness Analysis

Hearing Aid (half-concha)	Cost (retail)	Outcome Score (% improvement on CUNY-NST Test)	Cost per % Increase Outcome Score (cost-effectiveness)
Single-channel, single-program, dual-microphone, analog	$1104.42	24%	$46.02
Dual-channel, multiple-program, single-microphone, digitally programmable	$1,357.74	16%	$84.86
Multiple-channel, multiple-program, single-microphone, fully digital	$3,472.64	18%	$192.92

CUNY-NST, City University of New York–Nonsense Syllable Test.

one-channel linear hearing aid; a two-channel nonlinear hearing aid; and a multi-channel, multiband digital signal processing (DSP) hearing aid. The investigators found that the subjects scored higher on a speech recognition test with the DSP instrument, but no significant differences were found among the instruments on the self-report measure of benefit or satisfaction survey. The cost-effectiveness analysis revealed that it cost $49.67 for each percentage point improvement achieved with the single-channel linear hearing aid compared with $51.88 with the two-channel nonlinear instrument and $109.76 with the DSP.

Controversial Point

- A cost-effectiveness analysis revealed that it cost $49.67 for each percentage point improvement achieved with a single-channel linear hearing aid compared with $109.76 with a DSP instrument.

An HMO may use the results of the cost-effectiveness analysis in **Table 8–3** to determine which hearing aid technology an insurer will cover, or the maximum hearing aid allowance. However, these choices may not coincide with patient satisfaction. The outcome measure used in the analysis may not be the one of primary interest to the patient; for example, the patient may place a premium on cosmetics, the ability to change programs, or simply possessing the latest technology. As discussed earlier in this chapter, there is a large number of outcome measures from which to choose (objective performance measures of speech recognition and self-report measures assessing activity limitations and/or participation restrictions), any one of which may represent a better measure of outcome than percent correct, for example. Another limitation of cost-effectiveness analysis is that it cannot be used to make comparisons across programs. For example, although we may know that it costs $46.02 for each 1% improvement in intelligibility

with hearing aid A, and the same amount of money for each 1 mm reduction in blood pressure with medicine C, we know nothing about how the patient perceives the benefits of improved hearing in comparison to reduced blood pressure in improving that individual's quality of life, nor are we able to determine which $46.02 expenditure represents the better utilization of scarce health care dollars. Cost analyses that measure the association between cost and quality of life are best examined using cost-utility analyses.

Controversial Point

- Can the sale of digital hearing aids costing over twice as much as high-end analog instruments be justified if there is no significant difference in outcome between the two technologies?

Cost-Utility Analysis

A cost-utility analysis focuses on the quality of health outcome achieved by a particular intervention. The analysis typically involves determining (1) the costs of treatment, both direct and indirect, for each intervention approach; (2) the change in scores as a function of treatment on an HQoL instrument; and (3) the estimated quantity of years of life remaining that any treatment effects may influence HQoL (usually the life expectancy of the individual as indicated on actuarial tables). These data are then used to calculate the cost of treatment for different diseases or disorders per QALY. QALYs are used in a cost-utility analysis to put a monetary value on specified treatment protocols. Although cost-effectiveness and cost-utility analyses are similar from a cost perspective, they differ from an outcome perspective. Cost-effectiveness analyses examine the cost per unit of some specific outcome achieved; cost-utility analyses examine the cost per quality of life year gained.

Table 8–4 illustrates how cost-utility analyses may be used to examine the effects of various hearing aid

---

Table 8–4 Four Examples of Quality-Adjusted Life Year Calculations

QALY Example #1

Age of patient: 70
Cost of hearing aids: $2,000/pair
Benefit obtained: 25% (APHAB)
Life expectancy: 5 years

$$\text{Cost per QALY} = \frac{\$2,000}{25 \times 5} = \$1600.00$$

QALY Example #2

Age of patient: 70
Cost of hearing aids: $4,000/pair
Benefit obtained: 60% (APHAB)
Life expectancy: 5 years

$$\text{Cost per QALY} = \frac{\$4,000}{60 \times 5} = \$1,333.33$$

QALY Example #3

Age of patient: 5
Cost of implant: $50,000
Benefit obtained: 30% (open set monosyllables)
Life expectancy: 70 years

$$\text{Cost per QALY} = \frac{\$50,000}{30 \times 70} = \$2,380.95$$

QALY Example #4

Age of patient: 65
Cost of implant: $50,000
Benefit obtained: 70% open set monosyllables
Life expectancy: 10 years

$$\text{Cost per QALY} = \frac{\$50,000}{70 \times 10} = \$7,142.86$$

APHAB, Abbreviated Profile of Hearing Aid Benefit; QALY, quality-adjusted life year.

Table 8–5 Cost per QALY Provided by Cochlear Implants as Compared with Other Medical Devices and Services

Technology	Cost/QALY
Neonatal intensive care	$7,968
Cochlear implant	$9,325
Coronary artery bypass	$11,255
Coronary angioplasty	$11,485

QALY, quality-adjusted life year.

Source: Wyatt et al (1995).

intervention options on costs per QALYs. Examples 1 and 2 demonstrate that the cost per QALY for more expensive instruments may be lower if the improvement in outcome is high enough. Examples 3 and 4 illustrate that even a very large difference in outcome cannot overcome the effects of longevity when intervention is begun early enough (assuming the device does not need to be replaced). Such an analysis may be very useful for insurers and health care planners when determining what services to offer as part of a comprehensive health care plan. Wyatt et al (1995) conducted a cost-utility analysis on cochlear implants and compared the implant costs with those associated with other common medical interventions. The results of this analysis are summarized in **Table 8–5**. Cochlear implants compare very favorably with other high-cost medical interventions because of the age at which the patients received their implants and the benefits achieved from using the device. The power of early intervention is nicely illustrated with the neonatal intensive care example. This resource-intensive intervention can cost hundreds of thousands of dollars, but it may be considered a bargain when the costs and benefits are spread over an individual's lifetime. Cost-utility analyses have been used in several hearing aid–related studies. As previously noted, Abrams et al (2002) examined the cost utility of postfitting group AR treatment and found it more cost-effective than fitting hearing aids alone. Joore and colleagues (2003) calculated the cost per QALY among hearing aid recipients in the Netherlands and found the fitting of hearing aids to be a cost-effective health care intervention.

◆ Outcomes and Evidence-Based Practice

In examining the available evidence for hearing aid outcomes, Maki-Torkko et al (2001) noted a paucity of studies that provide high-quality evidence to guide the practitioner in determining candidacy, amplification characteristics, and rehabilitation plans for individuals with hearing loss. Rather, as Van Vliet (2005) points out, practitioners have tended to depend on clinical experience. The recent emphasis on EBP makes the measurement of hearing aid treatment outcomes of great importance on the national

health care stage. By routinely measuring clinical outcomes and engaging in carefully controlled clinical trials, audiologists can build a foundation for evidence-based clinical practice guidelines. To examine the current state of evidence for practices related to hearing aid rehabilitation in adults, the interested reader is referred to the American Academy of Audiology's (Valenti et al, 2006) *Proposed Guideline for the Audiological Management of Adult Hearing Impairment.* Clinical practice guidelines help to minimize variability in outcome, maximize treatment effectiveness, reduce risks, decrease waste, and improve patient satisfaction. The development and implementation of evidence-based clinical practice guidelines have the potential to elevate the profession of audiology among third-party payers, other health care providers, and, most importantly, current and future patients.

A key player in EBP guideline development is the Agency for Healthcare Research and Quality (AHRQ; www.ahrq. gov). The AHRQ is the health services research arm of the U.S. Department of Health and Human Services (HHS). One of its missions, through the National Guideline Clearinghouse (NGC), is to provide physicians and other health care professionals, health care providers, health plans, integrated delivery systems, purchasers, and others objective and detailed information on clinical practice guidelines and to further their dissemination, implementation, and use. In addition, the AHRQ reviews and synthesizes scientific evidence for conditions or technologies that are costly, common, or important to Medicare or Medicaid programs. To accomplish this goal, the AHRQ supports 13 EBP centers throughout the United States and Canada. There are several reviews and clinical practice guidelines that would be of interest to audiologists, including a review of the evidence on the effectiveness of universal hearing screening among newborns and EBP guidelines for the medical management of otitis media. Although there are EBP guidelines for contact lens care, there are no evidence reports related to hearing aids or the nonmedical management of hearing loss.

The AHRQ evaluates the evidence for a specific condition or technology across three major categories: the level of evidence, the grade of the evidence, and the strength of recommendations that can be made based on the evidence review and that often forms the foundation for a clinical practice guideline (CPG). Each of these categories is briefly described below.

Levels of Evidence

- ◆ Level 1 evidence results from large, randomized trials with clear-cut results where there is low risk of error.

- ◆ Level 2 evidence results from small, randomized trials with uncertain results (moderate to high risk of error).

- ◆ Level 3 evidence is collected from nonrandomized, contemporaneous controls.

- ◆ Level 4 evidence is from nonrandomized, historical controls and expert opinion.

♦ Level 5 evidence is the result of uncontrolled studies, case series, and expert opinion.

Grades of Evidence

♦ Grade A study requires level 1 evidence—randomized clinical trials.

♦ Grade B studies involve level 2 evidence—well-designed clinical trials that may not be randomized.

♦ Grade C studies involve levels 3, 4, or 5 evidence.

Strength of Recommendations

As a result of the review and grading of the evidence by AHRQ, recommendations are made for a particular intervention. Such recommendations become the basis of a CPG.

♦ Level I recommendations are usually indicated, always acceptable, and considered useful and effective (require grade A evidence).

♦ Level IIa recommendations are considered acceptable, of uncertain efficacy, and may be controversial. The weight of evidence is in favor of usefulness/efficacy (require grade B evidence).

♦ Level IIb recommendations are acceptable, of uncertain efficacy, and may be controversial. Level IIb recommendations may be helpful and are not likely to be harmful (require grade C evidence).

♦ Level III recommendations are not acceptable, of uncertain efficacy, and may be harmful.

Sources of Evidence

Although there are no audiologic-specific evidence reviews conducted by the AHRQ, there are numerous available sources of evidence to assist the audiologist with an EBP approach. These sources of evidence include books, non-peer-reviewed journals (e.g., *Hearing Review* and *Hearing Journal*), peer-reviewed journals (e.g., *Seminars in Hearing, Ear and Hearing, Trends in Amplification,* and *Journal of the American Academy of Audiology*), electronic bibliographic databases (e.g., Medline, PubMed, Cumulative Index to Nursing and Allied Health, and The Dome), and EBP Web sites (e.g., Clinical Evidence, Centre for Evidence-Based Medicine, and AHRQ). Cox (2005) presents a detailed outline of how to engage in an EBP review of a clinical question.

Critical Review of Evidence

Even without a systematic review of the audiologic evidence, research concerning the clinical efficacy of audiologic intervention is continually being conducted and reported. Not every article published necessarily represents good science or research. As a matter of fact, the AHRQ often rejects many articles in its evidence reviews due to poor quality research. Abrams et al (2005) and Cox (2005) delineate the criteria with which clinicians need to become familiar so that they can learn to distinguish higher quality from poorer quality research. These criteria include (1) knowledge of participant selection procedures; (2) whether or not participants were truly randomized into treatment arms; (3) the importance of "blinding" both participants and examiners to treatment arms; (4) the importance of having an adequate sample size to detect clinically meaningful effects; (5) a clear description of the therapeutic regimen, including descriptions of how the hearing instruments were selected and fit; (6) the use of well-selected outcome measures with known psychometric properties; (7) detailed information about study procedures; (8) discussion of withdrawals and study dropouts; (9) consideration of confounds and biases and, if discovered, how they were resolved; and (10) justification of statistical analyses, with results properly reported and interpreted.

♦ Summary

As the demand for EBP increases in health care, audiologists need to incorporate outcome measures such as those reviewed in this chapter as part of their standard clinical protocol. It is not enough for patients to simply express satisfaction with the services or devices they receive. Audiologists must be able to document the impact of those services through the use of standardized measures of objective and/or subjective benefit and satisfaction.

Measuring outcomes is nothing more than applying the scientific method to a clinical application. We develop a hypothesis that a particular hearing aid with specific features will have a certain effect on the activity and participation levels, as well as the quality of life, of a patient. We apply the chosen treatment to the patient, measure and analyze the results, and determine whether or not we have proven our hypothesis. In a sense, every clinical intervention is a scientific experiment.

Clinicians are probably familiar with many of the measures presented in this chapter and have likely used the data they provide to adjust hearing aid parameters, counsel patients, or assess satisfaction. **Table 8–6** illustrates how some of these measures can be applied to the WHO-ICF domains, the domains of HRQoL and satisfaction, as well as the common audiology terminology applied to these outcome measures. The measures selected for this table were chosen for their clinical practicability. They are easy to use, quickly administered and scored, and empirically tested. It is important for us to realize that these as well as many of the other outcome measures available to us can be used to demonstrate to administrators, insurers, referral sources, other health care providers, our patients, and their families that hearing aids are an effective and economical treatment for hearing impairment. As audiology continues to compete in the health care marketplace, we can demonstrate that our services have a positive impact on activity limitations, participation restrictions, and reduced HRQoL associated with hearing loss, and begin to do so using an evidence-based approach. "Neither unaudited experience

Table 8–6 Clinically Useful Measures to Assess Outcomes in the WHO, Generic, and Audiology Domains

WHO Domains	Generic Domains	Audiology	Outcome Measure
Impairment		Verification	2cc/REM functional gain
Activity limitations and/or participation restrictions		Validation	a. QuickSIN (objective) b. WIN (objective) c. HHIE (subjective—new users) d. APHAB (subjective—experienced users) e. COSI (subjective—new and experienced users) f. IOI-HA (subjective)
	HRQoL	Validation	HHIE (disease-specific) IOI-HA (disease-specific) WHO-DAS II (generic)
	Satisfaction	Validation	Selected items from MarkeTrak SADL HAUQ

HRQoL, health-related quality of life; QuickSIN, Quick Speech-in-Noise Test; WIN, Words-in-Noise Test; HHIE, Hearing Handicap Inventory for the Elderly; COSI, Client-Oriented Scale of Improvement; IOI-HA, International Outcomes Inventory–Hearing Aids; WHO-DAS II, World Health Organization–Disability Assessment Schedule II; SADL, Satisfaction with Amplification in Daily Life; HAUQ, Hearing Aid Users Questionnaire.

nor logical thought can replace controlled clinical trials, so until documentation of a procedure's effectiveness can be demonstrated, it should be considered a false idol and worship withheld."—Frank C. Wilson

Acknowledgments The authors wish to thank Dr. Rachel McArdle for her guidance in the completion of the section on objective speech recognition tests and Laural J. Portz for her assistance with tables and figures.

References

Abrams, H., Block, M., & Chisolm, T. H. (2004). The effects of signal processing and style on perceived value of hearing aids. Hearing Review, 11(13), 16–21.

Abrams, H., Chisolm, T., & Kenworthy, M. (2002, August 23). Utility approach to measuring hearing aid outcomes. Paper presented at the International Hearing Aid Research Conference, Lake Tahoe, NV.

Abrams, H., Chisolm, T. H., & McArdle, R. (2002). A cost-utility analysis of adult group audiologic rehabilitation: Are the benefits worth the costs? Journal of Rehabilitation Research and Development, 39, 549–558.

Abrams, H., McArdle, R., & Chisolm, T. H. (2005). From outcomes to evidence: Best practices for audiologists. Seminars in Hearing, 26(3), 157–169.

American National Standards Institute. (1997). Methods for the calculation of the Speech Intelligibility Index ANSI S3.5. New York: Author.

Beck, L. B. (2000). The role of outcomes data in health care resource allocation. Ear and Hearing, 21, 89S–96S.

Bentler, R. A., & Kramer, S. E. (2000). Guidelines for choosing a self-report outcome measure. Ear and Hearing, 21, 37S–49S.

Bergner, M., Bobbitt, R., Carter, W., & Gilson, B. (1981). The Sickness Impact Profile: Developments and final revision of a health status measure. Medical Care, 19(8), 57–67.

Besing, J. M., & Koehnke, J. (1995). A test of virtual auditory localization. Ear and Hearing, 16, 220–229.

Bess, F. H. (2000). The role of generic health-related quality of life measures in establishing audiological rehabilitation outcomes. Ear and Hearing, 21, 74S–99S.

Boothroyd, A. (1998). Hearing aids outcome evaluation. Paper presented at the Conference on Outcome Measurement for Hearing Aids, Los Angeles.

Byrne, D. (1992). Key issues in hearing aid selection and evaluation. Journal of the American Academy of Audiology, 3, 67–80.

Carhart, R. (1946). Tests for selection of hearing aids. Laryngoscope, 56, 780–794.

Chisolm, T. H., & Abrams, H. B. (2001). Measuring hearing aid benefit utilizing a willingness-to-pay approach. Journal of the American Academy of Audiology, 12, 383–389.

Cox, R. M. (1997). Administration and application of the APHAB. Hearing Journal, 50, 32–48.

Cox, R. M. (2005). Evidence-based practice in provision of amplification. Journal of the American Academy of Audiology, 16, 419–438.

Cox, R. M., & Alexander, G. (1995). The Abbreviated Profile of Hearing Aid Benefit. Ear and Hearing, 16, 176–186.

Cox, R. M., & Alexander, G. (1999). Measuring satisfaction with amplification in daily life: The SADL scale. Ear and Hearing, 20, 306–320.

Cox, R. M., & Alexander, G. C. (2002). The International Outcome Inventory for Hearing Aids (IO-HA): Psychometric properties of the English version. International Journal of Audiology, 41, 30–35.

Cox, R. M., Alexander, G. C., & Beyer, C. M. (2003). Norms for the International Outcome Inventory for Hearing Aids. Journal of the American Academy of Audiology, 14, 403–413.

Cox, R., Hyde, M., Gatehouse, S., et al. (2000). Optimal outcome measures, research priorities, and international cooperation. Ear and Hearing, 21, 106S–115S.

Demorest, M. E., & Erdman, S. A. (1986). Scale composition and item analysis of the Communication Profile for the Hearing Impaired. Journal of Speech and Hearing Research, 29, 515–535.

Department of Veterans Affairs. (1998). Tonal and speech materials for auditory perceptual assessment disc 2.0. Mountain Home, TN: VA Medical Center.

Dillon, H. (2001). Hearing aids. New York: Thieme Medical Publishers.

Dillon, H., Birtles, G., & Lovegrove, R. (1999). Measuring the outcomes of a national rehabilitation program: Normative data for the Client Oriented Scale of Improvement (COSI) and the Hearing Aid Users Questionnaire (HAUQ). Journal of the American Academy of Audiology, 10, 67–99.

Dillon, H., James, A., & Ginis, J. (1997). Client Oriented Scale of Improvement (COSI) and its relationship to several other measures of benefit and satisfaction provided by hearing aids. Journal of the American Academy of Audiology, 8, 27–43.

Drummond, M., O'Brien, B., Stoddart, G., & Torrance, G. (1997). Methods for the economic evaluation of health care programmes (2nd ed.). New York: Oxford University Press.

Feeny, D., Torrance, G., & Labele, R. (1996). Integrating economic evaluations and quality of life assessments. In B. Spilker (Ed.), Quality of life and pharmacoeconomics in clinical trials (2nd ed.). Philadelphia: Lippincott Williams & Wilkins.

Finney, D. J. (1952). Statistical method in biological essay. London: C. Griffen.

Flesch, R. (1948). A new readability yardstick. Journal of Applied Psychology, 32, 221–233.

Fletcher, H. (1950). A method of calculating hearing loss for speech audiogram. Journal of the Acoustical Society of America, 22, 1–5.

Furlong, W. J., Feeny, D. H., Torrance, G. W., & Barr, R. D. (2001). The Health Utilities Index (HUI®) system for assessing health-related quality of life in clinical studies. Annals of Medicine, 33, 375–384.

Gatehouse, S. (1992). The time course and magnitude of perceptual acclimatization to frequency responses: Evidence from monaural fitting of hearing aids. Journal of the Acoustical Society of America, 92, 1258–1268.

Gatehouse, S. (1999). Glasgow Hearing Benefit Profile: Derivation and validation of a client-centered outcome measure for hearing aid services. Journal of the American Academy of Audiology, 10, 80–103.

Gatehouse, S. (2000). The Glasgow Hearing Aid Benefit Profile: What it measures and how to use it. Hearing Journal, 53, 10–18.

Gatehouse, S., & Noble, W. (2004). The Speech, Spatial and Qualities of Hearing Scale (SSQ). International Journal of Audiology, 43, 85–99.

Harford, E. (1993, April 15). The impact of the hearing aid on the evolution of audiology. Carhart Memorial Lecture at the Annual Meeting of the American Auditory Society, Phoenix, AZ.

Hyde, M. L. (2000). Reasonable psychometric standards for self-report outcome measures in audiological rehabilitation. Ear and Hearing, 21, 24S–36S.

Johnson, C. E., & Danhauer, J. L. (2002). Handbook of outcomes measurement in audiology. Clifton Park, NY: Thomson Delmar Learning.

Joore, M. A., Potjewijd, J., Timmerman, A. A., & Anteunis, L. J. C. (2002). Response shift in the measurement of quality of life in hearing-impaired adults after hearing aid fitting. Quality of Life Research, 11, 299–307.

Joore, M. A., Van Der Stel, H., Peters, H., & Anteunis, L. (2003). The cost-effectiveness of hearing-aid fitting in the Netherlands. Archives of Otolaryngology—Head and Neck Surgery, 129, 297–304.

Kiessling, J., Pichora-Fuller, M. K., Gatehouse, S., et al. (2003). Candidature for and delivery of audiological services: Special needs of older people. International Journal of Audiology, 42(Suppl. 2), S92–S101.

Killion, M. C., Niquette, P. A., Gudmundsen, G. I., Revit, L. J., & Banerjee, S. (2004). Development of a quick speech-in-noise test for measuring signal-to-noise ratio loss in normal-hearing and hearing-impaired listeners. Journal of the Acoustical Society of America, 116, 2395–2405.

Kochkin, S. (1990). Introducing MarkeTrak: A consumer tracking survey of the hearing instrument market. Hearing Journal, 43(5), 17–27.

Lichtenstein, M. J., & Hazuda, H. P. (1998). Cross-cultural adaptation of the Hearing Handicap Inventory for the Elderly—Screening Version (HHIE-S) for use with Spanish-speaking Mexican Americans. Journal of the American Geriatrics Society, 46, 492–498.

Lopez-Vazquez, M., Orozco, J. A., Jimenez, G., & Berruecos, P. (2002). Spanish hearing impairment inventory for the elderly. International Journal of Audiology, 41, 221–230.

Maki-Torkko, E. M., Brorsson, B., Davis, A., et al. (2001). Hearing impairment among adults—extent of the problem and scientific evidence on the outcome of hearing aid rehabilitation. Scandinavian Audiology Supplementum, 54, 8–15.

McArdle, R., Chisolm, T. H., Abrams, H. B., Wilson, R. H., & Doyle, P. J. (2005). The WHO-DAS II: Measuring hearing aid outcomes in adults. Trends in Amplification, 9, 127–143.

Mulrow, C. D., Aguilar, C., Endicott, J. E., et al. (1990). Quality of life changes and hearing impairment. Annals of Internal Medicine, 113, 188–194.

National Institutes of Health. (1993). Quality of life assessment: Practice, problems, and promise. Bethesda, MD: Author.

Newman, C. W., Hug, G. A., Wharton, J. A., & Jacobson, G. P. (1993). The influence of hearing aid cost on perceived benefit in older adults. Ear and Hearing, 14, 285–289.

Newman, C. W., Weinstein, B. E., Jacobson G. P., & Hug, G. A. (1990). The Hearing Handicap Inventory for Adults: Psychometric adequacy and audiometric correlates. Ear and Hearing, 11, 430–433.

Newman, C. , & Sandridge, S. (1998). Benefit from, satisfaction with, and cost-effectiveness of three different hearing aid technologies. American Journal of Audiology, 7, 115–128.

Nilsson, M., Soli, S. D., & Sullivan, J. A. (1994). Development of the Hearing in Noise Test for the measurement of speech reception thresholds in quiet and in noise. Journal of the Acoustical Society of America, 95, 1085–1099.

Palmer, C. S., Niparko, J. K., Wyatt, J. R., Rothman, M., & de Lissovoy, G. (1999). A prospective study of the cost-utility of the multichannel cochlear implant. Archives of Otolaryngology—Head and Neck Surgery, 125, 1221–1228.

Palmer, C. V., Killion, M. C., Wilber, L. A., & Ballard, W. J. (1995). Comparison of two hearing aid receivers-amplifier combinations using sound quality judgments. Ear and Hearing, 16, 587–598.

Pavlovic, C. V. (1984). Use of the articulation index for assessing residual auditory function in listeners with sensorineural hearing loss. Journal of the Acoustical Society of America, 75, 1253–1258.

Pichora-Fuller, M. K., & Robertson, S. R. (1994). Hard of hearing residents in a home for the aged. Journal of Speech-Language Pathology and Audiology, 18, 278–288.

QuickSIN speech-in-noise test (compact disc). (2001). Elk Grove Village, IL: Etymotic Research.

Rankovic, C. V. (1997). Prediction of speech reception for listeners with sensorineural hearing loss. In Jestedt, W. (Ed.), Modeling sensorineural hearing loss (pp. 121–432). Mahwah, NJ: Lawrence Erlbaum.

Roberts, R., & Lister, J. (2005). Utility Measures for Audiology Application (UMAA) (computer software). Bay Pines, FL: VA Medical Center Bay Pines.

Sackett, D. L., Rosenberg, W. M., Gray, J. A., Haynes, R. B., & Richardson, W. S. (1996). Evidence-based medicine: What it is and what it isn't. British Medical Journal, 312, 71–72.

Saunders, G. H., & Jutai, J. W. (2004). Hearing specific and generic measures of psychosocial impact of hearing aids. Journal of the American Academy of Audiology, 15, 238–248.

Strom, K. E. (2005). The HR 2005 Dispenser Survey. Hearing Journal, 12, 18–36.

Sumner, W., Nease, R., & Littenberg, B. (1991). U-Titer: A utility assessment tool. In Proceedings of the 15th Annual Symposium on Computer Applications in Medical Care (pp. 701–705). Washington, DC: McGraw-Hill.

Tillman, T., & Carhart, R. (1966). An expanded test for speech discrimination utilizing CNC monosyllabic words. Northwestern University Auditory Test No. 6. Brooks Air Force Base, TX: USAF School of Aerospace Medicine Technical Report.

Turner, R. (1998). The hearing aid expert: Audiologist, dealer, or otolaryngologist? American Journal of Audiology, 7, 5–19.

Valente, M., Abrams, H., Benson, D., et al. (2006). Guidelines for the audiological management of adult hearing impairment. Audiology Today, 18(5), 44.

Van Vliet, D. (2005). The current status of hearing care: Can we change the status quo? Journal of the American Academy of Audiology, 16, 410–418.

Ventry, I. M., & Weinstein, B. E. (1982). The Hearing Handicap Inventory for the Elderly: A new tool. Ear and Hearing, 3, 128–134.

Walden, B. E., Demorest, M. E., & Hepler, E. L. (1984). Self-report approach to assessing benefit derived from amplification. Journal of Speech and Hearing Research, 27, 49–56.

Walden, B. E., Schwartz, D. M., Williams, D. L., Holum-Hardegen, L. L., & Crowley, J. M. (1983). Test of the assumptions underlying comparative hearing aid evaluations. Journal of Speech and Hearing Disorders, 48, 264–273.

Ware, J. E., & Sherbourne, C. D. (1992). The MOS 36-item short-form health survey (SF-36): 1. Conceptual framework and item selection. Medical Care, 30, 473–481.

Weinstein, B. E., Spitzer, J. B., & Ventry, I. M. (1986). Test–retest reliability of the Hearing Handicap Inventory for the Elderly. Ear and Hearing, 7, 295–299.

Wilson, R. H. (2003). Development of a speech in multitalker babble paradigm to assess word-recognition performance. Journal of the American Academy of Audiology, 14, 453–470.

World Health Organization. (1980). International Classification of Impairments, Disabilities and Handicaps – A Manual of Classification Relating to the Consequences of Disease. Geneva: World Health Organization.

World Health Organization. (2001). International Classification of Functioning, Disability and Health (ICF). Retrieved May 1, 2007, from http://www3. who.int/icf/

World Health Organization. Disability Assessment Schedule II (WHO-DAS II) 36-item interviewer administered version. Retrieved May 1, 2007, from http://www.who.int/icidh/whodas/index.html

Wyatt, J., Niparko, J., Rothman, M., deLissovoy, G. (1995). Cochlear implant cost effectiveness. The American Journal of Otology, 16, 52–62.

Yueh, B., Souza, P.E., McDowell, J. A., et al. (2001). Randomized trial of amplification strategies. Archives of Otolaryngology—Head and Neck Surgery, 127 1197–1204.

Zelski, R. (2000). Use of the Client Oriented Scale of Improvement as a clinical outcome measure in the Veterans Affairs National Hearing Aid Program. Unpublished doctoral dissertation, University of South Florida, Tampa.

Chapter 9

Documentation in Clinical Audiology: An Information Management Perspective

David A. Zapala

Data are not facts

Facts are not information

Information is not knowledge

Knowledge is not truth

Truth is not wisdom. . . .

Poem by James Autry, reprinted by permission

Over the years, there have been several chapters written on the topic of report writing and documentation in audiology (see, e.g., Gonzenbach, 2000; Stach, 1998). The focus of this chapter differs from those in several respects. First, the practice of audiology is changing at a rapid pace: technological innovations and practice settings have evolved, the scope of services provided by audiologists has expanded, and our ability to contribute to patient care is increasingly recognized in the health care setting. We bear greater responsibility for the effectiveness of our services. Consequently, we are becoming more evidence based and outcome oriented (Cox, 2005; see also Chapter 8). With this evolution, our documentation efforts must also change. Our documents need to be patient focused, capturing the logic of our assessment and management efforts, and not merely test focused. One of the primary objectives of this chapter is to arm the audiologist with tools to recognize when reports should focus on test results and when they should focus on patient management.

The second reason why this chapter's focus differs from earlier efforts is that the health care system is changing in profound ways. Computers and information technology have proved themselves invaluable in improving the quality and decreasing the cost associated with patient care. In a simple sense, using a computer to automate the generation of a paper report saves time and transcription costs. However, consider that it has been estimated that 10% of the information typically included in a paper-based hospital record cannot be located, and that 11% of laboratory tests are duplicated because the original data cannot be found (Goldenberg and Couch, 2005). An electronic medical record (EMR) is a computer network–based replacement for the paper record (Kohane et al, 1996). All medical information is placed into the EMR as it is developed; it is searchable and available to all health care providers simultaneously. This allows for greater collaboration and teamwork with fewer errors (Agency for Healthcare Research and Quality, 2001; Centers for Medicare and Medicaid Services and the Veterans Health Administration, 2005; Institute of Medicine, 2001; Valenti, 2000). Audiologists will be documenting in this digital environment. To understand how these systems can be leveraged to improve patient care and clinical services, the audiologist must learn to think in terms of medical information management, not just report writing.

Changes in the practice of audiology, changes in the health care system, and the implementation of the EMR and other health care information management initiatives will all affect how we approach documenting clinical encounters. This chapter provides a conceptual framework to introduce the audiologist to report generation from an information-processing point of view.

Special Consideration

- It is been estimated that 10% of the information typically included in a paper-based hospital record cannot be located, and that 11% of laboratory tests are duplicated because the original data cannot be found (Goldenberg and Couch, 2005).

◆ Problem-solving and the Clinical Process

Why document in clinical practice? The primary reason is to reinforce memory. It is impossible to remember everything, and well-written notes will remind us as audiologists of where we are in our relationships with patients.[1] We also create records for other caregivers, present or future, who may provide services to patients. These caregivers may be audiologists, physicians, nurses, social workers, or other health care professionals. Each will have a different level of understanding about what audiology does and how to interpret our reports. We write to satisfy various auditors of health care services, who look for documentation to support the diagnosis and treatment, justify entry into or continued treatment, describe progress and response to interventions, and justify discharge from care (Joint Commission on Accreditation of Health Care Organizations, 2005; Paul–Brown, 1994). Finally, we may be writing for patients themselves, as they are the true owners of their own health care information.

It is impossible to write directly to the needs of such a diverse group of consumers. As we shall see, in some situations, it is not even necessary to do so. However, when necessary, a well-written, well-structured report allows the reader to clearly understand why the patient came to the encounter, what was discovered, and what should happen next. Stated another way, the report captures the clinical decision making and problem-solving that occurred on behalf of the patient. Physicians and other "diagnosing" health care professionals are trained to think about the clinical process in a structured way, and that is how they write (Kasper et al, 2005; Mark, 2005). Most caregivers understand how clinical reports are structured and know where to look to find information of interest. This structured way of thinking and writing is the currency by which we contribute to coordinated

patient care as members of the health care team. Consequently, it is important that we master this form of thinking and communicating. This chapter is not about clinical thinking. However, it is important to recognize that we will document what we perceive to be important, so the process of clinical thinking and clinical writing cannot be separated.[2]

The Clinical Process

The practice of audiology is a professional endeavor. Individuals seek the services of professionals because they have problems to be solved. The solutions require knowledge and judgment that exceed the individuals' personal abilities. It is the professionals who must understand the individuals' problems and apply their own unique professional knowledge and judgment to suggest or offer solutions. So, for instance, individuals consult physicians for advice on matters of personal health, audiologists for advice on matters involving hearing problems and communication, and tax specialists for advice on matters concerning tax returns.

To offer an opinion, the professional must obtain or develop information about the nature of the consulting individual's problem. The professional must then distinguish between competing courses of action. This implies a definition of information that will be important for us in future discussion. We will define the term *clinical information* to mean an understanding of the likely cause of a patient's problem that is sufficiently detailed to support the choice of a subsequent management plan. Clinical information is actionable. From this perspective, the audiologic evaluation can be thought of as a formal method of developing clinical information about a patient's auditory capability with enough detail to decide upon a logical or rational management step.

Pearl

- Clinical information is actionable. This means the clinician has developed an understanding of the underlying cause of a patient's problem sufficient enough to explicitly state the problem and develop a rational management plan.

At its core, structured clinical documentation captures the evidence and logic behind any decisions made on the patient's behalf. In some settings, such as in private practice, the audiologist makes decisions about patient management. In other settings, the audiologic evaluation is used as evidence to support the medical decision making. The structure and composition of the audiologic report depend entirely on whether the

---

[1] In this chapter, the word *patient* is used to refer to a person who is seeking health care–related professional services. This usage implies a health care provider–patient relationship, not a physician–patient relationship.

[2] The textbook by Robert Baloh entitled *Dizziness, Hearing Loss, and Tinnitus* (1998) is a good reference that presents a structured approach to the assessment of ear-related medical disorders. Structured clinical thinking of audiologic problems, meaning problems using hearing in the functional sense, is the topic of audiologists' graduate education. This chapter assumes proficiency in audiologic management and assumes that the reader understands enough of the process of medical diagnosis to know when to refer patients for medical evaluation and management.

audiologist is making a clinical decision about patient management or merely offering evidence in support of a medical evaluation. The first task, then, in developing a documentation strategy for a given patient encounter is to determine who is managing the patient. If the audiologist is managing the patient, a formal structured clinical report will be necessary. If another health care provider is managing the patient, the audiologist contributes to that health care provider's documentation by submitting the elements of the audiologic evaluation as part of the physical examination. This will become clearer as we review the schema for the clinical process.

Pearl

- The first task in developing a documentation strategy for a given patient encounter is to determine who is managing the patient.

The clinical process is the basic schema that underpins the clinician-patient encounter. This schema is shown in **Fig. 9–1**. The clinical process starts with the patient's recognition that he or she is experiencing a problem. Following the classification of function by the World Health Organization (WHO; Stephans, 2003; Tang, 2000; WHO, 2001; see also Chapter 8 in this volume), the patient may be aware of impairment in a body function or structure (e.g., hearing loss) and possibly be experiencing difficulty in the performance of activities as a result (e.g., communicating, listening, and speaking). The point is, within the world of the patient, there is a perception that "something is wrong." Exactly what is wrong may or may not be evident to the patient. From the patient's perspective, the goal is to "get better" (the ideal outcome, or part 6 in **Fig. 9–1**). In medicine, the task of the clinician is to establish exactly what is wrong (diagnosis) and how bad it is (severity), estimate the expected time course of the condition (prognosis), and determine if something can be done to improve the prognosis (treatment) (Kasper et al, 2005). Audiology follows this model to some degree, but the audiologist's aims are not medical diagnosis and treatment. Rather, the audiologist's goals are to identify the cause of a patient's hearing or balance problem in the perceptual and communicative, as well as physiologic, domains and to determine how best to help the patient use residual or restored function. This is sometimes referred to as audiologic diagnosis and treatment. However, the word *diagnosis* has two meanings. In the medical realm, *diagnosis* specifically relates to the identification of disease. In the more general sense, it refers to the ability to assess the cause of a problem. It is the logical, cognitive process embodied in the latter definition that is the focus of this text. To clarify meanings: *medical diagnosis* refers to the process of distinguishing the presence of specific diseases, and *audiologic diagnosis* refers to the process of identifying the cause of hearing difficulties from the perceptual or communicative sense. When *diagnosis* or *treatment* occurs alone in this chapter, reference is to general usage of the terms and not specifically to medical diagnosis or treatment. Otherwise, the terms *assessment, clinical impression,* and *problem list* are employed in lieu of *diagnosis,* and *management* or *plan* in lieu of *treatment.* In all cases, it is the logic that underpins clinical decision making and documentation efforts that is important, not the domain in which the logic is applied.

Sources of Information or Knowledge

Regardless of the discipline, the professional or clinician must delve into three specific sources of knowledge in any encounter where a clinical decision is made. These knowledge sources are the patient, the discipline, and the profession.

Patient Self-Report The first source of information is the patient. The clinician must be able to listen to and understand the patient's specific problem. The patient is the only source of this information (represented by the top row of **Fig. 9–1**). The clinician will use this knowledge to form a "chief complaint" or problem(s) to be addressed, as understood from the patient's point of view. Impacting the problem to be

Knowledge Domain	Encounter Sequence >>>					
Individual Case	(1) Presenting Problem					(6) Outcome
Professional Knowledge		Collecting Evidence		(4) ASSESSMENT: Problem List, Clinical Impressions, "Diagnosis"	(5) PLAN: Treatment or Management	
		(2) SUBJECTIVE: Chief Complaint, Symptoms, History	(3) OBJECTIVE: Physical Signs, Special Tests			
Discipline Knowledge		(7) Learned Theories of Cause and Effect				

Figure 9–1 The clinical process. This schema captures the process by which a clinician's problem-solving efforts are organized on behalf of a patient. The figure is organized into two columns. The left-hand column designates the knowledge domain from which clinical information can be developed. There are three knowledge domains available to the clinician: knowledge gleaned from the patient, which is unique to that patient's life situation and experience (individual case); knowledge gleaned from professional assessment and management processes (professional knowledge); and knowledge gleaned from prior training and experience (discipline knowledge). The broad column on the right shows how these knowledge domains are systematically queried by the clinician as he or she interacts with the patient (encounter sequence). Each cell in the encounter sequence is numbered for reference purposes. Note that the middle row captures the clinical process by which the clinician systematically queries each knowledge source. Not only does this process underpin clinical decision making, but it also serves the basis for the common SOAP notation structure discussed later in the chapter. See text for additional details.

addressed from the patient's point of view is the ultimate outcome of the clinical process.

Discipline-specific Knowledge of Audiologist   Science is predicated on the assumption that the world is rational, that there are cause-and-effect relationships that are knowable. Scientific disciplines such as chemistry, physics, social science, and political science reflect bodies of knowledge where cause-and-effect relationships have been observed and documented. Different professionals have mastered different disciplines, and understand different systems of cause and effect. Medicine and audiology are such disciplines, and both focus on their unique systems of cause and effect, although there is certainly overlap as well. In the case of audiology, discipline-specific knowledge emanates from the scientific study of how humans use hearing on a day-to-day basis, and how hearing problems may cause perceptual or communicative disorders. Practicing audiologists refer to this mastered body of knowledge at various stages in the clinical process as they problem solve on behalf of their patients (part 7 in **Fig. 9–1**).

Professional Knowledge and Skill of Audiologist   Discipline–specific knowledge underpins the audiologist's ability to assess and manage a patient's hearing problem. However, even this is not sufficient for the clinician to be effective. The additional core skill that the practitioner must possess is the ability to discern, from the patient's description of the problem and formal test results, information pointing to the probable cause of the patient's complaint. Once the underlying cause is understood, a management plan can be developed. This ability to discern a cause (assessment/clinical impression/diagnosis) and select an effective management plan is the knowledge of the practicing professional. We refer to this as "professional knowledge and skill," so as to distinguish it from the more general and academic discipline knowledge. Activities related to professional knowledge are shown in the middle row of **Fig. 9–1**.

Professional knowledge and skill are used in several clinical activities. These activities include the task of collecting and organizing facts gleaned from the patient (part 2 in **Fig. 9–1**), physical examination, and special test results (part 3 in **Fig. 9–1**); developing one or multiple hypotheses about the cause of the patient's problems (assessment, impression, or diagnosis; part 4 in **Fig. 9–1**); and developing a management or treatment plan (part 5 in **Fig. 9–1**). To accomplish these activities effectively, the audiologist is always delving into the knowledge of the discipline, as well as relying on his or her ability to analyze and synthesize acquired facts into actionable information.

Ultimately, the effectiveness of any management plan provided by an audiologist is an outcome measured from the patient's perspective (part 6 in **Fig. 9–1**). In successful assessment and management efforts, the patient's problems are managed in a way that enables the patient to use his or her hearing more effectively in day–to–day situations. If efforts are less than successful, the clinical process must be revisited, cycling through the processes of **Fig. 9–1** again, beginning with step 1 in the encounter sequence.

Understanding the clinical process schema is helpful from several perspectives. Certainly, audiologists should be able to organize every step in the process for each type of patient presentation (e.g., infant hearing assessment, pediatric assessment, educational audiology assessment, auditory site of lesion assessment, adult hearing assessment, and vestibular and balance assessment). Beyond this, the key to quality report writing is to understand that the document is a record of how the practitioner worked through the clinical process in the specific clinical encounter. As we will see, the document may not be lengthy or complicated. However, there is a logic to the structure that must be followed to make the rationale behind the management plan understandable to others.

Documenting the Process: SOAP Notes

SOAP is a mnemonic for a way of structuring documentation of the clinical process (Kasper et al, 2005; Rakel, 2002; SEER's Web-based Training Modules, 2005). A SOAP note has four critical elements, each shown in **Fig. 9–1**: the *subjective* component (chief complaint, symptoms, and history; part 2) derived from the patient's self-report; the *objective* component, derived from observation and examination of the patient and test results (part 3); the *assessment* (problem lists, clinical impressions, and diagnosis; part 4), a clear statement of the problem as understood by the caregiver; and the *plan* (treatment or management; part 5) for addressing the problem. Many experts now also include an outcome step (part 6), to encourage the development of evidence for future evidence–based improvement of practice.

The chart note in **Fig. 9–2** shows the logic of the SOAP structure in a simple clinical encounter. The note starts with demographic information in the header: (1) the patient's

---

Patient Name: Mrs. Margaret Soandso

D.O.B.: 10/19/1948

Chart No.: 4157682

11/05/2007: S: Hearing aid suddenly stopped working. O/A: Inspection: occluded ear mold. Otoscopy: minimal wax in the ear canals (non-occluding). P: The ear mold was cleaned. Electroacoustic performance was checked and found to be identical to the final fit performance at the time of the last visit. Patient expressed satisfaction with the sound of the hearing aids.

David Zapala, Ph.D.

Figure 9–2 Simple chart note. Note that the SOAP structure—subjective component (S), objective component (O), assessment (A), and plan (P)—is maintained in this brief notation.

name and date of birth and (2) the chart number. These identifiers are used to ensure that the document corresponds to a unique patient record. Although this may seem redundant, a clinic may have two "Mary Smiths" as patients. The redundancy helps to resolve any ambiguity and avoid documentation errors if one patient identifier is nonunique (Agency for Healthcare Research and Quality, 2001; Institute of Medicine, 2001; Joint Commission on Accreditation of Health Care Organizations, 2005; Rothenberg, 2005).

The remaining sections of this brief note are self-explanatory. The logic of the SOAP documentation structure is apparent. One can work backward from outcome to subjective complaint, and notice a logical relationship between each sentence in the note. The patient expressed satisfaction with the repair (outcome) as a result of the cleaning of the earmold and the reestablishment of the prescribed hearing aid characteristics (management plan). The earmold was cleaned because the assessment impression (diagnosis) was that the mold was plugged with wax. It was established that the mold was plugged with wax through visual inspection of the mold (objective findings and assessment), and the symptom and time course of the complaint (subjective chief complaint or reason for visit).

The logical relationship between succeeding sections of the SOAP note reveals the underlying thought process used by the clinician in the clinical encounter. Any good documentation of a patient encounter will demonstrate this logical relationship. The outcome always relates back to the treatment plan. The treatment plan always relates back to the assessment impression. The assessment impression always relates back to findings in the subjective and objective part of the evaluation. Thinking in a structured way is a discipline that requires practice. A few moments spent applying the structure to even the briefest notes helps focus clinical thinking and makes the notes easier to understand.

Pearl

- A simple strategy for checking the completeness of a SOAP note is to read the report in reverse order. The outcome always relates back to the treatment plan. The treatment plan always relates back to the assessment impression. The assessment impression always relates back to findings in the subjective and objective part of the evaluation.

A more detailed example is given in **Fig. 9–3**, containing a chart note documenting the assessment and treatment of a patient referred for canalith repositioning of suspected benign paroxysmal positional vertigo (BPPV).

Patient: Jason C. Whirling

Date of birth: 06/14/1950

Chart number: 745621

Date of service: December 10, 2007

Audiologist: David A. Zapala, Ph.D.

Referring Physician: H.P. Sneed, M.D.

Reason for Referral: Assessment and management of transient positional vertigo

Mr. Jason C. Whirling is a 57-year-old local entrepreneur and physical fitness enthusiast who slipped and hit his head during a morning jog four weeks ago. He did not think that he hurt himself at that time. A few days later, however, he awoke in the middle of the night to the sensation of severe vertigo, apparently provoked when rolling onto his right side. He became nauseous. However, he was able to fall back asleep and slept soundly until the next morning. When he first awoke, he felt normal. However, when he moved to get out of bed, he experienced a second severe attack of vertigo that lasted about a minute, and left him feeling unsteady for the rest of the morning. He has since experienced recurrences of this dizziness when tilting his head back, or bending down to pick something up. Meclizine has not helped his symptoms. Dr. Sneed, his internist, suspects benign paroxysmal positional vertigo and referred Mr. Whirling for this appointment to see if canalith repositioning would help.

Mr. Whirling has good hearing by report, and has not noticed any change in hearing, tinnitus, aural pain, aural pressure or fullness. He denied diplopia, dysarthria, dysphagia, dysphonia or any change in strength, movement, or sensation.

EVALUATION: Eye movements appeared grossly intact, and there was no gaze nystagmus noted in room light nor under Frenzel lenses. Head thrust tests were normal. Romberg was normally accomplished. Neck hyperextension without tilting the head did not provoke dizziness. Neck range of motion appeared adequate for Dix-Hallpike and repositioning purposes. The Dix-Hallpike was positive for the right ear down, demonstrating a clockwise torsional nystagmus (relative to the patient), with latency, crescendo and gradual disappearance over the course of about 30 seconds. The nystagmus correlated with the patient's perception of dizziness. A transient nystagmus in the opposite direction was noted after the patient was returned to the sitting position. The positive Dix-Hallpike response diminished with subsequent trials. The left Dix-Hallpike maneuver and head rolled maneuvers were negative.

IMPRESSION: Right posterior canal benign paroxysmal positional vertigo, canalithiasis variety.

TREATMENT: A Gans maneuver was used twice. No nystagmus was observed, nor vertigo reported in any position during the second cycle.

FOLLOW-UP PLAN: Benign paroxysmal positional vertigo was explained in detail to the patient and he was given a written description of the problem. He was also given written post canalith repositioning instructions (clinic form 2000), which I reviewed with him in detail. He was given a neck collar to use for the remainder of the day. He verbalized understanding of the follow-up protocol and will return in one week if he experiences a relapse in transient positional vertigo between now and then. A follow-up appointment was made. He will cancel this if he is asymptomatic.

Figure 9–3 Example of an encounter documenting the evaluation and treatment of benign paroxysmal positional vertigo (BPPV).

The example in **Fig. 9–3** also follows the SOAP structure. The patient was treated with a Gans maneuver because he was thought to have right posterior canal BPPV because he had a positive Dix-Hallpike test on the right with no signs or symptoms pointing to a competing otologic or neurologic cause that might be underpinning his dizziness. Furthermore, his history was in keeping with BPPV, including age, antecedent head trauma, time course, and progression of symptoms. The details may not be meaningful to the uninformed reader, but the logic behind the decision making, what occurred during the contact, and the next step in the process are all identifiable.

The SOAP structure in **Fig. 9–3** can be broken down a little more. The first two paragraphs in the report reflect the subjective step in the clinical process. The onset and progression of symptoms are noted. Associated symptoms (nausea) and absent symptom (hearing loss, tinnitus, etc.) are noted as well. The audiologist asked questions to screen systematically for the presence of otologic or neurologic symptoms. Hearing and balance problems may emanate from benign, dangerous, or potentially life-threatening causes. Audiologists may feel comfortable treating the benign conditions, but they should always exclude the latter. The referring physician may sometimes complete the exclusion process. If this is the case, it should be noted in the report. If the audiologist considered case history information and observations from a physical examination in the decision process, it should be included in the report as evidence used to support subsequent decision making.

Special Consideration

- Audiologists routinely recognize and treat the symptoms of benign conditions such as presbycusic hearing loss or BPPV. However, to do so, active otologic or neurologic disease must be excluded. The audiologist must remain vigilant for signs and symptoms of active disease and refer appropriately.

Table 9–1 lists common symptoms associated with otologic and neurologic diseases. The table is not exhaustive, but is offered as a guide to organize the topics that may be addressed in the chief complaint, history, and physical examination sections of the report. Each patient is different. The audiologist must remain vigilant for signs and symptoms of active disease and refer appropriately.

In the "Evaluation" section of **Fig. 9–3**, the objective assessment stage of the encounter is documented. Here physical signs, observable by the examiner, are inventoried. In this case, eye movements were inventoried. These needed to be normal before subsequent head movement–induced eye movements could be ascribed to vestibular causes. Signs for acute loss of vestibular function were assessed (head thrusts, spontaneous nystagmus, and Romberg tests). Neck hyperextension and range of motion were assessed to protect the patient against harm during the assessment

(Dix-Hallpike test) and treatment (Gans maneuver) stages. In the assessment process, "what is working" can be as important as "what is not working."

In summary, the subjective and objective components present the evidence for the impression. The final confirmation can be found in the description of the positive right Dix-Hallpike test, which is exactly what would be expected for right posterior canal BPPV.

Controversial Point

- The American Academy of Audiology's scope of practice recognizes audiology's autonomous role in assessing and managing the symptoms of medically benign conditions such as presbycusic hearing loss and BPPV. These conditions are highly prevalent, not associated with significant morbidity or mortality, and can be cost–effectively evaluated and treated by audiologists. However, other professional medical organizations, such as the American Medical Association, have not always endorsed the value of evaluation and management of benign conditions by audiologists. According to the United States Department of the Treasury, as of June 28th, 2006, the national debt was $8,345,809,036,548.55 (http://www.publicdebt.treas.gov/opd/opdpenny.htm; assessed on 7/2/2006), a large part of this debt is driven by the cost of healthcare expenditures. We may be fast approaching the time when audiologist based evaluation and management of medically benign conditions is no longer optional. Careful, complete documentation, reflecting accurate clinical decision making will be required to accomplish this.

Figure 9–4 provides a simpler alternative to the lengthy note shown in **Fig. 9–3**. The logic of what was done, why, and the result remain in this second note, with much less detail. In this case, Dr. Sneed made the diagnosis, simplifying the decision-making burden of the audiologist. A long discourse is not required to follow the SOAP structure. There is a cost in terms of time and expense in writing longer notes, particularly if the services of a transcriptionist are used. When documenting clinical encounters, it is important to weigh the length and quality of the report against the cost in terms of time and money required to generate and read that report. Regardless of the level of detail, the decision making and writing must be explicit and clear, for both may come under scrutiny.

Pearl

- One must weigh the length and quality of the report against the cost in terms of time and money required to generate and read that report. Regardless of the level of detail, the decision making and writing must be explicit and clear, for both may come under scrutiny.

Table 9–1 Signs and Symptoms of Active Disease Processes and Benign Conditions Associated with Hearing or Balance Disorders

1. Signs and symptoms of active disease processes
   a. Onset and progression
      i. Acute onset (typically within 72 hours)
      ii. Rapid onset (typically within 90 days)
      iii. Progressive symptoms
      iv. Fluctuating symptoms, such as hearing loss, tinnitus, imbalance, and dizziness
      v. Location
         1. Unilateral unexplained symptoms (not from firearm use)
         2. Accompanying symptoms: symptoms potentially involving multiple branches of the eighth cranial nerve (CN VIII): hearing, dizziness, tinnitus, and imbalance
         3. Symptoms associated with other cranial nerve deficits
         4. Symptoms associated with other head and neck deficits
      vi. Aural pain (otalgia)
      vii. Aural pressure or fullness
   b. History
      i. Head or ear trauma
      ii. Ototoxic medication use
      iii. Infections or conditions that may affect hearing (example: torch infections or hyperbilirubinemia in newborns)
      iv. Family history of hearing loss prior to 30 years of age
   c. Physical examination
      i. Structural abnormalities in the ear, head, or neck (branchial arch defects, congenital malformations, and traumatic changes)
      ii. Abnormal or atypical finding on ear canal or tympanic membrane inspection
      iii. Discharge from the ears (otorrhea)
   d. Audiologic testing
      i. Signs or symptoms suggestive of a previously undiagnosed middle ear disorder
      ii. Signs or symptoms suggestive of an undiagnosed retrocochlear disorder
      iii. Any newly diagnosed sensorineural hearing loss of unknown etiology
      iv. Unexplained asymmetric hearing loss
2. Signs and symptoms consistent with benign hearing impairment
   a. Onset and progression
      i. Stable or long–standing
      ii. Congenital (previously evaluated medically)
      iii. Location
         1. Bilateral
      iv. Accompanying symptoms
         1. Bilateral symmetrical tinnitus in the face of bilateral symmetrical sensorineural hearing loss that is otherwise benign
   b. History
      i. Noise exposure
      ii. Familial hearing loss with aging (onset in the sixth decade or later)
      iii. Long standing problem, previously evaluated medically and unchanged
   c. Physical examination of the ear
      i. Within normal limits
   d. Audiologic testing
      i. No evidence of previously undiagnosed conductive or retrocochlear hearing loss
      ii. Signs and symptoms of bilateral cochlear hearing loss compatible with noise exposure or presbycusis
      iii. Hearing loss that has been previously evaluated medically and declared benign

For additional information, see Baloh, R. W. (1998). Dizziness, hearing loss, and tinnitus. Philadelphia: F. A. Davis; Ruckenstein, M. J. (1995). Hearing loss: A plan for individualized management. Postgraduate Medicine, 98, 197–214; and Ruckenstein, M. J. (1995). A practical approach to dizziness. Postgraduate Medicine, 97, 70–81.

Patient: Jason C. Whirling

Date of birth: 06/14/1950

Chart number: 745621

December 10, 2007

Audiologist: David A. Zapala, Ph.D.

Referring Physician: H.P. Sneed, M.D.

Reason for Referral: Particle repositioning for BPPV symptoms

S: Transient positional vertigo diagnosed as BPPV by Dr. Sneed

O: Positive right Dix-Hallpike; Negative left Dix-Hallpike and head roll tests

A: Right posterior canal BPPV

P: Particle repositioning x2 with no symptoms evident on the second trial. Patient will return as needed.

Figure 9–4 Simple version of a SOAP note for benign paroxysmal positional vertigo (BPPV) management and treatment.

◆ Objective Assessment in Audiology: From Data to Clinical Information

At its core, audiology is data driven. Audiologic data are the product of psychophysical, electrophysiologic, and psychometric measurements. Examples include thresholds on an audiogram (psychophysical measurement), pressure-compliance values on a tympanogram (electrophysiologic measurement), and subscale scores on a questionnaire (psychometric measurement). An audiologic report consisting of a listing of data points is uninformative. To be informative, data are interpreted, correlated, and placed in the context of the patient's presenting problem. It is important to understand this process for both report writing and information management purposes.

Tympanometric data provide an example. A tympanogram consists of a set of admittance or impedance values obtained at a set of ear canal pressures. With current automated tympanometers, as many as 200 data points may be sampled to derive the shape of the tympanogram, but each individual data point is not interpreted in isolation. Rather, the data are typically grouped by the shape of those 200 data points using the common Jerger classification: type A, type B, type C, and so on. This classification system is linguistically based and categorical. The categories capture the shape of the acquired data set in a way that is salient and efficient for most clinical purposes.

In the realm of information theory, classifying data sets into linguistically labeled categories is the process of turning a data set into a "fact." Categorizing a data set into a factual category reduces complexity, making it easier to see relationships across multiple measurements. The system we use to classify a set of data into a fact depends on what we recognize as important (Bouthillier and Shearer, 2002; Sveiby, 1998).

Audiologists routinely analyze data sets and classify them into facts, as seen in the following example summarizing a basic preemployment audiologic evaluation:

> Ear canals were clear, and the tympanic membranes appeared within normal limits; tympanograms were a normal type A, bilaterally. Pure-tone audiometry suggested hearing sensitivity to be within normal limits; acoustic reflexes were present at normal levels without decay, and word recognition was excellent bilaterally.

With the exception of the otoscopic inspection description, all of the facts in this example were generated by reducing a data set into a classification or category. The value of classifying data into categories of facts is that the salient features of each data set can be evaluated and communicated efficiently. However, a classified test result, in isolation, is seldom sufficient to determine a treatment plan. We cannot capture meaning or act on a type B tympanogram, for example; other facts need to be known. And even if we have other facts, a disparate assemblage of facts is not really information in the clinical sense of the word.

Facts must be organized using the knowledge of the discipline to define relationships between facts and to generate understanding of their meaning. It is only when test results are placed in the context of the patient's presentation and organized by the professional's knowledge of the discipline that actionable clinical information is developed. No test result stands alone. (See Lee, 2004, for more on the use of tests in clinical decision making.)

In the above example, the facts can be organized into this result statement: "Normal audiologic evaluation, no evidence of peripheral hearing impairment." If this finding occurs in the setting of a preemployment hearing test, it is consistent with the patient's presentation without auditory or communicative complaints. However, if this finding occurs within the context of a patient's complaining of significant auditory or communicative problems, the mismatch between the complaint and the audiologic results is informative: other factors must account for the patient's problem. In either case, we have reached the level of information.

Pearl

- Data sets are classified into facts, organized by discipline knowledge, and then interpreted in the context of the clinical encounter to produce clinical information.

Clinical information is the evidence used in decision making. It exists when there is sufficient understanding of the patient's circumstances to make a plan for treatment. In the context of a normal preemployment audiologic evaluation, as in the example above, one could logically state: "No communicative complaints and normal audiologic evaluation; retest next year." In the case of a normal evaluation in the context of communication difficulties, one could logically state: "Idiopathic or obscure auditory-based communication deficit (significant communicative complaints in the presence of a normal audiologic evaluation)—assess central auditory function or perhaps environmental communicative demands."

In a basic audiologic evaluation, audiogram data are classified by type, configuration, and severity; speech-recognition performance data as excellent, good, fair, and poor; and tympanograms by type, with acoustic reflexes either present, elevated, or absent. It is unlikely that the finding of a decreased 250 Hz pure-tone threshold carries weight in evaluating the probability that a patient has an acoustic neuroma. Rather, the evaluation is based on a review of the facts, for example, asymmetric hearing loss, poor speech discrimination, and elevated acoustic reflexes. To someone untutored in the field of audiology, such facts are meaningless. Only those with knowledge of the discipline can organize these facts into meaningful clinical information. In this example, the appropriate impression statement is that the presence of a retrocochlear lesion cannot be excluded in the involved ear. A common error in clinical report writing is assuming that the report's eventual reader has knowledge of the discipline of audiology. Because of this, audiologists may skip explicit statements summarizing facts that seem obvious to them. Such omissions tax the reader, however; clear, explicit impression statements are key to good communication.

Pitfall

- One of the common errors in clinical report writing is not including a clear, explicit impression statement, on the assumption that the consumer of the report has some background knowledge of audiology.

In summary, audiologists create information by collecting accurate data, classifying the data into sets of facts, and organizing the facts using their knowledge of the discipline. Creation of clinical information then leads to appropriate management decisions.

♦ Structuring the Audiologic Report

The audiologic evaluation changes structure depending on what elements of the clinical process are the responsibility of the audiologist. Some auditory or vestibular tests, for example, are performed solely for the purpose of aiding in otologic diagnosis. In these medical audiologic evaluations, patients are typically under the care of the referring physicians, who ask for supplemental auditory testing as an extension of their own physical examinations. In these cases, the structure of the reports will differ from situations where the audiologist is managing the patients independently. The differences will be discussed below.

Documenting Audiologic Services in the Medical Setting

Audiologists often work closely with physicians, typically otolaryngologists and neurologists, in part because the testing capabilities offered by the audiologist can play an important role in the medical diagnosis and treatment of ear or brain disease. Furthermore, effective treatment of ear disease includes the preservation or restoration of auditory and vestibular function whenever possible. Auditory and vestibular assessments thus become useful benchmarks in measuring the outcome of medical or surgical treatments of the ear. Finally, in large otolaryngology practices, a large proportion of the otologic caseload has residual or untreatable hearing or balance deficits that may be addressed through audiologic or vestibular rehabilitation efforts.

Depending on the role and division of labor between the physician and the audiologist, the audiologist may be responsible for all, part, or very few of the elements in the clinical process. The structure of any report thus reflects the understood division of labor. Regardless, the sum total of both the audiologist's and the physician's efforts must be comprehensive documentation of all elements of the clinical process. Consider the otolaryngological report in **Fig. 9–5**. In this example, the otolaryngologist captures every aspect of the clinical encounter sequence. The audiologic tests, which consisted of the basic comprehensive examination, constituted some of the evidence used to come to a clinical

impression. The documentation burden on the audiologist was limited to presentation of the acquired data and classification of the test results, which were copied over into the medical evaluation.

At a minimum, the following information should be contained in the report when the test data are to be used for medical evaluation purposes only:

1. Complete demographic information, including at least two unique identifying elements

2. A clear, brief description of the reason for referral

3. A description of the specific tests performed and a classification of the results (fact level description) with sufficient detail to accurately code the procedure using applicable Current Procedural Terminology (CPT) coding

4. Test data: Psychometric data with statement about the reliability or accuracy; electrophysiologic data with measurements and recording parameters

Items 1 and 4 need to be on the audiologic record; items 2 and 3 may be on the audiologic record or in the physician's notes.

Let's take the example of an auditory brainstem evoked potential study performed to assess retrocochlear status (**Fig. 9–6**). In this example, we assume that the referral was made because of other information gleaned in the clinical process that increases the likelihood of vestibular schwannoma or other retrocochlear lesion.

All of the elements described above are in this report: patient demographics with unique identifiers, referring physician, reason for referral, description of tests performed, clear impression statement, presentation of data evaluated and interpreted, and the attached raw traces with recording parameters (not shown).

The audiologist participated in clinical decision making for patient management in examples given in **Figs. 9–5** and **9–6**. The role was technical, supporting the physician's efforts to complete the clinical process. The task is more challenging when the physician and the audiologist share management prerogatives, as addressed in the next section.

The Basic Comprehensive Audiologic Evaluation

Pure-tone and speech audiometry, often supplemented with tympanometry measures, comprise the basic comprehensive audiologic evaluation. This is the bedrock evaluation for audiologic and otologic diagnoses. The same test data may be interpreted from different perspectives, depending on the discipline of the interpreter. From an otologic point of view, the audiologic evaluation points to the site of lesion, supplementing the physical exam in differentiating among different diseases affecting the ear. From the audiologic perspective, the type and severity of hearing loss strongly predict auditory–based communication deficits. The evaluation results may be interpreted within the context of either or both perspectives, depending on the needs of the patient.

CHIEF COMPLAINT: Ringing in the ears

HISTORY OF PRESENT ILLNESS: This 58-year-old man has had about a 1 1/2 year history of intermittent ringing in his ears, worse on the left side than on the right. It is not a pulsating sound. It is sometimes worse when he exercises or when he is diving (he likes scuba). The noise is not getting worse - it has been persistent. He has no other sensory dysfunction, such as a lack of coordination or balance, disturbances of smell or taste, or change in vision.

He has worked in a mill for many years and has used earplugs to protect himself from noise. He has been exposed to hunting and practice using shotguns.

He has borderline high blood pressure, which he has treated with diet, avoiding salt as much as possible. He drinks about 3 cups of coffee daily. He does not use tobacco or alcohol.

He has had routine physical examinations by his private physician and thinks he has normal blood sugar, thyroid and cholesterol.

His hearing is good, although his wife accuses him of "selective hearing."

OTORHINOLARYNGOLOGY REVIEW OF SYSTEMS AND PAST MEDICAL AND SURGICAL HISTORIES: Completely unremarkable.

GENERAL REVIEW OF SYSTEMS AND PAST MEDICAL AND SURGICAL HISTORIES: Obtained from the patient and from his referring physician. He takes no prescription medications. He has no medication allergies.

PHYSICAL EXAMINATION:

EARS: the external auditory canals and eardrums are normal. Hearing is grossly normal.

OTONEUROLOGIC: no nystagmus. Normal cranial nerves, carotid pulses, gait.

NOSE: normal septum inter permits. Mucosa pink. No discharge. Normal anterior and posterior rhinoscopy.

ORAL AND PHARYNGEAL: normal oral structures and temporal mandibular joints. No masses palpated in the base of the tongue or floor of the mouth. Salivary ducts and secretions are normal.

Mirror examination of the nasopharynx: hypopharynx and larynx normal. Vocal folds are mobile and approximate at midline. Voice is normal.

HEAD AND NECK: no masses or areas of tenderness or swelling over the face and head. No abnormal masses in the lymph node chains of the anterior and posterior cervical triangles. No thyromegaly.

AUDIOGRAM: audiogram performed today shows him to have bilaterally symmetric, neural sensory hearing loss in the 4 kHz range. This is compatible with noise induced hearing loss. There is no conductive component. Speech discrimination scores are excellent. Tympanometry is completely normal, as are all acoustic reflex tests.

IMPRESSION:

1. Tinnitus atrium, benign.
2. Noise induced, bilateral neural sensory hearing loss.

RECOMMENDATIONS: I gave the patient information regarding tinnitus and the discussion suggesting reduction of caffeine in his diet. He should also have routine laboratory examination including cholesterol, triglycerides, thyroid, and blood sugar.

Figure 9–5 Example of an otolaryngological evaluation report.

Organizing the Basic Comprehensive Evaluation as Part of a Medical Evaluation

The organization of the medical audiologic report should be structured to facilitate communication between the audiologist and the referring physician. The first step in determining the appropriate organization is to understand why the patient was referred. From this knowledge, the audiologist can ascertain what facts are important to develop in the course of the evaluation. The presentation of test results can thus be structured to allow the physician to focus quickly on the elements pertinent to the clinical problem.

There are three basic structures for organizing test results in a medical report. The first is test-based. In this structure, the results of each test are organized based on the equipment used. The following example represents test results organized by test type:

Reason for referral: Hearing loss and tinnitus: site of lesion evaluation

Audiometry: Audiogram demonstrated a symmetrical, sloping mild to moderate sensorineural hearing loss

bilaterally; speech discrimination was excellent (90%) for the right ear, good (84%) for the left ear.

Tympanograms: Normal type A patterns bilaterally; acoustic reflexes were present at levels consistent with cochlear hearing loss, and there was no reflex decay evidenced.

Auditory brainstem evoked potentials: Absolute and interpeak latencies for waves I, III, and V were well within normal limits bilaterally.

Impression: Results consistent with sloping mild to moderate cochlear hearing loss bilaterally; no evidence of retrocochlear involvement.

The second organizational structure is anatomically based. In this type of structure, the test results are grouped by the part of the auditory system assessed, moving from distal to proximal. For example:

Reason for referral: Hearing loss and tinnitus (site of lesion evaluation)

Evaluation summary: Ear canals appeared clear; tympanic membranes appeared intact with normal light reflexes. Tympanograms demonstrated normal type A tracings bilaterally. The audiogram demonstrated a symmetrical

Patient: John A. Doe

Age: 50 years

Date of Birth: 6/22/1956

Chart Number 123456

Date of Evalution: 1/16/2007

Audiologist: T. Paulatt, Au.D.

Referring Physician: Sidney Harvard, M.D.

Evaluation : Auditory brainstem evoked potentials

Reason for Referral: Unilateral hearing loss and tinnitus on the right side; disequilibrium—assess site of lesion

Impression: Abnormal evaluation, result consistent with right retrocochlear involvement

Waveform Quality: Good

Results:

Right Ear	Left Ear
I: 1.80 msec	I: 1.80 msec
III: 4.80 msec	III: 3.80 msec
V: 6.80 msec	V: 5.80 msec
I–V IPL: 5.0 msec	I–V IPL: 4.0 msec
Rate change: 4.0 msec	Rate change: 1.0 msec
Interaural wave V latency difference: 4.0 msec @ 51.1 cps (abnormal on the right)	

Figure 9–6 An example of an auditory brainstem response report.

sloping mild to moderate sensorineural hearing loss with excellent speech discrimination (90%) for the right ear and good (84%) discrimination for the left ear. Acoustic reflexes were present at levels consistent with cochlear hearing loss, and there was no reflex decay. Auditory brainstem evoked potentials demonstrated absolute and interpeak latencies for waves I, III, and V well within normal limits.

Impression: Results are consistent with a sloping mild to moderate cochlear hearing loss bilaterally, with no evidence of retrocochlear involvement.

A third organizational structure may be necessary when a potentially significant test result or test pattern needs to be brought to the attention of the referring physician, which often happens in hospital chart notes. This organizational approach might be called "priority based." The following is an example documenting the result of a request to assess a patient's hearing following a fall while in the hospital.

13:00 Audiology consult (audiogram placed in chart)

Reason for referral: Subjective loss of hearing in the right ear

Pertinent history: Middle ear surgery in the right ear 10 years ago with restoration of hearing. From patient's description, this sounded like a middle ear reconstruction of some form.

Findings:

Right ear: Signs possibly consistent with post-traumatic ossicular discontinuity and perilymph fistula. Evidence: moderate flat conductive hearing loss with pressure-induced nystagmus and subjective vertigo noted during tympanometry (Hennebert's sign).

Left ear: Test results essentially within normal limits.

Recommend: Otolaryngology consult for evaluation of signs and symptoms possibly consistent with perilymphatic fistula.

In this example, the organization of the note still follows a SOAP structure. However, the objective and assessment results are merged to present the most important clinical information first. This priority-based structure allows the referring physician to determine quickly what is important.

Making Audiologic Recommendations in the Medical Report

Figure 9–7 presents an example of an audiogram with some comments made by the audiologist. This was part of a medical evaluation of hearing in an otolaryngology office. The audiologist classified the data presented on the audiogram: slight sensorineural hearing loss to the speech frequencies, with a high-frequency notching-type sensorineural hearing loss; speech discrimination was good. The audiologist recommended hearing aids bilaterally. This example raises the following points:

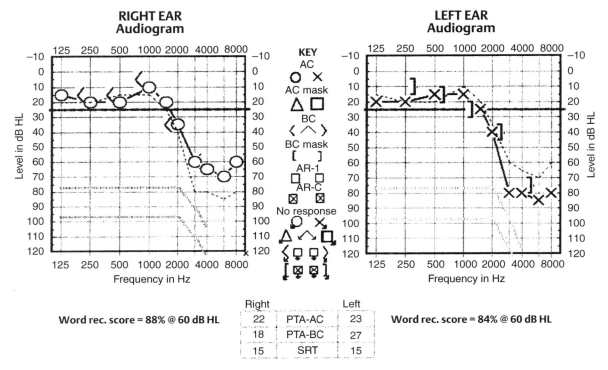

Word rec. score = 88% @ 60 dB HL

	Right		Left
	22	PTA-AC	23
	18	PTA-BC	27
	15	SRT	15

Word rec. score = 84% @ 60 dB HL

IMPRESSION : Bilaterally, hearing sensitivity is in the slight range through the speech frequencies; there is a high frequency notching type sensorineural hearing loss; speech discrimination is good bilaterally.

Recommend hearing aids bilaterally.

Figure 9–7 Example of an audiogram, with the audiologist's recorded impression.

♦ The audiologist clearly interpreted the data to the level of a set of facts: slight hearing loss, with good discrimination.

♦ These facts could be integrated into a physician's clinical process to develop a medical diagnosis, but they are not in themselves diagnostic—they do not rise to the level of clinical information when considered in isolation.

♦ The site of lesion and severity of hearing loss are not sufficient to organize treatment from an audiologic (perceptual or communicative) point of view. Although they are evidence for an auditory-based communication problem, they remain facts that must be organized into a larger "picture" before an assessment and treatment plan can be formulated.

♦ This report presents the common error in audiologic documentation mentioned earlier: there is such a strong relationship between the presence of high-frequency hearing loss and difficulty understanding speech that the audiologist may have assumed that the patient was experiencing hearing problems significant enough to warrant the use of bilateral hearing aids; hence the recommendation for amplification.

♦ No evidence is presented in the audiologic report to support the recommendation for hearing aids. There

may not be any subjective hearing problem recognized by the patient. Without evidence to suggest that the patient is having a hearing problem, it is premature to suggest bilateral hearing aids based solely on a test result. If there is no perceived hearing problem prior to treatment, how can the outcome following the use of hearing aids improve?

Either the report documentation is incomplete, or the audiologist is treating a test result and not the patient's problem. There are two solutions to this dilemma. The first assumes that the physician is documenting the entire clinical process and has evidence to support the presence of an auditory-based communication problem from a patient's chief complaint and history. In this case, a statement such as "Patient may benefit from hearing aids if clinically indicated" makes sense. It then falls to the physician to make the determination whether hearing aids are indicated.

An alternative is for the audiologist to establish the presence of an auditory-based communication deficit experienced by the patient. The patient's description of the deficit should correlate with problems expected with a high-frequency hearing loss. If this is the case, then a logical argument can be made for the use of hearing aids.

Leaving the recommendation as written is not an option, because the treatment plan addresses a problem that may

Date: 1/19/2007 1400 hrs

SUBJECTIVE: Sudden onset of headache and severe dizziness with possible co-occurring right-sided hearing loss and tinnitus. Symptoms rapidly developed following the initiation of epidural anesthesia, and subsequent delivery. Headache and dizziness not thought to be the result of anesthetic effects.

OBJECTIVE: Bedside audiological exam:
- Otoscopy: Ear canals are clear, eardrums intact, light reflex evidenced
- Tympanometry: Normal type "A" " tracings
- Audiometry: Right ear: moderate, sloping sensorineural hearing loss with poor speech discrimination. Left ear: hearing sensitivity appears within normal limits with excellent speech discrimination
- Acoustic reflexes: Absent on the right side, present without decay of the left side

ASSESSMENT: Impression: right sided sensorineural hearing loss with poor word recognition

PLAN: Suggest auditory brainstem evoked potential study

David Zapala, Ph.D. Audiology

Figure 9–8 Example of a hospital chart note for a patient complaining of headache, hearing loss, tinnitus, and dizziness.

not exist. The example given in **Fig. 9–7** makes it appear that the process of selecting and fitting hearing aids and organizing audiologic rehabilitation can be determined from the pure–tone audiogram or from the presence of sensorineural hearing loss alone. By extension, therefore, involvement of the audiologist in the treatment decision making is unnecessary, which is not the case.[3] If it were, we could use an aided audiogram that demonstrated sound field hearing sensitivity in the normal range to be evidence of an acceptable outcome. Very few patients would tolerate that type of fitting, however.

From a logical point of view, the audiologist's note is improved as follows:

Impression: Bilaterally, hearing sensitivity falls in the slightly hard of hearing range through the speech frequencies; there is a high-frequency notching-type sensorineural hearing loss that is severe enough to affect speech understanding and common everyday listening situations, such as the patient reports experiencing.

Recommend: Hearing aid trial to improve auditory communication abilities

The inclusion of a statement correlating a communication deficit with the observed high-frequency hearing loss brings the clinical interpretation offered by the audiologist

to the level of information—the point at which the problem is defined in sufficient detail to lead to a treatment plan. Other readers of the report recognize that the rationale for offering hearing aids is to treat the underlying communication deficit. The appropriate outcome statement is now improvement in understanding speech in everyday situations. The impression statement now supports the hearing aid recommendation.

Pearl

- Any recommendation or treatment plan should address a problem explicitly stated in the impression or diagnosis section of a report.

Figure 9–8 is another example of a hospital chart note of an audiology consult requested by an otolaryngologist. The consult was for an audiologic evaluation of a patient with headache, hearing loss, tinnitus, and dizziness. The demographic and audiologic data are not shown, although those data would be incorporated into the hospital chart. This note follows the standard SOAP structure. The reason for referral is found in the "Subjective" section of the note. All procedures performed are listed and the results interpreted, adding greatly to the ability of physicians and other health care workers to understand what occurred in the audiologic evaluation. For example, this note provides evidence for subsequent billing because each test is explicitly stated and corresponds with a specific CPT code. The term *sensorineural hearing loss* corresponds with an International Classification of Diseases (ICD-9) code, which is required for many types of billing. So far, this appears to be a reasonably good chart.

---

[3] Consider the position of the American Academy of Otolaryngology—Head and Neck Surgery on hearing aids:"Hearing aids are a recognized treatment for sensorineural hearing loss." This rather benign sentence implies support for the use of hearing aids. However, it also is the basis for the position that the practice of fitting hearing aids is part of the practice of otolaryngology—the audiologic component is unrecognized. A more appropriate position would be to say that "sensorineural hearing loss does not preclude the use of hearing aids."

But there is a problem. In this example, why was the auditory brainstem evoked potential study recommended? It would be obvious to an audiologist that unilateral sensorineural hearing loss with absent acoustic reflexes and poor word recognition are signs suggesting retrocochlear involvement, particularly in the setting of unilateral tinnitus, headache, and dizziness. However, an audiologist's ability to recognize the signs results from specialized training. It is not obvious to nonaudiologists or nonotolaryngologists why the evoked potential study is indicated. Recommendations contained in the "Plan" section of the note must address problems explicitly stated in the "Assessment" section. A better statement would be:

Assessment: Right sensorineural hearing loss with signs pointing to retrocochlear/posterior fossa involvement

Plan: Clinical correlation by the referring physician required to determine the relative risk of retrocochlear involvement. Auditory brainstem evoked potentials may be helpful in this regard.

In this example, the audiologist still used the term *sensorineural* to describe the hearing loss, but also included a specific statement about the risk of retrocochlear involvement. This satisfies the requirement of explicitly stating a problem.

The "Plan" statement begins with the phrase *clinical correlation,* which indicates that the information derived from the audiologic evaluation must be placed in the context of the referring physician's clinical process before a clear diagnosis is made. It is possible that the test results do not reflect a retrocochlear or posterior fossa process. Every assessment, after all, has the possibility of developing a false-positive or false-negative outcome. This statement alerts the managing physician and other readers of this report to consider posterior fossa disease as part of the potential causes of the patient's problems, but it recognizes that additional evidence needs consideration before acting. When the stated problem pertains to medical diagnosis or treatment, the audiologist must recognize that the physician may have evidence gleaned from other steps in the clinical process and that all facts must be considered before a medical diagnosis is made. Consequently, it is best to place a statement in the report to the effect that "clinical correlation is required to determine the significance of the present findings" when the medical diagnosis is implicated in the test results. No single test result can be interpreted in isolation (Go, 1998; Lee, 2004). Making definitive statements based solely on test data may lead to overutilization of medical resources and increase malpractice exposure if the audiologist's impression is wrong. When the patient's problems are best managed from the discipline of audiology, it is necessary to go through every step in the clinical process before making strong assessment and management statements in the report. When medical problems are suspected, work as a team with physicians to develop facts, and completely document the clinical process.

In summary, when working as a member of a health care team, the audiologist may or may not be responsible for completing all elements of the clinical process. When test results are generated to augment a medical examination, the audiologist may choose to interpret the test results by classifying the results for the physician's interpretation with other information. In other cases, the audiologist will interpret the data, develop an audiologic diagnosis, and create a treatment plan.

Documenting Services in Autonomous Audiologic Settings

Audiologists practicing independently are responsible for all steps of the clinical process. There are two important issues that must be addressed early in the clinical process: medically significant problems must be recognized and appropriately referred as needed, and the environmental effects of the hearing loss must be described. In the former, appropriate referral is triggered by the identification of an active disease process (**Table 9–1**). In the latter, the life situation of the patient, his or her communication demands, and the specific situations in which the hearing ability is problematic are characterized. Clearly understanding the context in which hearing fails leads to a personalized treatment plan. It is thus the basis of audiologic diagnosis and management.

Classifying Aspects of a Hearing Complaint

Audiologic rehabilitation is directed at managing the impact of hearing impairment on a patient's ability to function on a social/communicative and ecological level. Two patients with audiometrically identical hearing losses may differ markedly in their ability to use their residual hearing on a day-to-day basis. Internal and external patient factors may affect communication ability and the effects of hearing impairment (Dobie and Van Hemel, 2004; Mendel and Danhauer, 1997). Internal factors include age, education level, cognitive abilities, coping abilities, and interests. External factors include family circumstances, vocation and specific job setting environments, and willingness of other people to modify their communicative approach to the patient. Problems addressed by audiologic rehabilitation are determined in part by the magnitude of hearing impairment, the interests and abilities of the patient, and the environments in which the patient lives on a day-to-day basis. This last component, originally referred to as *hearing disability*, is now called *activities limitation stemming from hearing impairment* (Dobie and Van Hemel, 2004; Stephans, 2003; WHO, 2001; see also Chapter 8 in this volume).

For the most part, audiologic rehabilitation is directed at improving the functional abilities of the person with communicatively significant hearing impairment. This means that diagnostic statements used to rationalize a specific management plan must include both impairment- and function-focused descriptions of the patient's auditory capabilities. The basic comprehensive audiologic evaluation provides an impairment-focused problem description. Supplemental information, derived in the case history or from formal questionnaires, such as the Hearing Handicap

Knowledge Domain	Encounter Sequence >>>					
Individual Case	(1) Presenting Problem: Difficulty understanding speech of family members and friends					(6) Outcome: Decreased noise exposure and no progression in hearing loss over years; uses hearing aids with benefit in speech understanding; family helps with communication misunderstandings; person participates in communication activities to a fuller extent
Professional Knowledge		Collecting Evidence		(4) ASSESSMENT: Noise induced (firearms) high frequency hearing loss; communication deficits and activity restrictions compatible with hearing loss; continued risk of noise induced hearing loss	(5) PLAN: Hearing conservation counseling; audiologic rehabilitation (hearing aids, effective use of residual hearing.)	
		(2) SUBJECTIVE: Slowly developing hearing problem primarily in background noise, limiting participation in family and outside activities. History: Right-handed hunter	(3) OBJECTIVE: High frequency "noise notch" type sensorineural hearing loss, more severe on the left side			
Discipline Knowledge		(7) Learned Theories of Cause and Effect: Effects of firearm noise exposure on hearing; audibility theory and the effects of hearing loss on speech perception				

Figure 9–9 Example of the audiologic clinical process.

Inventory for the Elderly (HHIE; Ventry and Weinstein, 1982), may be used to describe the patient's functional capabilities. In writing a report, there must be enough description of the patient's day-to-day listening difficulties in the subjective sections of the report to lend support for any subsequent recommendation for audiologic management. Impairment-level descriptions, such as mild to moderate sensorineural hearing loss, are inadequate because two patients with the same audiometric configuration can experience different activity limitations, and thus require different audiologic treatment plans. The audiologic diagnostic statement must be at a sufficient resolution level to support the management plan and outcome measurement.

Figure 9–9 shows how an audiologic evaluation can be parsed using the elements of the clinical process. **Figure 9–10** shows the audiologic report and audiogram for the same case. In the "Background and Related Information" section of **Fig. 9–10,** the patient's listening difficulties are described from the patient's point of view, with specific types of experiences listed. In this case, there is "difficulty understanding speech spoken in background noise or group conversation situations and over distances." There is also an HHIE score and classification, with social and emotional subscale scores. In the "Impressions" section, there is a clear statement that the auditory deficits are significant enough to interfere with the patient's ability to understand speech on a daily basis. From that section, the management plan, composed of hearing aid use, review of listening strategies, and hearing conservation services due to the history of noise exposure, are all supported.

The audiologist may choose any number of methods to describe the functional impact of any measured hearing impairment. Regardless of whether a self-report tool, such as

the HHIE, or informal interview methods are used, the report should demonstrate the evidence and underlying thinking process of the audiologist as he or she plans a rehabilitation strategy. The treatment plan follows rationally from the diagnostic statements, and the diagnostic statements are based on evidence developed earlier in the report. Although the specifics may change, this model may be applied to any type of clinical encounter.

◆ Audiology and Medical Informatics

Computers have long replaced typewriters. However, the full impact of the computer and computer networks is just beginning to be felt in the health care system overall (Centers for Medicare and Medicaid Services, 2006; Rakel, 2002; Tang, 2000), as well as in the practice of audiology. Creating and transmitting reports in digital form saves a lot of paper. However, the true value of the computer lies not in replicating what can be done with paper and pencil, but in using the decision-support tools that computer systems offer to enhance our ability to deliver safe, effective, and efficient patient care (Doebbeling et al., 2006; Institute of Medicine, 2001).

Computers and, more specifically, point-of-contact information management systems can provide information that augments clinical decision making, allowing team members to assess and share clinical information comprehensively in real time (Goldenberg and Couch, 2005; Mark, 2005). As these systems develop, what is documented and why will change. For example, audiologists have an impressive array of diagnostic tests and reference sources at their disposal in the form of journal articles,

Chief Complaint / Reason for Referral:
Gradually developing hearing loss and modest tinnitus bilaterally.
Difficulty understanding speech in everyday situations.

Background and Related Information:
Mr. B. R. is a 70-year-old gentleman who presents for evaluation of hearing loss and bilateral tinnitus. Overall, he reports having moderate problems understanding speech on a daily basis. He does note difficulty understanding speech spoken in background noise or group conversation situations and over distances. He also notes difficulty distinguishing the direction of sounds. He is interested in trying hearing aids. His self-assessed hearing handicap (HHIE) score was 30% ('S' scale = 38%, 'E' scale = 23%), consistent with mild to moderate auditory based communication difficulties.

Mr. R's history was positive for noise exposure (military—artillery, recreational firearm use). He denies: otalgia, aural pressure / fullness, otorrhea, dizziness / imbalance, loudness intolerance, significant ototoxic medication exposure, familial hearing loss, ear infections, or prior ear surgery. He was evaluated by a local otolaryngologist within the past two months and brings a medical release for amplification.

Audiological Assessment: See attached test results.

Impressions:
Bilaterally, hearing sensitivity was in the mild to moderate range through the speech frequencies; there was a high frequency sensorineural hearing loss (AAO loss = 37%; 40 dB average loss), greater in the left ear, consistent with presbyacusis and noise exposure history.

No clear evidence for retrocochlear loss; hearing asymmetry likely the result of military noise exposure. Nevertheless we will follow this to ensure there is no a progressive hearing problem.

Substantial auditory-based communicative deficit—patient is a good candidate for amplification (hearing aids and assistive devices).

Plan:
Hearing aid evaluation (scheduled).

Hearing conservation (discussed).

Reviewed simple communication strategies with patient, provided in "Hints for Improved Communication" pamphlet (R187)

Retest hearing in 6 months, sooner if there is a change in hearing, tinnitus or balance.

A

Figure 9–10 (A) Example of an audiologic report.

textbooks, laboratory normal values, e-mail, and list server contacts with other medical specialists. It is impossible for a single practitioner to know how to interpret all possible medical tests or to identify all possible diagnostic conditions. Information systems, consisting of electronic medical records with linked "knowledge bases," can assist the audiologist in making decisions by automatically evaluating test results and providing situation–specific reference information (Kohane et al, 1996; Valenti, 2000). Automated algorithms can be developed to estimate the probabilities that various disorders are present based on the constellation of acquired test results (Kohane et al, 1996). In short, our documents are becoming "smart." A practical example of a simple smart document is the audiogram form found in **Fig. 9–10**. This was generated with software developed by the author and used at the Mayo Clinic in Jacksonville, Florida. The expected normal ranges for the acoustic reflexes, speech discrimination scores, tympanometry static volumes, and so on, are all presented on the form. These values change based on the patient's age, type of hearing loss, and other factors. The computer calculates normal reference ranges based on prior data collected from the audiology clinic. Modeling speech intelligibility performance using the Speech Intelligibility Index (American National Standards Institute, 1997, R2002) is another example of using the computational power of the computer for clinical decision-making purposes. These are examples of how storing and analyzing local data can improve test accuracy. Without computers, a test result is classified as normal or abnormal based on judgment calls or normal values in the literature, which are not clinic specific. By using the computational power of the computer, classification of test results can become more systematic and accurate (Go, 1998; Lee, 2004).

Medical informatics refers to the rapidly growing merger between computer-based information management systems and health care (Goldenberg and Couch, 2005). Information technology can be applied to all aspects of health care, including research, education, patient care, and practice management. Medical informatics focuses on improving patient care and safety by improving organization and management systems; providing secure, reliable, and accessible information; and delivering that information at the right time and at the right location for decisions to be made.

Health care information management systems are evolving on three levels (Gerberding, 2006; Goldenberg and Couch, 2005; Kohane et al, 1996):

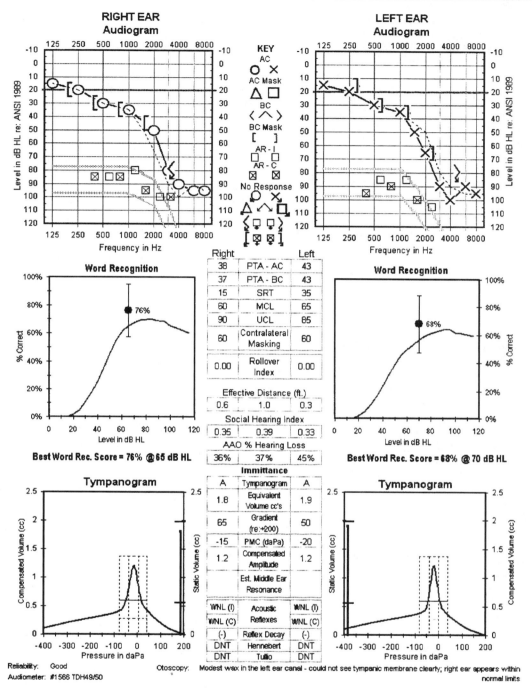

RIGHT EAR Audiogram

LEFT EAR Audiogram

KEY

	Right		Left
38	PTA - AC	43
37	PTA - BC	43
15	SRT	35
60	MCL	65
90	UCL	85
60	Contralateral Masking	60
0.00	Rollover Index	0.00

Effective Distance (ft.)

0.6	1.0	0.3

Social Hearing Index

0.35	0.39	0.33

AAO % Hearing Loss

36%	37%	45%

Immittance

Right		Left
A	Tympanogram	A
1.8	Equivalent Volume cc's	1.9
65	Gradient (re:+200)	50
-15	PMC (daPa)	-20
1.2	Compensated Amplitude	1.2
	Est. Middle Ear Resonance	
WNL (I)	Acoustic Reflexes	WNL (I)
WNL (C)		WNL (C)
(-)	Reflex Decay	(-)
DNT	Hennebert	DNT
DNT	Tullio	DNT

Word Recognition — 76%

Best Word Rec. Score = 76% @ 65 dB HL

Word Recognition — 68%

Best Word Rec. Score = 68% @ 70 dB HL

Tympanogram (Right)

Tympanogram (Left)

Reliability: Good

B Audiometer: #1566 TDH49/50

Otoscopy: Modest wax in the left ear canal - could not see tympanic membrane clearly; right ear appears within normal limits

Figure 9–10 *(Continued)* **(B)** Example of an audiogram.

Local level Practitioners need to make decisions about patient care and practice performance (Tang, 2000). The information management systems in these settings include office- and clinic-based networks. The software tools implemented on the systems focus on patient care decisions (e.g., EMR), financial performance, and coding and billing functions. Audiology-specific examples include the NOAH system, developed by the Hearing Instrument Manufacturers' Software Association (www.himsa.com),

and the various front- and back-office management applications used to run the business of audiology. Software designed to automate report generation, store and retrieve patient records, and test data also fall into this category.

Institutional/regional level Hospitals, multidisciplinary clinics, and multisite practices may track patient outcomes, assess financial performance, and maintain institution-wide electronic medical records (Gerberding,

2006; Goldenberg and Couch, 2005; Kohane et al, 1996). These systems may be used to organize and measure the performance of health care units (floors, clinics, departments, services, and disciplines), institutions, and regional systems.

Societal level   Information management systems focus on the organization of the overall health care system or large regional systems (Gerberding, 2006; Goldenberg and Couch, 2005; Kohane et al, 1996). These information management systems may be used by government agencies and insurance companies. They focus on the decision-support for the finance and allocation of resources and ultimately the utilization of services.

These systems are evolving and merging, so that information can be shared across levels. By tracking outcomes, health care information management systems can monitor the performance of health care organizations on a patient or practitioner level or on larger systems levels (Gerberding, 2006). The implications for evidence-based practice and the delivery of health care overall are enormous. We can or soon will be able to measure health care effectiveness in ways that have never been done before. Decision making, clinical outcomes, resource utilization, and costs are all traceable in the information age. The payoff is that practitioners and systems alike can learn what really works and what does not work within the context of their own unique approaches to patient care. Perhaps the most observable thrust of this effort is the move toward a universal digital electronic patient record. The Health Insurance Portability and Accountability Act of 1996 (HIPAA) is an important external force pushing for the adaptation of the personal EMR (Lusk and Herrmann, 1998). All of a patient's health care information developed over the course of his or her life, perhaps including the patient's genetic profile, would be stored on a single chip that could be read into the record of health care providers consulted by the patient. This would allow a greater understanding of the health and medication status of the patient and minimize duplicative services. Moreover, the patient's health, the types of services he or she uses, and the outcomes of those services can be tracked on a local, regional, or societal level.

As complex and remote as the evolving societal-level medical information management may seem to the average audiologist, the system will have significant impact on the future of audiology. At present, many of the services we provide are invisible to health care policy makers, in large part because the activities of health care providers can only be monitored by their billing activity through Medicare and other large third-party payers. Among audiologists working in nonautonomous environments, physicians will often require that audiologists bill their services "incident to" physicians. This means that the work of audiologists is coded and billed under a physician's or employer's provider number. When policy makers review health care utilization trends, the services provided by these audiologists appear to be provided by their employers. Similarly, because of payment rules, many of the treatments offered by audiologists, such as cerumen management and canalith repositioning for BPPV, must be billed "incident to" a physician to be paid.

Again, these services appear to be performed by the physician and not by the audiologist.

This cloaking of audiologic services will be reduced and eventually eliminated when all three levels of information management are fully integrated and providers' activities are monitored through information management systems that are independent of the billing practice. This will only occur, though, if the local information management system accurately reflects the audiologists' activities. Audiologists in training will be the ones who build these local information management systems. The larger implications of these activities must be understood so that accurate information can be recorded on such systems.

A formal discussion of all of the aspects of medical informatics is beyond the scope of this text. However, understanding the concepts already presented in this chapter will go a long way toward implementing the audiologic component of the electronic medical record and larger health-care information management system. For example, computerization allows a process of data entry and analysis to be combined with the process of generating a clinical report. With a fully automated EMR, audiologic data are stored, classified into clinical facts, then organized into meaningful clinical information in the form of a patient-focused clinical document. At the same time, the locally stored audiologic data may be used for other quality improvement purposes (within the limits of HIPAA regulations). For example, in **Fig. 9–11**, static ear canal volumes are plotted as a function of patient age using a specific brand of clinical tympanometer and a specific sweep speed. The data were captured from normal or sensorineural cases that were digitally stored in the process of analyzing and producing clinical reports. These data were used to generate regression equations that describe the mean and 95% limits for ear canal volumes in a specific clinic. The 95th percentile limits were then integrated into the report-writing software so that age-specific normal tympanogram values, unique to the device and recording protocol of the clinic, are displayed. These clinic-specific normal values allow classification of ear canal volumes with greater accuracy than is possible using more general literature-based references. This approach for generating clinic-, protocol-, and equipment-specific normal data has always been possible. However, with pen-and-paper-based reports, the time required to collect, analyze, and publish these types of analysis were prohibitive. When report writing and data analysis are combined, these analyses become much easier. This approach may be applied to multiple measures in routine audiologic practice. The result is more accurate classification of clinical facts from acquired data.

From a local perspective, raw audiologic test data can be useful and are likely worth the cost of data storage. However, these data are not likely to be useful on a regional or societal level. Every audiology clinic has different test equipment, protocols and clinical norms. Consequently, the criteria used to classify test results are based on local clinical norms and may not be generalizable across clinics. Regional systems would not be able to use locally generated data without strong standardization

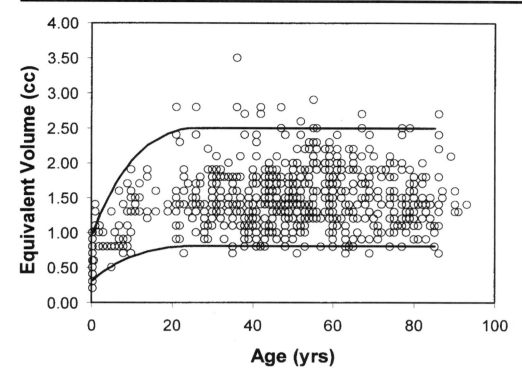

Figure 9–11 Normal values for equivalent ear canal volume by age for one type of clinical tympanometer. This was generated from a local clinical database using an information management system that generates audiologic reports and stores clinical data in the same application. Only normal and sensorineural impaired ears were analyzed.

efforts. In contrast, once test results are classified into facts, they are likely to be generalizable across clinics. As a result, local- and possibly regional-level information management systems may be interested in the set of facts generated by an audiologist or clinic. Analysis of test results may underpin the study of asset utilization and billing performance, clinical decision-making performance, and safety monitoring (as in the early detection of adverse events associated with a procedure or device). Clinical information covering assessment, management, and outcomes is important at all levels of the health care system. Locally, clinical information forms the backbone of patients' EMRs. Furthermore, information allows systems to measure the quality of health care services on an individual, regional, and societal level.

It is vitally important that audiology-derived information and services are accurately reflected in the EMR, so that the audiologist's contribution to patient care is recognized. For example, in a review of audiology standards used by the Social Security Administration, it was noted that there is virtually no information on how different degrees of hearing impairment affect a person's ability to function in different types of work settings (Dobie and Van Hemel, 2004). Acquiring this information may pave the way for greater societal support of hearing-related health care services. We might be better able to answer these types of questions in an integrated health care information management system.

Pearl

- Data, facts, and clinical information are the building blocks of the audiologic encounter. Generally, local information management systems that focus on clinical decision support will store all of these building blocks. Regional-level systems will be more interested in clinical facts and information. Societal-level systems will focus almost exclusively on information.

◆ Summary

This chapter reviewed clinical documentation from the perspective of medical information management. It covered the clinical process, translating data into information, and writing reports that are logically organized and that accurately reflect procedures and the decision making behind treatment. There is no way to anticipate all of the types of clinical reports that audiologists will be required to generate in the future. However, using the SOAP approach will help report writers to maintain a logical order to the presentation of information. The discipline of thinking about the clinical process in an organized structure goes a long way toward the goal of providing rational and effective treatment, as well as documenting what we did for the patient, and why.

References

Agency for Healthcare Research and Quality. (2001). New federal patient safety data system: National Summit on Patient Safety Data Collection and Use. Retrieved from http://www.ahrq.gov/qual/taskforce/gerber. htm

American National Standards Institute. (1997, R2002). Methods for the calculation of the Speech Intelligibility Index (S3.5). New York: Author.

Audry, J. A. (1991). Love and profit: The art of caring leadership. New York: Avon Books.

Baloh, R. W. (1998). Dizziness, hearing loss, and tinnitus. Philadelphia: F. A. Davis.

Bouthillier, F., & Shearer, K. (2002). Understanding knowledge management and information management: The need for an empirical perspective. Information Research, 8(1).

Centers for Medicare and Medicaid Services. (2006). Hospital quality information initiative. Retrieved June 22, 2006, from http://www.cms.hhs.gov/quality/hospital/hqii.asp

Centers for Medicare and Medicaid Services and the Veterans Health Administration of the Department of Veterans Affairs. (2005). Fact sheet: VistA-Office EHR. Baltimore, MD: Author.

Cox, R. M. (2005). Evidence based practice for provision of amplification. Journal of the American Academy of Audiology, 16, 419–438.

Dobie, R. A., & Van Hemel, S. (2004). Hearing loss: Determining eligibility for Social Security benefits. Washington, DC: Committee on Disability Determination for Individuals with Hearing Impairments, National Research Council/National Academy of Sciences Press.

Doebbeling, B. N., Chou, A. F., & Tierney, W. M. (2006). Priorities and strategies for the implementation of integrated informatics and communications technology to improve evidence-based practice. Journal of General Internal Medicine, 21(Suppl 2), S50–S57.

Gerberding, J. L. (2006). A patient safety network: Proposal from DHHS Patient Safety Task Force for Stakeholder Consideration, National Center for Disease Control and Prevention. Retrieved March 19, 2006, from http://www.ahcpr.gov/qual/taskforce/gerberdi.ppt

Go, A. S. (1998). Refining probability: An introduction to the use of diagnostic tests. In D. J. Friedland (Ed.), Evidence based medicine: A framework for clinical practice. Stamford, CT: Appleton & Lange.

Goldenberg, D., & Couch, M. (2005). Medical informatics and telemedicine. In C. W. Cummings, et al (Eds.), Otolaryngology: Head and neck surgery (4th ed; pp. 497–510). St. Louis: C. V. Mosby.

Gonzenbach, S. (2000). Preparing the clinical report. In H. Hosford-Dunn, R. J. Roeser, & M. Valente (Eds.), Audiology: Practice management (pp. 231–255). New York: Thieme Medical Publishers.

Institute of Medicine. (2001). Crossing the quality chasm: A new health system for the 21st century. Committee on Quality of Health Care in America, Institute of Medicine. Washington, DC: National Academy Press.

Joint Commission on Accreditation of Healthcare Organizations. (2005). Comprehensive accreditation manual for hospitals: The official handbook. Oakbrook Terrace, IL: Author.

Kasper, D. L., Braunwald, E., & Fauci, A. S. (2005). The practice of medicine. In Harrison's principles of internal medicine (16th ed.). New York: McGraw-Hill.

Kohane, I. S., Greenspun, P., Fackler, J., Cimino, C., & Szolovits, P. (1996). Building national electronic medical record systems via the World Wide Web. Journal of the American Medical Informatics Association, 3, 191–207.

Lee, T. H. (2004). Interpretation of data for clinical decisions. In L. Goldman & D. Ausiello (Eds.), Cecil textbook of medicine (22nd ed.). New York: W. B. Saunders.

Lusk, R., & Herrmann, K. (1998). The computerized patient record. Otolaryngologic Clinics of North America, 31, 289–300.

Mark, D. B. (2005). Decision-making in clinical medicine. In Harrison's principles of internal medicine (16th ed.). New York: McGraw-Hill.

Mandell, G. L., Bennett, J. E., & Dolin, R. (2005). Principles and practice of infectious diseases (6th ed.). Philadelphia: Churchill Livingstone.

Mendel, L. L., & Danhauer, J. L. (1997). Audiologic evaluation and management and speech perception assessment. San Diego, CA: Singular Publishing Group.

Paul-Brown, D. (1994). Clinical record keeping in audiology and speech-language pathology. ASHA, 36(5), 40–43.

Rakel, R. E. (2002). The problem–oriented medical record. In R. E. Rakel (Ed.), Textbook of family practice (6th ed.). New York: W. B. Saunders.

Rothenberg, J. D. (2005, August 30). Medication error prevention. Paper presented at the Mayo Clinic, Jacksonville, FL.

Ruckenstein, M. J. (1995a). Hearing loss: A plan for individualized management. Postgraduate Medicine, 98, 197–214.

Ruckenstein, M. J. (1995b). A practical approach to dizziness. Postgraduate Medicine, 97, 70–81.

SEER's Web–based Training Modules. (2005). The composition and organization of a medical record. Retrieved April 30, 2007, from http://training.seer.cancer.gov/module_abstracting/abstracting_home.html

Stach, B. A. (1998). Clinical audiology: An introduction. San Diego, CA: Singular Publishing Group.

Stephans, D. (2003). The World Health Organization's International Classification of Functioning, Disability and Health (ICF) and its relevance to audiology. AAS Bulletin, 28, 40–41.

Sveiby, K.-E. (1998). What is information? Retrieved November 19, 2005, from http://www.sveiby.com/articles/Information.html#Info%20or%20 Knowledge

Tang, P. C. (2000). Computer-based patient record system. In E. H. Shortliffe (Ed.), Medical informatics (pp. 327–358). New York: Springer.

Valenti, W. M. (2000). Errors in medicine: Problems and solutions for managed care. AIDS Reader, 10(11), 647–651.

Ventry, I. M., & Weinstein, B. E. (1982). The hearing handicap inventory for the elderly: A new tool. Ear and Hearing, 3, 128–134.

World Health Organization. (2001). International Classification of Functioning, Disability and Health (ICF). Retrieved June 22, 2006, from http://www3. who.int/icf/

Chapter 10

Infection Control

A. U. Bankaitis and Robert J. Kemp

Infection control refers to the conscious management of the clinical environment for purposes of minimizing or eliminating the risks of cross-contamination and the potential spread of disease (Bankaitis and Kemp, 2003). The management process begins with the mind-set that every patient is an assumed carrier of a potentially infectious disease. This mind-set is important in that audiologists are never in a position to fully know the overall health status of patients; furthermore, it influences how audiologists should conduct diagnostic and rehabilitative services in a manner that is consistent with minimizing cross-contamination in the clinical environment.

The nature of audiology inherently exposes both the clinician and the patient to a variety of microorganisms. Although many may be innocuous, a percentage of microorganisms encountered in the patient care environment will be opportunistic and potentially infectious; under the right conditions, these types of microorganisms may eventually lead to any number of health issues in more susceptible patient populations. These health issues may range from manageable, localized infections to more serious, life-threatening illnesses. The onset of disease manifestations may occur rapidly or at a later date, following a relatively long period of dormancy by the opportunistic microorganism.

Currently, health care workers, including audiologists and doctor of audiology (Au.D.) students, are responsible for implementing and following federally mandated infection control directives (Bankaitis and Kemp, 2003, 2004). It is the ethical and legal responsibility of audiologists and Au.D. students to learn and consistently execute issued infection control guidelines within the context of the clinical environment. Unfortunately, the literature, although limited in scope, suggests that audiologists do not adhere to basic infection control requirements. As reported by Almani (1999), for instance, the overwhelming majority of surveyed audiologists believe that the audiology clinic is not a setting associated with high exposure to communicable disease. The same study revealed that minimal infection control procedures, if any, were rarely implemented in audiology clinics. This degree of apathy most likely stems from multiple sources; however, a significant factor contributing to infection control indifference by audiologists may be attributed to the lack of exposure to infection control principles and guidelines during their graduate or doctoral studies or the lack of emphasis of infection control throughout professional practice. For example, although 74% of audiologists in this same study reported knowing the difference in basic infection control terms, as many as 45% responded incorrectly to basic terms (Almani, 1999). In the absence of formal training or practical application of infection control principles in the current environment, even the most experienced audiologists may not recognize the relevance of infection control to the clinical environment, particularly if the principles are not practically applied.

215

From these perspectives, the primary goal of this chapter is to provide foundational information on infection control. Specifically, this chapter will provide current and future audiologists with (1) a justification of infection control for the audiology clinic, (2) an introduction to regulatory agencies governing and monitoring various aspects of infection control, (3) a general review of the process of microbial transmission, and (4) practical infection control recommendations for application in the audiology clinic.

◆ Relevance of Infection Control to Audiology

Audiologists must be diligent in their efforts to control the spread of disease within the context of the clinical setting for a variety of reasons. Infection control is a federally mandated requirement set forth by the Occupational Safety and Health Administration (OSHA). OSHA mandates, oversees, and enforces infection control programs in health care settings to ensure compliance with current regulations (Bankaitis and Kemp, 2003, 2004). Infection control is the law; failure to comply with OSHA's directives and other federally mandated infection control responsibilities can result in citations and significant fines. More importantly, failure to implement basic infection control practices during audiologic assessments and vestibular testing or while fitting hearing instruments or cochlear implants can potentially put the patient or the clinician at risk for disease, particularly when considering the nature of the audiology profession.

Nature of Audiology Practice

The provision of diagnostic and rehabilitative audiologic services involves a significant degree of direct and indirect patient contact with multiple patients, multiple hearing aids, and various instruments, some of which require insertion into the external auditory canal (Bankaitis and Kemp, 2003). Inherently, the nature of what audiologists do in the clinical environment is associated with an increased risk of cross-contamination. Necessary infection control precautions must be recognized and appropriate protocols applied to minimize inadvertent exposure to potentially infectious bodily substances and opportunistic microorganisms.

Patient Population Served: Immunocompromised and Susceptible to Opportunistic Infections

Audiologic services are sought by a wide range of patients who vary across several factors, including age, nutritional status, exposure to past and current pharmacological interventions, and socioeconomic status. Each of these factors directly influences the overall integrity of the immune system (Bankaitis and Kemp, 2002). Patients with various forms or degrees of immunodeficiency remain susceptible to microorganisms that may not otherwise cause disease in healthier persons. These microorganisms often lead to opportunistic infections. By definition, opportunistic

infections originate from ubiquitous organisms that reside in relative abundance throughout the environment and on common surfaces. The organisms associated with opportunistic infections rarely cause disease or infection in healthy individuals; however, the hallmark of immunosuppression is susceptibility of individuals to these otherwise innocuous organisms. For example, *Staphylococcus* is found in large quantities on skin surfaces and has been recovered consistently from hearing aid surfaces (Bankaitis, 2002; Sturgulewski, 2005). Because it is found abundantly throughout the environment, its somewhat expected presence on hearing aid surfaces may be misconstrued by audiologists as insignificant from an infection control standpoint. On the contrary, despite its ubiquitous nature, *Staphylococcus* accounts for a high percentage of nosocomial, or hospital-acquired, infections (Murray et al, 1994). Many patients in hospitals will exhibit some form of immunodeficiency. Immunocompromised patients, whether due to illness, age, nutritional, or socioeconomic status, are susceptible to microorganisms, including *Staphylococcus*, that typically pose no threat to individuals with healthy, intact immune systems.

The principle of opportunistic infection applies to the audiology clinic as well. In the absence of infection control procedures, audiologists who handle hearing aids with their bare hands or reuse listening stethoscopes between patients without properly cleaning and disinfecting the instruments will inadvertently expose patients to bacteria and other dangers associated with contaminated instruments, objects, or equipment. Because audiologists often provide services to patients with some form or degree of immunocompromise, infection control is an important and necessary aspect of clinical practice. A proactive strategy must be implemented to minimize or reduce the possibility of the inadvertent spread of disease.

Contaminated Cerumen as an Infectious Substance

Cerumen is a bodily substance and considered potentially infectious when contaminated with blood, dried blood, blood by-products, mucus, or ear drainage (Kemp et al, 1992). Cerumen may not always be contaminated with these substances; however, given the color and viscosity of cerumen, it is not possible to determine whether or not it is contaminated. Because audiologists are not in a position to determine with predictable accuracy whether or not cerumen contains blood, blood by-products, or other forms of ear drainage, cerumen must be treated as a potentially infectious bodily substance (Bankaitis and Kemp, 2006).

Special Consideration

- Cerumen is a potentially infectious bodily substance when contaminated with blood, blood by-products, mucus, or other secretions. Because it is difficult to visualize the presence or absence of blood or other secretions within cerumen, audiologists must treat it as a potentially infectious substance.

External Auditory Canal as a Susceptible Route of Microbial Transmission

The external auditory canal is a natural orifice, providing microorganisms a portal of entry into the body. Despite the presumed antimicrobial properties of cerumen, the canal remains more prone to bacterial infection than other skin surfaces (Jahn and Hawke, 1992). Furthermore, it has been postulated that the efficacy of cerumen in inhibiting microbial growth is uniquely challenged for hearing aid wearers (Bankaitis and Kemp, 2002, 2003, 2004). Occlusion of the external auditory canal with a hearing instrument or earmold creates a darker and moister internal environment. As the ear canal retains moisture, the canal's pH level changes to more neutral or more alkaline levels that are more conducive to facilitating bacterial and/or fungal growth (Jahn and Hawke, 1992).

Unlike most other skin surfaces, the skin lining of the external auditory canal adheres directly to the perichondrium or periosteum (Alvord and Farmer, 1997). The absence of the subcutaneous padding creates a skin surface that is very thin. For example, the thickness of skin at the cartilaginous portion of the external auditory canal ranges from ~0.5 to 1.0 mm, whereas the skin at the osseous portion is only 0.2 mm thick (Lucente, 1993). This makes the external auditory canal extremely vulnerable to scratches, lacerations, or bruises (Bankaitis and Chaiken, 2005). Given the profuse blood supply to the ear canal, this region also is particularly susceptible to bleeding (Alvord and Farmer, 1997). Lastly, the anteroinferior portion of the external auditory canal contains a small series of transverse clefts underneath the canal skin called the fissures of Santorini (Kelly and Mohs, 1996). Although the fissures provide the cartilaginous canal with increased flexibility, this anatomical characteristic provides easy access for infection to pass between the external auditory canal and the nearby parotid gland (Kelly and Mohs, 1996). Taking into consideration the sensitivity of the external auditory canal and its vulnerability to injury and infection, audiologists working at the level of the canal must integrate necessary infection control procedures during patient care procedures to minimize the potential of microbial transmission.

Contaminated Hearing Instruments as a Mode for Microbial Transmission

In recent years, several studies specifically addressing microbial contamination in the hearing instrument dispensing environment have documented the presence of bacterial and fungal growth on hearing aid and earmold surfaces (Bankaitis, 2002; Sturgulewski, 2005). Although some of the recovered microorganisms were consistent with what would be expected to be found in the external auditory canal, the majority of the recovered microorganisms were not. Several microorganisms recovered from hearing aid surfaces are considered extremely virulent (e.g., *Staphylococcus aureus*, *Pseudomonas aeruginosa*), and others are exceptionally unhygienic (Bankaitis, 2005). For example, some hearing aids were contaminated with light to heavy amounts of bacteria (*Enterococci*) specifically found in fecal matter (Bankaitis, 2002). From this perspective, clinicians must be diligent in their infection control not only in the dispensing environment but also in every aspect of the clinical setting.

Special Consideration

- Recent studies have documented the presence of a variety of microbial growth on hearing aid surfaces. Although some of the microorganisms were consistent with normal ear canal flora, the majority of microorganisms were not and are considered either extremely virulent (e.g., *S. aureus*, *P. aeruginosa*) or exceptionally unhygienic (e.g., *Enterococci*). Audiologists should consider wearing gloves while handling hearing aids and earmolds. Hearing aids are often contaminated with cerumen and, technically, should be sterilized; however, because these instruments contain electronic circuitry, they cannot be immersed in a cold sterilant. Minimally, hearing aid surfaces should be properly cleaned and then disinfected before audiologists proceed to handle them with their bare hands.

◆ Regulatory Agencies Involved with Infection Control

Several federal and state agencies are responsible for developing standards and guidelines related to infection control in health care settings. These agencies are listed in **Table 10–1**. The foundation of these guidelines is based on regulations set forth by OSHA. In addition, each state enforces its own set of guidelines, although all states must minimally enforce the federal standards established by OSHA. The role of several other federal or independent agencies with influence in infection control policies will also be reviewed.

Occupational Safety and Health Administration

OSHA is a federal agency governed by the U.S. Department of Labor. The mission of OSHA is to regulate the workplace to ensure safe and healthful working conditions by enforcing or authorizing enforcement of the standards developed under the Occupational Safety and Health Act of 1970. OSHA assists states in establishing and enforcing safe and healthful working conditions; provides training, information, and education; and conducts research in the area of occupational safety and health (Bankaitis and Kemp, 2003, 2004; Kemp et al, 1992). To accomplish its mission, OSHA relies on the collaborative efforts of state agencies. In conjunction with state agencies, OSHA establishes and enforces occupational protective standards to prevent injury and to protect the health of American workers. To enforce its standards, OSHA conducts unannounced inspections of work sites.

Table 10–1 Regulatory Agencies Involved in Infection Control

Agency	Function
Occupational Safety and Health Administration (OSHA)	Regulates workplace to ensure safe and healthful work conditions
Joint Commission (formerly the Joint Commission on Accreditation of Healthcare Organizations, JCAHO)	Independent, nonprofit accrediting body for health care organizations
Commission on Accreditation of Rehabilitative Facilities (CARF)	Standard-setting commission for organizations providing services to individuals with disabilities
Environmental Protection Agency (EPA)	Protects human health and safeguards natural environment
Food and Drug Administration (FDA)	Consumer protection agency responsible for ensuring safety of foods, cosmetics, medicines, medical devices, and drugs

In response to the concerns of potential exposure to human immunodeficiency virus (HIV) in the workplace, in August 1987 OSHA announced the intent to develop guidelines for protecting health care workers from cross-infection of bloodborne diseases. In addition, OSHA proposed to develop cross-infection guidelines specifically geared toward health care workers and to monitor the safety of health care treatment personnel. Based on the recommended universal precautions issued by the Centers for Disease Control and Prevention (CDC), OSHA submitted a program that was outlined in the *Federal Register* on May 30, 1989. By 1991, the final standard was published. Through the power of federal law, OSHA mandates, oversees, and enforces infection control programs. Field inspectors randomly visit and inspect health care settings to ensure that such settings are in compliance with current regulations. Failure of an institution to comply with regulations results in citations and fines.

Joint Commission

The Joint Commission (formerly the Joint Commission on Accreditation of Healthcare Organizations, JCAHO) is an independent, nonprofit organization representing the nation's predominant accrediting body in health care. The mission of the Joint Commission is to improve the quality of health care provided to the public, as well as care accreditation and related services that support performance improvement in health (JCAHO, 1998). The commission establishes standards and conducts voluntary accreditation programs for hospitals, psychiatric facilities, substance abuse treatment and rehabilitation programs, community mental health centers, organizations providing services for the mentally and developmentally disabled, long-term care facilities, ambulatory health care facilities, and home health care organizations. Its accreditation is recognized nationwide as a symbol of quality, reflecting that an organization meets specific performance standards; to earn and maintain such accreditation, an organization must undergo an on-site survey by the Joint Commission every 3 years. Although endorsement is voluntary, many health care organizations seek accreditation because it assists centers in improving quality care, enhances community confidence and medical staff recruitment, expedites third-party payment, including Medicare and Medicaid eligibility, and favorably influences liability insurance premiums (JCAHO, 1998). With regard to

infection control, the Joint Commission sets general guidelines based on OSHA standards, which may vary depending on the facility. The facility then creates specific protocols for each department. Each department is usually delegated the responsibility of creating specific programs and protocols based on the general guidelines.

Commission on Accreditation of Rehabilitation Facilities

The Commission on Accreditation of Rehabilitation Facilities (CARF) is sponsored by 31 rehabilitation/habilitation organizations. This commission sets standards for organizations providing services to persons with disabilities such as spinal cord injuries, chronic pain, and emotional disorders. Like the Joint Commission, CARF issues general standards based on universal precautions that are then customized by each department in a facility. Membership in the Tucson, Arizona–based organization is voluntary.

Environmental Protection Agency

The mission of the Environmental Protection Agency (EPA) is to protect human health and to safeguard the natural environment. Specifically, the foundation of EPA's development was to ensure (1) that all Americans are protected from significant risks to human health in the environment where they live and work, (2) the implementation of national efforts for the reduction of environmental risk to humans and the ecosystem based on the best available scientific information, and (3) the fair and effective enforcement of federal laws that protect human health and the environment (EPA, 1998a).

Through the Office of Pesticide Programs (OPP), the EPA is responsible for protecting public health and the environment from the risks posed by pesticides and to promote safer means of pest control (EPA, 1998b). As such, the EPA directs, executes, and oversees the Federal Insecticide, Fungicide, and Rodenticide Act (FIFRA). Under FIFRA, the EPA registers all chemical disinfectants and sterilants intended for use on inanimate objects and/or environmental surfaces. The registration procedures are very comprehensive and specific. For a sterilant to earn registration rights, a substance must demonstrate a 100% kill of a large quantity of resistant spores that have been carefully applied and dried on the surfaces of 360 replicates. Repeat testing must be conducted, with a 100% kill recorded for the second time; otherwise, the product is not granted approval. Without a registration number displayed on a product's label, sale of a sterilant product in the United States is illegal and strictly prohibited (Kemp et al, 1992). In addition, the EPA has the responsibility of reviewing toxicological and hazards data, product literature, and other company information to determine the benefit versus risk ratio of a qualified product. In other words, even if a sterilant meets required criteria, if the product poses a significant risk to human health and the environment, the EPA has the right to deny registration of such a product. These procedures are necessary to ensure that products meet EPA standards.

Food and Drug Administration

The Food and Drug Administration (FDA) is a consumer protection agency governed by the U.S. Department of Health and Human Services. The FDA is responsible for ensuring the safety of foods, cosmetics, medicines, medical devices, food and drugs for pets and farm animals, and radiation-emitting consumer products, such as microwaves (FDA, 1998). The FDA also ensures that product labels are accurate and specific enough so that the contents may be used properly. In addition, the FDA operates the National Center for Toxicological Research, which is involved in researching and documenting biological effects of chemicals, including sterilants and disinfectants (FDA, 1998). This responsibility overlaps with the jurisdiction of the EPA, and oftentimes both agencies operate jointly and exchange information.

♦ Microbial Transmission Process

In order for microorganisms to gain access to the body, two events must occur. First, the microorganisms must have a mode of transmission or a means of migrating throughout the environment. Second, it must have a route of transmission. There are four principle modes of microbial transmission summarized in **Table 10–2** and provided in more detail in the following sections.

Mode of Transmission

Contact Transmission

Contact transmission represents the most frequent means of disease transmission in the health care setting and refers to a manner of potentially spreading disease through microbial exposure by way of touching or coming in contact with infectious objects. This category may be further subdivided into three subcategories: direct contact, indirect contact, and droplet contact. Direct contact transmission involves exposure to microbes via direct contact without intervening persons, barriers, or conditions. It occurs when a microbe is physically transferred from its resting place directly to a susceptible individual. Within the context of the audiology clinic, direct contact transmission may occur when a clinician touches a patient's ear with an unwashed hand. In this instance, the microbes residing on the surface of the audiologist's unwashed hand are directly transferred to the surface of the patient's ear.

Indirect contact transmission occurs when an individual comes in contact with a microbe that has already been transferred from its original resting place to a secondary surface. An example would be contact with a contaminated instrument or piece of testing equipment. This type of transmission can occur when an audiologist reuses a contaminated immittance probe tip or a contaminated listening stethoscope. In these cases, any microbial growth residing on instrument surfaces will be inadvertently transferred when other objects or items come in contact with the contaminated surfaces.

Droplet contact transmission occurs when infectious microbes come in contact with the mucosal lining of the eyelids, nose, or mouth of a susceptible individual. This typically occurs when an individual coughs, sneezes, or breathes upon another individual or on a work area surface.

Pitfall

• Contact transmission represents the most common mode of microbial transmission in the audiology clinic. Without appropriate infection control procedures, the risk of cross-contamination significantly increases.

Table 10–2 Modes of Microbial Transmission and Associated Subcategories

1. *Contact transmission*   A manner of spreading disease through microbial exposure by way of touching or coming in contact with potentially infectious objects
   a. *Direct contact transmission*   Microbial exposure occurs by coming in direct contact with potentially infectious microbes without intervening persons, barriers, or conditions
   b. *Indirect contact transmission*   Microbial exposure occurs by coming in secondary contact with contaminated objects
   c. *Droplet contact transmission*   Microbial droplets expelled briefly in the air come in direct or indirect contact with mucous membranes lining the eyelids, nose, and mouth
2. *Vehicle transmission*   A manner of potentially spreading disease through ingestion of or exposure to contaminated substances, including food, water, blood, and bodily fluids
3. *Airborne transmission*   A manner of spreading diseases through microbial exposure suspended in the air as droplet residue or dust particles.
4. *Vector-borne transmission* A manner of spreading disease whereby insects or animals carrying a pathogenic agent transfer disease by interacting with a susceptible host

Source: From Auban, Inc. Reprinted with permission.

Vehicle Transmission

Vehicle transmission refers to the transfer of potentially infectious microbes via ingestion or exposure to contaminated food or water. For instance, food poisoning can occur as a result of ingesting food items contaminated with *Salmonella* or drinking water contaminated with legionellosis.

Airborne Transmission

Airborne transmission involves the distribution of microorganisms by air in the form of either droplet nuclei (residue of evaporated droplets that may remain suspended in the air for long periods of time) or dust particles. Airborne transmission is differentiated from droplet contact transmission in that the latter involves exposure droplet nuclei that travel less than ~3 feet. In the case of airborne transmission, infectious organisms may remain suspended in the air or on surfaces for long periods of time and then be widely dispersed by air currents before being inhaled by or deposited on the susceptible host.

Vector-borne Transmission

Vector-borne transmission occurs when an animal or insect carries the pathogen and infects the susceptible host. The most recognized examples of vector-borne transmission include ticks transmitting Lyme disease and mosquitoes transmitting malaria.

Route of Transmission

Once a microbe approaches its host by one of the four modes of transmission, the second step involved in microbial transmission involves a route of transmission. Microbes require a portal of entry into the human body. Natural orifices of the body, including the nose, eyes, ears, and mouth, serve as common portals. Although the human body's skin, mucosa, and other resistive coverings and linings provide nonspecific defenses against microbial invasion, cuts, scrapes, nicks, and scratches, as well as chapped and cracked hands, are common routes for microorganisms to enter the body.

Special Consideration

- The external auditory canal represents a natural portal for microorganisms to gain access into the human body. It has been suggested that cerumen provides some level of antimicrobial protection to the external auditory canal. Despite the presumed antimicrobial properties of cerumen, however, the canal remains more prone to bacterial infection than other skin surfaces (Jahn and Hawke, 1992). It is critical for audiologists to ensure that reusable instruments (e.g., curets for cerumen removal, immittance probe tips) are cleaned and sterilized properly prior to reuse. Furthermore, appropriate hearing aid infection control procedures must be implemented to eliminate the potential of cross-contamination of equipment used with such instruments (i.e., listening stethoscopes) between patients.

♦ Infection Control Process

When a microorganism gains access to the human body, a cascade of events must take place in order for that particular microorganism to manifest as a localized infection or a systemic disease. The focus of infection control is not whether or not the microorganism eventually leads to a disease state; rather, it is on controlling microbial transmission at the level of the clinical environment, prior to the microbe gaining access into the human body. Audiologists must take into consideration the various modes and routes of disease transmission that may occur during the provision of clinical services and modify standard diagnostic and rehabilitative procedures such that the potential risk of cross-contamination is minimized. The first step toward developing an infection control plan is to become familiar with universal precautions.

Universal (Standard) Precautions

In the 1980s, the CDC issued several recommendations and guidelines for minimizing cross-infection of bloodborne diseases to health care workers. These guidelines were based on the principle that every patient is assumed to be a potential carrier of and/or susceptible host for an infectious disease. Eventually, these pronouncements were officially formalized as the Universal Blood and Bloodborne Pathogen Precautions (CDC, 1989).

More commonly referred to as universal or standard precautions, the Universal Blood and Bloodborne Pathogen Precautions were originally intended to protect health care workers from blood; however, these precautions have since subsequently been interpreted to safeguard workers against all potentially infectious body substances. Although the universal precautions specifically mention exposure to blood, semen, vaginal secretions, and other bodily fluids containing visible blood (CDC, 1989), audiologists handing devices or instruments potentially contaminated with cerumen should treat devices and instruments as potentially infectious. Furthermore, all patients should be considered potential carriers of or susceptible hosts to infectious disease. As such, infection control is regarded as standard care for every patient.

The universal precautions developed and made available by the CDC are relatively straightforward. To integrate infection control principles effectively, it is useful to consider the application of precautions within the context of the audiology clinic. The following section reviews each guideline and how that guideline pertains to audiology practice.

Appropriate Personal Barriers

Appropriately fitted gloves, either latex or nonlatex, must be incorporated in an infection control program. Gloves are considered one-time use items; they should not be reused, nor should the same pair be used during two separate patient appointments. After use, gloves should be properly removed and disposed of. Unless grossly contaminated with blood or other bodily fluids, gloves may be disposed of in the regular trash.

Pearl

- For those individuals allergic to latex, nonlatex products in the form of nitrile gloves are available.

Pitfall

- Latex gloves interact with silicone impression material, interfering with curing. Do not wear latex gloves when handling uncured silicone impression material during the initial phases of making an earmold impression. Once the material has cured in the ear canal, latex gloves may be used and should be used during the earmold removal process.

Audiologists involved in intraoperative monitoring or working in the operating room must wear gloves during patient preparation and needle electrode insertion and while conducting similar procedures within the surgical environment. Needle electrodes may cause bleeding in the insertion area, and it is important for audiologists to protect their hands from potential exposure to blood when further securing the needle electrodes in place. During the course of surgical procedures, it may be necessary to conduct specialized testing procedures (e.g., electrode impedance testing for cochlear implants) that will involve handling items that have made contact with blood and other bodily fluids.

Gloves are also appropriate in the clinical environment. There is general agreement that wearing gloves is indicated when hands are likely to become contaminated with potentially infectious material, such as blood, bodily fluids, and secretions (Bankaitis and Kemp, 2003). Although not visible, cerumen is often contaminated with blood, blood by-products, and/or secretions, and must be treated as a potentially infectious substance. Gloves should be worn during those procedures where contact with cerumen is anticipated or probable, including cerumen removal procedures, while handling cured earmold impressions that have been removed from patients' ears, and when handling hearing instruments. The only exception to wearing gloves while handling hearing instruments is in those cases where the hearing instrument has been properly cleaned and then disinfected with either a disinfectant towelette or with hearing aid/earmold disinfectant spray.

As shown in **Fig. 10–1**, safety glasses and disposable masks are necessary when there is risk of splash or splatter of potentially infectious material, or when clinician or patient is at risk of airborne contamination. For example, safety glasses should be worn when working with a grinding or buffing wheel, as this will reduce the risk of microbes or microbial by-products gaining access through the eye. It is recommended that masks also be worn to prevent particles of plastic from being inhaled. Regarding apparel, at minimum, it is highly recommended that clothing be protected by a standard laboratory coat. During vestibular testing and similar situations, a disposable gown would be appropriate due to the potential of patients becoming nauseous and potentially sick.

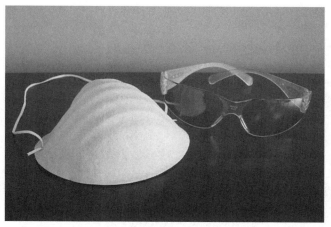

Figure 10–1 Safety glasses and molded masks are examples of appropriate personal barriers that audiologists should have readily available when performing diagnostic and/or rehabilitative procedures that may expose the clinician to various opportunistic or infectious microorganisms.

Hand Hygiene

Hand hygiene represents the single most important procedure for effectively limiting the spread of infectious disease. It is one of the most critical components of a basic infection control program. Exhaustively listing every potential circumstance that may require execution of hand hygiene procedures would be a significant and somewhat arbitrary task; indications for hand hygiene depend on the specific task or activity (Bankaitis and Kemp, 2003, 2004). Generally, superficial contact with an object that is not suspected to be contaminated does not require hand hygiene, whereas prolonged and intense contact with any patient warrants hygiene procedures (CDC, 2002). The CDC also indicates hand hygiene procedures prior to the initiation of invasive procedures, before providing services to patients, and after glove use, particularly when microbial contamination of the covered hands has likely occurred or when contact with mucous membranes, blood and bodily fluids, and secretions or excretions has been made (CDC, 2002). In addition, hand hygiene is an important component of the personal hygiene of all audiology practice personnel.

Pearl

- Hand hygiene is one of the most important parts of an infection control program. When hands are washed as often as they should be, the skin may experience temporary dryness or chapping. To minimize or eliminate this effect, use medical-grade liquid soaps to wash hands. These products contain special emollients that will help keep hands from drying or chapping.

Hand hygiene may be accomplished in one of two ways. Preferably, hands should be washed with medical-grade liquid soap and running water. At the time universal precautions were issued, washing hands with soap and water was

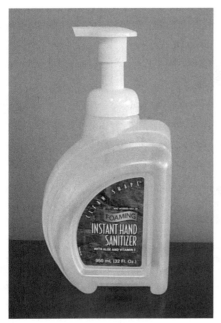

Figure 10–2 An example of a no-rinse hand degermer product that may be incorporated into an alternative hand-hygiene procedure to traditional liquid soap and running water.

the only recognized hand washing technique (Bankaitis and Kemp, 2003). The CDC has since endorsed the use of antimicrobial "no rinse" degermers as an alternative method to hand washing when access to a sink with running water is not available or easily accessible (CDC, 2002). **Figure 10–2** illustrates an example of a no-rinse hand degermer product. Because the CDC has recognized both procedures as meeting the definition of hand washing, the term *hand hygiene* is now used to refer to either technique (Bankaitis and Kemp, 2003).

"Touch" and "Splash" Surfaces Cleaning and Disinfecting

A touch surface refers to an area that may potentially come in direct or indirect contact with hands (Bankaitis and Kemp, 2003, 2004). Horizontal surfaces such as countertops, workbenches, service areas, tables, and the armrests of chairs are considered touch surfaces. A splash surface is an area that may be hit with blood, bodily fluids, or other secretions from a potentially contaminated source (Bankaitis and Kemp, 2003, 2004). Examples of splash surfaces are a work surface that a patient may potentially sneeze on and a surface that may come in contact with materials splattered from a grinding or buffing wheel during an earmold or hearing aid modification.

After each patient appointment, all touch and splash surfaces must be cleaned and disinfected. Cleaning is an important prerequisite to disinfecting and refers to procedures in which gross contamination is removed from surfaces or objects without killing germs **(Table 10–3)**. In contrast, disinfection refers to a process in which germs are killed. This process is appropriate for those objects that do not make contact with blood or other potentially infectious sub-

stances, including work areas and patient touch surfaces. The degree to which germs are killed depends on the level of the disinfectant. Household disinfectants kill a limited number of germs commonly found in the household. In contrast, hospital-grade disinfectants are much stronger and kill a larger number and variety of germs. As such, hospital-grade disinfectants should be incorporated in infection control protocols implemented in patient care settings, including clinics and private practice facilities (Rutala, 1990).

> **Pitfall**
>
> - Alcohol and bleach should be avoided as disinfectants in the audiology clinic because these agents chemically denature and destroy acrylic, plastic, rubber, and silicone materials that are typically used in manufacturing audiologic equipment and hearing instruments.

Critical Instruments Sterilizing

Sterilization involves killing 100% of vegetative microorganisms, including associated endospores **(Table 10–3)**. Whereas disinfection may kill some germs, sterilization, by definition, kills all germs and associated endospores each and every time. Instruments categorized as "critical" must be cleaned first and then sterilized prior to reuse. Critical instruments typically refer to those instruments introduced directly into the bloodstream (i.e., needles); however, they also include noninvasive instruments that come in contact with intact mucous membranes or bodily substances (blood, saliva, mucus, and pus) or that from use or misuse can penetrate the skin (Bankaitis and Kemp, 2003, 2004). Within the confines of the audiology clinic, reusable items that come in contact with cerumen and are intended to be reused with multiple patients should be cleaned and then sterilized, including but not limited to immittance probes, reusable specula, curets used for cerumen removal, and tools used to clean hearing aid ports. The only exceptions to sterilization are hearing instruments, as standard sterilization techniques would ruin such devices. In these cases, hearing instruments must be cleaned and then disinfected with either a disinfectant towelette or hearing aid/earmold disinfectant spray.

In general, there are two sterilization techniques: the autoclave and cold sterilization. The autoclave involves pressurized heat for sterilization. Because most hearing aid instruments would melt, this process is not recommended.

Table 10–3 Comparison of Definitions of Common Terms Used in Infection Control Procedures

Term	Definition
Cleaning	Removal of gross contamination
Disinfecting	Killing a percentage of germs
Sterilization	Killing 100% of germs, including endospores

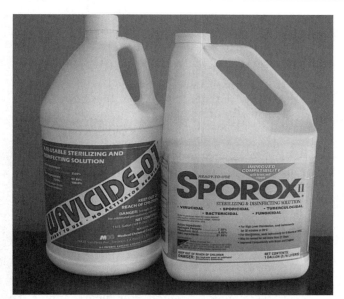

Figure 10–3 Two examples of commercially available cold sterilants for use in the audiology clinic. Wavicide-01 is a glutaraldehyde-based solution; Sporox II is a hydrogen peroxide–based solution.

Cold sterilization involves soaking instruments in EPA-approved liquid chemicals for a specified number of hours. Glutaraldehyde solutions in concentrations of 2% or higher or 7.5% or higher levels of hydrogen peroxide (H_2O_2) are the only chemicals approved by the EPA for cold sterilization. **Figure 10–3** shows two examples of commercially available cold sterilants. Gas sterilization is also an option; however, it is not readily available at all facilities.

Special Consideration

- Glutaraldehyde, an effective sterilant and high-level disinfectant, must be handled carefully. This chemical should never come in contact with skin or clothing. Persons who handle it should wear gloves and safety glasses. In addition, glutaraldehyde that has been poured into soaking trays must be placed in a well-ventilated area, as the associated fumes may irritate the eyes and nose and can cause respiratory problems. Soaking trays should have lids such that the tray can be kept closed when the tray is not being used. Glutaraldehyde should never be used in an ultrasonic cleaner because the cavitation created by the machine generates additional fumes.

Disposing of Infectious Waste

For the audiology clinic, most waste contaminated with ear discharge or cerumen can be placed in regular receptacles and discarded through normal disposal procedures. In the event that certain waste may be contaminated with excessive cerumen or mucus, the material should be placed in a separate, impermeable bag and only then discarded in the regular trash. This practice will separate the contaminated waste from the rest of the trash and minimize the chance of maintenance or cleaning personnel coming in casual contact with it. It is not anticipated that materials containing significant amounts of blood or bodily fluids would be encountered in the hearing aid clinic. In such an unlikely circumstance, materials containing significant amounts of blood should be disposed of in impermeable bags labeled with the symbol for biohazard waste and disposed of by a waste hauler licensed for medical waste disposal.

Cold disinfectants and sterilants are considered toxic, and disposal must be made in accordance with local and federal regulations. Disposal methods are generally stated in the manufacturer's specifications. Disposables that can cause injury, such as scalpel blades used in hearing aid modifications, should be placed in puncture-resistant, disposable containers more commonly known as sharps containers, as shown in **Fig. 10–4**. Ideally, the sharps container should be located where these items are used until final disposal.

Other Infection Control Requirements

Infection control plans must incorporate several additional elements as defined by OSHA. These additional applications are as follows.

Engineering and Work Practice Controls

Audiologists are responsible for developing and implementing both engineering and work practice controls. The term *engineering controls* refers to items or procedures specifically designed to isolate or remove bloodborne pathogen hazards from the workplace. Incorporating the use of a designated, closed-off, and tamper-resistant container to house used objects throughout the day is an example of an engineering practice control. This arrangement minimizes the

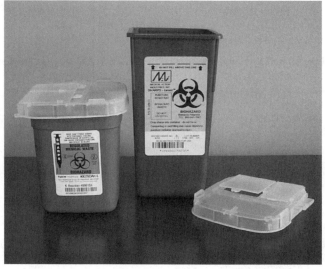

Figure 10–4 Sharps containers are red, puncture-resistant containers labeled as regulated medical waste. They come in a variety of sizes and represent an important component in an infection control program in terms of appropriate disposal of sharp instruments.

risk of inadvertent cross-contamination in several ways. First, the container isolates the contaminated specula from the workplace, eliminating or significantly reducing the risk of someone coming in direct contact with the contaminated instruments. Second, it reduces the risk of inadvertently reusing a contaminated object. This engineering control allows the audiologist to conveniently store used items until the end of the day, when the container can be transported to the designated room for cleaning and sterilization.

Work practice controls are also designed to reduce the likelihood of exposure to potentially infectious fluids, substances, or agents; however, these controls apply specifically to diagnostic and/or rehabilitative service procedures provided to the patient by the audiologist. Developing step-by-step procedures on how the front-office personnel are to manage drop-off hearing aids such that the instruments are not touched or handled by the staff's bare hands is an example of a work practice control. Work practice controls must be applied to the various diagnostic and/or rehabilitative services provided in the audiology clinic. Once these procedures are developed, they must be implemented and applied to each and every patient.

Written Infection Control Plan

OSHA requires each facility to have a written infection control plan. This plan is to be made available to all workers and must provide protocols to be used in the office for infection control. Although most hospitals and major health care centers typically have an infectious diseases department that handles the organizations' general infection control plan strategy, the department or division of audiology must have its own infection control plan that specifically outlines processes and procedures that have been designed to eliminate or at least minimize the potential for cross-contamination. This individualized infection control plan serves as the foundation of the department's infection control initiative. In accordance with OSHA's Bloodborne Pathogens Standard (29 CFR 1910.1030), the infection control plan must be in written form and contain specific sections, as reviewed described here.

Employee Exposure Classification   Each employee is classified on the basis of potential exposure to blood and other infectious substances. A classification category should be assigned for each employee and recorded in an infection control plan. There are three categories:

- *Category 1*   Personnel whose primary job assignment exposes them to cross-infection with bloodborne diseases or other potentially infectious microbes. This category includes physicians, nurses, physician assistants, paramedics, dentists, hygienists, and others whose primary job assignment requires that they participate in patient treatment or handle potentially contaminated instruments or items on a regular basis.

- *Category 2*   Personnel whose secondary job assignment potentially exposes them to cross-infection. This category is most appropriate for those professionals dispensing hearing aids, as some job-related procedures may

involve blood, ear drainage, or mucus/saliva contact. Any office personnel involved in cleaning of instruments or surfaces that may be contaminated with infectious microbes or substances would also fall into this category.

- *Category 3*   Personnel whose job requirements in the office never expose them to blood or other bodily fluids. Such persons do not clean instruments or treatment areas and are not involved in treatment procedures.

Hepatitis B Virus Vaccination Plan and Records of Vaccination
Employees who may encounter blood or other infectious substances are to be offered the opportunity to receive a hepatitis B virus (HBV) vaccination. The HBV vaccination must be offered to all category 1 and 2 workers free of charge. The employee is not required to accept the offer of vaccination, but a waiver must be signed noting the refusal of the offered vaccine. The vaccination should be administered by a trained medical professional and be given according to current medical standards. OSHA requires that this record be retained for length of employment plus 30 years (Kemp et al, 1992).

Plan for Annual Training and Records of Training   Each office is to conduct and document completion of annual training in infection control. Specifically, training must be provided at the time of initial assignment and must take place at least annually thereafter. Although the standard does not specify length of training, OSHA's standard does list the elements that must be included in the training program, including explanations of symptoms and modes of transmission of bloodborne diseases, location and handling of personal protective equipment, information on the HBV vaccine, and follow-up procedures to be taken in the event of an exposure incident. During the course of the year, if an update or new procedure is to be implemented, appropriate training must be conducted in a timely fashion to ensure that the new or updated procedure is understood and implemented. Records of training sessions should be filed with the infection control plan in a designated location.

Additional training should be provided when changes such as modifications of tasks or procedures or institution of new tasks or procedures affect the employee's occupational exposure. In this case, the additional training may be limited to addressing the newest information or change in procedure or policy and does not have to cover all the topics included in the initial training. Established employees changing exposure classification categories should be trained within 90 days of the hire or change in classification category.

Plan for Accidents and Accidental Exposure Follow-up   All infection control programs should plan for accidents. This includes the steps that will be taken when an accident occurs that can expose individuals to bloodborne pathogens or other potentially infectious agents. When an accident occurs, such as a patient falling, getting a nosebleed, or someone getting sick and vomiting, every member of the office staff should know what to do. This usually includes directions to avoid touching blood or other bodily fluid while administering appropriate aid.

Accidental exposures to bloodborne pathogens require follow-up. Although these will be extremely rare in the hearing aid clinic or private practice, an emergency plan should be created. As dictated by OSHA, if the exposure involves a percutaneous or mucous membrane exposure to blood or other bodily fluids, or a cutaneous exposure to blood when the worker's skin is chapped, abraded, or otherwise broken, the source patient must be informed of the incident and tested for HIV and HBV after consent is obtained. If the patient refuses consent or if he or she tests positive, the worker must be tested for HIV antibodies and seek medical evaluation for any acute illness that occurs within 12 weeks of exposure. HIV seronegative workers must be retested in 6 weeks and 6 months after exposure.

As stated above, an exposure occurs when a potentially infective substance comes in contact with a potential route of entry, such as the eyes, ears, nose, mouth, cuts, scrapes, and chapped hands. In an accidental exposure, the goals are to confirm that a disease has or has not been transferred and, in the event of a transfer, to treat the disease effectively and efficiently. Accidental exposures and the follow-up treatment should be recorded, and the circumstance of exposure, route of exposure, and source of the individual, including, if possible, the health status of the source, should be noted.

Implementation Protocols   Implementation protocols refer to infection control policies and procedures that have been designed to minimize exposure to infectious substances during routine clinical procedures. Most hospitals have an infection control department that generates general infection control protocols; however, audiologists must develop profession-specific protocols that address how clinicians will perform audiologic procedures associated with potential exposure to blood or bodily fluids and/or exposure to opportunistic microorganisms. Audiology-specific infection control protocols addressing cerumen removal, intraoperative monitoring, hearing aid dispensing, cochlear implants, and diagnostic testing are readily available, and the reader is referred to those sources for more specific information (Bankaitis and Kemp, 2003, 2004, 2005).

Postexposure Plans and Records   In the event that a medically treatable exposure occurs, the office must document the treatment that has taken place and the outcome. The OSHA requirements need to be reviewed, implemented, and documented individually for each employee.

◆ Summary

Infection control is an important aspect of audiologic practice. Recommended procedures and guidelines are not complex; however, infection control protocols do require diligence and consistency. When taken for granted, insufficiently executed, incorrectly applied, or completely ignored, potential consequences often put the health of patients and audiologists at considerable risk. The information covered in this chapter should provide audiologists with a basic understanding of infection control principles and the necessary guidelines to initiate clinic-specific infection control procedures.

References

Almani, A. M. (1999). Current trends and future needs for practices in audiologic infection control. Journal of the American Academy of Audiology, 10(3), 151–159.

Alvord, L. S., & Farmer, B. L. (1997). Anatomy and orientation of the human external ear. Journal of the American Academy of Audiology, 8, 383–390.

Bankaitis, A. U. (2002). What is growing on your patient's hearing aids? Hearing Journal, 55(6), 48–56.

Bankaitis, A. U. (2005). Hearing aids: Lick 'em and stick 'em? Sticking hearing aids in the mouth is not a good idea. Audiology Today, 17(6), 2–3.

Bankaitis, A. U., & Chaiken, R. (2005). The external auditory canal. In A. U. Bankaitis & S. Kelso (Eds.), Cerumen management (pp. 19–43). St. Louis: Auban.

Bankaitis, A. U., & Kemp, R. J. (2002). Hearing aid–related infection control. In M. Valente (Ed.), Strategies for selecting and verifying hearing aids (2nd ed., pp. 369–383). New York: Thieme Medical Publishers.

Bankaitis, A. U., & Kemp, R. J. (2003). Infection control in the hearing aid clinic. Boulder, CO: Auban.

Bankaitis, A. U., & Kemp, R. J. (2004). Infection control in the audiology clinic. Boulder, CO: Auban.

Bankaitis, A. U., & Kemp, R. J. (2005). Infection control during cerumen removal. In A. U. Bankaitis & S. Kelso (Eds.), Cerumen management (pp. 85–96). St. Louis: Auban.

Bankaitis, A. U., & Kemp, R. J. (2006). Infection control in the audiology clinic (2nd ed.). St. Louis: Auban.

Centers for Disease Control and Prevention. (1989). Guidelines for prevention of transmission of human immunodeficiency virus and hepatitis B to health-care and public safety workers. MMWR Morbidity and Mortality Weekly Report, 38(Suppl. 6), 1–38.

Centers for Disease Control and Prevention. (2002). Guideline for hand hygiene. MMWR Morbidity and Mortality Weekly Report, 51(RR16), 1–44.

Environmental Protection Agency. (1998a). EPA's mission. Retrieved June 6, 2003, from http://www.eipa.gov/epahome/epa.html

Environmental Protection Agency. (1998b). Office of pesticide programs. Retrieved June 6, 2003, from http://www.epa.gov/opp00001/regleg.html

Food and Drug Administration. (1998). Frequently asked questions. Retrieved June 7, 2003, from http://www.fda.gove/opacom/faqs/genfaqs.html

Jahn, A. F., & Hawke, M. (1992). Infections of the external ear. In C. Cummings et al. (Eds.), Otolaryngology—Head and Neck Surgery (2nd ed., pp. 2787–2794). St. Louis: TK.

Joint Commission on Accreditation of Healthcare Organizations. (1998). Facts about the Joint Commission on Accreditation of Healthcare Organizations. Retrieved June 6, 2003, from http://www.jcaho.org/about_jc/jcinfo.html

Kelly, K. E., & Mohs, D. C. (1996). The external auditory canal. Otolaryngologic Clinics of North America, 29(5), 725–739.

Kemp, R. J., Roeser, R. J., Pearson, D. W., & Ballachandra, B. (1992). Infection control for the professions of audiology and speech-language pathology. Olathe, KS: Iles Publishing.

Lucente, F. E. (1993). Fungal infection of the external ear. Otolaryngologic Clinics of North America, 26, 995–1006.

Murray, P. R., Kobayashi, G. S., Pfaller, M. A., & Rosenthal, K. S. (1994). Staphylococcus. In P. R. Murray et al. (Eds.), Medical microbiology (2nd ed., 166–179). St. Louis: Mosby-Year Book.

Rutala, W. A. (1990). APIC guideline for selection and use of disinfectants. American Journal of Infection Control, 18(2), 99–117.

Sturgulewski, S. (2005). Microorganisms and hearing aids: Considerations for infection control. Doctoral dissertation, Rush University, Chicago.

Chapter 11

Cerumen Management

Ross J. Roeser and Phillip L. Wilson

The ear canal is the primary acoustic pathway to the auditory system. Because of its fundamental role in audition, audiologists are required to have a thorough understanding of all aspects of ear canal anatomy, physiology, and pathophysiology. They must be able to examine the ear canal properly and identify normal structures and abnormal conditions. Cerumen management is now commonplace in audiologic practice.

This chapter covers the rationale for cerumen management, discusses the normal and abnormal aspects of ear canal anatomy and physiology, and describes the procedures for cerumen extraction.

♦ Rationale for Cerumen Management in an Audiology Practice

The presence of occluding cerumen in the ear canal is a pathological condition; it can cause conductive hearing loss, as well as tinnitus, vertigo, and skin irritation with accompanying itching and pain. Cerumen removal will result in immediately improved hearing; in fact, if sensorineural sensitivity is normal, cerumen removal will restore hearing sensitivity to normal levels.

Figure 11–1 illustrates audiometric data from a 58-year-old patient with impacted cerumen. As shown in this figure, a severe hearing loss is present with impaction. Following cerumen removal, thresholds improved by ~30 to 35 dB to a moderate hearing level.

This case study clearly demonstrates the effect of impacted cerumen on threshold sensitivity and provides an example of the potential improvement in communication abilities that can result when cerumen is removed. Because preexisting sensorineural hearing loss was present for this patient, reducing the additional hearing loss resulting from ear canal occlusion had a greater importance.

Beyond removing occluding cerumen to prevent hearing loss and other possible sequelae, routine audiologic procedures require that the ear canal be reasonably clear of cerumen; some procedures require that the ear canal be completely free from cerumen. These procedures include:

- Making earmold impressions for hearing aids
- Probe microphone measures
- Using insert earphones
- Electrocochleography (ECochG)
- Electronystagmography (ENG)

AUDIOGRAM

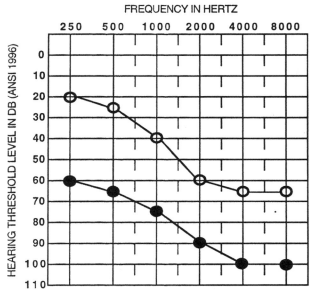

Figure 11–1 Audiometric data from a 58-year-old male with and without impacted cerumen. Before cerumen removal, results showed a severe hearing loss (solid points). Following cerumen removal, thresholds improved to a moderate loss (open points).

- Immittance measures

- Otoacoustic emissions (OAE)

The degree to which the ear canal is required to be free of cerumen depends on the audiologic procedure to be performed. For example, fitting a completely in the canal (CIC) hearing aid requires taking a deep impression of the ear canal. Because of the sensitivity of the canal and the need for an excellent fit for this style of amplification, the canal must be completely free of cerumen. Placing an otoblock near the tympanic membrane also requires that the canal be completely free of cerumen because the otoblock may cause the cerumen to be moved against the membrane. An inaccurate impression, caused by the presence of cerumen in the ear canal, may lead to a hearing aid that is either uncomfortable or likely to create feedback. Cerumen management is often required prior to taking impressions for CIC hearing aids. The necessity for a completely clear canal is not as great when taking impressions for in-the-ear (ITE) and in-the-canal (ITC) hearing aids or behind-the-ear (BTE) earmolds. However, for any type of hearing aid, the more accurate the impression, the more likely the device will fit properly. Real ear measurement of hearing aid characteristics requires the placement of a probe microphone in the ear canal near the tympanic membrane. The small diameters of the probe tubes can easily be clogged with cerumen, which will confound results. Additionally, excessive amounts of cerumen may create unusual resonances, not representative of hearing aid performance at the tympanic membrane (Ballachanda, 1995). For these reasons, a clean ear canal is essential for accurate and effective probe microphone measurement of hearing aid performance.

The use of insert earphones has several advantages in audiometric testing (see Chapter TK in the *Diagnosis* volume of this series). As a result, the use of insert earphones is becoming more popular in standard audiology practice, not only for routine threshold audiometry but also in the performance of auditory brainstem response (ABR) and ECochG. Cerumen within the ear canal can change the output characteristics of earphones and response characteristics of the ear canal (Ballachanda, 1995; Gerling et al, 1997; Gerling and Goebel, 1992). In addition, as with the insertion of an otoblock for taking ear impressions, placing an insert earphone into the ear canal may force cerumen toward the tympanic membrane, increasing ear canal blockage. Excessive or impacted cerumen may even fill the opening of the insert earphone, which would significantly reduce the sound pressure level of the stimuli reaching the tympanic membrane.

ENG relies on the ability of the examiner to direct a flow of air or water directly against the tympanic membrane. The presence of excessive or impacted cerumen may result in inaccurate readings. Cerumen extraction is required prior to testing when an excessive amount of cerumen is present.

When performing immittance measures and OAE, a probe tip is placed into the external ear canal. If significant amounts of cerumen are present, the probe tip can clog with excessive cerumen, resulting in invalid findings. For example, with immittance measures, test results indicating a flat tympanogram with absent reflexes would be found. Ear canals with enough cerumen to clog immittance and OAE instrument probe tips must be cleaned in order for reliable test results to be obtained.

Cerumen management is an important part of the hearing health care delivery system and should be part of standard audiologic care. If an audiologist instead refers a patient to a physician for cerumen management, a delay in diagnosis and treatment may occur. In addition, the patient may have questions regarding the audiologist's level of training and skills, or even competence. Furthermore, referring a patient with excessive/impacted cerumen to a physician may result in less than effective treatment. Survey data show that cerumen is typically removed in physicians' offices by individuals who have little or no formal training in the anatomy of the ear canal or in the procedures and precautions necessary for safe and effective cerumen removal (Sharp et al, 1990). Mahoney (1993) reports in a study of cerumen impaction among nursing home residents in Massachusetts that it was often difficult to get physicians to respond to requests for cerumen removal. She noted that the physicians responsible for the care of these elderly residents apparently assumed the patients had permanent age-related hearing loss and did not feel that the removal of impacted cerumen was of enough importance to warrant the time involved to clear the impaction. More significant from Mahoney's study was the finding that of those individuals who did receive treatment for impacted cerumen, the vast majority of ears remained impacted after treatment. This information does not necessarily imply that physicians do not have the knowledge and skills necessary to successfully manage excessive cerumen. It does imply, however, that very often physicians believe that cerumen management is a low priority and that the procedure is often relegated to other personnel who may or may not have the necessary skills.

Audiologists have the academic training and requisite skills to perform cerumen management. Over the last decade the American Speech-Language-Hearing Association (ASHA), the American Academy of Audiology (AAA), and the Academy of Doctors of Audiology (ADA; formerly the Academy of Dispensing Audiologists) have included cerumen removal as part of the scope of practice for audiologists. At the same time, many state licensing laws have been rewritten to include cerumen management as a recognized procedure to be performed by licensed audiologists. Improved opportunities in graduate training programs and heightened awareness of the need for cerumen management by audiologists have significantly increased the number of audiologists who are practicing cerumen management routinely.

Some audiologists choose not to practice cerumen management, which is their clinical prerogative. It appears that uncertainty regarding the appropriate procedures and the fear of liability of patients being injured are the primary deterring factors (Primus and Skordas, 1996).

The issue of liability is important in this discussion. As with other clinical procedures, audiologists must recognize that there are risks involved in cerumen management. These include injury to the ear canal, perforation of the tympanic membrane, exacerbation of chronic middle ear disease, and possible damage to the ossicular chain (Sharp et al, 1990). Primus and Skordas (1996) surveyed 500 audiologists on their cerumen management practices. For those audiologists choosing not to manage cerumen, patient injury and the audiologist's liability for injury were among the main concerns. Every procedure performed in an audiologist's practice potentially can result in a malpractice lawsuit. A successful outcome is not guaranteed when any procedure is performed. An audiologist's protection in the event of litigation is to have demonstrable knowledge, skill, and experience to perform the procedure. Practitioners increase their chances of success in these situations by using their knowledge, skill, and experience to consider all aspects of the procedure, to perform the procedure with care, and to document the procedure accurately.

Whether a specific audiologic procedure is covered by an insurance carrier is not always clear, and contacting the carrier will not necessarily clarify procedures or practices that are covered and/or the extent to which they are covered. A typical response from an insurance carrier when asked whether a specific procedure is covered will be vague and indicate that the procedures are covered if they do not violate existing law and are included as part of normal audiologic practice (Manning, 1992). Clinicians are individually responsible for ensuring they are practicing according to the standard of care within the scope of their practice.

Audiologists can perform cerumen management safely and effectively by taking a thorough case history, understanding the contraindications for cerumen management, and selecting the method most likely to achieve the desired result. If this general series of actions is taken, the risks in removing cerumen are as minimal as for most of the other procedures audiologists routinely perform.

◆ Composition and Types of Cerumen

Figure 11–2 shows a cross section of the human ear. The S-shaped ear canal is a membranocartilaginous structure that begins at the pinna and terminates at the tympanic membrane. The outer one third to one half of the ear canal is cartilaginous and is covered with relatively thick skin. The remaining portion of the ear canal is bony and is covered with a thin layer of skin that is sensitive to pain. A narrowing of the canal, named the isthmus, is located at the boundary between the cartilaginous and osseous portions of the ear canal. This narrowing at the isthmus sometimes restricts the ability to visualize the tympanic membrane.

Pearl

- Practitioners should be particularly careful not to scrape the deep portions of the ear canal with cerumen removal instruments, as it may cause pain for the patient and is more likely to result in bleeding.

Cerumen is primarily composed of secretions from two types of glands found in the cartilaginous portion of the ear canal. Sebaceous glands produce a fatty substance called sebum, and modified apocrine (ceruminous) glands produce apocrine sweat. Sebum and apocrine sweat combine with desquamated epithelial cells, dust, other small foreign bodies, and shed hair to make up cerumen (Perry, 1957).

The two types of cerumen are "dry" or "rice bran" and "wet" or "sticky." The dry type of cerumen is found in 78 to 87% of Asian populations (Matsunaga, 1962). Asians have a tendency to underproduce cerumen, resulting in dryness of the external ear canal (Meyers, 1977; Perry, 1957). This clinical observation suggests a scarcity of sebaceous and apocrine glands (Perry, 1957). The dry type of cerumen is

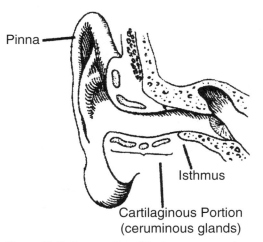

Figure 11–2 Cross section of the human ear canal.

odorless because of a reduced number of apocrine sweat glands, with apocrine sweat being primarily responsible for the odor of cerumen (Matsunaga, 1962). An odor accompanying cerumen is of diagnostic significance, as it often indicates the presence of an accompanying pathological condition (Matsunaga, 1962).

The wet or sticky type of cerumen is found in 95 to 98% of Caucasians and Negroid racial types (Petrakis, 1969). Provided no pathology is present, the distinction between the two types of cerumen is so clear that distinguishing between them can be made by a simple inspection of the ear canals.

Chromatographic analysis of wet and dry cerumen samples has shown that cerumen type is due to differences in quantity and composition of ear wax lipids. Dry cerumen contains squalene, triglycerides, free fatty acids, cholesterol, nonlipid substances, stearyl esters, and wax esters. Wet cerumen does not contain nonlipid substances, stearyl esters, and wax esters (Inaba et al, 1987).

Dry cerumen is brittle, appears ashlike and flaky, and ranges in color from light gray to brownish gray. As it is exposed over time to air, bacterial activity, oxidation, and dehydration change its color from golden brown to almost black (Matsunaga, 1962). Clinicians must be aware of the normal color variations of cerumen types when examining ear canals and have familiarity with the association between the color and consistency of cerumen and race. The decision to remove cerumen from an ear canal must be based on the conclusion from otoscopic examination that the material in the ear canal is, in fact, cerumen and not some other substance, such as blood or purulent material.

Pearl

- Clinicians must be aware of the normal color variations of cerumen and have familiarity with the association between the color and consistency of cerumen and ethnicity.

Cerumen type is inherited as a simple Mendelian trait, with the dry-type allele (mutational gene group) being recessive to the wet type (Bass and Jackson, 1977). The genetically based polymorphic nature of cerumen has been used to study both genetics and anthropology (Matsunaga, 1962).

◆ Functions of Cerumen

Although the physiological factors that control the sebaceous glands in the ear canal are not fully known, the function of the apocrine (ceruminous) sweat glands has been well established. Perry (1957) studied cerumen production by direct visualization of the skin of the distal portion of the ear canal in 150 subjects. Production of apocrine sweat increased in the presence of smooth muscle stimulants (Pitocin), adrenergic drugs (epinephrine and norepinephrine), and the emotional states of anxiety, fear, and pain.

Ceruminous glands also increased production when the canal wall was cleaned or rubbed in an action called "mechanical milking." Perry (1957) found in some cases that vigorous chewing caused ear canal distortions, resulting in the same milking effect.

Cerumen cleans, lubricates, and protects the ear canal. The cleaning function is the result of epithelial migration. Cerumen produced in the ear canal migrates toward the ear canal entrance. Dust and other small particles adhere to the cerumen and are cast off as the cerumen is extruded. Alberti (1964) studied this "conveyor belt" process by quantifying the growth, migration, and desquamation of the skin covering the tympanic membrane and deep ear canal in 62 human subjects. Weekly estimates of rate and migration patterns were made from dye spots placed on the ear drumhead for each subject using handmade sketches and serial photography. Migration was found to be centrifugal from the umbo spreading to all quadrants of the tympanic membrane. Near the umbo, the rate of migration was equivalent to the rate of fingernail growth. The rate of migration accelerated as the markers moved away from the umbo, with the most rapid migration taking place on the anterior wall of the external ear canal.

Jaw motion also helps to clean the ear canal. Debris attached to the ear canal wall is dislodged during speech and chewing as the jaw rotates vertically and horizontally about the terminal hinge axis of the temporomandibular joint, which makes up the inferior portion of the ear canal (Edwards and Harris, 1990).

The lubricating function of cerumen occurs because of the high lipid concentration of sebum, the substance produced by the sebaceous glands. This high lipid concentration accounts for its hydrophobic properties, as it acts as a natural emollient. Harvey (1989) used chromatography to analyze lipid concentrations in wet-type human cerumen and found the major constituents to be cholesterol, squalene, and several series of long-chain fatty acids and alcohols. Bortz et al (1990) reported similar findings.

Pearl

- Allowing the patient to see the amount of cerumen removed from the ear canal may encourage the patient to schedule regular cerumen management, especially if multiple cerumen-related hearing aid repairs have been needed.

Cerumen's cleaning and lubricating function is better understood than its antibacterial properties. Literature reports that cerumen protects the ear canal from bacteria, fungi, and insects (Adams et al, 1978; Caruso and Meyerhoff, 1980; Hawke, 1987). Some controversy exists, however, as some histological and histochemical studies have failed to support cerumen as a bactericide. Creed and Negus (1926) found that freshly secreted cerumen contained no bacteria, but became bacteria-contaminated in a short time. They concluded that cerumen's protective function was to prevent the entrance of dust and insects into the ear canal, acting like a type of "fly paper." Perry and Nichols (1957) supported this finding by observing that cerumen did not inhibit the growth of *Pseudomonas aeruginosa* when this bacterium was cultured from the ear canals of 45 healthy adult volunteers. After examining the effect of cerumen on the organism's growth, it was determined that there was no inhibition. More recent evidence in patients with recurrent otitis externa provides no evidence of cerumen's bactericidal effectiveness against common microorganisms when compared with patients from a healthy population (Pata et al, 2003).

Despite contradictory evidence, other studies have found that cerumen is effective against certain bacteria. Chai and Chai (1980) found that the viability of *Haemophilus influenzae, Escherichia coli* K-12, and *Serratia marcescens* was reduced by more than 99%, and the viability of two *P. aeruginosa* isolates (*E. coli* K-1 and *Streptococcus*) and two *Staphylococcus aureus* isolates was reduced by 30 to 80%. Stone and Fulghum (1984) also showed that a suspension of cerumen in a buffered medium inhibited the growth of certain bacteria (*S. aureus, Staphylococcus epidermidis, Streptococcus pyogenes, Streptococcus* sp. L-22, *E. coli, S. marcescens, Propionibacterium acnes,* and *Corynebacterium* spp. JOM 125 and 138). Based on the more recent studies, it can be concluded that cerumen most likely provides some bacterial protection against some strains of bacteria. The presence of cerumen in the ear canal acts as an oily barrier, preventing the ingress of microorganisms into the skin, and contains antimicrobial substances, including isozyme, immunoglobulin A (IgA), and fatty acids (Osborne and Baty, 1990).

The warm, dark, moist conditions in the ear canal are conducive to the growth of fungus. Hawke (1994) called the ear canal the "greenhouse of the human body." A study by Megarry et al (1988) documented the antifungal properties of cerumen. It was shown that human cerumen inhibited the growth of *Candida* and *Aspergillus,* two species of fungi commonly encountered in otomycosis. The growth of fungus requires an environment with low acidity; the presence of fatty acids in cerumen may inhibit fungal growth (Osborne and Baty, 1990).

♦ Excessive Cerumen

Presence in Certain Populations

Although the amount of cerumen in ear canals varies widely, more striking is the variation in the amount of cerumen across certain populations. **Table 11–1** provides data from children and adults and from two special populations: individuals with mental retardation and the geriatric population. In children, two studies found the prevalence of excessive cerumen to be ~10% (Bricco, 1985; Roche et al, 1978). Based on clinical experience, the 10% prevalence found in these studies appears to be high and may be due to the low number of subjects in the samples. Clinical experience would suggest that the prevalence of excessive cerumen in normal children is similar to adults and ranges from ~3 to 5%.

Table 11–1 Prevalence of Excessive/Impacted Cerumen in Different Populations *

Author(s) (Year)	Sample Size	Prevalence (%)
Children		
Roche et al (1978)	224	10.0
Bricco (1985)	349	10.0
Adults		
Lebensohn [Q56] (1943)	794	2.5
Lebensohn (1943)	3258	8.0
Perry (1957)	111	17.0
Hopkinson (1981)	500	4.0
Foltner (1984)	100	9.0
Cooper (1985)	587	5.0
Gleitman et al (1992)	892	5.0–34.0*
Individuals with Mental Retardation		
Nudo (1965)	494	36.0
Fulton and Griffin (1967)	191	28.0
Brister et al (1986)	88	22.0
Dahle and McCollister (1986)	18	31.0
Crandell and Roeser (1993)	121	28.0
Geriatric Population		
Mahoney (1987)	133	34.0–57.0†
Lewis-Cullinan and Janken (1990)	226	35.0
Mahoney (1993)	104	25.0–42.0‡

*The prevalence was age dependent, with the older subjects having a higher prevalence.
†Thirty-four percent of the subjects were found to have impacted cerumen, and an additional 23% had moderate to large amounts of cerumen, for a total of 57% with excessive/impacted cerumen.
‡Twenty-five percent of the subjects were found to have impacted cerumen, and an additional 17% had moderate to large amounts of cerumen, for a total of 42% with excessive/impacted cerumen.
Source: Adapted from Roeser, R. J., Adams, R. M., Roland, P. S., & Wilson, P. L. (1992). A safe and effective procedure for cerumen management. Audiology Today, 3(3), 20–21, with permission.

As shown in **Table 11–1**, data from seven studies found the prevalence of excessive cerumen in adults to be from 4 to 34%. Lebensohn (1943) studied the largest sample of adults. In two groups of naval personnel, ages 20 to 50, results showed occluding cerumen in 2.5% of 794 reserve midshipmen and in 7.7% of 3258 officers. No hypothesis was given for the sizable difference between the two groups. Methodological differences and sample size may account for some of the variability in prevalence rates shown in **Table 11–1**. There is a general tendency for the studies with the larger sample sizes to have lower prevalence rates. However, these data also suggest that there may be complex interactions accounting for occluding cerumen.

Histochemical studies were performed on cerumen samples from 90 subjects with normal and excessive cerumen to determine if excessive accumulation resulted from failure of normal migration, individual physiology, or hyperactivity of the ceruminous glands (Mandour et al, 1974). Enzymatic histochemical examination on biopsies of ear canal skin strips was performed. Results showed the lumina of the glands were distended in those with excessive cerumen, with the appearance of secretion in the apical parts of the lining of cells, indicating increased secretory activity. This finding suggests that in this study population, excessive cerumen is due primarily to an increased activity of the ceruminous glands.

Although Robinson and colleagues (1990) agree that increased cerumen production may account for excessive cerumen in some patients, they argue that cerumen type affects the process. In two studies, Robinson et al (1990) analyzed hydrated cerumen plugs taken from cerumen samples of 28 individuals and found that those with wet-type cerumen of the hard variety more commonly had chronic and recurrent cerumen impaction. Hard cerumen plugs also contained more sheets of keratin than soft cerumen plugs. From their results, they concluded that patients with chronic and recurrent cerumen impaction have a disorder of keratinocyte separation, resulting in a failure of the individual keratinocytes to break up or separate as they normally would. This condition reduces the integrity of the outwardly migrating sheets of epithelium (Robinson et al, 1990). Taken together, the results of the Mandour and Robinson studies suggest that excessive cerumen is related to a complex interaction of multiple factors.

Several studies suggest no apparent gender difference in the chemical makeup or amount of cerumen in the ear canal (Cipriani et al, 1990; Mandour et al, 1974; Roche et al, 1978; Yassin et al, 1966). Seasonal factors and marked racial differences in the appearance and chemical composition of cerumen have been reported. Cipriani et al (1990) studied cerumen over a 9-month period (November–July) and found decreasing triglyceride production as the seasons progressed from the winter to the summer months. It is suggested in this study that there is a relationship between seasonal diet and triglyceride levels in the ear canal, and a correlation is postulated between ear canal infectious pathology and triglyceride levels.

As shown in **Table 11–1**, patients with mental retardation and geriatric patients are two populations that clearly have a high prevalence of excessive cerumen. Nudo (1965) was

among the first to document that patients with mental retardation are more likely to have excessive cerumen than the general population. He found that 34% of 178 individuals in a residential center for mentally retarded adults had abnormal amounts of cerumen or foreign bodies in their ear canals, and that 23% exhibited hearing loss. Fulton and Griffin (1967) reported that 55 of 191 subjects (29%) had impacted cerumen, with 29 (53%) of those having bilateral impaction and 26 (47%) having unilateral impaction. Comparing otoscopic results from 44 mentally retarded adolescents to a typically developing control group matched for age and sex, Brister et al (1986) found a prevalence of excessive cerumen in 34% of the subjects with mental retardation; none of the normal controls was found to have excessive or impacted cerumen.

Crandell and Roeser (1993) studied longitudinal data from 117 adults with mental retardation (20–67 years of age) living in a privately owned residential center to document prevalence rates of excessive and impacted cerumen. Retrospective data analysis was performed by examining annual audiologic and otoscopic records from a 12-year period. Results from otoscopy were categorized as nonoccluded (< 50% occluded), excessive cerumen (50–80% occluded), and impacted cerumen (> 80% occluded). Of the 586 otoscopic examinations performed, 165 (28%) revealed excessive or impacted cerumen. Another significant finding was that recurrence of excessive and impacted cerumen was seen in 54% of those with excessive cerumen on the first examination and 66% of those with impacted cerumen on the first examination. These findings clearly show that individuals with mental retardation have a propensity to have excessive cerumen on serial examinations. The specific reason for abnormal cerumen accumulation and this propensity for serial problems is unknown. Clearly, regular otoscopy and ear canal management is a necessity for this population, and health care professionals working in these settings must be aware of the negative effect of excessive and impacted cerumen on the hearing health of those afflicted.

As individuals age, the secretion of the ceruminous glands decreases, as does the actual number of ceruminous glands. This results in a drier type of cerumen. This fact, coupled with an increase in the number and coarseness of hairs in the ear canal, especially in males, causes an increase in the percentage of geriatric patients who have excessive cerumen (Ruby, 1986). Gleitman et al (1992) clearly demonstrated the relationship between age and increased occurrence of excessive and impacted cerumen when they compared the extent of impaction to the chronological age of 892 subjects. A linear relationship was found in data, showing that 5% of the youngest age group (26–44 years) had excessive cerumen, whereas 34% of the oldest age group (65–74 years) had excessive cerumen.

Mahoney (1987) screened 133 elderly subjects and found that 82 (34%) had impacted cerumen, and an additional 56 (23%) had moderate to large amounts of cerumen. In a follow-up investigation of 104 nursing home residents, 62 to 100 years of age, 25 to 42% were found to have ears with moderate to large amounts of impacted cerumen (Mahoney, 1993).

Lewis-Cullinan and Janken (1990) performed otoscopic examinations on a random sample of 226 individuals 65 years of age or older. In addition, a four-frequency screening was performed at 40 dB hearing level (HL) on all subjects. If excessive cerumen was found during otoscopy, a follow-up rescreen was performed after cerumen removal. Thirty-five percent of the subjects had occluding cerumen, and hearing was shown to improve on the screening test following cerumen management. These figures clearly suggest the need for routine management of the ear canals of the geriatric population.

Pathophysiology

Complications of excessive cerumen in the ear canal include tinnitus, vertigo, itching, pain, external otitis, and hearing loss (Adams et al, 1978; Bricco, 1985; DeWeese and Saunders, 1973). Chronic cough has also been reported (Raman, 1986). The larynx is innervated by the vagus nerve, and the auricular branch of the vagus nerve serves the posterior and inferior wall of the ear canal and concha area of the pinna. Reflex coughing and sometimes sneezing can occur when the ear canal is manipulated during procedures, such as cerumen removal, because of this innervation.

Pearl

- Because of vagal nerve innervation of the ear canal and the possibility of cardiac arrhythmia (syncope), during ear canal manipulation patients should be seated in a chair with surrounding support in the event they lose consciousness.

Vagus nerve connections between the ear canal and tympanic membrane and the cardiac muscle also explain why cardiac depression has been seen during ear canal irrigation (Prasad, 1984). Although cardiac depression is rare, clinicians should take note of the possibility during ear canal manipulation (cerumen management, ear impression taking, ENG testing, etc.), and be aware that loss of consciousness may result when it occurs. Patients must be seated with proper support during ear canal manipulation so that loss of consciousness does not result in head trauma.

Myers et al (1987) reported one case of pseudodementia, a deterioration in mental and behavioral functions that simulates dementia, associated with impacted cerumen. Although this is an isolated report, it reinforces the discomfort that long-term occlusion of the ear canal can cause, which might be associated with abnormal behavioral manifestations.

Excessive cerumen affects auditory thresholds by gradually decreasing high-frequency sensitivity as the amount of cerumen increases; only when complete occlusion occurs are low-frequency thresholds attenuated. The data in **Figure 11–3** are from Roeser et al (2005) and show this effect. It is clear that thresholds below 1000 Hz are only slightly decreased until complete occlusion occurs. The

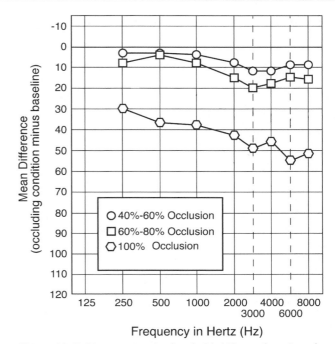

Figure 11–3 Mean pure-tone threshold shift as a function of percentage of ear canal occlusion. (From Roeser, R. J., Lai, L., & Clark, J. (2005). Effect of earcanal occlusion on pure tone threshold sensitivity. Journal of the American Academy of Audiology, 16(9), 740–746, with permission.)

decrease of low-frequency sensitivity explains why patients complain of sudden onset hearing loss when complete occlusion occurs. These patients likely had gradually increasing amounts of high-frequency loss as the occlusion increased, but it was not until the loss affected hearing in the speech frequencies that the behavioral consequence of the loss had its full impact. Of particular importance is that these data are in agreement with Chandler (1964).

In the 40 to 60% and 60 to 80% partially occluded conditions, thresholds decreased by an average of 7.5 and 13.0 dB, respectively. At frequencies above 1000 Hz, the average threshold shifts for the two partially occluded conditions were 10.0 and 16.8 dB, respectively. These findings have significant implications, especially when data are compared for serial audiometric testing, such as for industrial hearing conservation. Otoscopy and cerumen management are a prerequisites for valid threshold data when ear canals are occluded by 40 to 60% or more. In addition, it must be emphasized that the threshold shifts occurring when the ear canal is partially or completely occluded would be added to any preexisting sensorineural hearing loss (as shown in **Fig. 11–1**).

In contrast to excessive cerumen, asteatosis is a condition in which cerumen is underproduced or absent in the ear canal. Because of a lack of proper lubrication and accompanying dryness of the ear canal, patients with asteatosis will complain of ear canal itching. Prescriptive and over-the-counter (OTC) topical ointments are helpful for these patients.

◆ Excessive Cerumen Management

Knowledge and Skills Required

Because a procedure is within the scope of practice of an audiologist does not necessarily mean that the audiologist should perform the procedure. Professional ethical codes stress the competency of the practitioner and the safety of the patient. ASHA's Ad Hoc Committee on Advances in Clinical Practice (ASHA, 1992) addressed the education, training, knowledge, and skills necessary to perform cerumen management, as well as the precautions each audiologist should consider prior to undertaking cerumen management procedures (see **Table 11–2**). As shown in **Table 11–2**, ASHA recommends that audiologists have education and training in otoscopy, knowledge of abnormal conditions of the ear canal and tympanic membrane, and supervised experience in cerumen removal. Precautions include actions that may protect the audiologist from potential liability-producing procedural omissions. ASHA suggests that audiologists question regulatory bodies about limitations on their scope of practice, inquire with liability insurance carriers about their position on this procedure, examine specific institutional restrictions at the audiologist's place of employment, follow the universal precautions of the Centers for Disease Control and Prevention (CDC; 1988; see also Chapter 10 in this volume), institute an emergency medical assistance plan, and obtain the informed consent of the patient.

Infection Control

> **Pearl**
>
> • Hand washing is the most effective way to prevent the spread of infection and disease.

Chapter 10 in this volume covers the topic of infection control in detail. As pointed out in that chapter, cerumen is not a medium for infectious diseases, including acquired immunodeficiency syndrome (AIDS; ASHA, 1990). However, because of the possibility of skin lacerations and the potential for cerumen to contain blood, the universal precautions to prevent the risk of disease from bloodborne pathogens must be followed carefully when managing cerumen (CDC, 1988). Whether gloves should be used routinely for cerumen management as an infection control procedure is an individual decision. Some practitioners will choose to wear gloves, whereas others will not. However, whenever blood is present or when dealing with certain patients, such as those who are immunocompromised, gloves become a necessity.

Table 11–2 Education and Training, Precautions, and Knowledge and Skills Recommended for Cerumen Management by the ASHA Ad Hoc Committee on Advances in Clinical Practice

Education and Training

1. Use of pneumatic otoscopy, recognition of the canal and tympanic membrane condition, and removal of cerumen
2. Knowledge of medical conditions that might have an impact on the safe performance of cerumen management
3. Supervised experience in these procedures

Precautions

1. Inform institution and/or regulatory bodies (state licensure boards) that these procedures are within the scope of practice of audiology.
2. Check with appropriate state licensure board(s) to determine whether there are any limitations on the scope of audiology practice that restrict the performance of these procedures.
3. Check professional liability insurance to ensure that there is no exclusion applicable to these procedures.
4. Check medical policy, institutional insurance coverage, and delineation of practice privileges for the specific institution to ensure that there are no restrictions applicable to an audiologist performing these procedures.
5. Follow the universal precautions (ASHA, 1990; Centers for Disease Control and Prevention, 1988) to prevent the risk of disease from bloodborne pathogens.
6. Know who to contact in the event of an emergency or if medical assistance is needed.
7. Obtain informed consent by explaining the procedures to the patient, and maintain complete and adequate documentation.

Knowledge and Skills

1. Otoscopy: obstruction/medical conditions
2. Otoscopy: T mobility of eardrum
3. Otoscopy: status of ear canal and tympanic membrane
4. Otoscopy: cerumen verification/proceed to remove or refer
5. Pinna inspection/otoscopy for abnormal conditions
6. Emergency procedures needed
7. Cerumen removal methods and need for referral

Source: From American Speech-Language-Hearing Association. (1992). External auditory canal examination and cerumen management. ASHA, 34(Suppl. 7), 22–24, with permission.

Pearl

- Washing hands in front of the patient and using gloves when appropriate will increase the patient's confidence in the clinician's knowledge and skill as a practitioner. Additionally, instruments should be cleaned after use in each ear to prevent the possibility of spreading infection and disease.

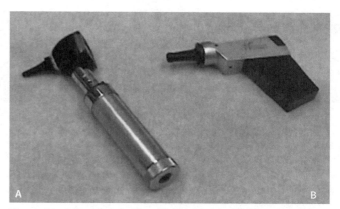

Figure 11–4 Two types of handheld otoscopes: **(A)** the Welch Allyn (Welch Allyn Inc., Skaneateles, New York) Model 25020 and **(B)** [Q47] the [Q48]Hotchkiss.

Procedures

Published procedures for safe and effective cerumen management are available (Ballachanda and Peers, 1992; Bradley, 1980; Burgess, 1977; Carne, 1980; Graber, 1986; Larsen, 1976; Manning, 1992; Marshall and Attia, 1983; Mawson, 1974; Roeser et al, 1992; Salomon, 1967). As pointed out by these reports, when proper techniques are followed, effective cerumen management is a relatively simple and safe procedure. In fact, cerumen management can be performed as a self-management procedure using an OTC ceruminolytic to soften the cerumen and irrigation with a rubber bulb to remove it from the ear canal (Jurish, 1991). The American Academy of Otolaryngology–Head and Neck Surgery (AAO-HNS, 1991) even recommends patient use of OTC ceruminolytics and irrigations when it can be established that the tympanic membrane is not perforated.

To ensure minimum risk and maximum efficiency, audiologists who manage cerumen must carefully follow accepted procedures. Accepted procedures require the preliminary steps of taking an appropriate case/medical history and performing an otoscopic examination of the ear canal. Some clinicians also perform premanagement audiologic and/or immittance tests and use a ceruminolytic to soften the cerumen. The removal of cerumen is accomplished using any one or a combination of several different procedures, including mechanical removal, irrigation of the ear canal with an oral jet irrigator, and suction.

Preliminary Steps

Examine the Ear Canal Visual examination of the ear canal and tympanic membrane (Sullivan, 1997) is an essential preliminary step in all audiologic procedures, from simple screening to comprehensive diagnostic evaluation. During cerumen management, examination of the ear canal is performed as a preliminary step to ensure that the material in the ear canal is, in fact, cerumen. Historically, otoscopy has moved from direct observation without the aid of special lighting or special instruments, to handheld otoscopes, to the use of video-otoscopes. Video-otoscopes have a miniature video camera that projects a highly defined color image of the ear canal and tympanic membrane on a television monitor (Sullivan, 1997).

Pearl

- The decision to remove cerumen from an ear canal must be based on the conclusion from examination of the ear canal that the material in the ear canal is, in fact, cerumen and not some other substance, such as blood or purulent material.

Figure 11–4 shows two types of handheld otoscopes. The Welch Allyn (Welch Allyn Inc., Skaneateles, New York) Model 25020 is in common usage and features a rechargeable battery and disposable specula. The Hotchkiss otoscope allows for easy insertion of an instrument into the ear for the removal of cerumen without the parallax error common with conventional otoscopes.

Pearl

- During ear canal examination and cerumen management, the patient's head should be at the same level as the examiner's head.

The development of fiberoptics and the miniaturization of video camera components provided for the development of the video-otoscope. The first models were introduced to audiologists in 1983 by Jedmed Instrument Co. (St. Louis, Missouri; Sullivan, 1997). An example is shown in **Fig. 11–5**. The video-otoscope facilitates examination of the ear canal, patient education, referral of abnormal conditions to physicians, and treatment of occluding or excessive cerumen.

Examination of the ear canal is essential prior to performing audiologic procedures to identify conditions that might complicate or contraindicate the procedure. The presence of excessive or occluding cerumen is a finding that might

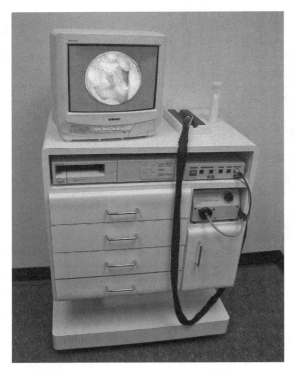

Figure 11–5 Example of a video-otoscope. [Q49]

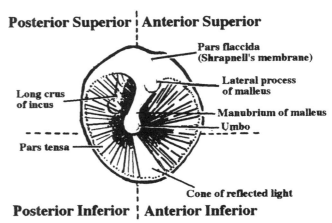

Figure 11–7 The landmarks of the normal tympanic membrane.

necessitate postponing an audiologic procedure until cerumen removal has been accomplished. **Figure 11–6** shows an example of a normal ear canal and one with a cerumen occlusion that would prevent many audiologic procedures without cerumen removal first. Otoscopic examination should determine if there are any unusual conditions requiring otologic referral. The tympanic membrane should be examined carefully, and normal landmarks should be noted (**Fig. 11–7**). If the tympanic membrane does not appear healthy, appropriate referrals should be made. When occluding material obscures the tympanic membrane, the audiologist first must make sure that the material is cerumen. The presence of abnormalities in the ear canal that might represent purulent drainage, blood, or other foreign bodies should be referred for medical examination. Procedures for removal of the cerumen must then be considered based on its type, consistency, texture, and location. The otoscopic exam also enables the audiologist to view and incorporate the patient's individual ear canal characteristics into any treatment plans. It is important to note the size and shape of the ear canal, locate the relative position of the tympanic membrane, and determine any ear canal turns or bends that deviate from expected patterns. If cerumen management is to be performed, the otoscopic examination also must be made to locate the blockage precisely to assist in developing a strategy for the removal of the cerumen. Based

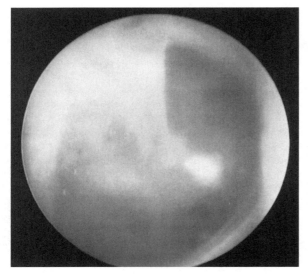

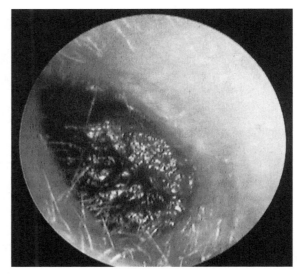

Figure 11–6 (A) A normal ear canal and **(B)** an ear canal occluded with wet-type cerumen.

on this thorough visual inspection of the ear canal, the audiologist can proceed with planned audiologic procedures, referral for medical examination, or treatment to remove cerumen deemed to interfere with planned procedures.

Obtain an Appropriate Case History   Perforation of the tympanic membrane or the presence of myringotomy (pressure equalization; PE) tubes are universal contraindications for cerumen management by ear canal irrigation. Good clinical judgment must be used to determine if patients should be referred to their physicians (or otolaryngologists) for cerumen management when any of the following are present:

♦ Recent earache

♦ History of ear surgery

♦ Drainage

♦ Dizziness

♦ Diabetes mellitus

♦ AIDS (ASHA, 1990)

♦ Blood-thinning medications

♦ Any other possible condition that would put the patient at risk

Irrigating the ear canal is contraindicated in the presence of diabetes mellitus and AIDS due to the possible development of malignant external otitis (*Pseudomonas* osteomyelitis), a life-threatening disease precipitated by external otitis. Trauma to the ear canal that is possible from irrigation may result in an innocuous infection of the squamous epithelium of the ear canal. This infection can progress to the underlying soft tissue, cartilage, blood vessels, or bone and eventually lead to cellulitis, chondritis, or osteomyelitis of the temporal bone. If untreated, invasive external otitis may lead to osteomyelitis of the base of the skull, multiple cranial nerve palsies, meningitis, and even death (Zikk et al, 1991). Because of the serious consequences, it is clear that the medical history must include questions about diabetes and/or AIDS; patients having either condition should be referred to their physician for cerumen management. For these patients, ear canal irrigation is contraindicated in favor of mechanical removal or suctioning under direct (microscopic) visualization (Zikk et al, 1991).

Optional Steps

Premanagement Audiometric and Immittance Data   This step is especially important when the tympanic membrane cannot be visualized by otoscopy. Cerumen management with water irrigation is contraindicated when the ear canal is partially occluded (not impacted), obscuring the tympanic membrane, and any of the following are present:

♦ A conductive component on the audiogram

♦ The inability to maintain a hermetic seal when performing immittance measures

♦ A flat (type B) tympanogram and a high ear canal physical volume

Any of the above findings would suggest tympanic membrane perforation and/or middle ear pathology.

Pearl

• Performing tympanometry before and after cerumen removal verifies that the tympanic membrane is intact. This procedure will help decide whether to proceed with irrigation and will document the status of the tympanic membrane after the procedure for medicolegal purposes.

Ceruminolytic   A softening agent (a ceruminolytic, mineral oil, or another recognized softening agent) should be placed into the ear canal prior to irrigation (see **Fig. 11–8**). It is best if the softening agent is used 2 or 3 times daily for 3 to 5 days prior to cerumen extraction. However, if a period of 3 to 5 days before the procedure is not possible, then using the softening step for as long as possible (30–45 minutes) before the removal process should prove beneficial. For dry and hard cerumen, a longer softening process will be mandatory (Marshall and Attia, 1983).

Special Consideration

• Softening cerumen with a ceruminolytic for 2 or 3 days is a requirement if the ear canal is occluded with hard, dry, long-term cerumen impaction.

If a softening agent is not used, cerumen removal may be impossible with irrigation. Furthermore, the ear canal may be left abraded, sore, and possibly bleeding, which would make it difficult or impossible to perform any further audiologic testing that requires a clear ear canal.

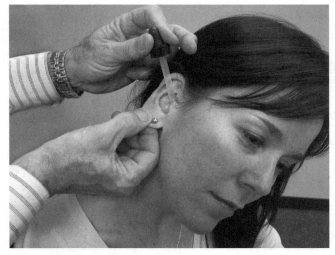

Figure 11–8 Using a ceruminolytic before cerumen management softens the debris and may facilitate cerumen removal.

Table 11–3 Summary of Commercially Available Ceruminolytics and Other Products Used for Softening Cerumen

Brand Name	Type	Composition
Audiologist's Choice	OTC	Carbamide peroxide (6.5%) and glycerine
Auro Ear Drops	OTC	Carbamide peroxide (6.5%) and glycerine
Bausch & Lomb	OTC	Carbamide peroxide (6.5%) and glycerine
Cerumenex Drops	Rx	Triethanolamine polypeptide, oleate condensate
Debrox	OTC	Carbamide peroxide (6.5%) and glycerine
Murine Ear Drops	OTC	Carbamide peroxide (6.5%) and glycerine
Other Products for Softening Cerumen		
Baby oil		
Colace liquid (docusate sodium)		
Hydrogen peroxide (3%)		
Mineral oil		
Sodium bicarbonate		
Virgin olive oil		

OTC, over the counter; Rx, by prescription.

Table 11–3 is a list of the commercially available ceruminolytics as well as several other common agents that have been used to soften cerumen. As shown, the composition of the OTC ceruminolytics is identical across the various brands that are available. Other products for softening cerumen are baby oil, Colace liquid, hydrogen peroxide, mineral oil, sodium bicarbonate, and virgin olive oil. All of these products have been reported to be effective in softening cerumen.

Several studies comparing the efficacy of different ceruminolytics and other agents have been reported. Three studies in particular assessed the effectiveness of ceruminolytics by measuring the amount of water needed to irrigate the ear canal successfully following the use of the ceruminolytic. Bailes et al (1967) found the ceruminolytic Waxsol (Norgine Ltd.) more effective than Cerumol (Laboratories for Applied Biology Ltd.). However, Burgess (1966) and Chaput de Saintonge and Johnstone (1973) failed to note any major differences between the preparations they evaluated. Included were olive oil, Xerumenex (Viatris), maize oil, and Dioctyl-medo [Q23] ear drops (a wetting agent). In vitro evaluations of Cerumol, olive oil, Waxsol, sodium bicarbonate, Cerumenex, and Dioctyl ear capsules have shown mixed results (Fraser, 1970; Horowitz, 1968). Fraser (1970) concluded that in vitro studies are inadequate as a means of assessing the efficacy of wax solvents because they do not consider skin irritation and because they do not provide actual information on the process of cerumen removal. Fahmy and Whitefield (1982) reported data from a multicenter trial comparing Exterol (Dermal Laboratories), Cerumol, and glycerol. Although their conclusion was that Exterol is markedly superior to the other ceruminolytics, their data were not compelling.

Robinson and Hawke (1989) found that a 10% solution of sodium bicarbonate was a more effective ceruminolytic than any of several organic liquids, including glycerine, olive oil, Cerumenex, Auralgan (Wyeth-Ayerst), and alcohol. The action of sodium bicarbonate disintegrated experimental 250 mg blocks of actual human cerumen in a matter of

minutes, as compared with several days for some of the organic liquids. The authors indicated that cerumen underwent significant swelling after treatment with the solution of sodium bicarbonate. It was also noted that the ceruminolytic used would depend upon the type of removal procedure that was contemplated. More recently, a randomized clinical trial compared the use of a docusate (a stool softener), triethanolamine polypeptide, and irrigation with a saline solution to determine their effectiveness in relieving cerumen obstruction in children. Neither ceruminolytic provided improved tympanic membrane visibility over saline irrigation (Whatley et al, 2003).

Overall, results from the above studies do not support using any one ceruminolytic over another, although ceruminolytics containing sodium bicarbonate appear to have some disintegrating advantage. The choice of whether to use a ceruminolytic or not will be made by individual clinicians. Reports on the clinical application of ceruminolytics have shown that when ears have hard, dry, impacted cerumen, the process of removal is significantly facilitated by administering a ceruminolytic for 2 or 3 days prior to removal (Roeser et al, 1991, 1992).

Informed Consent   Prior to cerumen management, the procedure should be explained to the patient, and permission should be obtained. For patients with hearing impairment, it is advisable to have printed materials describing the procedure and the risks.

♦ Cerumen Extraction Procedures

Cerumen management can be accomplished using mechanical removal, suction, or water irrigation. The following describes the procedures used for each technique. However, it should be pointed out that in routine practice, it is not unusual to use a combination of these approaches.

- During cerumen management, illuminating the ear canal with a head mirror, head lamp, or otoscope is very important.

Mechanical Removal

Mechanical removal is, by far, the most common procedure for removing cerumen when the ear canal is partially occluded and the ear canal debris is not adhering tightly to the skin of the ear canal. The following instruments, equipment, and supplies (some of which are shown in **Fig. 11–9**) are needed to carry out the procedure:

- Various sterile instruments, including wire loops, dull ring curets, forceps, and alligator forceps
- 4 × 4 gauze pad for cleaning instruments
- Otoscope specula to improve precision of instrument use

- When inserting any instrument into the ear canal, to avoid injury to the patient if sudden movement occurs, the clinician's hand should be braced on the patient's head.

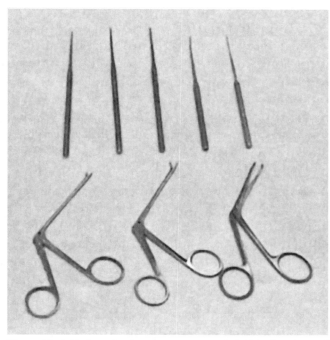

Figure 11–9 Various-sized cerumen curets and alligator forceps used for mechanical removal of cerumen.

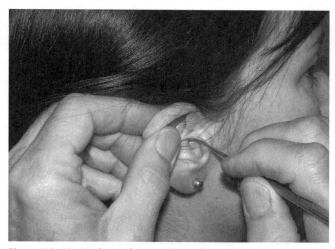

Figure 11–10 Mechanical removal is performed by bracing the hand holding the instrument against the patient's head and carefully inserting the instrument into the ear canal, while straightening the canal by lifting the pinna with the opposite hand.

A step-by-step procedure for mechanical removal of cerumen is as follows:

1. Based on findings from the otoscopic examination, the instrument to be used is selected.

2. The patient's ear canal is straightened with the examiner's free hand by gently pulling the pinna slightly backward and upward. The examiner's free hand and forearm are used to steady and control the patient's head by having him or her press against them.

3. The use of a fiberoptic otoscope as a light source, the use of both eyes to achieve depth perception, and insertion of an instrument through the speculum to guide the position of the curet and to improve depth judgment (**Figs. 11–10** and **11–11**) are recommended.

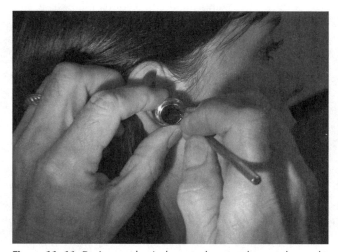

Figure 11–11 During mechanical removal, a speculum can be used to straighten the ear canal and keep it open while the instrument is used to remove debris.

4. The instrument is inserted into the ear canal against the cerumen, either on the lateral or superoposterior position, and the cerumen is gently dislodged and removed from the ear canal. When curets are used, loosening the debris and gently rolling it laterally is the goal in most situations. If a speculum is used, removal of the speculum and curet simultaneously will prevent the cerumen from "fouling" the speculum and blocking the vision of the examiner.

5. Cerumen that is hard and dry may adhere to the skin lining of the canal. Removal of cerumen in this case may cause patient discomfort and injury to the canal wall, as well as bleeding. The use of a ceruminolytic for 30 to 45 minutes to soften the debris may provide a better result.

6. If the majority of the cerumen has been successfully removed, but a cleaner canal is needed for a procedure, such as probe microphone measurements, it may be advisable to use suction or irrigation, rather than risking injury to the patient by scraping the canal wall.

Suction

Suction equipment is typically available through medical supply companies; an example of a suction system is shown in **Fig. 11–12**. Appropriate-sized suction tips must be chosen based on the patient's ear canal shape and size.

Pearl

• To be effective, a suction instrument with at least 21 inches/Hg vacuum is needed.

Cerumen extraction using suction is particularly appropriate when the cerumen is very soft or semiliquid and can be found near the entrance to the canal (Ballachanda and Peers, 1992). There is a possibility that the suction device may become clogged during the procedure. Manning (1992)

suggested that a warm cup of water be available to suction through the tip periodically to keep the pathway clear. Large pieces of cerumen should not be suctioned through the apparatus, as these also are likely to cause clogging of the line.

There is some indication that the sound created by the suction device may create temporary threshold shifts. Young children are often frightened by the loudness of suctioning; for this reason, suction may not be as well tolerated by this population.

The step-by-step procedure for ear canal suctioning is as follows (Manning, 1992):

1. Before the procedure begins, the patient should be instructed about the sound of the suction in the ear canal to prevent surprised discomfort.

2. A 4 × 4 gauze pad and cup of water should be available in a convenient location to clean the internal and external portion of the suction tip and tubing when necessary.

3. Using the knowledge gained from a thorough otoscopic examination, identify the location of the cerumen in the ear canal, and insert the suction tip through a speculum, held in place by the hand braced against the head, onto the surface of the cerumen.

4. Increased suction pressure can be achieved by using the thumb to cover the suction hole on the suction tip.

5. Vacuum the cerumen from the ear canal by gently moving the suction tip into the cerumen.

6. Sometimes a piece of cerumen may attach itself to the suction tip without being vacuumed through the system. If this happens, remove the suction tip and the speculum simultaneously, and clean the tip with the 4 × 4 gauze pad.

7. Large and/or hard cerumen that is not suctioned from the ear canal may need to be extracted with either mechanical removal or irrigation.

Irrigation

Water irrigation is preferred with more complete occlusions and when the cerumen is hard and dry. Irrigation typically results in a cleaner canal, but water may be present following irrigation and must be removed prior to carrying out many audiologic procedures.

Figure 11–13 shows several of the instruments needed to perform aural irrigation:

♦ An irrigation tool: ear syringe, oral jet irrigator (WaterPik), or earwash system (Welch Allyn Ear Wash System)

♦ A kidney-shaped basin to catch the water

♦ Aural bulb or syringe

♦ Cerumen curets or spoons

Also needed are a plastic sheet to cover the patient, towels to wipe up excess water, and cotton swabs.

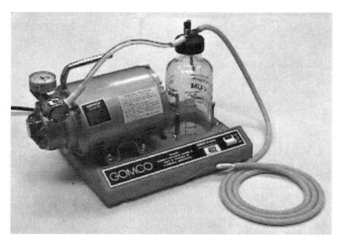

Figure 11–12 Example of a system used for suctioning cerumen. [Q51]

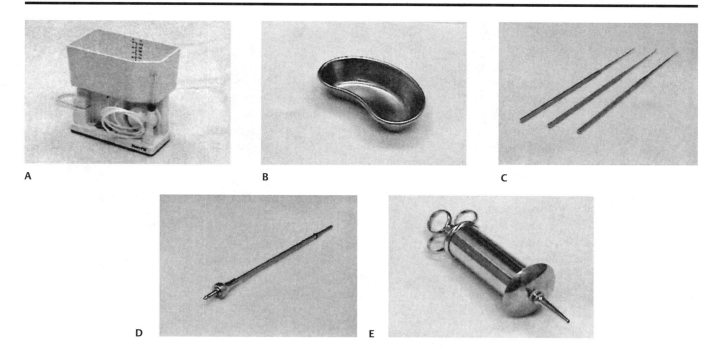

Figure 11–13 Irrigation of the ear canal is accomplished with **(A)** an oral jet irrigator, **(B)** a kidney-shaped bowl, and **(C)** cerumen curets or spoons. Also shown **(D)** is an alternate attachment for the oral jet irrigator. The alternate attachment specifically directs the water flow away from the tympanic membrane. An aural bulb or an aural syringe **(E)** can also be used.

Irrigation must be performed carefully, as damage to the ear (iatrogenic hearing loss and vertigo) can result (Bapat et al, 2001.) Using an oral jet irrigator has the advantage of providing a constant, controlled pulsating pressure stream, whereas the pressure produced by an ear syringe is highly variable. However, oral jet irrigators can produce extremely high water pressures, and severe damage to the ear can result unless low pressure settings are used (Roeser et al, 1992; Seiler, 1980). Bailey (1983) stated that external otitis and perforation of the tympanic membrane with a secondary purulent otitis media can result from using an oral jet irrigator in the ear canal. In addition, he speculated that frequent use could result in cochlear damage. However, he later acknowledged that oral jet irrigators can be employed without complications if patients have strong, healthy tympanic membranes (Bailey, 1984).

Controversial Point

- Using an oral jet irrigator to manage cerumen has been deemed unacceptable by some practitioners because high pressures will cause damage to the tympanic membrane. However, when used at proper pressure settings, oral jet irrigation of the ear canal is safe and highly effective.

The most compelling data on the potential hazards of using oral jet irrigators for cerumen management are from Dinsdale et al (1991). Case studies were presented of three patients who had suffered otologic insult from the use of an oral jet irrigator for cerumen management. All three patients had perforations of the tympanic membrane with associated hearing loss. Moreover, vertigo, ataxia, nausea, and vomiting were present in two of the patients. In addition to these case studies, Dinsdale et al (1991) reported data from irrigating the ear canals of "fresh" cadavers with an oral jet irrigator at full power and at one-third power. Tympanic membrane perforations were created in three (6%) of the 50 ears: 2 at one-third power and 1 at full power.

Pitfall

- Never turn the oral jet irrigator on while the irrigator tip is in the ear canal. Always physically feel the water stream from the irrigator tip for pressure and temperature before inserting it into the ear canal.

It is clear that there are potential hazards associated with using an oral jet irrigator for cerumen management. However, if used properly, an oral jet irrigator is safe and effective. It is very important to use a low pressure setting (no more than one fourth of the maximum); higher settings can cause damage to the ear. All precautions should be taken to prevent setting the pressure adjustment at higher levels.

The Welch Allyn Ear Wash System was specifically designed for ear irrigation (**Fig. 11–14**). The system regulates water pressure and warm water temperature. The water is delivered to and suctioned from the ear canal by the probe using a closed loop system.

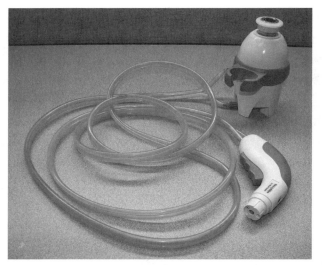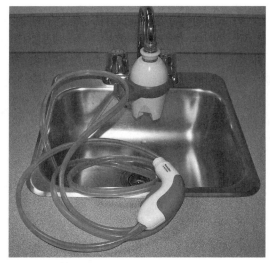

A **B**

Figure 11–14 The Welch Allyn (Welch Allyn Inc., Skaneateles, New York) Ear Wash System was specifically designed for aural irrigation. **(A)** The system consists of a regulator, two plastic tubes used as a closed loop system, and pistol-like irrigator. **(B)** The regulator is attached to a standard faucet.

The step-by-step procedure for ear canal irrigation is as follows:

1. A plastic sheet is used to keep the patient dry during the irrigation procedure.

2. The oral jet irrigator is filled with lukewarm water. A thermometer can be used to ensure that the water is at body temperature (37°C, 98°F). Cold or hot water cannot be used because the vestibular reflex may be triggered, causing dizziness and possibly vomiting.

3. The patient is asked to hold the kidney-shaped basin firmly against the side of the face immediately below the ear, with the head tilted slightly downward **(Fig. 11–15)**.

4. The patient's ear canal is straightened with the examiner's free hand by gently pulling the pinna slightly backward and upward. The free hand and forearm are used to steady and control the patient's head by having him or her press against them.

5. The oral jet irrigator is turned on, and the tip is placed into the kidney-shaped basin. Once it has been established that the pressure from the irrigator is not too high, the tip is inserted into the ear canal.

6. The stream of water from the oral jet irrigator is directed against the wall of the ear canal not obscured by the occluding cerumen; usually the jet will be aimed at the superior ear canal wall. If there is complete occlusion, the stream is directed at the superior wall of the ear canal at the edge of the cerumen plug. This procedure will build up a slight pressure behind the cerumen plug, fragment it, and force it out. Directing the stream at or against the cerumen plug should be avoided, as this may force the cerumen deeper into the ear canal.

7. Care is taken to ensure that the tip of the instrument is inserted just at the entrance of the ear canal so that there is space to allow drainage of the irrigating fluid. If the entrance is blocked, fluid cannot drain, a pressure buildup will occur, and damage to the ear is possible. Also, care must be taken that the tip of the instrument is not inserted too deeply, because the inner half of the ear canal is sensitive.

8. The ear canal is irrigated for 20 to 30 seconds. After each irrigation, the ear is checked with an otoscope to determine progress in removing the cerumen. Irrigation continues until the tympanic membrane is sufficiently visible for examination. If the cerumen does not dislodge after several attempts at irrigation, clinical judgment should be used to determine if further softening for 3 to 5 days will be required before additional irrigation is attempted or if the ear presents with a difficult condition that will require medical referral. If

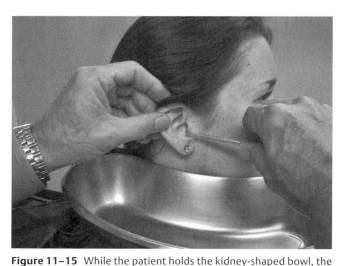

Figure 11–15 While the patient holds the kidney-shaped bowl, the tip of the oral jet irrigator is inserted into the ear canal, allowing space for the water to exit. The water jet should be directed toward the superior margin of the debris, which will allow water to fill the backspace and force the debris from the canal.

medical referral is chosen, the continued use of a softening agent will make the removal process easier during the office visit. It is not advisable to use the softening agent for more than 3 to 5 days.

9. A blunt ear curet or a wire curet (cerumen spoon) is used to remove cerumen that is dislodged through irrigation but remains and partially occludes the ear canal. When using the curet, adequate lighting is provided with a head mirror or head lamp. The procedure used is to place both hands on the patient's head to stabilize the head and neck. With the curet between the thumb and forefinger, the curet tip is slowly inserted into the ear canal just beyond the dislodged cerumen plug. The cerumen is gently spooned or rolled out. Extreme care is taken not to put undue pressure on the skin of the ear canal.

10. Once the cerumen is removed, the ear canal is examined with an otoscope to verify that the canal is cerumen free and there is no bleeding. The ear canal and possibly the tympanic membrane may be slightly reddened.

11. If the ear canal is clear and there is no bleeding, the canal is dried by placing several drops of 50% vinegar 50% alcohol or 70% alcohol solution (at body temperature) into it. After using the solution, the patient's head is inclined for 15 to 25 seconds to allow any liquid to drain away.

12. The pinna and outer portion of the ear canal are dried with a towel.

13. As a final step, the ear canal is checked with an otoscope to make sure that all of the fluid is drained from it and that there is no bleeding. Bleeding is rare, but should it occur, a cotton swab is used to absorb the small amounts of blood. If the bleeding is excessive, referral to a physician is needed.

14. The procedure and outcome are documented in the patient's chart, including a description of the otoscopic examination both pre- and postmanagement, as well as follow-up audiometric findings.

Nontraditional Procedures

Ear Candling

Ear candling, also known as "ear coning" or thermoauricular therapy, uses a hollow tube made of rolled fabric soaked in beeswax to resemble a candle. The candle is put through a hole in an aluminum plate, which protects the ear from hot wax and burning debris. With the patient lying on his or her side with the affected ear up, one end of the candle is placed into the patient's ear canal, and the aluminum plate is positioned against the ear. The other end of the candle is then lit, and the material is allowed to burn down slowly (~10–15 minutes) until it reaches the aluminum plate near the ear canal. After the candle is extinguished, the remaining material is removed from the ear canal. In theory, the candle is supposed to draw cerumen from the ear canal employing capillary forces produced by the burning candle (the "chimney effect").

Despite numerous anecdotal claims, no reliable effectiveness data exist for ear candling. Moreover, concern has been raised regarding safety. A survey of 122 otolaryngologists in the United Kingdom revealed that 14 physicians had treated patients with complications from the use of ear candles, including 13 with burns, 7 with occlusions of the ear canal, 6 with temporary hearing loss, 3 with external otitis, and 1 with tympanic membrane perforation (Seely et al, 1996).

Ototek Loop

The Ototek loop (Earest Inc., Columbia, Missouri) was designed by an otologist as an inexpensive cerumen extraction tool. The device has a cerumen loop at the end of a plastic probe; a shield prevents the probe from penetrating the eardrum. The looped end is inserted along the edge of the ear canal, and the tip is moved to the opposite side, allowing debris to be scooped out.

◆ Summary

This chapter reviews the physiology and pathophysiology of cerumen and describes issues and procedures for cerumen management. Cerumen is the product of two types of glands in the ear canal: sebaceous and modified apocrine. Two types of cerumen, dry and wet, are genetically determined. The function of cerumen is to cleanse and lubricate the ear canal, and it has some protective properties. Although cerumen normally builds up and falls from the ear canal, it can become excessive or impacted, a finding that is common in individuals with mental retardation and in the elderly. Cerumen management has risks associated with it that can be minimized through proper extraction techniques. The procedures for cerumen management include mechanical removal, suction, and irrigation.

References

Adams, G., Boies, L., & Papparella, M. (1978). Fundamentals of otolaryngology. Philadelphia: W. B. Saunders.

Alberti, P. W. (1964). Epithelial migration on the tympanic membrane. Journal of Laryngology and Otology, 78, 808–830.

American Academy of Otolaryngology–Head and Neck Surgery. (1991). Earwax: What to do about it. Washington, DC: Author.

American Speech-Language-Hearing Association. (1990). Report update: AIDS/HIV implications for speech-language pathologists and audiologists. ASHA, 32, 46–48.

American Speech-Language-Hearing Association. (1992). External auditory canal examination and cerumen management. ASHA, 34(Suppl. 7), 22–24.

Bailes, I. H., Baird, J. W., Bari, M. A., et al. (1967). Wax softening with a new preparation. Practitioner, 199, 359–362.

Bailey, B. J. (1983). Impacted ear wax and a water-pick instrument. Journal of the American Medical Association, 250, 1456.

Bailey, B. J. (1984). Editorial reply to "Removal of cerumen." Journal of the American Medical Association, 251(4), 1681.

Ballachanda, B. B. (1995). The human ear canal. San Diego, CA: Singular Publishing Group.

Ballachanda, B. B., & Peers, C. J. (1992). Cerumen management: Instruments and procedures. ASHA.

Bapat, U., Nia, J., & Bance, M. (2001). Severe audiovestibular loss following ear syringing for wax removal. Journal of Laryngology and Otology, 115, 410–411.

Bass, E. J., & Jackson, J. F. (1977). Cerumen types in Eskimos. American Journal of Physical Anthropology, 47, 209–210.

Bortz, J. T., Wertz, P. W., & Downing, D. T. (1990). Composition of cerumen lipids. Journal of the American Academy of Dermatology, 23, 845–849.

Bradley, M. E. (1980). Appliance: A new aid for ear syringing. Journal of Laryngology and Otology, 94, 457–459.

Bricco, E. (1985). Impacted cerumen as a reason for failure in hearing conservation programs. Journal of School Health, 55, 240–241.

Brister, F., Fullwood, H. L., Ripp, T., & Blodgett, C. (1986). Incidence of occlusion due to impacted cerumen among mentally retarded adolescents. American Journal of Mental Deficiency, 91, 302–304.

Burgess, E. H. (1966). A wetting agent to facilitate ear syringing. Practitioner, 197, 811–812.

Burgess, E. H. (1977). Earwax and the right way to use an ear syringe. Nursing Times, 73(40), 1564–1565.

Carne, S. (1980). Ear syringing. British Medical Journal, 280, 374–376.

Caruso, V. G., & Meyerhoff, W. L. (1980). Trauma and infections of the external ear. In M. Papparella & D. Shumrick (Eds.), Otolaryngology: The Ear (Vol. 2, pp. 1345–1356). Philadelphia: W. B. Saunders.

Centers for Disease Control and Prevention. (1988). Morbidity and mortality weekly report: Perspectives in disease prevention and health promotion (p. 37). Atlanta: Author.

Chai, T. J., & Chai, T. C. (1980). Bactericidal activity of cerumen. Antimicrobial Agents and Chemotherapy, 18, 638–641.

Chandler, J. R. (1964). Partial occlusion of the external auditory meatus: Its effect upon air and bone conduction hearing acuity. Laryngoscope, 74, 22–36.

Chaput de Saintonge, D. M., & Johnstone, C. I. (1973). A clinical comparison of triethanolamine polypeptide oleate-condensate ear drops with olive oil for the removal of impacted wax. British Journal of Clinical Practice, 27(12), 454–455.

Cipriani, C., Taborelli, G., Gaddia, G., Melagrana, A., & Rebora, A. (1990). Production rate and composition of cerumen: Influence of sex and season. Laryngoscope, 100, 275–276.

Cooper, S. J. (1985). Relationships of hearing protector type and prevalence of external auditory canal pathology.

Crandell, C. C., & Roeser, R. J. (1993). Incidence of excessive/impacted cerumen in mentally retarded individuals. American Journal of Mental Retardation, 97, 568–574.

Creed, E., & Negus, V. E. (1926). Investigations regarding the function of aural cerumen. Journal of Laryngology and Otology, 41, 223–230.

Dahle, A. J., & McCollister, F. P. (1986). Hearing and otologic disorders in children with Down syndrome. American Journal of Mental Deficiency, 90, 636–642.

DeWeese, D., & Saunders, W. (1973). Otolaryngology. (4th ed.). St. Louis: C. V. Mosby.

Dinsdale, R. C., Roland, P. S., Manning, S. C., & Meyerhoff, W. L. (1991). Catastrophic otologic injury from oral jet irrigation of the external auditory canal. Laryngoscope, 101, 75–78.

Edwards, J., & Harris, K. S. (1990). Rotation and translation of the jaw during speech. Journal of Speech and Hearing Research, 33, 550–562.

Fahmy, S., & Whitefield, M. (1982). Multicentre clinical trial of Exerol as a cerumenolytic. British Journal of Clinical Practice, 36, 197–204.

Foltner, K. A. (1984). The case for otoscopic screenings in industrial hearing conservation. Hearing Journal, 37(6), 27–30.

Fraser, J. G. (1970). The efficacy of wax solvents: In vitro studies and a clinical trial. Journal of Laryngology and Otology, 84, 1055–1064.

Fulton, R. T., & Griffin, C. S. (1967). Audiological-otological considerations with the mentally retarded. Mental Retardation, 5(3), 26–31.

Gerling, I. J., Boester, K., & Yu, J. H. (1997). The transient effect of cerumen on the external ear resonance. Paper presented at the annual conference of the American Academy of Audiology, Ft. Lauderdale, FL.

Gerling, I. J., & Goebel, J. J. (1992). Interaural variability in external ear resonance: The effect of debris. Paper presented at the annual convention of the American Speech-Language-Hearing Association, San Antonio, TX.

Gleitman, R. M., Ballachanda, B. B., & Goldstein, D. P. (1992). Incidence of cerumen impaction in general adult population. Hearing Journal, 45, 28–32.

Graber, R. F. (1986). Removing impacted cerumen. Patient Care, 20, 151–153.

Harvey, D. J. (1989). Identification of long-chain fatty acids and alcohols from human cerumen by the use of picolinyl and nicotinate esters. Biomedical and Environmental Mass Spectrometry, 18, 719–723.

Hawke, M. (1987). Clinical pocket guide to ear disease. New York: Gower Medical Publications.

Hawke, M. (1994). The human ear canal. Seminar presented at the annual meeting of the American Academy of Audiology, Dallas, TX.

Hopkinson, N. (1981). Prevalence of middle ear disorders in coal miners. Cincinnati, OH: U.S. Department of Health and Human Services.

Horowitz, J. I. (1968). Solvents for ear wax. British Medical Journal, 4, 583.

Inaba, M., Chung, T. H., Kim, J. C., Choi, Y. C., & Kim, J. H. (1987). Lipid composition of ear wax in hircismus. Yonsei Medical Journal, 28, 49–51.

Jurish, A. (1991). Hearing trouble? Maybe it's earwax. Prevention, 43(10), 113–117.

Larsen, G. (1976). Removing cerumen with a water-pick. American Journal of Nursing, 76(2), 264–265.

Lebensohn, J. E. (1943). Impacted cerumen: Incidence and management. United States Naval Medical Bulletin, 41, 1071–1075.

Lewis-Cullinan, C., & Janken, J. K. (1990). Effect of cerumen removal on the hearing ability of geriatric patients. Journal of Advanced Nursing, 15, 594–600.

Mahoney, D. F. (1987). One simple solution to hearing impairment. Geriatric Nursing, 8(5), 242–245.

Mahoney, D. F. (1993). Cerumen impaction: Prevalence and detection in nursing homes. Journal of Gerontological Nursing, 19, 23–30.

Mandour, M. A., El-Ghazzawi, E. F., Toppozada, H. H., & Malaty, H. A. (1974). Histological and histochemical study of the activity of ceruminous glands in normal and excessive wax accumulation. Journal of Laryngology and Otology, 88(11), 1075–1085.

Manning, R. (1992). Cerumen management. Lexington: Eastern Kentucky Speech and Hearing Clinic.

Marshall, K. G., & Attia, E. L. (1983). Disorders of the ear. Boston: John Wright–PSG.

Matsunaga, E. (1962). The dimorphism in human normal cerumen. Annals of Human Genetics, 25, 273–286.

Mawson, S. R. (1974). Diseases of the ear (3rd ed.). Baltimore: Williams & Wilkins.

Megarry, S., Pett, A., Scarlett, A., Teh, W., Zeigler, E., & Canter, R. J. (1988). The activity against yeasts of human cerumen. Journal of Laryngology and Otology, 102, 671–672.

Meyers, A. D. (1977). Practical ENT: Managing cerumen impaction. Postgraduate Medicine, 62, 207–209.

Myers, B. A., Siegfried, M., & Pueschel, S. M. (1987). Pseudodementia in the mentally retarded: A case report and review. Clinical Pediatrics, 26, 275–277.

Nudo, L. (1965). Comparison by age of audiological and otological finding in a state residential institution for the mentally retarded: A preliminary report. In L. Lloyd & R. Frisina (Eds.), Audiological assessment of the mentally retarded: Proceedings of a national conference (pp. 137–277). Parsons, KS: Parsons State Hospital and Training Center.

Osborne, J. E., & Baty, J. D. (1990). Do patients with otitis externa produce biochemically different cerumen? Clinical Otolaryngology, 15, 59–61.

Pata, Y. S., Ozturk, C. O., Akbas, Y., Gorur, K., Unal, M., & Ozcan, C. (2003). Has cerumen a protective role in recurrent external otitis? American Journal of Otolaryngology, 24, 209–212.

Perry, E. J., & Nichols, A. C. (1957). Studies on the growth of bacteria in the human ear canal. Journal of Investigative Dermatology, 27, 165–170.

Perry, E. T. (1957). The human ear canal. Springfield, IL: Charles C. Thomas.

Petrakis, N. L. (1969). Dry cerumen: A prevalent genetic trait among American Indians. Nature, 222, 1080–1081.

Prasad, K. S. (1984). Cardiac depression on syringing the ear: A case report. Journal of Laryngology and Otology, 98, 1013.

Primus, M. A., & Skordas, J. D. (1996). Cerumen management in audiological practice. Poster session presented at the annual meeting of the American Academy of Audiology, Salt Lake City, UT.

Raman, R. (1986). Impacted ear wax: A cause for unexplained cough? Archives of Otolaryngology—Head and Neck Surgery, 112, 679.

Robinson, A. C., & Hawke, M. (1989). The efficacy of ceruminolytics: Everything old is new again. Journal of Otolaryngology, 18, 263–267.

Robinson, A. C., Hawke, M., & Naiberg, J. (1990). Impacted cerumen: A disorder of keratinocyte separation in the superficial external ear canal? Journal of Otolaryngology, 19, 86–90.

Roche, A. F., Siervogel, R. M., & Himes, J. H. (1978). Longitudinal study of hearing in children: Baseline data concerning auditory thresholds, noise exposure, and biological factors. Journal of the Acoustical Society of America, 64, 1593–1601.

Roeser, R. J., Adams, R. M., Roland, P. S., & Wilson, P. L. (1992). A safe and effective procedure for cerumen management. Audiology Today, 3(3), 20–21.

Roeser, R. J., Adams, R. M., & Watkins, S. (1991). Cerumen management in hearing conservation: The Dallas (Texas) Independent School District Program. Journal of School Health, 61(1), 47–49.

Roeser, R. J., Lai, L., & Clark, J. (2005). Effect of earcanal occlusion on pure tone threshold sensitivity. Journal of the American Academy of Audiology, 16(9), 740–746.

Roeser, R. J., & Roland, R. (1992). What audiologists must know about cerumen and cerumen management. American Journal of Audiology, 1(5), 27–35.

Ruby, R. R. (1986). Conductive hearing loss in the elderly. Journal of Otolaryngology, 15, 245–247.

Salomon, J. L. (1967). New technique for rapid ear irrigation. Journal of Occupational Medicine, 9(11), 576–577.

Seely, D. R., Quigley, S. M., & Langman, A. W. (1996). Ear candles, efficacy and safety. Laryngoscope, 106, 1226–1229.

Seiler, E. R. (1980). Ear syringing. British Medical Journal, 280, 1273.

Sharp, J. F., Wilson, J. A., Ross, L., & Barr-Hamilton, R. M. (1990). Ear wax removal: A survey of current practice. British Medical Journal, 301, 1251–1253.

Stone, M., & Fulghum, R. S. (1984). Bactericidal activity of wet cerumen. Annals of Otology, Rhinology and Laryngology, 93, 183–186.

Sullivan, R. F. (1997). Video otoscopy in audiologic practice. Journal of the American Academy of Audiology, 8(6), 447–467.

Whatley, V. N., Dodds, C. L., & Paul, R. I. (2003). Randomized clinical trial of Docusate, triethanolamine polypeptide, and irrigation in cerumen removal in children. Archives of Pediatrics and Adolescent Medicine, 157, 1177–1180.

Yassin, A., Mostafa, M. A., & Moawad, M. K. (1966). Cerumen and its microchemical analysis. Journal of Laryngology and Otology, 80, 933–938.

Zikk, D., Rapoport, Y., & Himelfarb, M. Z. (1991). Invasive external otitis after removal of impacted cerumen by irrigation. New England Journal of Medicine, 325(13), 969–970.

Chapter 12

Supervision

Gyl A. Kasewurm and Kris English

While serving as president of Williams College (1836–1887), Mark Hopkins described his vision of the optimal learning/teaching environment: a learner sits at one end of a log, an instructor sits on the other end, and each has the other's undivided attention during the instructional process (Maeroff, 2003). To some degree, this concept of "a classroom of one" describes how an audiologist supervises graduate students and assistants. The audiologist may have only one student or assistant to consider, and during the workday he or she can focus on that one supervisee's development. What does not apply is the part about "undivided attention," because the average audiologic practice or clinic tends to be hectic and requires the practitioner's involvement with patients, technology, and other aspects.

Overseeing the development of a student or assistant puts the audiologist into a teaching role, although most audiologists lack formal training in instruction or evaluation. In 1978, Rassi observed that audiology had "largely ignored the training of supervisors" (p. 2). Unfortunately, little has changed since then. A few valuable materials have been written, notably Anderson's (1988) classic textbook and two chapters by Rassi and McElroy (1992a,b), but a review of doctoral (Au.D.) programs in the United States indicates that only ~10% include coursework or training in supervision, and virtually no research is being conducted on this topic (Martin and Seestedt-Stanford, 2003).

To make up for this shortcoming, this chapter will draw upon materials from other fields (e.g., business management, psychology, and teacher education), as well as the limited information available in our field.

♦ The Tasks of Supervision

Supervising in audiology involves the following tasks: online teaching of topics such as applications of theory to practice, data interpretation, policies, and procedures; promoting growth by giving feedback; and evaluating competencies. The following sections will provide background and suggestions for each task.

Online Teaching

We mentioned the concept of a "classroom of one" at the beginning of the chapter, but the reader is fully aware that teaching in a clinical setting has little resemblance to teaching in a classroom. Unlike the classroom, clinical settings require students and assistants to apply their knowledge and skills directly, all while using technology and interacting with patients and their families. In addition, supervisees are adults, whose learning styles are different from those of children and adolescents. To be an effective teacher, then, it is helpful to consider how adults learn.

Principles of Adult Learning

In the 1960s, education theorist Malcolm S. Knowles considered the differences in learning approaches as demonstrated by adults and children, and felt that because the two groups learn differently, they should be taught differently. He coined the term *andragogy* to describe the approach to teaching adults, as opposed to *pedagogy,* or the approach to teaching children (Rall and Brunner, 2006). He proposed that, whereas children might be described as "empty vessels" into which instructors "pour" knowledge, adults learn differently because they are no longer "empty." In fact, they present with a collection of lifetime experiences to which they regularly refer (a highly interactive process). Adults, by virtue of their age, have a deeper and broader repository of life experiences than children, and use that repository to give meaning to what they learn.

Because their approach to learning is pragmatic, adults want to know why they are learning something. If they are not informed of the "why," they are not as motivated to acquire new knowledge or skills. The "how" of learning is also important to consider: adults usually prefer a hands-on, problem-solving approach to learning, as opposed to a didactic, lecture-based style. The hands-on experiences support the transfer of new skills and knowledge from theory to practice. Without that experience, retention is not as likely to occur.

Knowing how adults learn should guide our thinking as supervisors. We can ask ourselves these questions: Does our instruction explain *why* this information is needed? Do we provide problem-solving approaches to learning, or do we orally instruct or provide a relevant article, with no follow-up discussion to support the transfer process? Do we find ways to provide immediate application of a concept to a clinical practice, to help connect new knowledge to previous knowledge? Do we engage the learner actively, or do we expect him or her to take a passive role?

Following is an example of how a supervisor can choose one of two teaching approaches. The situation involves the arrival of new instrumentation purchased by the clinic.

"Empty Vessel" Approach   The supervisor gives a technical manual accompanying a new piece of office equipment to a supervisee and requests that he learn how the equipment operates. She fails to provide the following: a why (her plan to have the supervisee train the rest of the staff by the end of the week) or a how (release time for the supervisee to have hands-on practice, ideally with a learning partner). The supervisee therefore perceives the task as "busy work."

Outcome: At the end of the week, during a staff meeting, the supervisor calls upon the supervisee to conduct the training and is angry when she sees that the supervisee is not prepared. The supervisee, in turn, is upset for being put on the spot. He had read the manual, understood about half of it, but did not see the need to understand the rest of it.

Adult Learner Approach   The supervisor gives the manual to the supervisee and requests that he work with another staff member to learn how the equipment operates, to train the rest of the staff (the why). A clear deadline is given as well as release time for practice for both trainers (the how).

Outcome: The supervisee and the more experienced staff member work together to learn how to use the equipment, and are prepared to train others at the end of the week. Working with a partner gave the supervisee experience in explaining what he knows and clarified what he does not understand.

Pearl

- Adults learn best when they understand why they are learning something and when they can immediately apply theory to practice.

Promoting Growth with Feedback

Supervisees require input on their performance, but they may not feel comfortable requesting it. Supervisors, too, may not be comfortable with providing feedback, perhaps because they equate feedback with negative criticism. The following rules for constructive feedback are designed to help the supervisee perceive feedback as "evidence to consider," rather than as criticism that can weaken working relationships (Weston and Brown, 2003). Each rule has a "do" and an associated "don't."

Pearl

There are three rules for providing constructive feedback.

1. Do describe specifically what you observe; don't evaluate.
2. Do focus on behaviors a person can change; don't focus on personal characteristics.
3. Do give feedback with advance notice; don't catch a supervisee off-guard.

Feedback Rule 1: Do Describe Specifically What You Observe; Don't Evaluate

Describe what was seen and heard and what was/was not accomplished, without judging the actions as "good" or "bad." For example:

"You met our goal for today of seeing all patients precisely at the time of their appointments. The one time you ran a few minutes late, you asked the front-office person to apologize for the delay and indicate how long the delay would be. This was consistent with our office's policy to respect patients' time."

This feedback is very specific: it describes the mutually agreed-upon goal, the behaviors observed, and the underlying policy for these behaviors. A student or assistant will experience no ambiguity about what went right and why. Additionally, there is no need to evaluate these procedures as "good": the supervisee can perceive for himself or herself that he or she met the supervisor's expectations and knows that he or she is mastering this competency.

Another example:

"You seemed flustered when the patient challenged your recommendation. You replied, 'I've successfully fit dozens of patients with these hearing aids.' This reply defended your position, but it did not uncover the patient's concerns. We still don't know what he was upset about. What would you do differently next time?"

Again, this feedback is very specific: it describes a situation and why the outcome was unfavorable. There is no need to evaluate this reply as "bad": when the supervisee's response is described, he or she can see that the outcome was not an optimal one. The subsequent question conveys the expectation that the learner is to make a change and needs to consider how to do so.

Nothing is less helpful than a vague acknowledgment at the end of the day that one "did fine." Feedback that is incident-specific gives the supervisee very clear direction on what he or she is mastering, and what he or she should do differently next time.

Feedback Rule 2: Do Focus on Behaviors a Person Can Change; Don't Focus on Personal Characteristics

This rule overlaps somewhat with rule 1, in that it focuses on describing behaviors; however, it encourages the supervisor to separate personality characteristics from behaviors, which helps the supervisee from feeling attacked. An example of equating behaviors with personality follows:

"You have been fussing with your hair all day. Your bangs are always in your eyes, and half of your face is covered. Patients with hearing loss need to see your face, but you are putting your vanity ahead of their needs."

This supervisee may have had no idea that her hair had been a distraction, and now she is been told she is vain and self-centered. In addition, she has been given no constructive steps to follow. Compare with the following feedback:

"I guess you are letting your bangs grow out. My concern is, it covers your eyes and much of your face, and I notice our patients are straining to watch your face. I don't think you are noticing that, though. Could you give some reasons as to why this might be a problem? During work hours, please use a clip to keep your hair back."

Feedback Rule 3: Do Give Feedback with Advance Notice; Don't Catch a Supervisee Off-guard

Feedback should be given with some advance notice, as part of a semiplanned event ("I took some notes on your testing procedures earlier; are you ready to confer now, or shall I save these notes for later?") or a specifically planned event ("Today is 'feedback day': plan on taking about 15 minutes at the end of the day for a conference"). If feedback is given without notice, it will usually be perceived as criticism (unless it is overt praise), and the supervisee may not learn as much from the input. The supervisee who is not open to the feedback at a particular moment will appreciate the opportunity to decide to postpone it; the supervisee who agrees to accept the feedback when offered is in "learning readiness" mode.

Describing a plan for providing feedback reduces the tendency for a supervisee to look for excuses to explain what went wrong. Developmentally, students or assistants may not have yet established an internal locus of control, that is, an assumption of responsibility for their actions. Supervisees who still operate with an external locus of control will find fault with others (patients or family members) or

technical problems for outcomes, instead of acknowledging their own role. Unexpected feedback can exacerbate that tendency; planned feedback gives the supervisee time to think and learn.

Pearl

- Effective feedback has often been described as resembling a sandwich. A "feedback sandwich" will conscientiously begin with a positive comment, follow up with a specific concern that needs to be addressed, then conclude with another positive statement of progress.

Feedback can address technical, performance-based skills and, although often overlooked by supervisors, essential "people" or interpersonal skills. The next section will describe both situations and provide suggestions on how to give feedback in each.

Providing Feedback on Technical Skills

Technical skills can be assessed in a hierarchical fashion, from "no skill demonstrated" to "emerging" to "proficient." Assessments can be individualized to give ongoing feedback on specific skills. For example, in assessing the skills needed for tympanometry, the following skills are rated: confirming the equipment is functioning with a biological check, obtaining an ear-tight seal in a variety of patients, obtaining a tympanogram, accurately interpreting the results, obtaining different reflexes, and interpreting the results. Each skill can be rated using a scale, such as that found in **Table 12–1**. **Table 12–1** also outlines the level of intervention provided by the supervisor. More sophisticated clinical procedures will require more complex task analyses.

Providing Feedback on Interpersonal Skills

Audiology students have reported that, although they receive ample feedback and evaluation of their technical skills, they rarely receive input about how they interact with patients (English and Zoladkiewicz, 2005). Supervisors are well aware that interpersonal skills are as important as technical ones, but it is likely that they lack the tools to evaluate these skills effectively, or they have not appreciated students' need for feedback in this area. Readers are referred to **Fig. 12–1** for a tool that can provide this kind of feedback. This form can be modified as needed.

Evaluating Competencies

Supervisors are accustomed to evaluating competencies, either at the end of a semester for graduate students or at the end of a training session for audiologist's assistants (described later). However, evaluations are enhanced when baseline data are collected upfront and when feedback is provided by all parties who interact with the supervisee (referred to as a "360-degree" assessment). The following sections describe both of these aspects of evaluation.

Table 12–1 Evaluating Technical Skills

Rating a Supervisee's Skill Levels				
0 *Absent:* Skill not evident	**1** *Emerging:* Skill emerging	**2** *Present:* Skill present; needs further development	**3** *Developed:* Skill developed; needs refinement and/or consistency	**4** *Consistent:* Skill well developed and consistent
Supervisor's Role				
Modeling intervention: Requires constant supervisory instruction, modeling, and intervention	*Frequent intervention:* Requires frequent supervisory monitoring	*Frequent monitoring:* Requires frequent supervisory consultation	*Infrequent monitoring:* Requires infrequent supervision	*Guidance:* Requires guidance only

Today's hearing evaluation was conducted by an audiology graduate student. Your evaluation of this clinician's communication and interpersonal skills will help in the clinician's development as well as the development of the training program.

Please take a couple of minutes to complete the following questionnaire. The clinician will NEVER KNOW who completed this questionnaire; this form will be combined with others, and all input will remain anonymous. THANK YOU.

1. The clinician introduced him/herself at the beginning of the appointment.

      Yes   No   Don't recall

2. The clinician listened attentively to the information you wanted to convey.

      Strongly Agree   Agree   Disagree   Strongly Disagree

3. The clinician asked you relevant questions.

      Strongly Agree   Agree   Disagree   Strongly Disagree

4. The clinician used effective nonverbal skills while listening.

      Strongly Agree   Agree   Disagree   Strongly Disagree

5. The clinician explained procedures clearly.

      Strongly Agree   Agree   Disagree   Strongly Disagree

6. The clinician explained results clearly.

      Strongly Agree   Agree   Disagree   Strongly Disagree

Other comments? (Please be constructive):

Figure 12–1 Example of a 360-degree assessment (to be completed by patient).

Establishing a Baseline

Assessment is most effective when a baseline has been established. It is difficult to measure progress over a month or a semester if the starting point has not been defined. One way to establish a baseline for assessment is to have the supervisee initially evaluate his or her own skills. For example, at the University of Pittsburgh, 4th year Au.D. students use a self-assessment tool to describe their skill levels at the beginning of their extern year and to indicate specifically the kinds of supervision they will need. This form was developed when externs reported experiencing some awkwardness in requesting specific supervision from their preceptor. To facilitate the discussion, students helped to create the Supervision Request Form, to indicate whether they will need help in using unfamiliar equipment, for example, or if they have had minimal exposure to a particular procedure and do not feel prepared to manage it independently. By evaluating their level of preparedness, the students themselves establish their "externship baselines" with their preceptors. The preceptors, as supervisors, cross-check a few of the items to determine if both parties agree to such definitions as "emerging" versus "mastered" skill.

Pitfall

- Collecting information on baseline performance is easily overlooked when faced with a busy schedule. However, Without a baseline, it is difficult to determine what goals have been met and what still needs to be accomplished.

360-Degree Assessments

Originally developed in the business world, 360-degree assessments are now being used in medical training (e.g., Joshi et al, 2004; Musick et al, 2003; Potter and Palmer, 2003) and in audiology training (**Fig. 12–1**). This process is based on the assumption that feedback is needed from all constituencies, not just the immediate supervisor. In audiology, collecting feedback from staff, patients, family members, physicians, laboratory workers, sales representatives, and others who interact with the supervisee can provide balance as well as multiple perspectives. Although we lack data to confirm the effectiveness of this kind of assessment approach in audiology, we can extrapolate from other fields that multiple inputs tend to agree across raters, and supervisees have reported benefit from this kind of feedback.

Special Consideration

- Evaluations are enhanced when baseline data are collected upfront by all parties who interact with the supervisee.

◆ Additional Concerns in Supervision

The Gender Gap: Differences in Communication

In any supervisory relationship, there is a risk of communication breakdowns because of gender differences. The differences between men's and women's communication styles have been examined for years, most recently by Baron-Cohen (2005), who submits an "empathizing-systematizing theory" as one possible model to account for the differences. He describes three "brain types": type E, more common in females (40%), may be hardwired for empathy; type S, more often found in males (60%), may be hardwired for understanding systems (rules, constructs, functionality); and type B may describe the brains of individuals who are balanced or equally expressive in both areas (20% of men and 40% of women). The differences are likely related to hormones; for instance, toddlers who had lower fetal testosterone have been shown to have higher levels of eye contact, which is related to sociability and empathy.

If a supervisor perceives that a gender difference underlies a communication breakdown, it is recommended that the supervisor make communication styles a topic of conversation. For example, a supervisor might say:

"I've noticed we say the same things differently. When I came into the office today, I said to the office staff, 'Is it cold in here, or is it me?' When you arrived a couple minutes later, you said, 'I'm closing this window; it's freezing in here!' Have you noticed that? I ask because it could affect how we communicate about supervision."

The supervisee in this example may or may not have noticed that she communicates differently than the supervisor, although she might readily agree that she seems to share vaguely defined "communication barriers" with her supervisor. To overcome these kinds of barriers, the supervisor should assume responsibility in acknowledging differences in communication styles and take the lead to ensure that both parties are attempting to bridge the differences.

Supervision and Stress

Mundy (2006) provides a thoughtful analysis of the kinds of stress involved in audiologic supervision. Stressors experienced by graduate students involve (1) academics, (2) finances, and (3) career choice. Not surprisingly, 1st year students report the greatest stress related to workload. Students also report stress due to exam anxiety, absence of leisure time, and the transition to greater clinical responsibilities. Depressive symptoms among graduate students in clinical programs are usually higher than in the general population, and twice as many females note depressive symptoms than males.

Supervisors also experience stress. Although students may assume that their supervisors have all the answers and are "finished" with professional training, the supervisors actually must keep abreast of new technologies, protocols, research outcomes, and other changes in the profession. Besides these stress factors, their workloads may not be adjusted to allow for the extra time needed to work with students who work slower than seasoned professionals, while workloads may not be adjusted to allow for the extra time needed. In busy clinical settings, supervisors may feel a "tug-of-war" between their job responsibilities to see a certain number of patients and their uncompensated responsibilities to train students. This conflict between the time required for student training and the fiscal discipline exercised by clinical programs can cause considerable stress for supervisors, who may be too busy to even analyze the problem.

Stressors for audiologist's assistants include providing services to patients without a set schedule, having a very broad job description that includes being proficient in a multitude of tasks, having the responsibility of satisfying patients' sometimes impossible demands, and being seen as subordinates by patients.

◆ Supervising Audiologist's Assistants

So far, this chapter has considered general supervision concerns, assuming supervisees are graduate students or assistants. The following section addresses concerns unique to the supervision of audiologist's assistants. As audiology transitions to a doctoral-level profession, and as patients obtain improved access to audiologists for hearing and balance health care, it has become necessary that members of the profession determine the continuum of education and personnel preparation needed to provide quality audiologic services. This includes the education, preparation, and supervision requirements for audiologist's assistants (Novak, 2004).

Most other medical and allied health professionals—physicians, nurses, optometrists, physical therapists, occupational therapists, dentists, and veterinarians—have well-developed support staff, including paraprofessionals and technicians. The comparable staff position in audiology is the audiologist's assistant. When appropriately trained, an audiologist's assistant can free the audiologist to be more productive. Today, audiologist's assistants are being successfully employed in practice settings, including the military, Veterans Affairs (VA) clinics, educational institutions, hospitals, industrial settings, and private practices.

Controversial Point

- Although audiologists may feel the use of audiologist's assistants is controversial, in fact it has been recommended by audiology professional organizations for over 30 years.

When minor time-consuming tasks such as analyzing and cleaning hearing aids and completing paperwork are removed from the audiologist's workload, additional time can be directed toward other vitally needed services, such as patient and family counseling, rehabilitative therapy, training, supervision, teaching, and research. Of course, the audiologist must maintain the clinical authority over more advanced cases, such as those involving special tests or difficult-to-test patients. Using audiologist's assistants can enable audiologists to spend more time performing tasks for which their extensive education has prepared them.

Changing demographics and a broadening scope of practice have affected the delivery of audiology services. An audiologist's day in the 1970s was devoted to performing pure tones, speech audiometry, tympanometry, and some aural rehabilitation. This contrasts with the workload of the average audiologist today: audiometry, electronystagmography, otoacoustic emissions, auditory brainstem response, electrocochleography, central auditory processing evaluations, posturography, hearing aid programming, vestibular rehabilitation, industrial audiometry, cochlear implant therapy, and hearing aid sales and service, to name a few tasks.

Background

The need for support personnel in audiology practice is not a new idea, but the concept has yet to be embraced by the majority of audiologists. More than 30 years ago, John Moncur, chair of the first Committee on Support Personnel appointed by the American Speech and Hearing Association (now the American Speech-Language-Hearing Association, ASHA), advocated the use of support personnel in audiology practice and determined that the matter needed immediate attention (ASHA, 1981). In 1989, the American Academy of Audiology (AAA) supported the idea of using support personnel, saying: "The role of the support personnel will be to relieve the audiologist so that more time is available for the decision processes inherent in diagnostic, educational and rehabilitative activities."

The Consensus Panel on Support Personnel in Audiology was developed in 1997 to further study the concept and included members from all of the professional audiology organizations. The panel determined that audiologists were, in fact, using support personnel in audiology service delivery programs to ensure both the accessibility and the highest quality of audiology care while addressing productivity and cost/benefit concerns (AAA, 1997a,b). The auspicious group of professionals concluded that audiology support personnel should engage in only those tasks that were planned, delegated, and supervised by an audiologist and acknowledged that specific roles of audiology support personnel would be influenced by the needs of the supervising audiologist.

Currently, there is no standard term to describe support personnel, and current state laws use a variety of titles to identify such employees. The most common title for support personnel is assistant, with 13 states using that identifier. Ten states use the title aide, and four use both assistant and aide (ASHA, 2006). Other commonly used titles are hearing health technician, audiology aide, audiology support person, audiometric technician, and audiometric assistant.

A recent position statement developed by the AAA (2006) advocated the title audiologist's assistant to describe these support personnel. and defined them as individuals who, after appropriate training, perform tasks that are prescribed, directed, and supervised by a professional, such as a licensed audiologist. The document advocates the use of assistants to ensure accessibility and the highest quality of care while addressing productivity and cost-benefit concerns (American Academy of Audiology, 2006). The role of the assistant is to support the audiologist in performing routine tasks and duties so that the audiologist is available for the more complex evaluative, diagnostic, management, and treatment required by the level of education and training of a licensed audiologist.

It is the position of AAA and ASHA that audiologist's assistants are vital to the future of the profession (AAA, 2006; ASHA, 1989). It has been established that these individuals can provide valuable support to audiologists in the delivery of quality services to patients. Position statements written and supported by these professional organizations strongly suggest that the duties and responsibilities of audiologist's assistants should be assigned only by supervising audiologists. The supervising audiologist maintains the legal and ethical responsibilities for all assigned activities that the audiologist's assistant provides. The needs of the consumer of audiology services and protection of the patient remain paramount. According to the most recent AAA document (2006), audiologists, by virtue of their education and training, are the appropriate and only qualified professionals to hire, supervise, and train audiologist's assistants.

The use of audiologist's assistants is increasing. At the time of writing, there are over 25,000 occupational hearing conservationists certified by the Council for Accreditation in Occupational Hearing Conservation. Since 1968, the U.S. military has used specially trained enlisted technicians to support audiologists (AAA, 2006). These observations suggest that, although the use of audiologist's assistants may not yet be not routine, they are currently being employed in many practice settings to enhance and support the work that audiologists perform.

A recent report from the Department of Veterans Affairs revealed that the number of audiology support personnel in VA hospitals increased 619% from 1996 to 2004. In the same time period, the ratio of audiologists to support persons decreased from 24:1 in 1996 to 5.26:1 in 2004 (Dunlop, 2005). The same study indicated that approximately one third of the work routinely done by audiologists could be handled by support personnel without compromising the quality of care to patients. A 2001 survey of audiologists indicated that 45% of audiologists employed assistants or had previously employed them in their practices (Hamill and Freeman, 2001). A survey of the AAA membership in 2004 revealed that ~28.4% of audiologists employed assistants in their practices (E. Sullivan, assistant deputy director, AAA, personal communication, July 24, 2004).

The duties and responsibilities assigned to an audiologist's assistant should be based on the training, available supervision, and facility needs of the specific work setting. The scope of practice of the supervising audiologist will also dictate the duties and responsibilities assigned to the assistant. The purpose of the audiologist's assistant is to improve access to patient care by increasing availability of audiologic services, increasing productivity by reducing wait times and enhancing patient satisfaction, and reducing costs by enabling assistants to perform tasks that do not require the skills of a licensed audiologist. Appendix 12–1 defines the tasks of an audiologist's assistance tasks

in some basic data collection. Some duties and responsibilities will require direct supervision, whereas others need only indirect supervision.

Examples of the types of services that an assistant can perform after appropriate training and demonstration of competency include

- ◆ Equipment maintenance
- ◆ Hearing aid repair
- ◆ Neonatal screening
- ◆ Patient preparation for testing
- ◆ Hearing conservation
- ◆ Testing assistance
- ◆ Record keeping
- ◆ Assisting in clinical research
- ◆ Clerical duties

Education and Training

The educational background required to become a registered or licensed audiologist's assistant varies greatly from state to state. Criteria range from a high school diploma with specialized training to a bachelor's degree with enrollment in a master's degree program. Generally, the accepted minimal education background for an audiologist's assistant has been a high school diploma and competency-based training. At present, 19 states regulate the use of audiology support personnel, although the requirements vary dramatically from state to state (ASHA, 2006).

The training received by an audiologist's assistant may be an intense, regimented program such as the technician program provided by the military; the Web-based audiologist's assistant course provided by Nova Southeastern University; or a competency-based training program developed by the audiologist who supervises the assistant. Regardless of the type and degree of training, it is the responsibility of the supervising audiologist to ensure that the assistant is competent to perform the duties assigned. The training should be well documented, and the assistant should be able to demonstrate duty-specific competencies. Examples of an assessment can be found in Appendix 12–2.

Furthermore, it is expected that annual continuing education be provided to maintain proficiency. The supervising audiologist is ultimately responsible for all the work performed by the assistant.

Patient Care and Safety

The audiologist who employs and/or supervises audiologist's assistants maintains responsibility for all services provided by the assistants. Training provided by a supervising audiologist should include specific instruction and demonstration of each task the assistant is to perform and continuous, direct observation by the audiologist until the assistant can demonstrate competency with the task. The assistant should not perform any task until the audiologist determines the assistant is fully competent.

Supervision and Evaluation

The supervising audiologist has the primary role in the clinical, technical, and administrative actions related to audiologist's assistants. It is the position of the AAA (2006) that services provided by an audiologist's assistant will be determined by the state-licensed audiologist as dictated by the facility where the services are to be delivered. Tasks assigned must not extend beyond the defined range of knowledge and skills of the assistant. The supervisor must also take responsibility for billing that is associated with services provided by an assistant. Some insurance carriers (e.g., Medicare) do not allow payment for services provided by support personnel, whereas other insurers recognize some services provided by support personnel that are billable. It is the responsibility of the supervising professional to determine when billing is appropriate and to advise patients of noncovered services under their insurance plans.

Once the assistant is trained in all aspects of appropriate services, the supervising audiologist should determine the level of day-to-day supervision and develop a monitoring strategy to help the assistant maintain accurate knowledge and skill level for his or her position. See Appendix 12–2 for an example of an evaluation format for audiologist's assistants. The audiologist will also determine the need for ongoing training to update the assistant's skills set and/or introduction of new procedures, techniques, and treatment options. As is true with employees of any organization, clear task direction is essential to maintain a high level of productivity in an organization. There should be a written description of policies and procedures so the assistant knows what is expected of him or her.

Pitfall

- When key "how to" knowledge is locked up in individuals' heads or buried somewhere—on "sticky" notes, in e-mails, or in out-dated, unused manuals—performance suffers and serious operations problems are common.

Although there is not an established standard that suggests the number of assistants supervised by one audiologist, each supervising audiologist should determine the number that will ensure provision of the highest quality patient care. At all times, the supervising audiologist should hold paramount the needs of the patient and entrust to the assistants only those services for which they are qualified.

◆ Summary

This chapter highlights key aspects of audiologic supervision. The audiologist who takes on the role of supervisor is responsible for teaching, providing feedback, and evaluating the supervisee's skills (technical and interpersonal). This process is inherently stressful, particularly when differences in communication styles occur. Although supervising students has always been part of our scope of practice, audiologists are now also being challenged to consider how best to supervise paraprofessionals (audiologist's assistants). As the profession of audiology continues to evolve, it might consider the value of providing training and specialty recognition for practitioners via continuing education. When audiologists enhance their supervision skills, they and their students will benefit.

Appendix 12–1

Example of Annual Patient Screening Form for Use by Audiologist's Assistants

Annual Hearing Aid Check-Up

Name_____Date_____Technician_____

INSTRUMENT LEFT RIGHT

Type_____

Purchase Date_____

Hearing 250 Hz 500 Hz 1000 Hz 2000 Hz 3000 Hz 4000 Hz

PREVIOUS_____

Left Ear_____

Change_____

Previous_____

Right Ear _____

Change _____

2 or more thresholds vary +10 dB?

Yes_____ No_____ Refer_____

Aided Discrimination @ 45 dB _____

# of hours worn per day _____

Discrimination varies by 10%?

Yes_____ No_____ Refer_____

Patient happy with current hearing aids? Yes_____ No_____

Is patient interested in new technology? Yes_____ No_____

Anything patient would like to discuss

with an audiologist? Yes_____ No_____

If yes to any question, refer_____

Would you like to extend L&D insurance? Yes_____ No_____

Appendix 12–2

Example of Evaluation for Audiologist's Assistants

Date of Review:_____

Employee's Name:_____

Manager's Name:_____

Job Title:_____

Department:_____

Review Period: From _____ To _____

Accomplishments/Results: Summarize the contributions the employee has made during the review period. Evaluate progress in meeting established performance goals and objectives, if applicable.

Evaluations are based on the following performance categories:

Outstanding   Performance far exceeds expectations.

Good   Performance usually exceeds expectations.

Average   Performance consistently meets expectations.

Fair   Performance does not meet expectations.

Knowledge of position: Employee exhibits proficiency in technical job skills. Demonstrates knowledge of what needs to be done and how to accomplish the tasks. Understands work environment, job requirements, and patients' needs. Works to learn new technologies and to acquire additional job-related skills and abilities.

Circle one:

Outstanding   Performance far exceeds expectations.

Good   Performance usually exceeds expectations.

Average   Performance consistently meets expectations.

Fair   Performance does not meet expectations.

Quality of work: Employee demonstrates a commitment to quality and produces reliable, accurate, and neat work. Employee strives to complete work correctly the first time and does not repeat mistakes once corrected.

Circle one:

Outstanding	Performance far exceeds expectations.
Good	Performance usually exceeds expectations.
Average	Performance consistently meets expectations.
Fair	Performance does not meet expectations.

Productivity: Employee's productivity is commensurate with job requirements. Uses resources appropriately and effectively and doesn't waste time.

Circle one:

Outstanding	Performance far exceeds expectations.
Good	Performance usually exceeds expectations.
Average	Performance consistently meets expectations.
Fair	Performance does not meet expectations.

Organization: Employee logically plans and organizes work activities to meet assigned objectives. Prepares appropriately for discussions, meetings, and presentations. Organizes and utilizes resources appropriately to maximize job performance.

Circle one:

Outstanding	Performance far exceeds expectations.
Good	Performance usually exceeds expectations.
Average	Performance consistently meets expectations.
Fair	Performance does not meet expectations.

Dependability: Employee arrives for work on time and meets schedules and other commitments on a timely basis.

Circle one:

Outstanding	Performance far exceeds expectations.
Good	Performance usually exceeds expectations.
Average	Performance consistently meets expectations.
Fair	Performance does not meet expectations.

Teamwork: Employee establishes and maintains cooperative and productive working relationship with other employees. Works effectively with others to meet company's objectives and contributes to team goals.

Circle one:

Outstanding	Performance far exceeds expectations.
Good	Performance usually exceeds expectations.
Average	Performance consistently meets expectations.
Fair	Performance does not meet expectations.

Communication: Employee expresses ideas and information concisely and effectively and shares ideas and listens to the ideas of others.

Circle one:

Outstanding	Performance far exceeds expectations.
Good	Performance usually exceeds expectations.
Average	Performance consistently meets expectations.
Fair	Performance does not meet expectations.

_____ _____
Employee's Signature   Date

_____ _____
Supervisor's Signature   Date

Salary adjustment_____

References

American Academy of Audiology. (1989). Audiometrist program. Audiology Today. 2(3), 3–5.

American Academy of Audiology. (1997a). Guidelines for the use of support personnel for newborn hearing screening. Audiology Today, 10(4), 16.

American Academy of Audiology. (1997b). Position statement and guidelines of the consensus panel on support personnel in audiology. Audiology Today, 9(3), 27–28.

American Academy of Audiology. (2006). Position statement: Audiologist's assistants. Audiology Today, 18(2), 27–28.

American Speech-Language-Hearing Association. (1981). Employment and utilization of supportive personnel in audiology and speech-language pathology. ASHA, 23(3), 165–169.

American Speech-Language-Hearing Association. (1989). Position statement and guidelines on support personnel in audiology. ASHA, 40(10), 12–13.

American Speech-Language Hearing Assiociation. (2006). Retrieved May 14, 2007, from www.asha.org/about/legislation-advocacy/state/state-licensure.htm#legs

Anderson, J. (1988). The supervisory process in speech-language pathology and audiology. Austin, TX: Pro-Ed.

Baron-Cohen, S. (2005). The essential difference: The male and female brain. Phi Kappa Phi Forum, 85(1), 23–24.

Dunlop, R. (2005). Support personnel in VA audiology. Report submitted to the Working Group on the Task Force on Supervision in Audiology.

English, K., & Zoladkiewicz, L. (2005). AuD students' concerns about interacting with patients and families. Audiology Today, 17(5), 22–25.

Hamill, T., & Freeman, B. (2001). Scope of practice for audiologists' assistants: Survey results. Audiology Today, 13(6), 34–35.

Joshi, R., Ling, F. W., & Jaeger, J. (2004). Assessment of a 360-degree instrument to evaluate residents' competency in interpersonal and communication skills. Academic Medicine, 79(5), 458–463.

Maeroff, G. I. (2003). A classroom of one: How online learning is changing our schools and colleges. New York: Palgrave Macmillan.

Martin, J., & Seestedt-Stanford, L. (2003). Research in audiology education: Into the abyss. Audiology Today, 15(3), 46–47.

Mundy, M. (2006). Stress management within audiology supervision. Seminars in Hearing, 27(2), 98–106.

Musick, D. W., McDowell, S. M., Clark, N., & Salcido, R. (2003). Pilot study of a 360-degree assessment instrument for physical medicine and rehabilitative residency programs. American Journal of Physical Medicine and Rehabilitation, 82(5), 394–402.

Novak, R. (2004). Thoughts on the development of our audiology profession. Audiology Today, 16(4), 18–19.

Potter, T. B., & Palmer, R. G. (2003). 360-degree assessment in a multidisciplinary team setting. Rheumatology (Oxford), 42(11), 1404–1407.

Rall, E., & Brunner, E. (2006). Mentoring in audiology. Seminars in Hearing, 27(2), 92–97.

Rassi, J. (1978). Supervision in audiology. Baltimore: University Park Press.

Rassi, J., & McElroy, M. (1992a). Clinical teaching: Delineating competencies and planning strategies. In J. Rassi & M. McElroy (Eds.), The education of audiologists and speech-language pathologists (pp. 301–335). Timonium, MD: York Press.

Rassi, J., & McElroy, M. (1992b). Education in the clinic. In J. Rassi & M. McElroy (Eds.), The education of audiologists and speech-language pathologists (pp. 175–196). Timonium, MD: York Press.

Weston, W., & Brown, J. B. (2003). Teaching the patient-centered clinical method: Practical tips. In M. Stewart, J. B. Brown, & T. Freeman (Eds), Patient-centered medicine: Transforming the clinical method (pp. 199–214). Oxon, UK: Radcliffe Medical Press.

Section III

Business Applications

Chapter 13

Writing a Business Plan

Gyl A. Kasewurm

Entrepreneurship runs deep in the American psyche (Timmons et al, 2004). Many of today's pop heroes are celebrated for their entrepreneurial achievements. The majority of people entering the workforce 40 years ago sought employment in large, established corporations in hopes of securing a job that would last a lifetime. If America has learned anything in the past 20 years, though, it is that job security is a myth. To succeed today, people need to be creative in designing their careers. For those with the entrepreneurial spirit, a well-developed business plan can serve as a priceless tool in evaluating success throughout the life of the business.

Business planning is the process of creating a model or picture of the owner's goals and expectations for the business. The business planning process is one of learning. It is a disciplined approach in which the writer asks questions, seeks answers, and plans for increasingly demanding market tests. The model, the business plan, provides essential information to outline what the organization will look like. A business plan describes the who, what, when, where, why, and how of a good adventure story. Although a business plan must present the facts, it should also stress the unique qualifications of the owner and the impact that they will have on the business and its potential customers. In other words, a good business plan should outline the business, forecast the future, and provide an inspiring story that will captivate and convince readers of the viability of the proposed business.

Pearl

- A well-written business plan provides guidance for the life of the business.

The strategic portion of the plan serves as the heart of the document and should cover in detail expectations for the first 12 months of the business and explain the next 2 to 5 years in lesser detail (McKeever, 1994). The process begins by identifying the aims of the organization, known as the vision, or mission, statement, and takes the reader through an analysis of the concept. This phase investigates the business environment, the organization's capabilities, the competitive advantage, and its basis for growth. The action steps involve setting objectives and developing strategies for key areas of the business, followed by an implementation process.

The business plan is a multipurpose tool, containing several different sections, that assists the writer in planning and operating a business. Although the business plans of major corporations can stretch to several hundred pages, many entrepreneurs' plans may be as short as 5 pages. The length of each section should be tailored to the particular needs of the individual business owner and the information needed to convince readers that the business will succeed. Detailed planning forces the naive business person to examine every aspect of the business before making a financial investment. The owner can easily change strategies, markets, or the nature of the business on paper without losing any hard-earned cash. These decisions will help determine the course of the business for years to come.

If the goal of the business plan is to obtain financing, the writer must remember that the financier may read hundreds of plans. The executive summary must captivate readers and motivate them to read on. For maximum efficiency, the plan should be short, concise, and easy to read. There is a common misconception that a business plan is used primarily for raising capital. However, the primary purpose of writing the business plan is to gain a deep understanding of the opportunity that the entrepreneur is envisioning. A good business plan tests the feasibility of the proposed venture (Timmons et al, 2004). The business plan process not only can prevent an entrepreneur from pursuing a bad opportunity, it can also help an entrepreneur reshape his or her original vision into a better opportunity.

One of the principal reasons for business failure is lack of planning. According to the U.S. Small Business Administration (SBA), ~1 million new businesses are established in America each year. Of these, ~200,000 will survive the first 5 years (Timmons et al, 2004). When pondering the concept of business planning, one critical fact seems to emerge: all businesses need a business plan. A well-written business plan provides the solid foundation for future growth. Federal Express, one of the largest venture capital investments in the United States, with more than $34 billion in annual sales, still prepares an annual business plan (Rich and Gumpert, 2004). Lenders are unlikely to grant a capital request without detailed information that will lead them to believe the business will succeed. The essential directive is to provide sufficient information to support the objectives, strategies, and tactics being developed without making the document so lengthy as to bore the reader. Detailed information that is of interest but not essential to the arguments supporting the document should be included in the appendixes. Initial preparation of the business plan may begin a year or more before the need to use it, allowing time to evaluate and critique the business venture. This painful but necessary exercise demonstrates that careful consideration has been given to the business's development, and the process affords a wonderful opportunity for the entrepreneur to investigate whether the potential business concept has what it takes to succeed. A well-written business plan clarifies the focus of the business and provides a logical framework from which the business can develop and grow during the subsequent 3 to 5 years (Hosford-Dunn et al, 1995).

In addition to probing existing strengths and weaknesses, the plan should paint a realistic picture of the expectations and long-term objectives of the business. It is better to abandon an idea in its infancy than to invest a lot of time and money before learning that the idea will not work. The annual *Hearing Review* and *Hearing Journal* surveys can serve as excellent resources for projected revenue for the business. Growth is implicit in entrepreneurship. However, it takes a long time for new companies to become established and grow. Historically, only two of every five new businesses survive 6 or more years, and few achieve substantial growth during the first 4 years (Timmons et al, 2004). The lesson is that entrepreneurs need to think big. Do not plan to create a job; plan to build a business.

◆ Deciding to Start a Private Practice

Private practice is a wonderful opportunity for many audiologists. However, not everyone possesses the drive or desire to start and run a business. Certain characteristics are helpful in maintaining a private practice. Successful entrepreneurs generally view obstacles as opportunities. Persistence is a common trait among entrepreneurs, and they operate from a mind-set of resourcefulness. Starting and sustaining a successful private practice means several years of long hours, hard work, and financial sacrifice with no guarantees of success. However, many entrepreneurs—audiologists who own their own practices are entrepreneurs—do not consider owning a practice work because they are making a profit while doing a job they love. Faced with the facts and a drive for autonomy, a motivated entrepreneur will view private practice as an outstanding opportunity for independence and financial rewards.

> **Pearl**
>
> • The hallmark of a successful entrepreneur is enjoying running a business.

The first step on the path to entrepreneurship is understanding personal goals and aspirations. The writer of a business plan should explore the answers to the following questions:

◆ Am I a self-starter? A small business owner must possess drive and initiative. Regardless of the number of employees a business has, the responsibility for getting the job done ultimately rests with the owner. It seems that people who are successful in any context possess certain common attributes: energy, passion, commitment, knowledge, and the ability to create a good team (Timmons et al, 2004).

◆ Do my career goals include owning my business and working more than 40 hours per week to reach my personal and professional goals? New owners know that they will have to devote long hours to establishing their business, being willing to have a "24/7" attitude toward work.

◆ Do I like and am I able to get along with people? Nearly all small businesses succeed because of interaction with people; in the case of an audiology practice, that means patients and employees. Individuals who dislike interpersonal contact on a regular basis are at a distinct disadvantage in a private practice.

- Do I have any experience or exposure to the workings of a small business? The most valuable experience for starting and establishing a business is working in someone else's. The small business environment is something that must be experienced to be appreciated, and that exposure is essential to making the decision to become an entrepreneur.

- What is at the heart of my reason to open a private practice? The most pervasive characteristic of entrepreneurs is that they do not enjoy working for someone else. These individuals enjoy making their own decisions and being the one in charge. It is important to define your passion and to make certain that the proposed business incorporates that passion.

- Do I have excellent organizational abilities? The ability to organize people and tasks is essential for a small business owner. A new business owner has to be able to juggle multiple roles while maintaining a sense of order and control. It has been my experience that a disorganized person is generally busy losing patients and money and has a difficult time figuring out what is going wrong.

- Do I have the ability to make decisions quickly and confidently? Unfortunately, a business owner may not have the leisure of waiting hours or days to decide how to resolve a conflict or how to handle financial issues that may arise.

Successful entrepreneurs have to believe in themselves and in their vision of the future. Starting a business is a very demanding endeavor that takes a great deal of time and energy. Before making the decision to establish a private practice, the writer of a business plan should sit down and chart perceived strengths and weaknesses of the prospective business, then analyze whether those will blend into a successful business opportunity. Successful entrepreneurs understand that a good idea is not necessarily a good opportunity.

Pitfall

- The business that fails to plan plans to fail.

◆ Contents of a Business Plan

The Cover Sheet

The cover sheet of the business plan is like the cover of a book. The image should be attractive and should contain the following information: company name; contact person and address; phone and fax numbers; e-mail address; names, titles, addresses, and phone numbers of the owners or corporate officers; date; and copy number. Most of this information is self-explanatory. The contact person for a new venture should be the president or another member of the founding team. The cover should also have a line stating

COVER SHEET

Audiology Associates
742 Ridgeway Drive
South End, MI 49917
(888)555-1212

John Jones, President
3516 Magnolia Lane
Saint Joseph, MI 49085

Sam Huston, Vice President
902 N. Aurilla Drive
Benton Harbor, MI 49022

Patrick Mensinger, Secretary
177 Conda Road
Stevensville, MI 49127

Wilma Beck, Treasurer
678 Nelson Road
Saint Joseph, MI 49085

Plan prepared June 2007 by the corporate officers

A

Financing Proposal
for
Audiology Associates

To be submitted to
Horizon Bank and Trust

John Jones
Audiology Associates
742 Ridgeway Drive
South End, MI 49917
(888)555-1212

B

Figure 13–1 (A,B) Sample cover sheets.

the copy number. Entrepreneurs maintain a log of who has copies of the business plan so that they can prevent unexpected or unwanted distribution.

The preceding information need not be presented in an elaborate fashion. However, if the plan is used to obtain financing, a new cover sheet should be used for each proposal. The cover should be eye catching, serving as the first glimpse of the proposed business. **Figure 13–1** gives examples of cover sheets, using fictional names.

The Executive Summary

The executive summary is the most important part of the business plan. This brief statement, also known as the statement of purpose, addresses and explains key elements of the business, stating the business objectives on the first page of the plan. This key synopsis of the business must capture the reader's attention and should present the most compelling aspects of the proposed business opportunity. The first sentence should hook the reader and convince him or her to read on. In addition, the statement should illustrate how the proprietor intends to use the plan once it has been developed and explain the current state of the company, what products or services it will offer, its market, its competition, and its finances. The executive summary is a quick overview of all aspects of the business in an attempt to introduce the company to the readers. If someone were to read only the executive summary—and many readers will never read past this point—he or she would learn the name and nature of the business, its legal structure, the amount of the loan request, and a repayment schedule. If the plan is for internal use only and not for the purpose of obtaining a loan, the statement would be a summary of the business and its goals for the future. Because this section introduces and summarizes the essence of the business plan, the writer must determine what he or she most wants the reader to know about the business idea. These ideas must be condensed into a few paragraphs that can be read and absorbed quickly and easily.

Pitfall

- The executive summary can make or break the business plan.

The executive summary presents an opportunity to convince the reader that the plan is worth reading, yet leave enough unsaid to require a deeper look. In this section, the writer emphasizes the positive aspects of the business idea and minimizes the negative aspects. For instance, if a unique market niche has been discovered, the entrepreneur should include this in the executive summary. However, the writer may want to eliminate the fact that he or she has no prior experience operating a business. Individuals who read the business plan are busy and probably have many specific questions that need to be addressed in the remainder of the plan. The reader will form an immediate impression of the prospective company from this section, and first impressions are lasting ones.

The statement of purpose appears at the beginning of the document but is usually put in final form after completion of most of the business plan. The statement of purpose conveys the focus of the business and justifies the venture into entrepreneurship. The entire plan should be thoroughly scrutinized before the statement of purpose is finalized to increase the likelihood that the writer is able to write it effectively and concisely. Entrepreneurs who attempt to write the statement of purpose first often end up with a vague and shallow communication. Although the statement of purpose need not border on the dramatic, it must succeed in generating immediate interest from the reader. Ending the summary on a personal note allows an opportunity to convey an assessment of the business's history to date (if there is one) and feelings about its future. For example: "The founders of Better Hearing Associates believe there is a need for audiologic services among the more than 30 million hearing-impaired persons in Berrien County...."

The short, businesslike summary will usually be no longer than one page, but it can be longer if necessary. A sample of an executive summary is found in **Fig. 13–2**.

Special Consideration

- Most business failures result from poor business management and not from a lack of knowledge of the profession.

Audiology Associates

Audiology Associates, an S Corporation established in 2001, is a private practice providing audiological care to the residents of southwestern Michigan. The business, located at 742 Ridgeway Drive in South End, Michigan, is seeking capital in the amount of $125,000 for the purpose of opening a second office in the nearby town of Stevensville, Michigan. Funding is needed in time for the new office to be opened in January of 2008.

The increased incidence of hearing loss has led to a 20% rise in revenue for each of the past two years. This increase has necessitated the addition of another office to better serve the growing number of patients at Audiology Associates. Repayment of the loan and interest can begin promptly within 30 days of the receipt of the requested funds. The loan can be further secured by company owned real estate that has a 2006 assessed value of $645,000.

Figure 13–2 Sample executive summary.

Table of Contents

Continuing the theme of making the document easy to read, a detailed table of contents is critical. The table of contents follows the executive summary, which is expanded and supported in the remainder of the business plan. The contents page helps a prospective lender understand the road map of the plan. As with any professional document, its appearance affects how others react to it. A professional look and feel further increase the chances of the plan being well received.

Every business plan should include the following main sections, along with subsections and supporting documents:

+ Description of the business

+ Financial information

+ Financing proposal

+ Risks

+ Conclusion

The contents page serves as an outline of the plan and should include these main sections, along with any subsections, exhibits, and appendixes. Because a business plan may be a lengthy document, the table of contents will guide the reader to sections of particular interest. In a way, the executive summary states the intended journey of the business, and the table of contents makes it easy to locate stops on the tour. If the purpose of the business plan is to seek a loan from a financial institution, the plan should be specific as to the use of the lender's money, and these uses must be supported in the remainder of the document.

Description of the Business

The description of the business summarizes the organizational structure of the business. This section should address questions such as What exactly is the business? How will it be run? Why will the business succeed? When describing the business operations, the writer should include appealing aspects of the business and any unique factors that may influence the success of the business (Pinson and Jinnett, 1996; see also **Fig. 13–3**).

Determining the central focus of the business and projecting goals for the business 5 years ahead are some of the most important decisions a business owner will make. A private practice can take many directions, and it is wise to decide the projected focus long before the doors open. If it is impossible to describe an idea clearly, the writer will want to take more time to create a plan for the future of the business. Throughout the business plan, it is important to inform the reader of all major factors, positive and negative, that may have an impact on organizational aspects of the operation. This section should provide the reader with the concept of how the business will work and why it will survive in a competitive marketplace.

Special Consideration

• The secret to successful writing is rewriting: edit, edit, edit.

Before writing the description of business section, it will be helpful to explore the answers to the following questions:

+ What business will I be in?

+ What is the status of the business? Is it a start-up or an expansion of an existing business? A takeover or a buyout?

+ What is the business's form: Sole proprietorship, corporation, or partnership?

+ What are the economic trends, and how will they contribute to the success of the business?

Audiology Associates is an audiology clinic that specializes in helping hearing impaired individuals to hear better. This clinic provides services to patients of all ages, including those who are handicapped and physically limited. During the coming year, Audiology Associates plans to expand the business by providing services to patients who have vertigo. Several local physicians have expressed a need for such services, and revenue is projected to increase by 20% from the vestibular evaluations.

Audiology Associates concentrates on providing excellent customer service by providing walk-in hours for patients who need hearing aid repairs and adjustments. Audiology Associates, which has been in business since 2001, is currently open Monday through Friday from 7:30 am until 5 pm. Audiology Associates specializes in dispensing and fitting digital hearing aid technology. The business, which presently serves over 8000 patients, is open year round and located at 742 Ridgeway Drive in South End, Michigan.

Figure 13–3 Sample description of business.

♦ Are there any local economic factors that will influence the business (e.g., does the location present a concentration of potential patients)? Have any major industries in the vicinity closed?

♦ Will the business contract with physicians, health maintenance organizations, hospitals, clinics, other dispensers, or industries that will contribute to its success?

♦ What kind of experience do I have in this type of business?

♦ How will the business be unique? What procedures will be used in an attempt to outshine the competition?

♦ Will the business have any special relationships with suppliers that may contribute to the success of the business?

By examining the central focus of the business, the writer can estimate possible sources of revenue. Once goals for revenue are determined, the owner can begin planning how to generate the needed revenue to operate profitably. Financial goals and projected revenues should be incorporated into the description of business.

Pearl

• A good business plan tests the feasibility of an idea.

Products and Services

In this section of the business plan, the writer must devote attention to the products and services that the business will provide. This is the place for the writer to be passionate about his or her vision for the proposed business. It is acceptable to use both quantitative data and emotional appeals that support the story that the plan is telling. The writer should describe in detail the products and services that the business will offer and qualifications needed to provide the services. This section of the plan should identify the competitive advantage of the proposed venture, clearly and forcefully explain why the proposed business is better than the competition, and outline the reasons that it will outperform the competition. Once again, the writer should seize every opportunity to discuss the uniqueness of the business and how it will differ from the competition (see example in **Fig. 13–4**).

Entrepreneurs are more familiar with their profession and the products and services they offer than the readers of the document are. Therefore, it is important that characteristics of the products and services be explained in a clear and concise fashion. The writer should state the stage of development the business is in and include any products or services that the business plans to offer in the future. Information should be given on extended warranty programs, proposed testing procedures, or unique service programs that the business offers or will offer. The writer may want to consider including case studies and projected outcomes to support these claims.

A detailed description of the core products the business will sell should be highlighted in this section of the business plan (Horan, 2004). The writer need not include each product that will be sold, but rather the types of products that the business will offer, such as directional hearing aids and assistive listening devices. The next step is to explain the services the business will sell and how those services will benefit the target market. For example, if a private practitioner dispenses hearing aids, peripheral services include the delivery, fitting, routine servicing, repairing, and annual evaluations of the units, in addition to annual hearing evaluations and hearing aid adjustments.

Because the average life of a hearing aid is 4 to 5 years (Kochkin, 2005), the products and services section of the business plan should explain how this life cycle will have an impact on the profitability of the business. For example, the writer should describe the average age of prospective buyers and calculate the projected lifetime value of the average patient. Hearing aid technologies continue to evolve, and this evolution will have an impact on hearing-impaired consumers and the future growth and profitability of the business. The plan should project peak sales months and when capital may be needed for key equipment purchases. The anticipated increase in the incidence of hearing impairment and the fact that 72% of consumers with aidable hearing losses fail to use amplification could have an impact on patient flow and business profitability (Horan, 2004).

One of the most important characteristics of a good business plan is its ability to convey to the reader the reasons that the target market will want to consume the products and/or services that the business will offer. The plan must explain why the projected business will be better equipped to satisfy the needs of the public and why the services offered will surpass those of the competition. Potential patients have needs, and the plan should successfully convey a variety of ways to meet those needs. Audiologists provide services and sell products that work hand in hand to benefit hearing-impaired consumers. Essentially, the business must present the products and services in such a way that consumers believe their communication needs can be satisfied.

Management and Personnel

This section of the business plan will characterize the unique qualifications of the business owner and the individuals who will play key roles in operating the proposed business. The management team will be responsible for the success or failure of the business venture. The SBA reports that many small businesses come and, unfortunately, go. According to the SBA definition of failure and its statistics, over 50% of small businesses fail in the first year, and 95% fail within the first 5 years. In his book *Small Business Management* (1983), Michael Ames gives the following reasons for small business failure:

♦ Lack of experience

♦ Insufficient capital

♦ Poor location

♦ Poor inventory management

Amplification systems, when properly fit and maintained, can provide significant benefit to persons with hearing loss. Improvements in hearing aid technology render a multitude of fitting options and flexibility.

Miniaturization of hearing aid circuitry and the ability to interface hearing aids with computer-based programs provide the user with the opportunity to use state of the art technology and offer a cosmetically acceptable alternative to the large behind-the-ear instruments. Improvements in fitting procedures have increased the accuracy of fitting frequency specific gain and compression characteristics. Automatic signal processing, digital processing and directional processing have the potential to increase user satisfaction by reducing the effects of background noise on the primary speech signal of speech.

In addition to prescribing and fitting hearing aid technology, Audiology Associates will offer comprehensive hearing aid fitting services. Patient satisfaction surveys will be used before and after fitting to assess the benefits of amplification in conjunction with target gain validation through the use of real ear measurements.

Audiology associates will offer comprehensive hearing, middle ear, and vestibular assessments for patient of all ages. Treatment for vestibular disorders will be based upon test results and will be provided through the use of a modified Epley maneuver. Studies have cited that 79–100% of patients with benign paroxysmal positional vertigo experience relief of their dizziness following therapy employing the Epley maneuver.

Figure 13–4 Sample products and services.

- Overinvestment in fixed assets
- Poor credit arrangements
- Personal use of business funds
- Unexpected growth
- Competition
- Low sales

These figures are not meant to discourage potential business owners. However, underestimating the difficulty of starting a business is one of the biggest obstacles entrepreneurs face. Success can be achieved if the owner is patient, willing to work hard, and well prepared for the venture.

The primary objective of a business plan is to sell the target audience on the business idea, and a large part of the sales job is convincing the reader that the entrepreneur is competent, talented, and has what it takes to run a successful business. Therefore, this section of the business plan should outline who will be responsible for specific duties and why the individuals are qualified to perform those duties. An important consideration in organizational structure is the culture that evolves to determine the values, beliefs, and patterns of behavior that will be acceptable and practiced by the organization's members (DeThomas and Grensing-Pophal, 2001). The culture that evolves will be, consciously or unconsciously, the result of the entrepreneur's management philosophy that will be stated in this section of the business plan.

An organization is defined as a structured group of human, physical, informational, and financial resources combined to accomplish specific goals (Rich and Gumpert, 2004). The organizational design that results from this effort will define the relationship and formal lines of authority that will exist between the various players in the organization. In general, the job-related attributes for each key position should include

Education This means the training that is directly related to the job or duties that will be performed. This may include formal education, on-the-job training, or the successful completion of executive development programs.

Qualifications   These include the tangible skills and intangible attributes needed to effectively perform a particular job.

Experience   This refers to the individual's exposure to the duties and responsibilities that are directly or indirectly related to a particular job. The key to what is appropriate experience is job-related exposure.

Successes   This refers to the career or job-related accomplishments that indicate an individual's ability to succeed. Included are such considerations as superior work performance that has been recognized, promotions, and awards received.

Health and energy   Lenders need to be assured that the entrepreneur is capable of the long hours required to start and survive in a small business.

This section of the plan should describe the key positions that must be filled in the future and the reasons these positions will contribute to the success of the organization. The description should identify each position by job title and outline the duties, responsibilities, and degree of authority for each position.

The business plan should include the names, responsibilities, and relationships of key employees and outside experts who will participate in managing the practice. It is unnecessary to discuss every employee and consultant in detail. However, it is essential to describe the characteristics listed above as they apply to the primary participants in the business. In many new private practices, the audiologist is responsible for performing most of the duties. It is important to realize that audiologists who are business owners should not fool themselves into thinking that they can be responsible for everything. Although new business owners may want to save costs by assuming responsibility for all roles, wise entrepreneurs tap legal, financial, technical, marketing, and other experts to share in the duties of the business. Most importantly, owners should focus efforts on what they are trained to do as audiologists and ask for assistance in areas in which they are unqualified or not interested. Organizations with formal structures and an organizational chart are better positioned to achieve their goals. An example of an organizational chart is found in **Fig. 13–5**.

Profile of the Target Market

This section of the plan sets the stage for the proposed business to enter and grow in the marketplace successfully. An entrepreneur needs to decide where his or her product or service will fit into the marketplace. The target market of the business can be defined as "that group of customers

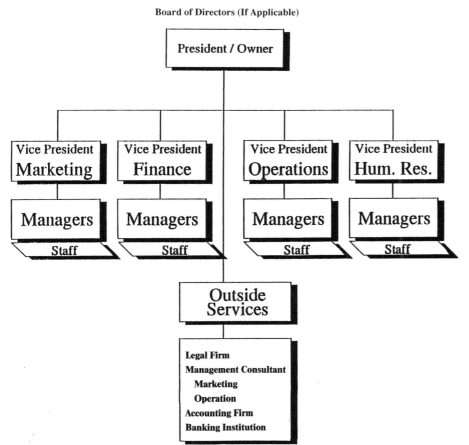

Figure 13–5 Sample organizational chart. Hum. Res., Human Resources.

with a set of common characteristics that distinguishes them from other customers" (Brandt, 1997). This section of the plan describes how the products or services will be differentiated from the competition. It is the job of the management team to identify the target market and to delineate the customer groups to which the business expects to sell. The plan's emphasis should be in the area that the audience sees as most critical, and the plan must offer to meet the measurable goals and objectives valued most by the target market.

By targeting customer groups with particular characteristics, business planners often discover new opportunities. A service business should define exactly how wide a geographical area it plans to cover. For most businesses, the area is dictated by a reasonable access time for the customer to travel to the office or for the professional to travel to the customer. Geographic proximity can be a key factor in determining the target market of the proposed business. For example, the farther a consumer must travel to reach the office, the less likely he or she may be to respond to the target marketing offer. The business planner must then decide whether enough customers are within the geographical area to support the business.

In the target market section of the business plan, the writer must state the potential consumers of products and services, the geographical size of the marketplace, and the anticipated growth potential of the target market. Once the demographic information is processed, the writer may want to add services or products that will cater to the needs of the target market. For instance, if the business is located next to a senior living facility, management may want to concentrate a segment of the business on providing assistive listening devices to older adults.

Pearl

- History shows that the only businesses that survive are those that meet the needs of consumers in the target market.

An established practice should begin by focusing on existing customers. Who are they, and what do they have in common? A new business should ask "Who will be our customers, and how will their needs best be met?" while an established practice may ask, "What are the average age and demographics of our patients, and what services are they lacking?" To survive, any business requires a steady stream of customers who desire the products and services the business offers. The reader will take the business plan more seriously once he or she realizes that the entrepreneur has identified the profile of his or her average customer and projected the business's earning potential from that target market. Based on the knowledge gleaned from the target market analysis, entrepreneurs need to position their practices accordingly. The business plan must address the very question of whether there is indeed a market for the services and products that the potential business will be offering.

Understanding the Competition

Pitfall

- It is unrealistic to believe that your business has no competition.

A business is unable to be strategic without knowing its competition, and strategic opportunity does not exist in the absence of competition. Competition comes from many sources. Some of the competition will be direct, such as other audiologists offering the same products and services. Direct competition refers to products or services that consumers treat as acceptable alternatives, such as McDonald's and Burger King (DeThomas and Grensing-Pophal, 2001). In the world of audiology, direct competition may be defined as two practices that offer the same products or services to the same market. Indirect competition refers to products or services that can be easily substituted for one another, such as automobile travel for air travel or movie rental for attendance at a movie. Indirect competition for an audiology practice may include offering audiometric services to different target markets. For example, audiologists who provide services to nursing home patients are indirect competition to audiologists who provide services to children through school systems.

When writing a business plan, the writer should explore the potential influences of both direct and indirect competition. An effective marketing strategy should produce products or services that are, in the minds of consumers, better choices than the available alternatives or substitutes. The writer of the business plan must investigate who and what the proposed business will be competing against to make a convincing case for why the proposed product or service makes a better choice for patients. Some factors of direct and indirect competition to explore include the following (DeThomas and Grensing-Pophal, 2001):

- Primary products and services supplied by the competition
- Potential patients
- Primary distribution channels
- Longevity of products and services
- Possible promotions and necessary investment

Once the research has been completed, the writer will want to investigate and invent new and unique ways to compete in the target market. Answers to the following questions will be helpful:

- What can the business do better than the competition?
- What can the business do differently than the competition?
- What will make the business stand out from the competition?

Every business must evaluate the competition and try to determine an untapped market for the practice. In addition, the competition can prove to be a valuable source of information: What do they do well? What could the proposed business do better? How does the competition satisfy their customers? What type of pricing structure does the competition maintain? Where and how do they advertise? The writer should compile competitive information that can give the practice the edge to survive in an aggressive marketplace.

The eventual performance of a prospective business is influenced by external factors over which the business has little or no control. In the case of competitors, the flow of competition will depend largely on barriers to entry into the marketplace, such as large capital requirements or slow and restrained growth of the market. In addition to expanding current markets and perhaps creating new markets, the owner of a new business will need to draw customers from the competition, and the business plan should include a strategy for maximum patient retention. Analyzing the competition will reveal who the competition is, where they are located, what products or services they offer, and how the new business can provide a unique and needed service to consumers. Technological change remains a force that drives the marketplace. However, state-of-the-art technology is not always the answer to securing a major portion of the marketplace. Often, ensuring that the business offers exceptional customer service and on-site repair facilities will be enough to carve out a section of the market. Defining the competition will enable the business to establish a battle plan for capturing and retaining its share of the target market.

Controversial Point

- In addition to expanding current markets and perhaps creating new markets, the owner of a new business will need to draw customers from the competition.

Marketing

In the marketing section of the business plan, the writer needs to convince the audience that a real opportunity exists and that the proposed business can capitalize on it. This section identifies what methods will be used to reach potential customers and how customers will be informed of the products and services that the business will offer. A marketing strategy should explain how the business will organize and implement its plans to achieve desired sales performance. Although meticulous detail is not necessary, the reader of the business plan must gain an understanding of how the business intends to market its products and services.

Pearl

- Marketing activities do not always yield immediate results.

A budget is simply a plan expressed in quantitative terms, such as estimated expenses, expected sales revenue, sales in units, the number of services performed, and estimated profit. Effective planning must include accurate cost projections and budget analysis. The marketing budget should detail estimated revenues and expenditures. The revenue estimates consist of forecast sales in units or numbers of service units performed and the selling price per unit. On the expense side, the budget should detail the dollar amount and timing of all marketing-related expenditures. The difference between forecasted revenue and expenses is the projected marketing profit goal.

Three commonly used approaches to budgeted marketing programs are the percent of sales, matching, and default or affordable methods (DeThomas and Grensing-Pophal, 2001). Both the percent of sales and matching methods operate on the assumption that marketing activities are the consequence of sales; that is, sales occur in the absence of effective marketing efforts. The reality, however, is that sales are the result of effective marketing efforts. Many businesses make the mistake of reducing marketing expenditures when sales decline, which is often counterproductive. When sales decrease, increased marketing efforts are often needed to boost lagging sales.

In the default or affordable approach, funds spent on marketing activities are considered an investment in the business. The amount spent on marketing activities is determined by the cash flow remaining after the company's mandatory obligations and management priorities are met. Planned marketing expenditures are expected to generate a return on investment (ROI) that justifies the funds used.

The expected rate of return on the dollars that will be invested in the marketing program, not how much money remains after spending priorities have been satisfied, should determine the amount actually spent. In theory, dollars should be committed to an investment as long as the expected return is greater than the cost of the funds invested. Monitoring the effects of various marketing efforts is essential, and the marketing budget should be reevaluated regularly to determine the use of future marketing dollars.

A marketing budget needs to include monies for signage, brochures, business cards, stationery, and everything that projects the company's image to the public. An important aspect of marketing is to make certain the message is consistent across media. For in-depth discussion of Marketing budgets and campaigns in audiology practices, refer to Chapter 5. Many established practitioners hire professionals to develop a consistent marketing campaign that meets the needs of the prospective target market. A leading cause of business failure can be directly attributed to the lack of effective marketing and promotion.

Pitfall

- Inconsistent marketing messages may create a marketing mess instead of a marketing mix.

Many methods are available to reach the market segment, including direct mail, television, radio, newspaper ads, educational seminars, and online marketing. Publicity is free media coverage, such as press releases, that can provide credibility for a business. When a business pays for an advertisement, the practice is telling customers that its product or service is good. When a member of the media or someone else outside the organization gives the business's products or services a boost, consumers may perceive it as impartial judgment, and the publicity may be worth several paid advertisements.

Business and community involvement through participation in civic events and membership in business organizations is another means of promotion. Most civic organizations have weekly programs and are looking for educated and interesting speakers. Although it may be difficult to find time to devote to public speaking, the effort can provide dividends for years to come.

In summary, the business planner should report how promotional dollars will be spent, why those avenues were selected, how the message will reach the target market, when the promotional campaign will begin, how much the marketing plan will cost, and what format the advertising will take. Timing is important. The marketing plan will require contacting promotional resources well in advance to determine publication schedules. For example, if a business is to open in July, and local telephone directories are published in September, you may need to place the telephone directory ad in April. At this point in the plan, it is a good idea to include a chart or table to track events and timing, as shown in **Table 13–1.** When working with a complex project, it may be appropriate to prepare a project schedule, showing the duration and progression of events and items over time and charting the scheduled and actual progress of projects.

Pricing

The pricing structure of the business is critical to its success and is determined through market research and analysis of financial considerations. Pricing is a challenging and controversial topic that requires more in-depth discussion than is available within the scope of this textbook. However, it is superficially addressed in this chapter for purposes of fleshing out the business plan. Different vantage points and opinions on pricing are presented in more depth in Chapters 5 and 15-17. Determining how to price the products and services

Profit and Loss Statement

Sales	$100,000
Cost of Goods Sold	30,000
Gross Margin	70,000
Expenses	35,000
Earnings Before Interest and Taxes	35,000
Interest Expense	1,000
Earnings Before Tax	34,000
Tax	7,000
Net Income	$ 27,000

Figure 13–6 Profit and loss statement.

that the business will offer is always difficult. Every small business wrestles with the question of how to set prices. There is no magic formula that will determine the best; the goal is to find the price at which profit is maximized. Some hearing health care professionals make the mistake of establishing a hearing aid pricing structure based on what the competition charges instead of basing pricing on the cost of operating their actual business.

A pricing strategy that may get a new business in trouble is to offer a low price in hopes of penetrating the marketplace and gaining market share rapidly. The problem with establishing a low price for products and services is that it may be impossible to raise the prices later after the business has developed an established patient base. A low price may also connote lower value versus the competition.

Pricing strategies can broadly include the following approaches:

Competitive pricing This is pricing based on what the competition charges. An inherent assumption of this strategy is that the products and services provided do not differ significantly from those of the competition.

Table 13–1 Timing and Tracking of Tasks

Task No.	Task Name	Person Responsible	Start Date	Completion Date
1	Finalize planning	John Jones	01/04/08	01/06/08
2	Apply for loan	John Jones	01/05/08	01/06/08
3	Finalize suppliers	Susan Brown	01/04/06	01/07/08
4	Meet with local referral sources	Mary Jones	01/05/08	01/07/08
5	Seek builders	David Jones	01/05/08	01/06/08
6	Tender information	David Jones	01/06/08	01/08/08
7	Supervise builders	David Jones	01/08/08	01/11/08
8	Plan office interior design	Mary Jones/Susan Brown	01/09/08	01/12/08
9	Determine marketing budget and date of execution	John Jones	01/10/08	01/12/08

Market penetration pricing This approach involves setting prices below the competition to increase the share of the market or gain entry into it.

High price strategies This is pricing to create an exclusive image separate from the general market.

Bundled pricing Pricing is based on "packages" that promote "extras" into a single priced bundle (Hirji, 1999).

There are several additional strategies that can be employed when making pricing decisions. The cost-plus pricing approach, long used in the retailing industry, calculates the cost of providing the product or service and adds what is judged to be an appropriate amount for profit. This method is frowned upon by some experts, who argue that pricing of products and services should be determined not simply by the costs but by market forces (Hirji, 1999). It is not unusual in an audiology practice to find a multiplier being applied to the cost of a product to arrive at a final price, and the multiplier typically varies based on the level of product with a higher multiplier being applied to a lower-priced product. The cost-plus approach can be problematic for a new business, as it will be difficult to determine actual cost accurately without a history. Because most entrepreneurs underestimate costs (Timmons et al, 2004), there is a tendency to underestimate the cost of the product or provision of a particular service.

The break-even analysis is another means of making pricing decisions. In this method, the break-even point (BEP) estimates the approximate profit or loss at different levels of predicted practice activity. In BEP analyses, fixed costs are the cost of operating the practice, and variable costs are the cost of goods. This information can be used to adjust the selling price to the patient based on a known or assumed mix of products and services. The break-even analysis is often used to represent the relationship between a business's costs, sales revenues, and profits. This analysis will indicate the level of revenue needed to cover the variable costs. It is important to establish the relationship between price and cost. A common planning error involves establishing a retail price that provides an adequate margin over cost, only to discover that most hearing aids are sold during an "open house," with accompanying pricing discounts on each unit sold. This can result in a lack of revenue to cover overhead expenses. Price and cost assumptions must be explicit in the plan and must be used as input to the financial projections.

A viable business operates between the price ceiling and the price floor. The price ceiling is the highest price a consumer will pay for a product or service on the basis of a perceived value. The price floor is the lowest amount at which the business is able to offer a product or service, meet all costs, and still make a desired profit. The difference between the two allows for discounts, bad debts, and returns. In addition to meeting all the costs of operating a business, the company must generate a profit. Reason would suggest that, in determining pricing, it is wise to know what the competition is charging. However, the pricing structure of a business should be made on the basis of profitability, not on what the competition is charging. The price of goods and services should reflect the products or services themselves and also an intangible image factor. Positioning or predetermining the perceived value in the eyes of consumers can be accomplished through promotional activities. To be successful, the owner must decide what the business offers that the competition does not. This unique benefit or service should be promoted to consumers.

Collections strategies are an important part of developing a pricing within the business plan. A business owner must decide what payment policies will be used and how the policies will be enforced. If a patient cannot pay cash for the purchase, credit card or financing options should be available. In most practices, delayed third-party insurance claims make up the largest percentage of accounts receivable. It is critical to assess reimbursement rates and then determine how many patients the practice can afford to see at those reduced prices.

In addition to delineating collection strategies, the business plan's financial section must also identify and integrate external pricing forces into its pricing structure, financial projections, and communications with patients and providers. Two examples are:

> Insurance companies (e.g., Medicare) typically determine the prices that are charged for particular services or products. If Medicare determines a "reasonable and customary" charge for a diagnostic service, and the practice will participate in the Medicare program, the owner must accept what the insurance allows for that service and cannot bill the patient more than the allowed amount. If the practice will not accept Medicare, it may be difficult to convince patients to pay more than the allowed fees. It is critical for the owner to determine the percentage of discounted services that the business can afford to provide.

> Medicare patients must be notified in writing that they will be responsible for the balance that their insurance carrier fails to pay. Medicare requires that a notice of exclusion from Medicare benefits (NEMB) waiver be given to patients when services are not covered. A copy of an NEMB is provided in Appendix 13–1.

Pitfall

- Lack of courage in pricing is an error that many business people make. Wal-Mart pricing does not work at Tiffany's.

Financial Information

The first sections of the business plan described the physical setup of the business and shared plans for finding and reaching potential customers. Investors routinely expect business plans to project sales, profits, and other key financial results 5 years into the future. This is not to say that investors, once they decide to back a company, simply accept its financial projections at face value. Many start-up companies fail to achieve the rosy projections posed by the writer. The various operational plans prepared by the entrepreneur indicate where the company is expected to go and how it will get there. The financial plan estimates and plans for the financing needed to implement these intentions. A convincing financial plan answers these key questions:

- What amount of financing is needed to make the plan feasible?

- In what form will the financing be needed?

- Who will provide the financing?

Pitfall

- Many small business owners are poorly prepared for their role as chief financial officer.

Generating convincing responses to these questions requires business knowledge, the factors that determine the success or failure of its operation, a basic understanding of the financial side of the business, and the ability to translate this information into a sound financial game plan. This section is the quantitative interpretation of everything stated in the text portion of the plan. Well-executed financial statements provide the means to look at the profitability of the business. The financial documents included in the plan are not just for the purpose of satisfying a potential lender or investor; they act as a guide during the life of the business. To be effective, the financial section of the business plan must be current. This means examining the financial statements periodically and measuring the actual performance against projections.

A business's financial statements are numerical representations of how well the business is doing. The idea beyond these statements is to portray a picture of what is happening within the company and between the company and the rest of the world. Because lenders and financial backers focus on dollars and cents, it is important to prepare competent, professional financial projections for the business. In terms of revenue, the business plan should begin with a forecast of how many of each particular product will be sold at what prices. When approaching a financial forecast, the business planner should project every product the business expects to sell and how much it expects to charge for those products and services. Annual reports published by *Hearing Review* and *Hearing Journal* may be helpful in determining the amount of revenue that the average private practice produces in a month.

A major error in the financial management of a practice is not planning for the future (Traynor, 2005). Financial projections should be broken down into monthly forecasts for years 1 through 5. The writer should build a budget to use as a guideline for the expenditure of any funds. Budgets are financial plans that include forecasting expenses, revenues, assets, liabilities, and cash flows based on a plan that is established in the business plan. A budget can greatly enhance the chance for success by forecasting future cash expenditures. A budget helps the owner to perceive problems before they

Profit and Loss
May 2007

	May '07
Ordinary Income/Expense	
Income	
Income	99,306.75
Income-Ind.	2,419.00
Total Income	101,725.75
Expense	
Acct Fees	75.00
Advertising	3,333.43
Auto Loan	1,626.86
Bank Chrg	90.88
Charity	300.00
Cleaning	340.00
Dues	50.00
Earmolds	30.25
Education	1,440.66
Entertain	450.00
Equipment	149.99
Equipment - Main	2,358.17
FICA - employer	1,710.77
Gifts	179.67
Hearing Aids	43,563.66
Insurance Health	289.07
Insurance-Disab	427.92
Medicare Witholding	400.09
Office Maint.	150.00
Office Util	296.03
Outside service	1,873.81
Payroll	
Gross	27,593.00
Total Payroll	27,593.00
Postage	116.00
Postage Lease	175.14
Rent	2,114.21
Returns	381.38
Supplies	1,158.91
Telephone	1,645.11
Travel-Bus	4,215.89
Total Expense	96,535.90
Net Ordinary Income	5,189.85
Net Income	5,189.85

Figure 13–7 Sample profit and loss worksheet.

occur and potentially alter plans to prevent those problems. Although this may seem a daunting task for the inexperienced audiologist, the process is relatively simple and painless if done properly. In many instances, it is wise to hire an outside expert to assist in the financial planning of the business venture. Once the financial spreadsheets have been completed, a two- to three-page explanation of the financials should be written and should precede the financial section of the plan. The business plan should include the following: profit and loss statement (**Figs. 13–6** and **13–7**), balance sheet (**Fig. 13–8**), and cash flow worksheet (**Fig. 13–9**).

Profit and Loss Statement

This document will be used to project revenues over time. The most important element in all the projections is the anticipated sales volume. The credibility of this forecast is so important that an entire section of the marketing plan may be devoted to supporting this projection. The owner must calculate the costs of goods and/or services, as well as the anticipated fixed overhead costs. The net difference of

BALANCE SHEET			
ASSETS		**LIABILITIES**	
Cash	$10,000	Accounts Payable	$10,000
Accounts Receivable	14,000	Taxes Payable	2,000
Inventory	12,000	Notes Payable Short term	12,000
Total Current Assets	36,000	Current Liabilities	24,000
		Long-Term Debt	18,000
		Total Liabilities	42,000
Fixed Assets			
Equipment	50,000		
Accum Depreciation	(10,000)	Total Capital/Equity	34,000
Total Fixed Assets	40,000		
		Total Liabilities	
Total Assets	$76,000	and Equity	$76,000

Figure 13–8 Sample balance sheet.

total revenue less total costs will determine the profit and loss of the business. This statement shows how much money a company will earn during an accounting period. Although no set of projections will be 100% correct, experience and practice tend to make the predictions more accurate. Even if the projections are inaccurate, they will provide a benchmark against which to measure short-term goals. Most income statements have a general form similar to that shown in **Fig. 13–6** and a specific form like the one shown in **Fig. 13–7**.

It is recommended that small businesses make 5-year projections for both planning purposes and income projections, whereas an existing business should include financial statements for the immediately preceding 2 years (Horan, 2004). In addition, the business plan for an established business should include copies of the past three tax returns to substantiate the projected financial claims. Including one or two dozen financial spreadsheets in the business plan is likely to provoke skepticism rather than confidence. Investors are aware that financial projections for a proposed business are usually overly optimistic. Take care not to bore the reader with too much detail. When detail is warranted, it is best placed in properly referenced appendixes to the main business plan document.

Special Consideration

- A lender's reason for denying a finance application can be valuable to a potential business.

The Balance Sheet

In simple terms, the balance sheet lists everything a company owns and everything it owes at a moment in time. The company's money comes from institutions that have lent money or extended credit in one form or another. These actions create a liability on the part of the company to pay the money back. Funds may also come from owners who have invested their own money in the company. Such investments by owners are called equity. A balance sheet has two sides. One side lists all the company's assets, the other all the company's liabilities. Balance sheets are designed to show how the assets, liabilities, and net worth of a company are distributed at any given time. In general, all companies, large or small, use the same categories arranged in the same order when composing a balance sheet. An example of a balance sheet can be found in **Fig. 13–8**.

The balance sheet gives a profile of the worth of the company's assets: cash, accounts receivable, inventory, equipment, property, and all the company's liabilities, such as accounts payable, notes payable, taxes and interest payable, and salaries. The differences between assets and liabilities constitute the company's net worth. If the business has a track record when the business plan is developed, the business sheet will show considerable equity. If this is a new venture, the balance sheet may show little or negative equity.

Cash Flow Statement

The cash flow statement shows the reader where the firm's money came from and what it was spent on during a specified period. Cash flow statements involve the inflow and outflow of cash. Inflows are usually represented by positive

---

CASH FLOW WORKSHEET

Cash Flow for the Period of _____ *to* _____

1) **Beginning Cash Balance**   _____
2) **Cash Receipts**
   a) **Cash Sales**   _____
   b) **Accounts Receivable collected** _____
   c) **Loans and Other Cash Income**   _____
3) **Total Cash Available (1+2a+2b+2c)**   _____

4) **Business Expenditures**
   a) **Products**   _____
   b) **Advertising**   _____
   c) **Insurance**   _____
   d) **Interest**   _____
   e) **Office Supplies** _____
   f) **Rent**   _____
   g) **Salaries**   _____
   h) **Telephone**   _____
   i) **Dues**   _____
   j) **Other Expenses**_____   _____
   k) _____   _____
   l) _____   _____

5) **Total Expenses (4a thru 4l)**   _____

6) **Loan Principal Repayments**   _____

7) **Other Cash Paid-Outs**   _____

8) **Total Cash Paid-Outs (5 + 6 + 7)**   _____

9) **Ending Cash Balance (3 – 8)**   _____

Figure 13–9 Sample cash flow worksheet.

numbers, whereas outflows are negative numbers. It is common practice to use parentheses rather than a minus sign to indicate negativity. A cash flow worksheet can be found in **Fig. 13–9**.

Cash and *profitability* are not synonymous terms. It is possible to have cash, yet be operating at a loss. Conversely, it is possible to be operating profitably, yet have no cash. The question that must be addressed is, How much cash is needed to be operating profitably? The first step in cash flow forecasting is to estimate how much the business is expected to sell or receive in income for a given period of time. If the business is dealing in products, the plan should forecast the number of units the office expects to sell and multiply this number by the cost per unit, then translate these figures into the expected dollar volume of sales.

The plotting of expected revenues, expenses, assets, liabilities, and equity forecasts the level of cash flow. Cash flow totals are a critical index of how successful the busi-

ness will be, and this forecasting estimates the timing of cash flowing into and out of the business. To assess the feasibility of a venture, the owner must assess how much cash is necessary to acquire the capital resources necessary to establish the business. This is known as fixed capital. The amount of cash needed to support the trading of the business until the proceeds of sales are received is known as working capital.

The cash flow forecast considers cash received into the business from all sources, including sales, capital funds, and loan funds. In addition, this forecast should include cash paid out by the business, including operating expenses, expenditures on capital items, and loan repayments. Obviously, it is essential that the amount of money flowing into the business exceeds the amount flowing out. If outflows exceed inflows, sooner or later the business will fail. Small businesses are especially vulnerable to cash flow problems because they tend to operate with inadequate cash reserves.

Gordon Hearing Aids is an audiological private practice that aims to provide quality services and superior products to the more than one hundred thousand consumers in Berry Count, Michigan, Marketing objectives include introduction of at least two new high technology products per year, direct mail advertising sent twice yearly to all residents of Berry County, and expansion of services into Vanna County, Michigan.

The business seeks to provide wealth for its owners through an annual net profit of 25%, which will allow reinvestment in the company to continually upgrade facilities and equipment. A human resource objective is to expand the skill base of company employees which will lead to an increase in personal productivity. The firm's key success factors have been modified as economic efficiency, maintenance of high standards of quality, increase of target market coverage, and customer satisfaction.

Gordon Hearing Aids is recognized as an industry leader. With very little marketing effort, it has maintained sales close to its capacity and at its current level of personal productivity. The business is financially sound and exemplifies execeptional customer service and high standards of quality in the market it currently serves.

Figure 13–10 Sample conclusion.

Break-even Analysis

A break-even analysis provides a sales objective, expressed in either dollar or unit sales, at which the business will be breaking even, that is, neither making a profit nor losing money. Once the break-even point is known, the business will have an objective target. Increased sales do not necessarily mean increased profit. For instance, doing a high volume of Medicaid work may mean a lot of "work" but very low profit margins and, consequently, very little profit.

Fixed costs are those costs that remain constant no matter what the sales volume may be. These include rent, salaries, benefits, and taxes. Variable costs are those costs associated with sales, including cost of goods, variable labor costs, and sales commissions. The net operating profit of an enterprise is represented by the gross revenue for the period less the total fixed costs for that period. The break-even point for a business is the point at which all of the variable and fixed costs are met, but no operating profit is achieved.

Financing Proposal

The purpose of this section is to assist the entrepreneur in turning a business plan into a financing proposal that fits the business and capital needs. Most financing deals rarely progress beyond the first screening. Therefore, the proposal must be attractive enough to warrant attention and tailored to the needs of the intended audience. If the business needs more equity than is available from the bank, the entrepreneur may search for a financier who routinely invests in small businesses, or contact parents, grandparents, or the richest living relative.

A bank loan consists of money that will be repaid over a period of time at an additional cost (interest). The money an owner invests in a business is equity, that is, money that will not be repaid unless a portion of the business is sold or a partnership is formed. Debt financing does not lead to sharing ownership of the business, whereas equity financing does. An owner who is unable to obtain financing should consider acquiring a partner who will share ownership of the business. From a banker's standpoint, the higher the debt, the riskier the deal, and short-term loans are generally less risky than long-term loans.

Every lender wants to answer one very basic question before approving a loan for a new business: Will the borrower be able to repay the loan and interest as planned? To answer that fundamental question, lenders may ask more detailed questions. When dealing with a local bank, the owner may want to emphasize the reliability of the past credit history and include supporting documents. First impressions are often lasting ones, so it is important to dress well and to have the documents available that the lender may request. If the loan request is denied, the entrepreneur may choose another lender in the area who may be more willing to finance the business venture. An example of a loan application can be found online at www.toolkit.cch.com/tools/downloads/loan.rtf.

Risks

Every new venture faces several risks that may threaten its survival. The plan needs to acknowledge the potential risks, or investors will believe that the entrepreneur is naive or untrustworthy. It is important for the writer to understand these critical risks because they most often are directly related to the assumptions that will drive the success or failure of the business. The following questions should be addressed in the plan:

♦ What happens if the owner becomes incapacitated or dies?

♦ Will consumers in the target market buy the product being sold for the price expected?

♦ What if a similar business is established in the target market?

♦ Is the business adequately insured if a patient sues the business?

Obviously, it is impossible to anticipate everything a new business may encounter. However, it is a good idea to provide a section that illustrates the planner has thought about the unexpected and has ideas on what to do if things do not go as planned. This is referred to as a contingency plan. The written business plan need not present the contingency plan in great detail. Rather, this detail must be in the mind of the business owner when the idea is presented to potential financial backers. The writer should identify the anticipated risks and propose the action that will result if the risk occurs. Critical assumptions vary from one company to another, but some common categories are market interest and growth potential, competitor actions and retaliation, time and cost of development, operating expenses, and availability and timing of financing (Timmons et al, 2004).

Pearl
♦ A common critical risk is market acceptance of the proposed business.

A good contingency plan has two parts. First, it spells out warning signals that may indicate the business is off course; second, it explains the actions needed to correct the problem. The problem with most new businesses is that the owner does not anticipate having difficulties until the business is already in trouble. This is especially true in small businesses, where running out of cash is often a problem.

Good business planning establishes a system to monitor operations so that the discovery time for problems is as short as possible. This process involves monitoring financial results and carefully analyzing the implications of any changes. A contingency plan should address the need to implement an action quickly and decisively. For example, if the

financial forecast projected selling 15 hearing aids per month in the first 6 months, and the business sold only 10 per month, how would the business meet its debt and payroll obligations? A system should be devised to establish when the business is beginning to slide into trouble. In this case, management may establish a policy that states if revenue is down $X\%$ for 2 consecutive months, adjustments will be made to compensate for the losses.

Some business plans do not include a section explicitly dealing with contingency planning; rather, the issue is dealt with in the financial section. The main purpose of the risk section is to convince the reading audience that time was spent considering problems that the business may face, and options are provided in case problems do occur.

Conclusion

The conclusion section of the business plan summarizes the key elements of the plan and demonstrates the consistency between the overall aims, the present position analysis, and the proposed business strategies. A well-constructed conclusion to a business plan may be comprised of the aims of the business, the key factors for success, the extent that the proposed business can satisfy the key factors for success, and any major challenges that the business may face.

A sample of a conclusion is found in **Fig. 13–10**.

♦ Preparing for the Future

Pearl
♦ Good planning and persistence breed success.

After completing the business plan, the writer should have a good idea of the services the business will offer, the products that will be sold, to whom they will be sold, who the competition is, how the business will be marketed, what the risks are, and what kind of finances will be involved in the business venture.

An initial step in the business planning process is to create a timeline. The timeline will establish the specific time frame of the operations and will assist in planning special events, such as the purchase of equipment, hiring of additional employees, seasonal highs and lows, and vacations. When starting a business, the owner is faced with a monumental set of tasks that can be organized and predicted through the completion of a timeline of events necessary to open the business by a certain date.

If the writer has created a well thought out business plan, he or she now has a check in hand and is ready to embark on the adventure of starting the business. Suddenly faced with a large sum of money, the business owner should take care not to spend the money carelessly or too quickly. The owner needs to prioritize and schedule purchases to ensure the business follows the path that the plan has paved. Success does not begin when the money begins flowing. Success begins long before, as the owner attacks and meets all necessary goals to get the business on the road to profitability.

Although nothing is easy, a private practice in audiology can be a lucrative and rewarding experience for the person who is willing to devote the time and energy needed to succeed. A sample of a business plan is included in Appendix 13–2.

Appendix 13–1

Notice of Exclusions from Medicare Benefits

There are items and services for which Medicare will not pay.

- ◆ Medicare does not pay for all of your health care costs. Medicare only pays for covered benefits. Some items and services are not Medicare benefits, and Medicare will not pay for them.

- ◆ When you receive an item or service that is not a Medicare benefit, you are responsible to pay for it, personally or through any other insurance that you may have.

The purpose of this notice is to help you make an informed choice about whether or not you want to receive these items or services, knowing that you will have to pay for them yourself.

Before you make a decision, you should read this entire notice carefully.

Ask us to explain if you don't understand why Medicare won't pay.

Ask us how much these items or services will cost you (**estimated cost: $_____**).

Medicare will not pay for _____.

❑ 1. Because it does not meet the definition of any Medicare benefit.

❑ 2. Because of the following exclusion[1] from Medicare benefits:

❑ Personal comfort items.

❑ Most shots (vaccinations).

❑ Hearing aids and hearing examinations.

❑ Most outpatient prescription drugs.

❑ Orthopedic shoes and foot supports (orthotics).

❑ Health care received outside of the USA.

❑ Services required as a result of war.

❑ Services paid for by a governmental entity that is not Medicare.

❑ Services for which the patient has no legal obligation to pay.

❑ Home health services furnished under a plan of care, if the agency does not submit the claim.

❑ Items and services excluded under the Assisted Suicide Funding Restriction Act of 1997.

❑ Items or services furnished in a competitive acquisition area by any entity that does not have a contract with the Department of Health and Human Services (except in a case of urgent need).

❑ Physicians' services performed by a physician assistant, midwife, psychologist, or nurse anesthetist, when furnished to an inpatient, unless they are furnished under arrangements by the hospital.

❑ Items and services furnished to an individual who is a resident of a skilled nursing facility (SNF) or of a part of a facility that includes a SNF, unless they are furnished under arrangements by the SNF.

❑ Services of an assistant at surgery without prior approval from the peer review organization.

❑ Outpatient occupational and physical therapy services furnished incident to a physician's services.

❑ Routine physicals and most tests for screening.

❑ Routine eye care, eyeglasses, and examinations.

❑ Cosmetic surgery.

❑ Dental care and dentures (in most cases).

❑ Routine foot care and flat foot care.

❑ Services by immediate relatives.

❑ Services under a physician's private contract.

[1] This is only a general summary of exclusions from Medicare benefits. It is not a legal document.

The official Medicare program provisions are contained in relevant laws, regulations, and rulings. Form No. CMS-20007 (January 2003)

Appendix 13–2

Sample Business Plan

The following example of a business plan was used by an audiologist who started a new private practice. Note that it contains most, but not all, of the business plan components discussed in this chapter.

AUDIOLOGY ASSOCIATES

January 2007

John Jones
President
488 E. Magnolia Lane
Saint Joseph, Michigan 49987
(555) 555–6549

Mission Statement for Audiology Associates

Audiology Associates (AA) was established to provide quality comprehensive audiometric services, including diagnostic audiometric assessments, vestibular assessments, vestibular rehabilitation for benign paroxysmal positional vertigo, hearing aid sales, and service to a diverse patient population. AA is a nondiscriminatory practice.

Statement of Purpose

AA is seeking $65,000 for the purpose of purchasing equipment and supplies, property rental located at 742 Ridgeway Drive in South End, Michigan, renovations and furnishings for the office space, and maintenance of sufficient cash reserves to operate an audiology practice offering diagnostic audiometric evaluations, hearing aid sales, vestibular assessments, and vestibular rehabilitation for benign paroxysmal positional vertigo. This sum, along with the $20,000 cash equity and $60,000 offered as collateral, will be sufficient to finance this company through the start-up phase of the business.

Description of Business

AA is an audiology practice specializing in diagnostic audiological assessment, hearing aid sales, including conventional and programmable technology, vestibular assessment, and rehabilitation for benign paroxysmal positional vertigo (BPPV).

According to the National Institutes of Health 2005–2006, the prevalence of chronic impairment as a result of dizziness affects more than 2 million people in the United States alone. Vertigo or dizziness is the most common reason for seeking medical care in the population older than 75. It is estimated that 15 to 23% of individuals older than 65 who experience falls do so as a result of vertigo. The most common balance disorder is BPPV.

BPPV is particularly amenable to therapy. Several treatment regimens have been suggested in the literature. AA will use a modified Epley maneuver to remove debris from the semicircular canals. Studies have cited efficacy rates of 79 to 100% successful after one treatment.

AA will provide the diagnostic testing for vestibular disorders on the referral from a physician. Treatment by means of a modified Epley maneuver will be suggested for those patients with BPPV (the most common cause of dizziness in adults younger than 50).

A key component in identifying balance disorders, communication disabilities, and pathological conditions of the ear is through a thorough diagnostic audiometric evaluation. Audiometric assessment can help determine the need for medical treatment or amplification.

According to the US Census Bureau, the fastest growing segment of the United States population is that of persons over the age of 85, and the incidence of hearing loss is highly prevalent in that population. Couple this with the fact that hearing loss is increasing in all age populations, especially in those of people over the age of 50, and the results equate to a burgeoning potential patient base.

Amplification systems, when properly fit and maintaind, can provide the hearing-impaired person with significant benefit. Improvements in hearing aid technology have opened up a multitude of fitting options and flexibility and the ability to introduce and dispense new technology to patients every 4 to 5 years.

Hearing aid technology has improved dramatically over the past few years, and patients with mild high-frequency losses can be successfully fit with amplification. This state-of-the-art technology offers cosmetically and acoustically acceptable options for patients. Improvements in fitting procedures and real world listening environments have increase the accuracy of fitting frequency-specific prescription. Directional and self-learning devices have increased user satisfaction which has caused a concomitant increase in patient referrals.

Personnel

Vestibular Assessment and Rehabilitative Audiologist—This position must be held by a certified audiologist. Past experience with electronystagmography (ENG) testing or special course completion for hands-on testing and assessment is necessary.

Lenore Halpin, Au.D., will be the primary service provider for vestibular services. Dr. Halpin has more than 10 years of experience with ENG testing and has completed two educational courses on assessment and treatment of BPPV offered by Dr. Susan Bauer and Dr. Marian Girardi.

Testing and rehabilitative services will also be provided by Darlene Lewis, Au.D., audiologist. Dr. Lewis has experience providing rehabilitation services for BPPV. She will be working part time at AAA.

Dispensing Audiologist—Duties will be to sell hearing aids, provide hearing aid rehabilitation and consultation, provide hearing aid repair, and remake services. This position must be filled by a licensed dispensing audiologist or an audiologist with a hearing aid trainee's license. A minimum of 2 years' experience with hearing aid selections and fittings is preferred.

Administrative Assistant—Duties will include patient scheduling, billing insurance companies, document accounts payable and receivable, filing, assisting with correspondence, and contacting patients for new and follow-up appointments. This candidate needs to have a clean and professional appearance. He or she must be able to interact with patients and other professionals with a courteous, friendly attitude. Knowledge of computer-based billing, word processing, and file management is preferred but not necessary if the candidate shows a willingness and ability to learn.

AA will offer comprehensive hearing aid fitting services. AA will be equipped with the latest technology available for fitting hearing aids and completing real-ear measurements and target gain assessments. This will ensure that patients get the professional services needed and the maximum benefits from amplification. Prefitting and postfitting patient satisfaction surveys will be used to quantify hearing aid fitting success in conjunction with target gain validation through the use of real-ear measures.

Marketing Plan

AA will target Berrien, Van Buren, and Cassopolis counties in Southwest Michigan. Services will be promoted to physicians and clients in these areas. Marketing highlights will market that AA employs two full-time doctors of audiology. The practice offers the world's first virtual reality hearing center. AA provides vestibular assessment, vestibular rehabilitation for BPPV, audiometric services, and hearing aid sales in one location. AA will participate with BCBS, Medicare, Medicaid, PPOM, Priority Health, and Blue Care Network. Physicians will be attracted by our insurance participation, ease in scheduling, comprehensive services, and Dr. Halpin's experience as an exceptional diagnostic audiologist. Patients will be attracted by our location, word of mouth reputation, insurance participation, services, and competitive prices. Information will be disseminated through advertisements in local newspapers, brochures sent to physicians, and flyers sent to previous hearing aid clients.

Competition

Saint Joseph currently has 4 hearing aid dispensing audiologists and 3 hearing aid dealerships offering hearing aid and related services. These companies are located in 12 different locations. The majority of the hearing aid dispensers are located in the southeast and southwest areas of Berrien County. In the northeast, competition will come from a Miracle Ear satellite office and Rapp Solartone, both located on Prainer Avenue. These locations do not employ an audiologist and are unable to provide comprehensive audiologic services, hence, no physician referrals. Neither of these locations provides vestibular assessment or rehabilitation services.

Three locations provide vestibular assessment at this time: St. John's Hospital, Drs. Harry and Byrns, and Baroda Ear Nose and Throat. None of these locations provides rehabilitation for BPPV. A physical therapy group is located at St. Mary's Hospital that provides vestibular rehabilitation, but it does not provide audiometric or vestibular assessments.

Financial Overview

AA is an audiology private practice offering diagnostic audiometric evaluations, hearing aid sales, vestibular assessment, and vestibular rehabilitation for BPPV. On the basis of data from similar businesses in the Saint Joseph area, it will take up to 8 months for AA to become a profitable corporation. The start-up costs for these first 8 months is projected to be $91,000, which includes an investment of approximately $65,000 in equipment.

A personal investment from David and Lenore Halpin in the amount of $60,000 and an approved line of credit for $40,000 will be sufficient to finance this company through the start-up phase and into the second year, when the company will be profitable. In addition, David will continue with his current employment as a civil engineer. A detailed budget estimate of the initial 2 years of operation, including projected expenses and revenues, is included.

Attached are **Figs. 13–A1** (profit and loss worksheet), **13–A2** (cash flow projection by quarter, year 2), and **13–A3** (business portfolio).

Profit and Loss
(Projected Income) Statement For Period Ended _____

Company Name _____

	Mo 1	Mo 2	Mo 3	Mo 4	Mo 5	Mo 6	Mo 7	Mo 8	Mo 9	Mo 10	Mo 11	Mo 12	Total	Ratio
Revenue														
1) Gross Sales (Total Revenue)														
2) Less Sales, returns & allowances														
3) Net Sales (1-2)														
Cost of Goods Sold														
4) Beginning Inventory														
5) Plus: Purchases														
6) Total Goods Available (4+5)														
7) Less: Ending Inventory														
8) Total Cost of Goods Sold (6-7)														
9) Gross Profit (Gross Margin (3-8)														
Operating Expenses														
10) Advertising														
11) Automobile														
12) Depreciation														
13) Dues/Subscriptions/Licenses														
14) Insurance														
15) Interest														
16) Legal and Professional														
17) Office Supplies														
18) Payroll Expenses (Taxes)														
19) Rent														
20) Salaries														
21) Taxes-Sales, etc.														
22) Telephone														
23) Travel & Entertainment														
24) Utilities														
25) Wages - Employees														
26) Other Expenses: _____														
27) _____														
28) _____														
29) _____														
30) TOTAL OPERATING EXPENSES (10+29)														
Profit Before Taxes (9-30)														
Taxes - Federal _____														
Taxes - State _____														
Taxes - Local _____														
Profit After Taxes														

Figure 13–A1 Profit and loss worksheet.

Cash Flow Projection by Quarter, Year Two

	A	B	C	D	E	F
1		1st Qtr.	2nd Qtr.	3rd Qtr.	4th Qtr.	Total
2	Cash Receipts					
3	Receivables	$3,200				$3,200
4	Wholesale	$38,900	$54,800	$76,500	$94,800	$265,000
5	Retail	$41,000	$37,400	$48,600	$53,000	$180,000
6	Other Sources			$12,000	$15,000	$27,000
7	Total Cash Receipts:	$83,100	$92,200	$137,100	$162,800	$475,200
8	Cash Disbursements					
9	Cost of Goods	$57,528	$66,384	$90,072	$106,416	$320,400
10	Variable Labor			$604	$2,196	$2,800
11	Advertising	$2,000	$2,305	$3,125	$3,695	$11,125
12	Insurance	$950	$950	$950	$950	$3,800
13	Legal and Accounting	$500	$500	$500	$500	$2,000
14	Delivery Expenses	$1,600	$1,844	$2,500	$2,956	$8,900
15	*Fixed Cash Disbursements	$12,630	$12,640	$12,640	$12,640	$50,550
16	Mortgage (rent)	$2,628	$2,628	$2,628	$2,628	$10,512
17	Term Loan	$1,602	$1,602	$1,602	$1,602	$6,408
18	Line of Credit			$12,140	$15,360	$27,500
19	Other					
20	Total Cash Disbursements:	$79,438	$88,853	$126,761	$148,943	$443,995
21						
22	Net Cash Flow:	$3,662	$3,347	$10,339	$13,857	$31,205
23						
24	Cumulative Cash Flow:	$2,424	$5,771	$16,110	$29,967	$54,272
25						
26	*Fixed Cash Disbursement					
27	(FCD)	Year Two				
28	Utilities	$2,640				
29	Salaries	$39,000				
30	Payroll Taxes and Benefits	$4,875				
31	Office Supplies	$360				
32	Maintenance and Cleaning	$360				
33	Licenses	$115				
34	Boxes, Paper, etc.	$800				
35	Telephone	$1,800				
36	Miscellaneous	$600				
37	Total: FCD/yr	$50,550				
38	FCD/qtr	$12,638				

This spreadsheet was prepared using the Excel spreadsheet program from Microsoft.

Figure 13–A2 Cash flow projection by quarter, year 2.

Capital Budget

Product Description	Current Est.	Month 1	Month 2	Month 3	Month 4	Month 5	Month 6	Month 7	Month 8	Month 9	Month 10	Month 11	Month 12	Total
Audiometer	$ -													$ -
Sound Booth	$ 3,700.00	$ 3,700.00	$0	$0	$0	$0	$0	$0	$0	$0	$0	$0	$0	
Tympanometer	$ 1,700.00	$ 1,700.00	$0	$0	$0	$0	$0	$0	$0	$0	$0	$0	$0	
Curets and Headlight	$ 300.00	$ 300.00	$0	$0	$0	$0	$0	$0	$0	$0	$0	$0	$0	$ 300.00
Otoscope	$ 200.00	$ 200.00	$0	$0	$0	$0	$0	$0	$0	$0	$0	$0	$0	$ 200.00
Procedure Table	$ 1,000.00	$ 1,000.00	$0	$0	$0	$0	$0	$0	$0	$0	$0	$0	$0	$ 1,000.00
Vestibular Testing Unit	$ 20,000.00	$ 20,000	$0	$0	$0	$0	$0	$0	$0	$0	$0	$0	$0	$ 20,000.00
Phonics Box w/ Real Ear	$ 2,500.00	$ 2,500.00	$0	$0	$0	$0	$0	$0	$0	$0	$0	$0	$0	$ 2,500.00
Grinding Wheel w/ Attachment	$0	$0	$0	$0	$0	$0	$0	$0	$0	$0	$0	$0	$0	
NOAH Software	$ 1,000.00	$ 1,000.00	$0	$0	$0	$0	$0	$0	$0	$0	$0	$0	$0	$ 1,000.00
Fax Machine	$ 300.00	$ 300.00	$0	$0	$0	$0	$0	$0	$0	$0	$0	$0	$0	$ 300.00
Copy Machine	$ 600.00	$ 600.00	$0	$0	$0	$0	$0	$0	$0	$0	$0	$0	$0	$ 600.00
Computer (2)	$ 5,000.00	$ 5,000.00	$0	$0	$0	$0	$0	$0	$0	$0	$0	$0	$0	$ 5,000.00
Printers (2)	$ 500.00	$ 500.00	$0	$0	$0	$0	$0	$0	$0	$0	$0	$0	$0	$ 500.00
Phone System	$ 2,000.00	$ 2,000.00	$0	$0	$0	$0	$0	$0	$0	$0	$0	$0	$0	$ 2,000.00
Furniture	$ 5,000.00	$ 5,000.00	$0	$0	$0	$0	$0	$0	$0	$0	$0	$0	$0	$ 5,000.00
Misc.	$ 2,000.00	$ 1,000.00	$0	$0	$0	$0	$0	$0	$ 1,000	$0	$0	$0	$0	$ 2,000.00
Total Capital Expenditures	**$ 44,800.00**	**$ 44,800.00**	**$0**	**$0**	**$0**	**$0**	**$0**	**$0**	**$1,000**	**$0**	**$0**	**$0**	**$0**	**$ 44,800.00**

Operating Expenses

Product Description	Per Year Estimate	Monthly Estimate	Month 1	Month 2	Month 3	Month 4	Month 5	Month 6	Month 7	Month 8	Month 9	Month 10	Month 11	Month 12	Total
ASHA, AAA, MAA Dues	$ 370.00	$ 30.83													$ 370.00
Dealers Exam	$ 740.00	$ 61.67	$ 400.00	$ -	$ -	$ -	$ -	$ -	$ -	$ -	$ -	$ 340.00	$ -	$ -	$ 740.00
Corporate Publications	$ 3,000.00	$ 250.00	$ 1,500.00	$ -	$ -	$ -	$ -	$ -	$ -	$ 1,000.00	$ -	$ 500.00	$ -	$ -	$ 3,000.00
Advertisements	$ 6,500.00	$ 541.67	$ 200.00	$ 2,500.00	$ 200.00	$ 200.00	$ 200.00	$ 200.00	$ 200.00	$ 2,000.00	$ 200.00	$ 200.00	$ 200.00	$ -	$ 6,500.00
Liability Insurance	$ 600.00	$ 50.00	$ 50.00	$ 50.00	$ 50.00	$ 50.00	$ 50.00	$ 50.00	$ 50.00	$ 50.00	$ 50.00	$ 50.00	$ 50.00	$ 50.00	$ 600.00
Employment Insurance	$ 1,200.00	$ 100.00	$ 100.00	$ 100.00	$ 100.00	$ 100.00	$ 100.00	$ 100.00	$ 100.00	$ 100.00	$ 100.00	$ 100.00	$ 100.00	$ 100.00	$ 1,200.00
Wages/FICA	$ 31,377.08	$ 2,368.08	$ 2,368.08	$ 2,368.08	$ 2,368.08	$ 2,368.08	$ 2,368.08	$ 2,368.08	$ 2,368.08	$ 2,368.08	$ 3,108.11	$ 3,108.11	$ 3,108.11	$ 3,108.11	$ 31,377.08
Lease w/ remodel	$ 21,000.00	$ 1,750.00	$ 1,750.00	$ 1,750.00	$ 1,750.00	$ 1,750.00	$ 1,750.00	$ 1,750.00	$ 1,750.00	$ 1,750.00	$ 1,750.00	$ 1,750.00	$ 1,750.00	$ 1,750.00	$ 21,000.00
Construction Cost															
Utilities	$ 2,400.00	$ 200.00	$ 200.00	$ 200.00	$ 200.00	$ 200.00	$ 200.00	$ 200.00	$ 200.00	$ 200.00	$ 200.00	$ 200.00	$ 200.00	$ 200.00	$ 2,400.00
Phone	$ 2,400.00	$ 200.00	$ 200.00	$ 200.00	$ 200.00	$ 200.00	$ 200.00	$ 200.00	$ 200.00	$ 200.00	$ 200.00	$ 200.00	$ 200.00	$ 200.00	$ 2,400.00
Supplies	$ 2,400.00	$ 200.00	$ 200.00	$ 200.00	$ 200.00	$ 200.00	$ 200.00	$ 200.00	$ 200.00	$ 200.00	$ 200.00	$ 200.00	$ 200.00	$ 200.00	$ 2,400.00
Maintenance/Cleaning	$ 1,200.00	$ 100.00	$ 100.00	$ 100.00	$ 100.00	$ 100.00	$ 100.00	$ 100.00	$ 100.00	$ 100.00	$ 100.00	$ 100.00	$ 100.00	$ 100.00	$ 1,200.00
Training/Education	$ 2,400.00	$ 200.00	$ -	$ -	$ -	$ -	$ -	$ 600.00	$ 800.00	$ 200.00	$ 200.00	$ 200.00	$ 200.00	$ 200.00	$ 2,400.00
Travel/Entertainment Exp.	$ 2,400.00	$ 200.00	$ 200.00	$ 200.00	$ 200.00	$ 200.00	$ 200.00	$ 200.00	$ 200.00	$ 200.00	$ 200.00	$ 200.00	$ 200.00	$ 200.00	$ 2,400.00
Lawyer Fees	$ 2,100.00	$ 175.00	$ 100.00	$ 100.00	$ 100.00	$ 100.00	$ 100.00	$ 100.00	$ 1,000.00	$ 100.00	$ 100.00	$ 100.00	$ 100.00	$ 100.00	$ 2,100.00
Corporate Fees/License	$ 500.00	$ 41.67	$ -	$ -	$ -	$ -	$ -	$ -	$ 500.00	$ -	$ -	$ -	$ -	$ -	$ 500.00
Accountant Fees	$ 2,000.00	$ 166.67	$ 500.00	$ 100.00	$ 100.00	$ 100.00	$ 100.00	$ 100.00	$ 500.00	$ 100.00	$ 100.00	$ 100.00	$ 100.00	$ 100.00	$ 2,000.00
Misc.	$ 2,400.00	$ 200.00	$ 200.00	$ 200.00	$ 200.00	$ 200.00	$ 200.00	$ 200.00	$ 200.00	$ 200.00	$ 200.00	$ 200.00	$ 200.00	$ 200.00	$ 2,400.00
Total Expenses	**$ 84,987.08**	**$ 6,836.68**	**$ 8,068.08**	**$ 8,068.08**	**$ 6,768.08**	**$ 6,768.08**	**$ 6,768.08**	**$ 6,968.08**	**$ 8,368.08**	**$ 8,768.08**	**$ 6,708.11**	**$ 7,648.11**	**$ 6,708.11**	**$ 6,708.11**	**$ 84,617.08**

Projected Revenue

Service/Sales	$ per test	Month 1	Month 2	Month 3	Month 4	Month 5	Month 6	Month 7	Month 8	Month 9	Month 10	Month 11	Month 12	Total
Vestibular Testing	$ 250.00	0	0	1	2	3	3	4	4	6	6	8	10	47
Vestibular Treatment	$ 120.00	0	0	0	0	1	1	1	2	2	2	3	3	15
Hearing Test	$ 70.00	0	8	12	16	20	20	20	25	25	25	30	30	231
Hearing Aid Sales	$ 500.00	0	4	4	6	8	10	10	14	14	16	20	20	126
Total Revenue		**$ -**	**$ 2,560.00**	**$ 3,090.00**	**$ 4,620.00**	**$ 6,270.00**	**$ 7,270.00**	**$ 7,620.00**	**$ 9,590.00**	**$ 10,490.00**	**$ 11,490.00**	**$ 14,460.00**	**$ 14,960.00**	**$ 92,720.00**

Figure 13–A3 Business portfolio. AAA, American Academy of Audiology; ASHA, American Speech-Language-Hearing Association; FICA, Federal Insurance Contributions Act (Social Security); MAA, Michigan Academy of Audiology. (Continued)

Net Income Projections	Month 1	Month 2	Month 3	Month 4	Month 5	Month 6	Month 7	Month 8	Month 9	Month 10	Month 11	Month 12	Total
Total Capital Expenditures	$ 44,800.00	$ -	$ -	$ -	$ -	$ -	$ -	$ 1,000.00	$ -	$ -	$ -	$ -	$ 45,800.00
Total Operating Expenses	$ 8,068.08	$ 8,068.08	5,768.08	$ 5,768.08	$ 5,768.08	$ 6,368.08	8,368.08	$ 8,768.08	$ 6,708.11	$ 7,548.11	$ 6,708.11	$ 6,708.11	$ 84,617.08
Total Liability	$ 52,868.08	$ 8,068.08	6,768.08	$ 6,768.08	$ 6,768.08	$ 6,368.08	8,368.08	$ 9,768.08	$ 6,708.11	$ 7,648.11	$ 6,708.11	$ 6,708.11	$ 130,417.08
Total Revenue	$ -	$ 2,660.00	3,090.00	$ 4,620.00	$ 6,270.00	$ 7,270.00	7,520.00	$ 9,990.00	$ 10,490.00	$ 11,490.00	$ 14,490.00	$ 14,950.00	$ 92,720.00
Net Income	$ (52,868.08)	$ (5,408.08)	(2,678.08)	$ (1,148.08)	$ 501.92	$ 901.92	(848.08)	$ 221.92	$ 3,781.89	$ 3,941.89	$ 7,781.89	$ 8,241.89	$ (37,697.08)

First 8 months cost = $ 102,744.64			First 8 months income = $ 41,320.00				First 8 months net = $ (61,424.64)					

Figure 13–A3 (Continued)

References

Ames, M. (1983). Small business management. St. Paul, MN: West Publishing.

Brandt, S. (1997). Focus your business (pp. 123–134). Friday Harbor, WA: Archipelago Publishing.

DeThomas, A., & Grensing-Pophal, L. (2001). Writing a convincing business plan. Hauppauge, NY: Baron's Educational Series.

Hirji, N. (1999). Business awareness for optometrists. Woburn, MA: Butterworth-Heinemann.

Horan, J. (2004). The one page business plan. Berkeley, CA: The One PAGE Business Plan Company.

Hosford-Dunn, H., Dunn, D., & Harford, E. (1995). The business plan. In Audiology business and practice management (pp. 55–76). San Diego, CA: Singular Publishing Group.

Kimbro, D. (2004). Think and grow rich. San Diego, CA: Aventine Press.

Kochkin, S. (2005). MarkeTrac VII: Hearing loss population tops 31 million people. Hearing Review, 12(7), 16–29.

McKeever, M. (1994). How to write a business plan. Berkeley, CA: NOLO Press.

Pinson, L., & Jinnett, J. (1996). Anatomy of a business plan. Chicago: Upstart Publishing.

Rich, S., & Gumpert, D. (2004) Business plans that win $$$. New York: Harper & Row.

Timmons, J., Zacharakis, A., & Spinelli, S. (2004). Business plans that work. Chicago: McGraw-Hill.

Traynor, R. (2005). Finance considerations in audiology practice. Audiology Today, 17(5), 42–45.

U.S. Small Business Association. (2006a). Starting your business: Business planning. Retrieved June 28, 2006, from http://www.sba.gov/starting_business/planning/writingplan.html

U.S. Small Business Association. (2006b). Starting your business: Startup basics. Retrieved June 28, 2006, from http://www.sba.gov/starting_business/startup/areyouready.html

Chapter 14

Designing an Audiology Practice

Jane H. Baxter, Deborah W. Clark, and Alan L. Desmond

Audiologists work in a range of settings: hospitals, private practices, schools, medical clinics and ear, nose, and throat (ENT) offices, hearing and speech centers, and universities. The inspiration to design a new practice may rise from several factors. Perhaps the existing space is too small, or parking is insufficient. Perhaps a hospital-based clinic is relocating due to overall reorganization of space. Maybe the practitioner is simply ready to work independently. Whatever the reason, the preparation and careful planning for this endeavor are of utmost importance. The work environment is as important as the home environment. The efficiency and aesthetics of the office will impact job satisfaction for all employees as well as the experience of the clients. Remember that most people who schedule an appointment arrive with some degree of anxiety or uncertainty. A professional environment that makes a statement about the quality of service provided will go a long way in ensuring that clients make return visits.

This chapter discusses the design process, from initial planning to the physical layout, with a focus on patient and staff needs. Also addressed in this chapter are such considerations as incorporating balance assessment in an audiology practice, the paperless office, networking, and ergonomics, as well as the privacy requirements of the Health Insurance Portability and Accountability Act (HIPAA) that affect the design of an office.

♦ The Design Process

The first step in designing a new audiology practice is planning. It is important to consider the demographics of the area in which the practice will be situated as well as the existing competition. Is the target population children, adults, or a combination of the two? Will the practice focus primarily on diagnostic services, rehabilitation, or both? Which professionals will refer to the practice? If there is competition in the area, what will this new practice have to offer that the established nearby practice does not provide?

Consider how staff and clients will move within the space. What will be the most comfortable flow in and out of the office for clients? Color schemes and decor will help define the image of your practice. As part of the planning process, it is important to consider location, layout, equipment, construction, and interior design. You also need to decide whether you will lease, rent, or purchase an office.

Pearl

- In the initial planning stage, think about not only how the practice is now but also how you expect it to be in 5 to 10 years. It is much more cost-effective to pay rent for extra space now than to be forced to move to a bigger location in a few years.

Planning

Once the decision has been made to design a practice, there are several things to consider. Now is the time to brainstorm about the "ideal" practice, with the understanding that compromises may need to be made later on. The focus of the practice will dictate many decisions. For example, if primarily diagnostic services are being offered, you must allow sufficient space for sound booths, electrophysiological tests, and otoacoustic emissions (OAE), in addition to audiometric and immittance procedures. Counseling space will also be necessary. If vestibular services are provided, there will be additional space requirements. If the focus of the practice is rehabilitation of hearing loss, there will be space requirements for real ear and electroacoustic evaluations of hearing aids, as well as basic diagnostic equipment. Sufficient space may also be necessary for assistive device displays and aural rehabilitation classes. A practice with a pediatric focus will have many considerations regarding specific equipment and a child-friendly decor.

Because it is not expected that audiologists have any formal training in architecture, real estate, space planning, or interior design, it is important to seek professional guidance from those with expertise in these areas. When planning a budget, include the cost of hiring these professionals. The money spent up front may keep you from losing money later on due to poor decisions made during the planning stage. For example, there may be regulatory considerations that an architect will be aware of. Hospitals, in particular, may have design or construction regulations that must be adhered to. (If an existing hospital-based practice is being moved to another location, the hospital may have contracted professionals available to provide assistance.) On the flip side, these professionals are unlikely to know anything at all about audiology. They will need to understand what an audiologist does and who receives services. If there is an existing practice, it might be helpful for these consultants to spend some time observing part of the daily routine. If a new practice is being opened, perhaps there is a nearby audiology practice, located far enough away so as not to be a competitor, that would allow observation in the office for a short time.

Selecting a Location

Selecting a location for a practice is one of the most important decisions to be made. Location refers to the general geographical region (state, county, city, and neighborhood) as well as the specific building site and the space within the building. Several factors will influence the decision regarding where to open or relocate a practice.

Professional considerations include the following:

- Is office space available that is affordable and desirable?
- Are referral sources nearby and plentiful?
- Are other audiologists in the community cordial and collaborative?

Economic considerations include the following:

- Is there growth potential to support a new practice?
- Is the audiologist/population ratio low?
- Are consumer credit and collection records good?
- Do fee schedules reflect rises in the cost of living?
- Is the patient mix (private pay, third-party, etc.) likely to be favorable?
- Are income levels and wages high?

Personal considerations include the following:

- Where do you want to live? Is moving to a new area an option, or is it better to stay in the same area?
- Is the residential area of the proposed location attractive, affordable, and available?
- Is the climate favorable?
- Is the community progressive and well managed?
- Are schools modern, and is the education level high?
- Do cultural and other activities agree with your interests and hobbies?

If you are flexible and searching for a major change in location, it is best to talk with experts about the environment (urban, suburban, or rural), climate, schools, cost of living, community, taxes, and other lifestyle issues that are important. Professionals (accountants, lawyers, audiologists, medical personnel, etc.) can assist in determining the risk factors in moving to a certain locale. **Table 14–1** lists characteristics to consider when selecting a community.

Neighborhood and Building Site

Once you have selected the community, the next step is to find the actual neighborhood and building site. The perception of the location is critical. If the practice is located in a shopping center, it may attract a different clientele than if it is in a professional building. Which setting is more congruent with the population you want to serve? Are there similar

Table 14–1 Characteristics to Consider when Selecting a Community

Characteristic	Attributes
Source of income in city	Professional; wholesale/retail; manufacturing; farming
Population size	Large; medium; small
Population trends	Well established; growing/reviving; stationary/permanent/stable; stagnant; declining; uncertain/high turnover; seasonal
Income stream of community	Multiple industries and income sources; positive business climate: new businesses; competition of a few industries; dependent on one industry
Income distribution	Wealthy; middle income; low income; evenly distributed
Competing services	Few; average; many; too many
Type of competition	Minimal service—price-sensitive, low-tech; average service and competence; full service—organized, high-tech; sophisticated delivery system, leading edge
Quality of life	Well-maintained homes; ample parks; attractive streets; churches; high-quality schools; adequate professional services: banks, lawyers, doctors, etc.; adequate transportation and utilities; satisfactory climate; convenient recreation/entertainment

Source: Adapted from Windmill, I., Cunningham, D., & Johnson, K. (2000). Designing an audiology practice. In H. Hosford-Dunn, R. J. Roeser, & M. Valente (Eds.), Audiology practice management (pp. 291–311) New York: Thieme Medical Publishers.

service-oriented businesses nearby? Is it preferable to be near a medical center, senior center, physician private practices, or university? Don't forget to evaluate the competition. Determine the number of other professionals and providers in the area that offer the same kinds of services your practice will be offering. It is time to talk with real estate, banking, and legal experts.

It is also important to be on the lookout for negative influences such as unsightly nearby buildings, noise, fumes, industry, fire hazards, safety concerns, and poor or difficult access. Check the flow of traffic near the site and the ambiance of the building. Because most audiology patients are typically pediatric or geriatric, it is helpful to have ground-floor space, near convenient (and handicapped-accessible)

parking. **Table 14–2** lists several qualities to consider when visiting building sites.

As you are evaluating the actual building site, check the common areas in the building. Is the lobby clean and professional? Is there visible and attractive signage for each unit (Baxter, 1994)?

Suite Space and Layout

Within the space, is the configuration compatible with the practice's needs? Are there enough rooms, and are they large enough? Are the windows, lighting, and electrical/telephone outlets adequate and well placed? Would remodeling be necessary to make the area efficient? Who will pay

Table 14–2 Comparative Qualities of Actual Building Site

Neighborhood	Building A	Building B
Building is conveniently located, easy to find (high visibility). Neighborhood is safe; sidewalks and roads are in good condition. Building is located in professional area, near referrals. Transportation and parking are convenient. Site is quiet and away from traffic and noise sources. Commercial stores are nearby for supplies, staff lunches, etc.		

Building	Building A	Building B
Construction is sound, and building is in good condition. Building will support a sound booth. Landscaping is attractive. Building (and suite) has daily janitorial service. Restrooms are well maintained and nearby. Site has flexibility for future expansion needs. Common areas and lobby are clean and professional. Signage is highly visible.		

Suite	Building A	Building B
Ambiance of space is positive, and layout is efficient. Windows provide nice view and adequate lighting. Floors and walls are in good condition or will be replaced. Ventilation, electrical, plumbing, and telephone outlets are ample. Suite is handicapped accessible. Storage is adequate.		

Table 14–3 Example of SWOT Techniques for Evaluating a Location

Strengths

- It is in an established community with older, educated population.
- Referrals are nearby
- Site is close to home.
- Space is available in central location, with good terms.

Weaknesses

- Market is very competitive, with several successful audiology practices.
- Rent is high.
- Noisy traffic: becomes congested in afternoons

Opportunities

- New medical building is being built across the street from site.
- One of the local audiologists is retiring next year.
- Retirement home is locating in the area.

Threats

- New medical building will eventually open audiology clinic with dispensing services.
- People in this area seem to prefer managed care insurance.

SWOT, strengths, weaknesses, opportunities, and threats.
Source: Adapted from Windmill, I., Cunningham, D., & Johnson, K. (2000) Designing an audiology practice. In H. Hosford-Dunn, R. J. Roeser; & M. Valente (Eds.), Audiology practice management (pp. 291–311). New York: Thieme Medical Publishers, with permission.

for necessary changes and upgrades? It is best to address these issues before you become too attached to a particular location.

To help in making these decisions, consider the SWOT (strengths, weaknesses, opportunities, and threats) technique. Analyze each location by considering SWOT characteristics, as given in **Table 14–3.** When comparing strengths and weaknesses, you need to collect more data to have a realistic understanding of the site's potential. For example, when looking at possible referrals in the area, contact existing clinics, physicians, schools, and other professionals to ask approximately how many referrals per month they might provide. Are these referral sources dependable, or will there be changes in the future (e.g., retirement, downsizing, moving)? This analysis will help reveal the differences between different locations.

Leasing, Renting, or Purchasing an Office

Most private practice audiologists rent their space. When looking for space, it is important to have an advocate who will represent the needs of the practice. There are usually two realtors involved in real estate transactions. One realtor represents the landlord (or building); the other represents the tenant (audiology practice). It is a good idea to have a real estate attorney present while you are negotiating the lease. Leases are generally written to protect the landlord and property. You and your attorney should review the lease prior to the meeting to determine what changes are wanted and what items need negotiation and revision. Sometimes the landlord will provide a build-out allowance to help make the space suitable for the tenant. In a build-out allowance, the landlord agrees to finance some of the remodeling costs. This typically covers walls, basic flooring,

and electrical and plumbing systems. The financial amount and items covered in the build-out are usually negotiable, so it is wise to discuss different options with experts before the meeting.

Purchasing an existing building is more complex and expensive upfront, but it may be a wise investment for the future. There are tax advantages and long-term appreciation benefits, but there are also more risks. You may need to rent out part of the building, which makes you a landlord. The upkeep of the building will be the owner's responsibility. Consider the costs, effort, time, and personal (and emotional) energy that will be necessary to manage a building. A tax or real estate attorney can help you decide which option is best.

Special Consideration

- The location of a practice is crucial to its success. Do research upfront to facilitate the decision-making process. Be completely honest when evaluating professional, economic, and personal goals.

Pearl

- Spending time and money on the right consultants will save time and money in the long run. Specialists to consult with may include realtor, attorney, architect, space planner, interior designer, accountant, other audiologists, potential referral sources, bankers, and the local chamber of commerce.

- When negotiating a lease (with help from your attorney), research to determine what a fair agreement is, then negotiate to get it. Make sure the details are clearly spelled out.

Creating an Office Layout

Providing for Services

Whether you are working with an existing space or moving into a new space, the first step in creating the layout of a practice is to list all audiologic services and procedures that will be offered in this office (Windmill et al, 2000). **Table 14–4** lists operations an audiologist might expect to include in a practice.

For each of these potential operations, there are specific questions that must be answered to create a layout that works efficiently and conveniently for all personnel. Diagnostic procedures, amplification/aural rehabilitation procedures, and business operations, as well as various miscellaneous operations, should be analyzed separately. In thinking about procedures provided, accompanying workspace should be planned for. Allow enough space not only for the equipment but also for audiologists to place charts and record results. Personal work styles of audiologists and other staff members are of great importance. Additionally, compliance with the Americans with Disabilities Act (ADA) is crucial.

Diagnostic Procedures A practice offering advanced diagnostics may need to plan space for OAE, immittance, evoked potentials, and/or vestibular tests, in addition to conventional audiometry. Some of the most important layout decisions for diagnostic procedures will depend on how the sound booth is used.

1. Will immittance, electrophysiological tests, and/or OAE be performed inside or outside the booth? If multiple procedures are performed inside the booth, patients do not need to be moved from one space to another. Many elderly people have difficulty getting in and out of chairs, so providing as many services as possible in one spot may be beneficial. If the additional equipment is inside the sound booth, a larger booth will be required. A disadvantage is that if the practice has more than one audiologist, staff may find they spend a lot of time waiting for equipment to become available. If more booths are needed, additional equipment will have to be purchased for each booth, which becomes an expensive proposition. If procedures are performed outside the booth, a smaller sound booth will allow more space for equipment to be placed on the perimeter. This also allows easier access for other audiologists during busy clinic time, and it is likely to be a less expensive option.

2. How many booths will be needed? If this is an established practice, such as a hospital-based practice moving to a new facility, the number of booths necessary will be determined based on the size of the practice and the number of audiologists. For a newly established private office, it may be best to start small and allow for future growth.

3. What size sound booths are needed? If services are provided for children, visual reinforcement audiometry and play audiometry will be performed. The size of the sound booth necessary will depend largely on the population served. Obviously, evaluating children requires a larger test

Table 14–4 Potential Operations in an Audiology Practice

Audiologic Operations	**Miscellaneous Audiology**
Audiometry, pure tones, speech	Cerumen management
Immittance	Interpreter services
Otoacoustic emissions	Client/parent education
Visual reinforcement audiometry	Storage (audiology supplies)
Play audiometry	
	Business Operations
Evoked Potentials	Coding
Vestibular Procedures	Filing
Electronystagmography	Billing and collections
Rotational testing	Computer services
Posturography	Reception
Vestibular rehabilitation	Accounting
	Waiting room
Central Auditory Processing Evaluations	Administrative operations
Amplification Procedures	
Consultation	**Miscellaneous Operations**
Real ear and electroacoustic evaluations	Kitchen
Fitting amplification	Break room
Assistive devices	Restroom
Hearing aid laboratory	Storage (cleaning supplies)
	Coat closets
	Computer network

Source: Adapted from Windmill, I., Cunningham, D., & Johnson, K. (2000). Designing an audiology practice. In H. Hosford-Dunn, R. J. Roeser, & M. Valente (Eds.), Audiology practice management (pp. 291–311). New York: Thieme Medical Publishers, with permission.

space for visual reinforcers, a table and chairs, toys, and so on. There are sound booth specifications for sound-field testing. (see "Obtaining Equipment"). It may also be necessary to provide extra space for a parent as well as a test assistant to sit inside the booth. Provisions must also be made for wheelchair access in the test space.

Amplification and Aural Rehabilitation Procedures

1. Will real ear and electroacoustic evaluations of hearing aids be performed inside or outside the sound booth? If outside noise is likely to interfere with these measures, it may be beneficial to perform them in a test booth. Disadvantages of performing multiple tests in the booth have already been discussed.

2. Will audiologists share equipment? This is discussed in detail in "Accommodating Personal Work Styles."

3. Where will consultations take place? A noisy or otherwise distracting environment will be particularly frustrating to new hearing aid users. Most people with hearing impairment struggle to hear even in quiet environments. Limiting potential distractions will enable patients to focus and better follow the conversation. Potential distractions include traffic noise from an open window, noise from children in a pediatric waiting room, and busy phones.

4. Where will assistive listening devices (ALDs) be displayed? Options include the waiting area and a specialized ALD demonstration room.

5. What is required for a safe and efficient hearing aid laboratory? If basic services such as cleaning hearing aids and minor repairs will be performed on the premises, having a well-organized laboratory is crucial. Access to a sink will be necessary. Many audiologists do shell repairs that require the use of certain chemicals. If this is the case, the hearing aid laboratory will need to be well ventilated. An exhaust fan may be necessary.

6. Where will client/parent education take place? Clients will receive most information regarding their hearing loss in designated diagnostic or consultation areas. Many audiologists realize the benefit of offering aural rehabilitation classes in topics such as speechreading and communication strategies. If classes are to be offered, a room with sufficient space for small groups should be part of the plan.

Pearl

• Consider installing a loop or other assistive device in consultation areas or teaching rooms.

Miscellaneous Audiology

1. Will cerumen management services be provided in a specialized room or in the diagnostic test area? A specialized room with a sink and chair that raises and lowers (e.g., a dental chair) will make cerumen removal easier. This room could also be used for making earmold impressions. The obvious downsides of a special room such as this are cost and the frequent moving of patients who may have ambulatory problems.

2. Where will audiology supplies be stored? This cannot be overestimated. A central storage area, in addition to smaller storage areas for each workroom, is recommended.

Special Consideration

• If the practice will be treating patients from different backgrounds whose first language is not English, you may need to consider interpreter services. Some hospitals provide a central interpreter service that can be linked in real time to a remote site. Special monitors may be necessary, and placement of these should be determined.

Providing for Business Operations

Most likely a bookkeeper and/or office manager, along with a receptionist, will be among additional staff personnel. Depending on the size of the practice, other support help may be necessary. Business operations will include coding, filing, billing and collections, computer services, reception, scheduling, accounting, and administrative operations. Make a list of the furniture and equipment the office staff will need (see "Obtaining Equipment"). Needless to say, appropriate space for these operations is necessary. If business operations are not efficient, this will have a negative impact on the overall practice. Input from staff regarding space requirements is essential.

The design of the waiting room is of utmost importance. If walk-in services are to be provided, such as hearing aid cleaning and basic repairs, a larger waiting area will be necessary than would be needed if patients were seen by appointment only. See the "Interior Design" section of this chapter for more information regarding the waiting room.

Providing for Miscellaneous Operations

Miscellaneous operations include a kitchen/break area, restroom facilities, storage for coats and cleaning supplies, and computer networking needs. An efficient and pleasant environment may reduce employee stress, but it cannot replace an adequate break area. Don't forget to provide space for employees to have lunch. A small refrigerator and microwave oven should be on the equipment list. An office with inadequate storage space will be a frustrating and cluttered environment. Include a coat closet in the storage plans. Regarding restrooms, a hospital or professional building may provide these in a lobby or hallway. If not, space for restrooms will have to be incorporated in the overall design plans. If multiple computers are networked, how much space is necessary for networking requirements?

Accommodating Personal Work Styles

The organization of an office will depend greatly on the personal work styles of the audiologist(s). Examples of layout options are illustrated in **Figs. 14–1A** and **B**. Assume audiologists A and B are both looking for office space for a two-person dispensing practice. They each find office space in a professional building. **Figures 14–1A** and **B** have identical dimensions. Audiologist A **(Fig. 14–1A)** prefers to share diagnostic and consultation rooms to keep "patient space" separate from "office space." Audiologist B **(Fig. 14–1B)** doesn't mind seeing patients in his or her office and likes the idea of having all services available in one area. There are clear advantages and disadvantages to each arrangement.

In **Fig. 14–1A**, each audiologist has his or her own office, and patients are not necessarily seen in this space. Diagnostic and rehabilitative space is shared. A clear advantage of this arrangement is economic, in that only one sound booth, audiometer, hearing aid analyzer, and so on need to be purchased. This may be necessary for a new practice with a limited budget. In this arrangement, there is also additional space available for a patient education/ALD room, as well as a cerumen removal/impression room with sink. Another option would include space for evoked potential or vestibular testing. The primary disadvantage of this arrangement is scheduling. If two audiologists are seeing patients, only one at a time can do a hearing evaluation or hearing aid fitting. Over time this could mean a loss of income if patients are not scheduled efficiently.

In **Fig. 14–1B**, each audiologist has his or her own office and workspace. The audiologist performs real ear, hearing aid electroacoustic evaluations, impression taking, and cerumen removal in his or her office. Patient privacy becomes a bigger issue. The audiologist may have current patient files in the office for easy access related to report writing, follow-up phone calls, and other activities. These files will need to be stored out of sight of other patients who will be in and out of the office. The start-up cost of this arrangement is obviously higher because twice the equipment will

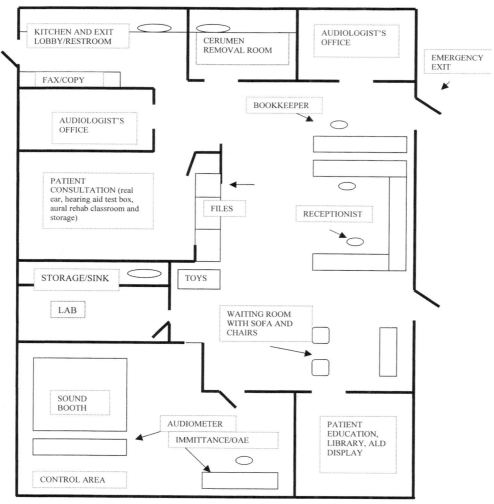

A

Figures 14–1 Potential office layouts that reflect personal work styles of individual audiologists. Although the basic floor plan and square footage are identical, **(A)** illustrates an office with much shared space. ALD, assisted living devices; OAE; otoacoustic emissions. (*Continued*)

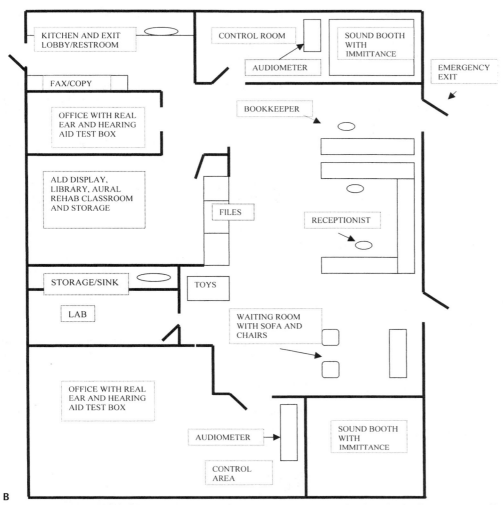

Figures 14–1 (*Continued*) **(B)** Illustrates an office in which each audiologist works individually. ALD, assisted living devices.

need to be purchased. Note also that the separate patient education room and cerumen removal room are lost. An advantage of **Fig. 14–1B** is scheduling. Each audiologist can see patients as time is available, with no concern regarding equipment availability. In addition, patients are not moved as frequently. This is helpful if there are a number of geriatric patients or others with mobility issues.

Although the basic layouts are very similar, each audiologist has designed a practice that is conducive to his or her own work style and habits. Patient flow will be very different in these two offices. The audiologists who work in the office illustrated in **Fig. 14–1A** will share much of the space and interact with each other often during the day. The audiologists who work in the space illustrated in **Fig. 14–1B** may not see each other much during the day at all but are able to organize their space in a way that works best for them individually. The pros and cons of each layout should be considered carefully, with attention to work style/habits versus budget issues.

Pearl

• Although sharing space and equipment may make good economic sense, scheduling patients will be more challenging. Personnel who schedule patients must be aware of these limitations.

Accessibility for People with Disabilities

Regardless of whether a pediatric or geriatric population will be served in the audiology practice, accessibility for people with disabilities must be planned for. The ADA requires adequate provisions for wheelchair access. For an audiology practice, specific areas for consideration are the entrance, sound booth, restrooms, and parking.

Entrance Having steps at an entrance can make the office inaccessible for people in wheelchairs or those with other mobility issues. Adding a short ramp or providing signage that directs persons to an accessible entrance is one solution. Additionally, door handles that require tight grasping, pinching, or twisting must be replaced with models that meet ADA requirements.

Sound booth   Will the sound booth be raised or recessed? (See "Construction" regarding the pros and cons of recessing the sound booth.) If the booth is raised, a wheelchair ramp will need to be constructed. Maneuvering space around the booth and door should be sufficient.

Restrooms   Are restrooms provided in a common area, as in a hospital or many professional buildings? If yes, ADA requirements for restrooms may have already been met. If no, the ADA has very specific requirements for wheelchair accessibility. Grab bars, sufficient maneuvering space, and accessible lavatories are just a few examples of ADA specifications. In planning a new office, consult the ADA to assure compliance. A contractor should also be very familiar with ADA requirements.

Parking   Once again, if planning an office in an existing professional building, hospital, or mall, parking spaces for persons with disabilities are likely to be in place already. If not, handicapped parking requirements as specified by the ADA must be well researched.

The information provided in this chapter should not be considered sufficient for planning an ADA-compliant facility. One resource, the *ADA Guide for Small Businesses* (1999) is available online through the U.S. Department of Justice.

Determining Operational Space Requirements

After producing a list of operations and equipment, the operational space requirements can be determined. Generate a list of rooms needed for the various operations, both clinical and business. By now a complete list of equipment and furniture (see "Obtaining Equipment") that will be used in each room should have been generated. It may be logical to combine various operations in one room, such as immittance and audiometry. If electronystagmography (ENG) and auditory brainstem tests share a computer, these two operations may need to occur in the same room. Be sure to obtain input from staff members who will be working in these various spaces. Other audiologists may have insight regarding patient flow and layout based on previous employment.

Once a decision has been made regarding the number of rooms needed and what equipment will go in each room, it is time to estimate square footage requirements. This may be more complicated than it seems. For example, you will know the exact dimensions of a sound booth based on the manufacturer's specifications. The surrounding space will be more complicated to determine. Sufficient space for doors to open will be necessary to accommodate typical movement patterns and wheelchair accessibility. Space for additional audiologic testing equipment (e.g., audiometer, compact disc player, and immittance equipment) will be needed. The supplies used for various business activities

will determine the need for storage and counter space. Don't forget printers, cleaning supplies, and sinks.

Unfortunately, it is not possible to look into a crystal ball to see into the future and plan for everything. Predictions regarding growth may or may not be accurate. Over time there will be changes in equipment or services, referral sources, or economic trends. Because it is not possible to predict every aspect of growth, it is recommended that ~20% more square footage be added onto each room estimate for unanticipated changes. This will allow accommodation of additional equipment and/or staff in the future. Furthermore, it is a good idea to add another 20 to 25% square footage overall to account for dead space (Windmill et al, 2000). Dead space includes closets, hallways, and restrooms. **Table 14–5** demonstrates how one might estimate space for a sample practice.

Using this formula, the total square footage may be quite surprising. If the square footage is more than the budget allows, a space planner may be able to help determine where cuts need to be made. This final analysis of square footage is, of course, closely tied to the decision about location.

After location has been identified and square footage determined, the layout should be sketched. If using existing space, start by sketching boundaries around fixed points. For example, the waiting area and sign-in desk/window will need to be next to the front entrance. From this point, think about the logical patient and staff traffic patterns. Could operations be maximized by having certain services close to each other or farther apart? It may work well to have the hearing aid fitting facilities near the bookkeeper in case clients have financial concerns or questions regarding their purchases.

Pearl

- When possible, it is helpful to have more than one entrance to the office. There should be an entrance the audiologists and other staff can use without passing by the waiting room. This allows employees to arrive at work and go on breaks without the disruption of seeing patients in the waiting area.

In the beginning of the planning process, it is important to think big. When it is time to get into the details of planning, you may have to scale things down or make compromises. Finding the balance between the perfect work environment and reality may be difficult. Choices will inevitably have to be made, but it is important that staff and patients are able to move about the space comfortably and safely. If the office is planned well, with the best service in the best location possible, that planned extra room for growth will fill quickly.

Obtaining Equipment

Equipment is a major investment in any new audiology practice. In developing the layout of the office, a list of procedures and equipment is generated. Some equipment is mandatory for opening a practice, and some can be added

Table 14–5 Example of Square Footage Calculations

Room Number/Title	Functions Included	Square Footage
Waiting	Seating for 10 persons	150
	End tables	4
	Coffee service	3
	Literature/magazine stand	3
	Approximate total	160 × 1.2 = 192
Reception/office staff	Desk/work area	60
	Filing rack (wall mounted)	10
	Fax	5
	Copy machine	5
	Supplies	20
	Approximate total	100 × 1.2 = 120
Audiometry I	Sound booth and control room	150
	Room for door swing	60
	Hall space	40
	Approximate total	250 × 1.2 = 300
Audiometry II	Immittance, otoacoustic emissions, video-otoscopy	100
	Approximate total	100 × 1.2 = 120
Evoked potentials	Auditory brainstem response, electronystagmography	120
	Approximate total	120 × 1.2 = 144
Hearing aid	Consultation and fitting, probe microphone unit, computer with NOAH software, earmold supplies, hearing aid supplies, chairs for family	150
	Approximate total	150 × 1.2 = 180
Business/office	Billing, collections, coding, filing	150
	Business manager	100
	Approximate total	250 × 1.2 = 300
Storage	Miscellaneous supplies	40
	Approximate total	40 × 1.2 = 48
Break room	Small kitchen	100
	Approximate total	100 × 1.2 = 120
Restroom	Restroom	20
	Approximate total	20 × 1.2 = 24
	Subtotal	**1548.0**
	Dead Space	**× 1.2**
	Total Estimated Square Footage	**1857.6**

Source: Adapted from Windmill, I., Cunningham, D., & Johnson, K. (2000). Designing an audiology practice. In H. Hosford-Dunn, R. J. Roeser, & M. Valente (Eds.), Audiology practice management (pp. 291–311). New York: Thieme Medical Publishers, with permission.

later. Obtain price quotes from several vendors regarding purchasing versus leasing equipment. **Table 14–6** lists some of the audiologic equipment you should consider when opening a practice.

Sound Booth

One of the most important decisions will be the specifics of the sound booth(s) purchased. As discussed in the layout section of this chapter, the size will be dictated, in part, by which procedures will be performed inside the booth as well as space limitations. There are many other characteristics on which to decide. Sound booths come in different sizes and have different insulation characteristics. Most private practices choose a single-walled sound booth for a variety of reasons:

- The building may not support the weight of a double-walled booth.

- Sound insulation is adequate: a single-walled booth will support sound-field testing up to 90 dB; this meets the needs of most private practices. A single-walled booth attenuates 50 to 60 dB.

- Cost is more reasonable.

- A single-walled booth requires less space.

Table 14–6 Audiologic Operations Equipment

Equipment	Specifics
Sound booth	Single, double walled, or custom. Pediatric testing requires 6 foot × 6 foot interior
Speakers	Pediatric testing requires 45 degree azimuth in relation to speaker
COR/VRA	Plexiglas cubes, video capability (LCD panel mounted on speakers)
Play audiometry	Dimmer for lights. Cabinet with doors so toys are out of sight. TV with VCR/DVD player for children to watch during OAE and immittance testing
Audiometer	Single, 1.5, or 2 channel. Options: Integrated PC-based system, extended frequency, various types of masking, patient response button
Transducers	Insert (ER-3A/5A), headphones (TDH-39, -49, or -50), bone oscillator
Monitor	Infrared or hard wired. Allows audiologist and test assistant to communicate
CD player	Multiple track for ability to switch CDs easily
Acoustic immittance	Options: screener and/or diagnostic, portable or desktop, multifrequency tympanometry, eustachian tube function, acoustic reflex latency, and contralateral and ipsilateral stimulation; printer options
OAE	Options: transient and/or distortion product, desktop or portable
Evoked potentials	Options: one versus two channel, various transducers and stimuli. Add ASSR for pediatrics
Vestibular equipment	Electronystagmography, rotational testing, platform posturography, vestibular rehabilitation equipment

ASSR, auditory steady-state response; CD, compact disc COR/VRA, conditioned orientation response/visual reinforcement audiometry; LCD, liquid crystal display; OAE, otoacoustic emissions.

If you will be doing cochlear implant testing or sound-field testing > 90 dB, a double-walled booth is necessary because sound will bleed through the walls and introduce feedback into the system. Most medical centers use double-walled booths partially because the booth may be located in a hallway or near a noisy area. If there is excessive ambient noise, some of it may leak into the booth, preventing adherence to American National Standards Institute (ANSI) standards for acceptable ambient noise levels.

> **Pearl**
>
> • To determine if a single- or double-walled booth is needed, have a noise survey (octave band analysis) done prior to ordering a sound booth. Ambient noise can be measured in the area during times when testing will be performed.

Some audiologists decide that a custom sound booth is their best option because of space issues or design concerns. An engineer is needed to determine acceptable angles of surfaces. An architect can design a soundproof wall easily, but doors, windows, and panel jacks allow sound to leak in. Several manufacturers now offer plug-in doors and windows that are compatible with custom walls. The cost of a custom booth is likely to be much more expensive.

Pediatric testing requires consideration of specialized equipment. The traditional setup with conditioned orientation response (COR) toys behind Plexiglas can be enhanced by adding multicolored chaser lights around the border of the Plexiglas. This allows for three stages of reinforcement:

♦ Chaser lights blinking

♦ Light flashing showing animal inside Plexiglas

♦ Light flashing and movement of animal or toy inside Plexiglas

Another option in visual reinforcement is the use of video. A flat-panel liquid crystal display (LCD) screen is mounted above the speaker and connected to a DVD player. The audiologist can reinforce with a video or still pictures. This can be customized for each child depending on his or her interests.

Some audiologists prefer to use insert phones rather than supra-aural phones to further attenuate outside noise. There are two types of inserts available: 3A and 5A. Many years ago, 3A insert phones were introduced to provide greater interaural attenuation (helpful with masking dilemma cases), to ensure more accurate test results with collapsing ear canals, and to provide more comfort for the patient. Insert phones are often easier to use with children because headphones fit smaller heads poorly or create uncomfortable pressure on the ears. Insert 3A phones are lightweight, but the long tube can transfer sound. If the tube is attached to the collar, and the patient rubs his or her finger on the tube, the rubbing noise can be transferred through the tube. This interferes with testing. The newer 5A insert phones do not transfer sound through the tube, but they are heavier and can pull the foam earpiece loose. The 5A insert phones cannot be used with auditory brainstem response (ABR) equipment.

Supra-aural TDH-39, -49, or -50 earphones are necessary when testing atretic, stenotic, or draining ears (Frank, 2000). Some audiometers allow you to switch easily between headphones and insert phones and provide calibration for each. Some older audiometers can only be calibrated for one type of earphone, so corrections will need to be made when switching phones. A switch box can be added so the audiologist can switch easily between inserts and headphones without unplugging anything or going into the booth. Special circumaural earphones are required for testing ultra-high frequencies (above 8 kHz.).

The standard for most audiology clinics is the 1.5-channel audiometer. This meets the needs of audiologists performing a variety of diagnostic testing. Two-channel audiometers

Table 14–7 Amplification Equipment

Equipment	Specifics
Real ear	Response options: REUR, REIR, REAR, RECD, speech mapping, directional microphone, and occlusion. Stimulus options: ICRA, male, female, child, live speech. Sometimes integrated with HA analyzer.
Hearing aid analyzer	Possible features: ANSI specs for measurement of hearing devices, FM systems, and cochlear implants. Other options: ability to measure T-coils, battery drain, directional microphones, noise reduction, and other digital parameters. Display: graphs versus numerical.
Hearing aid computer	Check with individual manufacturers and HIMSA regarding hardware requirements. Networking capability. serial port is required if using Hi-Pro.
Hi-Pro or NOAH link	Cables and connectors from each manufacturer. Consider storage of cables. Hanging them from hooks prevents tangling and enables quick access.

ANSI, American National Standards Institute; FM, frequency modulation; HA, hearing aid; HIMSA, Hearing Instrument Manufacturers' Software Association; ICRA, International Collegium of Rehabilitative Audiology; REAR, real ear aided response; RECD, real ear-to-coupler difference; REIR, real ear insertion response; REUR, real ear unaided response.

were popular in the past and are being reintroduced via personal computer (PC)–based systems. A PC-based audiometer is unmatched in flexibility, data storage, and the transferring of data (see Chapter 18). One system positions the audiometer inside the booth on the wall in place of the jack panel. It connects to a PC outside the booth. This is an integrated system that features a universal serial bus (USB) connectivity to accommodate advancements in computer technology. It includes an audiometer, a real ear system with speech mapping that is compatible to the NOAH software system from the Hearing Instrument Manufacturers' Software Association, and add-on modules for tympanometry and video-otoscopy (see "Saving Space: The Paperless Office"). Miniaturization of equipment is changing the amount of desk space needed. The smaller "footprint" (surface space taken up when the equipment is in position) allows more flexibility in arranging the work area.

There are many options regarding real ear equipment and hearing aid analyzers. **Table 14–7** lists equipment needed for the hearing aid and rehabilitation part of a practice. Several manufacturers combine the two functions into one piece of equipment. This is more economical and saves valuable desk space. A real ear system is currently available that is the size of the palm of one's hand. This portability is very convenient. Consider using a speaker on a movable arm or pedestal so that directional microphones can be assessed during real ear measurements.

Special Consideration

- Decide which equipment should be portable (so that it can be used by different audiologists in different locations) and which should have a designated space. Which computer should be used for a single function, and which should be integrated for multipurpose use?

Pearl

- Leasing equipment requires less money upfront and allows the practice to replace equipment with newer models as they are introduced.

Hearing Aid Laboratory

Hearing aid laboratory space is central to any dispensing audiology practice. See **Table 14–8** for some suggestions of items that are useful in the laboratory. Ample storage, electrical outlets, plumbing (sink), and superior lighting are crucial for an organized and efficient hearing aid laboratory.

Pearl

- Clear plastic containers with small compartments are handy for tiny components, tubing, earhooks, vent plugs, and so on. These can be stored behind closed doors to keep the laboratory looking clean and orderly.

Pitfall

- Be sure to attend to detail when planning the hearing aid laboratory. A laboratory with inadequate storage or an inefficient setup will be disorganized and frustrating for employees to use.

Office Furniture

The business end of an audiology practice requires several pieces of furniture and equipment. The style of furniture you select will add to the ambiance of the office. (See "Interior Design" and "Ergonomics" sections for specifics.) **Table 14–9** lists some examples of furniture and equipment needed to set up a practice. You can open a practice with minimal furniture and add to it as the practice grows. Chairs, desks, and a telephone system are needed immediately; however, an ALD display can be added later.

Pearl

- Use graph paper to make a dimensionally accurate drawing of each room. Create cutout drawings representing desks, tables, filing cabinets, chairs, and so on. It is easy to move the "furniture" around to determine the most efficient arrangement. Software is available to help with this.

Table 14–8 Hearing Aid Laboratory Equipment and Supplies

Equipment	Specifics
Bench drill, grinder, and polisher	Accessories: burs, bits, fine sandpaper, buffing compound, light and Plexiglas shield to protect face and eyes from debris
Ultrasonic cleaner	Cleans earmolds, immittance, and OAE tips. (*Tip:* Beakers can be used to keep earmolds separated; this allows for cleaning more than one set of molds at a time.)
Hearing aid restoration system	Vacuum, suction, and drying chamber to clean microphones and receivers and to dry out hearing aids
Magnifying otoscopes	Allows staff to see into receivers and microphones and to read small serial numbers
Magnifying lamp	Swivel arm for individual adjustments
Electric air blower	Used to bend tubing/removal cords and lessen drying time for repairs
Sterilizer	Used for soaking tools, tips, and other supplies that are in direct contact with earmolds and custom products, and during cerumen removal

Supplies	Specifics
Organizer for hearing aid supplies	Spare parts: volume controls, hooks (filtered and unfiltered), potentiometer/programming covers, wax springs/guards, battery doors, wind screens, microphone covers, nail polish for right/left markings
Organizer for earmold supplies	Variety of tubing (medium, thick, double-walled, 3 to 4 mm horn, CFAs, moisture-proof tube, etc.), vent plugs, reamer, superglue, cement, etc.
Hearing aid repair kit	Patch kit for damaged custom hearing devices
Personal safety	Make sure laboratory is OSHA compliant for employee safety: safety glasses and gloves; ventilation; lighting; vision, hearing, and skin protection
Tools	Screwdrivers, needle-nose pliers, tubing expanders, tubing inserter, blunt-tip scissors, tweezers (blunt and pointed), penlights, small brushes
Battery tester	Shows variety of voltages from 1 to 9 V
Ear impression supplies	Impression material, syringes, measuring spoons, putty knife or mixing utensils, ear dams, timer, lubricant for dams, leveler to mark impressions for directional microphones, cerumen removal tools, boxes for shipping and storing molds, order/repair forms. (*Tip:* Use portable containers so they can be transferred to various treatment rooms.)
Hearing aid stethoscopes	Allow for listening check of hearing aids. Options: variety of tips for different canal sizes, dampers for power aids
Stock earmolds	Custom molds and noncustom sponge molds for temporary/demo use
Loaner hearing aids	Several varieties and styles (BTE, noncustom canal, demos). Catalog each aid and devise a check-in/out procedure
Dehumidifying kit	Variety: microwaveable, electric, travel
Patient hearing aid supplies	Air blowers, dehumidifying kits (see above), wax guards, battery testers, battery holders, hearing aid storage boxes, lubricant, wax removal kits, disposable wipes and cleansers
Pediatric accessories	Hearing aid retainers (Huggies), alligator clips, tamper-proof battery doors (and tools to open)

BTE, behind the ear; CFA, craniofacial abnormality; OAE, otoacoustic emissions; OSHA, Occupational Safety and Health Administration.

Table 14–9 Office Equipment and Furniture

Equipment	Furniture
• Telephone system • Computers (see Chapter 18) • Printer(s) (see Chapter 18) • Fax and copier • Paper shredder • File system (closed vs open) • Typewriter (for forms/envelopes) • Calculator or adding machine • Credit card machine • Microwave oven • Refrigerator	• Ergonomic chairs for staff and waiting room • Desk/workstation for reception area and audiologists' work areas (audiometer, acoustic immittance, real ear, etc.) • Pediatric table and chairs for inside booth and waiting room • Magazine rack and table for waiting room • Lighting • Storage for office and audiologic supplies • Book shelves and brochure holders • ALD cabinet and display area • Storage (open or closed) to display items for sale (batteries, dehumidifying kits, lubricants, etc.)

ALD, assistive listening device.

Construction

Once the location and building are selected and the design plans are worked out, it is time to focus on the actual construction. An architect and space planner will assist during this phase. Establish a realistic timeline for construction. The space needs to be configured to meet the practice's specific operational needs. The floor plan previously developed will formalize the details of the construction. Every detail must be analyzed, including

Walls   Type of material, insulation, and soundproofing should be considered

Flooring   Material used (carpet, wood, tile, linoleum, etc.). Consider patient stability; mobility of wheelchairs, walkers, and strollers; staff comfort; sound absorption; wear and tear; and ease of maintenance.

Electrical   Location of outlets and light fixtures to allow proper lighting for detailed work. Prepare for expansion and rearrangement of furniture.

Plumbing   Location of pipes and sinks are important so hands, equipment, tools, and hearing devices can be easily cleaned

Workspace   Consider counter height when planning the sink and counter areas. Ergonomically, it makes sense to have raised counters so personnel will not develop back strain.

Heating/cooling/ventilation   The thermostat needs to be in a convenient location for staff members. Locate the vents so air does not blow directly on clients or staff. Check the noise level of the ventilation system, and be sure that the system can disperse fumes properly.

Soundproofing   Ideally, this covers doors, walls, pipes, floor, ceiling, and ventilation system. Outside sounds can interfere with audiologic tests.

Networking   Determine the location of the network control room, and be sure that the network cables are installed prior to drywall.

Sound Booth

In the early stages of construction planning, it is important to think about the requirements of the sound booth or booths. It is better to have a recessed booth so that patients do not have to step up to enter the booth. This also eliminates the need for ramps for patients in wheelchairs. Ramps can be prohibitively expensive if the floor is a concrete slab or if the office space is not on the ground floor. An alternative to the recessed booth is to build the floor up into a gradual ramp so there is no step into the booth. Consider carefully the location of the booth within the room, as sound booths are rarely moved. Conferring with the installers and the manufacturer at this stage can save you time and money. The ventilation system and the actual outside dimensions of the booth should be considered. The installers often use forklifts and need large openings to install the booth. Decide which way the door should open and

where the window should be located. See "Obtaining Equipment" for details on sound booths.

It is important to stay informed of all meetings and decisions at this stage. It cannot be stressed enough how crucial it is for the managing audiologist to oversee the operation and to communicate continually with the architect. Be aware that storage cabinets, sinks, and counters add significantly to the overall construction costs. It is worthwhile to make the space as attractive and efficient as your budget will allow. The architect needs to be reminded of the budget as plans are developed.

Floor plans should be finalized only after you are confident that they will meet the practice's needs. Making changes after construction has begun is very expensive and causes delays. Once construction has begun, pay close attention to details. Compare the actual work with the plans. If you notice deviations, contact the construction supervisor immediately.

As a real-life example, an audiologist met with the project's electrician and expressed a desire for extra electrical outlets. The electrician said he would install "plenty." The audiologist was not available on the day they were installed, and she later discovered that all eight of the outlets were placed in one corner of the exam room. The thermostat was placed on the wall where the file cabinets were intended. The architect and space planner had this information on the plans but did not notice the actual location of the installed thermostat. The lesson? Visit the construction site daily, if possible.

Pitfall

- Catch mistakes as soon as possible. It is very costly to change things once construction has been completed. Evaluate how a particular "mistake" will affect the daily function of the practice. Sometimes it is less expensive in the long run to correct the mistake now than to live with it as an annoyance or inefficiency.

Pearl

- Visit the construction site daily, if possible. Check and recheck all details, especially the location of electrical and phone outlets, plumbing, and ventilation systems. Be sure to get more electrical outlets than you think you will need.

Interior Design

At this point in the process, decisions have been made regarding audiologic services, patient flow, and efficiency. Most likely there also have been many decisions made about the overall image of the office. The interior design will support this image. An expert in interior design is most helpful at this point. Interior design decisions include general atmosphere, waiting room specifics, patient population needs, and staff needs.

Atmosphere

Soon after walking through the door, a patient will start to form an opinion of the office. Patients and their families expect a professional atmosphere. A calming atmosphere will make them feel more at ease. Whether the primary population served is geriatric or pediatric, the colors and furniture chosen will go a long way to set the proper atmosphere.

Waiting Room

The waiting room should be a place that is not only calm and professional but also visually interesting. Consider the effect of an "open area" waiting room versus a more separated design. When a waiting area is open to the rest of the office, and there is friendly interaction taking place between employees and clients, the clients in the waiting room will start to have a positive impression before their appointment begins. If the waiting room is isolated, the clients may perceive the environment as less friendly.

Take time to select artwork that complements the environment and is pleasant to look at. The waiting room may be the best place to hang diplomas, although these could also be hung in a diagnostic or consultation area. A fish tank with brightly colored fish can be soothing. A video monitor with informational programs can be added to help keep clients occupied while in the waiting area. Some audiologists like to provide a coffee area within the waiting room. If there are likely to be several children seen, the safety of this may render it a poor idea.

The waiting room is an excellent place to keep brochures that patients can peruse. A magazine rack is a must. Proper and sufficient lighting is necessary for comfortable reading. A waiting room with plenty of natural light may meet this need if patients are seen primarily in daylight hours. If there is little natural light, well-placed area lamps will warm and soften the atmosphere of your waiting room when used in conjunction with fluorescents. Place them in a way that they can allow for a comfortable reading environment.

Patient Population Needs

Furniture should, first of all, be comfortable. The furniture selected should complement the overall color scheme and style of the office. Most importantly, it should be easy for elderly clients or others with mobility limitations to use. Chairs should be sturdy, with arms that allow people to support themselves when rising. Generally, chairs are a better option than a sofa or loveseat for this purpose. If the patient population is solely pediatric, comfortable chairs for both children and adults will be necessary. If a combination of young and old will be seen in the office, it is preferable to have a separate pediatric area with small chairs, toys, and so on.

From a practical standpoint, proper signage is very important. There may be areas, such as a hearing aid laboratory, where it is unsafe or unwise to allow patients. Directions to restrooms should be easy to see. Any special signage for wheelchair access should also be posted and easily visible for those needing to know the correct route.

Signs should not only be clear and easy to read but also convey a professional image and complement the overall atmosphere.

Staff Needs

Selection of furniture for business and audiology staff will be affected, in part, by the personal work style of the individuals. For both audiologists and business personnel, comfort and efficiency are key. This is discussed in greater detail in the "Ergonomics" section of this chapter.

Audiologists will require sufficient space for all audiologic equipment and supplies. Chairs and tables that raise and lower will be helpful when seeing both children and adults so that equipment can be adjusted to optimal height. It may be helpful to have patient chairs on rollers so that patients can be easily moved short distances (i.e., a few feet or inches). One disadvantage of rollers is that they make chairs less stable as people sit down and rise from them. Staff members are likely to spend more time in front of computers, so ergonomic considerations as they relate to computer use should be well researched.

Patient privacy issues are important for both audiologists and staff (see "Health Insurance Portability and Accountability Act Requirements"). Proper storage of charts not only keeps them out of sight of other patients but also adds to the impression of an organized office. Computers with patient data should be situated so that patients cannot easily see someone else's personal information.

◆ Adding Balance Assessment to an Audiology Practice

The diagnosis and treatment of vestibular disorders are a natural fit for an audiology practice. Vestibular disorders are common in the geriatric population, and the most effective treatments do not include medicine or surgery. Management of vestibular disorders is within the scope of practice and licensure for audiology, and the Current Procedural Terminology (CPT) codes applicable to vestibular testing are billable by audiologists. Most clinics are already equipped to perform hearing evaluations, and comprehensive audiometric evaluation is an essential component of the workup for vestibular dysfunction.

Competent management of vestibular disorders requires training, alliances, equipment, and space in addition to that required to perform hearing health care. The practice commitment is substantial in terms of both time and expense. There are different levels of vestibular management that may be offered. Practitioners are obligated to investigate the various diagnostic protocols and treatment techniques available, determine the level of vestibular management they will offer, and inform their patients as to the capabilities and limitations of the services offered.

The five main categories to consider when planning a vestibular clinic are training, alliances, equipment, office layout, and patient flow.

Table 14–10 Differences between Infrared Video and Electro-Oculography

Calibration   The corneoretinal potential, which is the basis for EOG recordings, changes over time as a result of light exposure. VNG recording is unaffected by light exposure.

Artifact   Eye blinks and eyelid flutter can be mistaken for vertical nystagmus with EOG or VNG. VNG allows direct visualization of the eye throughout the examination.

Rotary nystagmus   EOG and most VNG record in the vertical and horizontal axis only, and rotary nystagmus may not be recordable through either technique. VNG allows direct visualization of the eye throughout the examination.

Bell's phenomenon   The eyes roll superiorly and distally when they are closed. This can inhibit nystagmus response. The eyes stay open, but in darkness, with VNG.

Cost-effectiveness   Because of time spent on electrode application and darkness adaptation, EOG testing generally takes longer than VNG testing. A few dollars per test can be saved on the cost of electrodes.

EOG, electro-oculography; VNG, videonystagmography.

Training

The major equipment manufacturers sponsor regional courses that serve as an introduction to current research and vestibular management techniques. Workshops and instructional courses at professional academy meetings provide the opportunity for interaction with more experienced specialists.

Alliances

There are aspects of vestibular management that fall outside the scope of practice of audiology. Comprehensive evaluation and treatment of the dizzy or balance-disordered patient require a multidisciplinary approach, minimally including a medical director, audiologist, and physical therapist. Not all patients need the services of all these specialists, but some need the services of all three.

With the proper alliances, offering vestibular services does not have to be an all-or-nothing proposition. Miller (2003) suggests a "hub and spoke" arrangement, in which many patients can be effectively managed at smaller, less-equipped practices that refer them on to a "hub" clinic when more comprehensive evaluation is indicated. It may be prohibitive for an existing or start-up audiology clinic to offer a full range of vestibular testing and treatment. By forming referral alliances, audiology practices can add vestibular services to their practice in a more cost-effective manner. Offering ENG/videonystagmography (VNG), rudimentary posturography, canalith repositioning, and home-based vestibular exercises provides sufficient evaluation and effective treatment for many vestibular patients. Patients who are unresponsive to treatment and those who do not have a firm diagnosis after ENG/VNG are referred to a fully equipped specialty clinic.

Equipment

Most vestibular specialty clinics are in major teaching hospitals associated with large universities and medical schools, chiefly because of high equipment costs (these can exceed $200,000). In these facilities, the standard triad of vestibular test equipment is

- Computerized ENG
- Rotary chair testing
- Computerized dynamic platform posturography

Equipment manufacturers now provide lower cost alternatives to encourage audiology practices to offer vestibular management. As a result, there are many equipment options to consider. **Tables 14–10** through **14–12** summarize categories of equipment and various considerations for their purchase and use.

A practice may wish to add only certain aspects of vestibular management, such as ENG/VNG. The equipment-purchasing decisions that need to be made are ENG versus VNG, caloric irrigator stimulus (air, open loop water, or closed loop water), and examination chair or table. **Table 14–10** describes the differences to consider between ENG and VNG. The more technically correct term for electrode-based recording of eye movements is *electro-oculography* (EOG); however, with the advent of infrared video recording, the two techniques are often described as ENG (electrode based) or VNG (video based). **Table 14–11** outlines the pros and cons of the different irrigators.

Controversial Point

- Limiting the evaluation of the dizzy patient to audiometrics and ENG/VNG may result in many patients with treatable vestibular disorders incorrectly being told they have normal vestibular function.

Pitfall

- Infrared video requires eyes open, which may be difficult for elderly or medicated patients when in total darkness or when vertigo is induced. Patients who have very small eyes or poor contrast between the pupil and the iris and sclera are better suited for EOG recordings.

Table 14–11 ENG Caloric System

Type of ENG Caloric System	Advantages	Ongoing Costs	Disadvantages
Open loop	More consistent irrigation	Sterile distilled water	Water bottle storage
Closed loop	No water spillage	Replacement balloons	Difficult with narrow ear canals
Air	No water spillage	None	Periodic maintenance

ENG, electronystagmography.

> **Pearl**
>
> • Some commercially available infrared systems offer the option of EOG recording capabilities, which can be used on an as-needed basis.

ENG alone is insufficient to evaluate many patients with vestibular dysfunction; rotational testing is an important component of a balance clinic test battery. Studies indicate that rotational tests are significantly more sensitive to vestibular pathology than is the caloric portion of the ENG exam (Arriaga et al, 2005; Jacobson, 2002; Saadat et al, 1995; Shepard and Telian, 1996). Rotary chair and active head rotation (AHR) test different aspects of the vestibular response. The ideal situation would enable vestibulo-ocular reflex (VOR) testing for the full range of frequencies, from as low as that evaluated by ENG (0.003 Hz) to as high as can be generated by the patient (typically 3 to 6 Hz).

> **Special Consideration**
>
> • Bilaterally absent caloric responses might be misinterpreted as absence of vestibular function if higher frequency rotational tests are not performed (Goebel and Rowdon, 1992). This type of information is critical to designing a customized vestibular rehabilitation program, as therapy for patients with total loss of vestibular function differs from that for those with residual vestibular function.

Table 14–12 Attributes and Costs of Vestibular and Balance Equipment

Test	Advantages	Disadvantages	Cost
ENG/VNG VOR at 0.003 Hz (most common test method)	• Records nystagmus and voluntary eye movements • Removes visual fixation • Tests one labyrinth at a time • Screens for some CNS disorders • Tests for most common pathology: BPPV	• Caloric test evaluates only horizontal canal • Caloric test simulates very slow movements, below the range of normal head speeds • Does not record rotary nystagmus • No measure of functional ability • Minimal information on central compensation	$18,000–$30,000
Infrared video recording	• Easier and more stable calibration • Captures rotary nystagmus on video • Reduced artifact	• Requires eyes open • At the time of writing, vertical channel recordings may not be reimbursed by Medicare	$25,000–$30,000
EOG	• Eye movements recorded while eyes closed • Vertical electrode recordings reimbursed by Medicare	• Increased likelihood of test administration errors	$18,000–$20,000
Rotary chair VOR at 0.01 to 0.64 Hz	• Physiologic stimulus at several frequencies • More sensitive than caloric test	• Cannot test labyrinths separately • High equipment cost	$60,000–$120,000
AHR VOR at 1 to 6 Hz	• Tests VOR at more real-life head speeds • Low equipment cost • Takes no additional space • Short test time	• Questionable test–retest reliability • Some consider it experimental • At the time of writing, Medicare reimbursement inconsistent by region	$13,000–$15,000
Posturography	• Measures visual and somatosensory inputs for balance • Helps customize rehabilitation programs • Provides objective data for outcome measures	• Cannot diagnose vestibular disorder • High equipment cost • Reimbursement inconsistent by insurance carrier	$60,000–$80,000

AHR, active head rotation; BPPV, benign paroxysmal positional vertigo; CNS, central nervous system; ENG, electronystagmography; EOG, electro-oculography; VNG, videonystagmography; VOR, vestibulo-ocular reflex.

Table 14–13 Vestibular Therapy Equipment and Supplies

Equipment	Function	Cost
Balance beam	For hip strategy exercises	$85–$125
Foam mat (8 inches thick, 4 × 8 feet)	Compliant surface while walking and patient safety	$115–$230
Nonglass, lightweight, full-length mirror	Provides patient with safe visual feedback	$250–$370
Mini trampoline	Compliant surface and vertical VOR stimulus	$60–$140
Physioballs (large and small)	For hip strategy and vertical VOR stimulus	$15–$22
Lightweight rubber ball (12 inches)	For ball toss and kick exercises	$1–$2
Safety belt	To support patient during exercises	$25–$35
Metronome	To time head and eye movements	$15–$25
Kitchen timer	To time exercises	$1–$5
Balance board	For hip strategy exercises	$75–$150
Exam table	For repositioning maneuvers	$270–$400
Training software (e.g., Balance Master)	Provides visual feedback for weight shifts	$10,000–$25,000

VOR, vestibule-ocular reflex.

For most portions of the ENG/VNG examination, a manual reclining chair (e.g., JedMed ENT chair; JedMed Instrument Co., St. Louis, Missouri) is an excellent choice because it reclines quickly for positional testing, is easily set to a 30-degree angle for caloric testing, and elevates or lowers for better access to the patient for canalith repositioning. However, a standard examination table is required if a Semont maneuver is included as a treatment option.

The equipment **(Table 14–13)** needed for performing vestibular rehabilitation is relatively inexpensive. A larger room is preferable, but nearly all activities can be performed in a 10 × 10 foot space, as long as there is a long unobstructed hallway available for walking exercises. Of course, patient privacy may be a concern if the hallway is used by other staff members or patients. The therapy room should be equipped with a monitoring camera and VCR to record all therapy sessions. The tapes should be stored in a locked, private area consistent with HIPAA regulations. The tape can be given to the patient upon discharge.

> **Pearl**
>
> • Patients are often surprised and pleased when they can view their progress on video beginning with the initial therapy session.

> **Special Consideration**
>
> • Keep patients' videotapes in permanent, secure storage to guarantee patient privacy rights.

Office Layout

Fully equipped vestibular practices are rare due to start-up expenses and ongoing personnel expenses. For the same reason, they must stay very busy to achieve profitability. To be successful, full-service vestibular practices need to see more than one patient at a time, using separate rooms dedicated to different portions of the vestibular evaluation. For some existing practices, adding vestibular services may not be possible because of the amount of space required. An existing audiology practice could expand to include full-service vestibular services by adding test rooms: one for ENG/VNG and AHR, one for rotational chair and posturography, and a third for vestibular rehabilitation therapy. The ENG/VNG room should be isolated from the waiting room (in case patients panic or become nauseous) and away from the audiometric suites (secondary to loud conversations and equipment). With certain aspects of the ENG/VNG exam, patients must be in darkness or have their eyes closed, and hearing instruments must be removed. This can make for difficult communication. Having an ALD available can minimize shouting.

The room for ENG/VNG testing can be fairly small, but large enough for patients to be placed in a supine position, to allow the audiologist or technician to maneuver around a patient during repositioning, and to accommodate an observer or family member. AHR testing takes up no additional space. Minimally, the room should be 8 × 10 feet and, ideally, should contain a sink if water calorics will be used. ENG requires a darkened room to eliminate changes in calibration when the eyes open. VNG can be performed in a lighted or darkened room. The room used for rotational chair and posturography must be larger (12 × 16 feet), simply to accommodate the larger equipment. Depending on the type of equipment purchased, it may be necessary to control light in the room. The specific manufacturer can offer guidance in this regard.

Patient Flow

The arrangement of the test rooms is dictated by the logical order of the test battery typically used for dizzy patients. The case history interview and audiometric evaluation should be performed first to assess (1) the health and integrity of the ear canal and tympanic membrane prior to caloric irrigation, (2) auditory sensitivity and symmetry, and (3) possible presence of retrocochlear pathology. Inspection for gaze and spontaneous nystagmus must take place before any other vestibular tests, because their presence will affect all other tests. The oculomotor test battery is usually performed prior to positional or caloric testing because the task is similar to the calibration procedure, and it is unlikely to provoke vegetative symptoms that may prevent completion of remaining scheduled tests.

Positional and positioning (Dix-Hallpike) testing should be performed before caloric irrigation, which could inadvertently provoke positional vertigo when placing the patient in the 30-degree supine position. Additionally, a positive Dix-Hallpike and appropriate canalith repositioning may resolve the patient's complaints, and caloric testing may not be required. If caloric testing is planned, it should be scheduled after any other tests planned for that day, as patients occasionally become nauseous and refuse any additional testing. This is also true, but much more infrequent, with rotational chair testing. Posturography may be done at any time that is convenient for the clinic. A full battery of tests can take up to 3 hours. Many elderly patients become fatigued, which can affect test performance. The evaluation can be broken up over two visits.

Pearl

- In a busy practice, it is inevitable that the infrared camera used for VNG will be dropped. Carpeted floors minimize damage to the camera.

Vestibular evaluation and treatment present an opportunity for existing or start-up audiology practices to expand into new patient populations and increase services for their current patients. The commitment in terms of training, space, and expense is considerable, but, like most investments, diversification builds a stronger foundation.

♦ Saving Space: The Paperless Office

After developing the layout, it may become clear that the "dream" office is simply not attainable because of costs. One way to gain a little more space (and be more environmentally friendly in the meantime) is to design a paperless office. In reality, a true paperless office is not really "paperless." About 70% of the paper generated in an office is read once and either filed or discarded (Halpin, 2004). A paperless office can significantly reduce clutter and the amount of paper stored.

If the decision has been made for a paperless office, you and your staff will need to be computer literate and proficient. An up-to-date computer system is necessary (see Chapter 18). Flat-screen monitors are available that will take up less space. It is also essential to have a reliable scanner/printer. A scanner with a document feeder is

highly recommended. A laser printer is preferable over an ink-jet printer.

Other essential components of a paperless office are a hard drive/backup device, a high-speed Internet connection, an up-to-date operating system that meets the requirements of the software, a good office suite package (word processing and spreadsheet) that allows a user to transmit files in portable document format (PDF), and e-mail and antivirus/firewall software. The importance of backup and virus protection cannot be stressed enough. It is also a good idea to have a secondary backup unit, such as a CD or DVD burner, that will allow staff to copy files on a regular basis. These files can then be stored off site or in a fireproof safe. More information on the paperless office can be found in Halpin (2004).

Several audiometers have software that can store audiogram data and be linked to other devices inside or outside the clinic. The results can be customized and put into reports, then exported into electronic patient journals. If the office is networked, the data can be transferred to NOAH and real ear equipment to be used later during the hearing aid fitting and rehabilitation appointments. Records can be shared with referring physicians or other audiologists, then digitally reported to health care plans for electronic reimbursement. Audiologists attempting to create a paperless office are pleased with this option, as a lot of paper is eliminated. Time is saved and patient care is streamlined because the data are entered only once. The information can be recalled at later appointments.

♦ Networking

Computers are a necessary part of most work environments. Many businesses have found that the office runs more efficiently if the computers can communicate with each other. A computer network enables a practice to have one database that can be shared by many audiologists and front-office personnel. A network consists of a server and one or more user clients. The server can have multiple functions (e.g., NOAH server and data backup server) but should be stand-alone and not used by audiologists or other office staff during the day. Using the server as a workstation creates the potential for computer crashes, which could bring down the entire office (see Chapter 18). When planning, it is a good idea to have dedicated space set aside for the server and wiring closet. This is the central point of the network.

You should investigate the pros and cons of wireless versus hardwired networks. A wireless network avoids the effect of retrofitting an existing space with cables (see Chapter 18). If the space is already completed, it may be difficult or impossible to install wires. However, a wireless system can get interference from radio waves that will cause intermittency. This interference can come from other parts of the building. It is very frustrating to be working with a patient and suddenly not be able to complete the test or task because the connection is lost. Another disadvantage of wireless is that it requires security measures. With wireless, anyone can tap into the system.

A wired network is generally faster than a wireless one. If you are customizing the building space, the wires can be installed before the walls are erected. A network consultant can design and install the network. The disadvantage of wire is that it is permanent, so moving equipment can be more difficult. Care must be taken when rearranging furniture because the location of outlets and wires determines the configuration of the office.

The voice (telephone) and data network can use the same physical network. If you are designing a new office, this will save you a lot of money. A data network can handle all computers and data, from NOAH stations to front-office patient information and billing, hearing aid tracking, and so on. The same network can serve both IBM-compatible and Apple computers.

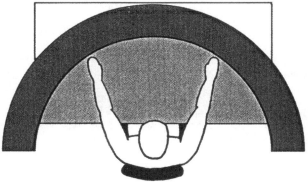

 Frequent use area (High priority area)

Occasional use area (Lower priority area)

Figure 14–2 Materials at your desk should be placed according to priority and frequency of use. (From Donkin, S. W. (2002). Sitting on the job. Laguna Beach, CA: Basic Health Publishing, with permission.)

Pitfall

- The best computer system is only as good as the backup system. It is wise to back up files daily and to keep a copy of the data off site.

Special Consideration

- Decide if the practice will have two or more databases for office management and audiologic care (e.g., NOAH), or if patient information will be shared in one database. If all patient information is shared, be aware of HIPAA regulations. Different levels of access may be necessary for audiologists and front-office personnel.

♦ Ergonomics

Ergonomics in the workplace refers to matching the work environment to people's bodies. The body is like a machine. Balance is important for this "machine" to obey the basic laws of physics and engineering. To be balanced, the upper body must be positioned directly over the legs, the spine is straight, and the shoulders are centered over the torso. Frequent deviation from balance can cause aches and pains. Usually the body will adapt to compensate for imbalance caused by poor posture or work habits. However, when the body is out of balance for prolonged periods of time, nerves can become irritated, causing pain or discomfort.

Chair and workstations should be ergonomic, that is, comfortable and safe. For maximum support and comfort, the chair should be slightly padded so the cushion can evenly distribute body weight. The best sitting posture will vary from person to person depending on body type and the kind of work done. For example, if a person's work requires a great deal of reading or writing at a desk, he or she will lean forward. The seat pan of the chair should be tilted slightly forward so that the thighs angle down. However, if the person is working at a computer terminal and keyboard, the seat pan should be tilted slightly back to take advantage of lumbar support in the backrest. Overtilting can also cause problems.

The height of a chair will depend on the height of the work surface, the person's body, and the task performed. At a computer keyboard, forearms should be at an angle of ~90 to 110 degrees to the upper arms. If the task involves frequent use of phone or other deskwork, forearms should be allowed to rest on the work surface. When sitting, the feet should comfortably touch the floor without pressing on the chair seat with the back of the thighs. If this does not occur, use a small footstool. Legs should fit comfortably under the desk. Chairs that can be easily adjusted for height, back support, and seat pan will allow multiple users to work comfortably at a variety of tasks.

If used frequently, the telephone should be kept in easy reach. If the staff often write or type when using the phone, consider attachments or headphones. Headphones are particularly helpful for staff members who have multiple responsibilities.

Workstation implements (computer mouse, telephone, keyboard, etc.) should be positioned according to priority and frequency of use. Items used most often should be placed in easy view or access to avoid excessive twisting and bending (**Fig. 14–2**). For computer use, exact eye-to-screen distance should take visual acuity into consideration. A user's head should be held in a normal posture when looking at the computer screen. Only the eyes should be moved to see characters on the screen. As a general rule, position the screen so the center is at approximately chin level.

Proper lighting is an important factor in an ergonomically comfortable office. Lighting should enable staff to focus on the work at hand without being distracted. Poor lighting can cause fatigue and eye strain. The light should not be too bright, which might cause squinting. Reflections from strong lighting can interfere with the ability to see materials. More information about ergonomics in the workplace can be found in Donkin (2002).

> **Pearl**
>
> • A common high-risk activity for audiologists is the frequent bending over that is needed to look into patients' ears or to make earmold impressions. This type of repetitive activity can cause significant discomfort. Adjustable chairs and tables are available; additionally, work surfaces should be positioned at a proper height to reduce excessive bending.

An ergonomics specialist can help in the designing of the office. Ergonomically friendly chairs, work surfaces positioned at the proper height, careful consideration of computer placement, and placement of frequently used tools will significantly reduce the risk of on-the-job injuries and increase productivity.

♦ Health Insurance Portability and Accountability Act Requirements

The passage of HIPAA in 1996 (Torres, 2001) meant that audiology practices, like all other medical practices, had to protect the privacy of patients' records. When evaluating a site, be aware of patient confidentiality requirements. Will there be a private space to discuss personal information with patients (face to face or over the telephone) so that other patients and staff do not hear? Patients' charts must be stored in a secure place so that nonauthorized personnel and other patients do not have access to private information. At night these files must be locked up. Fax and copy machines need to be positioned so that patients walking by do not see private information. Computer monitors should have privacy screens or face away from patient areas. Incoming and outgoing mail needs to be kept away from patient areas. Patient invoices, reports, and phone messages should also be out of sight. Computer backups need to be locked in a secure space as well.

It is important to think of patient privacy as you are planning the layout of the space. Small changes in design and arrangement of furniture and equipment can have a major impact on privacy. See the discussion of HIPAA in Chapter 7.

♦ Summary

Designing an audiology practice begins with a vision of what could be and ends with the realization of your dreams. There are several overlapping phases during the design process, each requiring careful research and attention to detail. During the planning phase, evaluate different locations and layouts to determine which setting will be best for the practice. Once construction is under way, decide which equipment and furniture will be needed. The ambiance of the office will be reflected by interior design decisions. When the process is complete, the reward will be an ideal work environment that provides a pleasurable experience for audiologists, staff, and patients alike.

References

Arriaga, M. A., Chen, D. A., & Cenci, K. A. (2005). Rotational chair (ROTO) instead of electronystagmography (ENG) as the primary vestibular test. Otolaryngology—Head and Neck Surgery, 133, 329–333.

Baxter, J. (1994). Locating and equipping an audiology practice. In Development and management of audiology practices (pp. 15–23). Rockville, MD: American Speech-Language-Hearing Association.

Donkin, S. W. (2002). Sitting on the job. Laguna Beach, CA: Basic Health Publishing.

Frank, T. (2000). Basic instrumentation and calibration. In H. Hosford-Dunn, R. J. Roeser & M. Valente (Eds.), Audiology diagnosis (pp. 181–225). New York: Thieme Medical Publishers.

Goebel, J. A., & Rowdon, D. P. (1992). Utility of headshake versus whole-body VOR evaluation during routine electronystagmography. American Journal of Otology, 13(3), 249–253.

Halpin, M. R. (2004). The practical paperless office using Microsoft, Adobe, and some sage advice [electronic document]. Louisville, KY: Transformata Publishing LLC.

Jacobson, G. (2002). Development of a clinic for the assessment of risk of falls in elderly patients. Seminars in Hearing, 23(2), 161–178.

Miller, E. (2003). Spending wisely. Advance for Audiologists, 5(5), 27–29.

Saadat, D., O'Leary, D., Pulec, J., & Kitano, H. (1995). Comparison of vestibular autorotation and caloric testing. Otolaryngology—Head and Neck Surgery, 113(3), 215–222.

Shepard, N. T., & Telian, S. A. (1996). Practical management of the balance disorder patient. San Diego, CA: Singular Publishing Group.

Torres, J. P. (2001). How to comply with HIPAA and the HHS regulations. Overland Park, KS: Veterans Press.

U.S. Department of Justice. (1999). ADA guide for small businesses. Retrieved from November 14, 2005, at http://www.usdoj.gov/crt/ada/ smbusgd.pdf

Windmill, I., Cunningham, D., & Johnson, K. (2000). Designing an audiology practice. In H. Hosford-Dunn, R. J. Roeser, and M. Valente (Eds.), Audiology practice management (p. 291–311). New York: Thieme Medical Publishers.

Chapter 15

Practice Accounting

Joy Colle Benn and Robert M. Traynor

Accounting may be viewed as an onerous burden that has little to do with engaging in the work of audiology, and audiology students do not often see the relevance of accounting to their own career objectives. For audiologists embarking on careers as autonomous doctoring professionals, however, participation in the financial oversight of their work setting has never been more important or more appropriate. The obligation of financial oversight is no longer restricted to those audiologists engaged in traditional private practice. On the contrary, today's audiologist-employee must be increasingly willing to take an active role in the financial aspects of the workplace. Whether self-employed or an employee of a not-for-profit agency, a public school, a hospital, a physician-owned practice, or a specialty rehabilitation clinic, a successful career will undoubtedly include at least some oversight and management of the financial aspects of the practice. Knowledge of accounting is necessary to make financial decisions from purchasing equipment and supplies to expanding services and determining salaries.

This chapter will be a valuable resource for persons engaged in

♦ Writing a business plan

♦ Borrowing business start-up funds

♦ Acquiring a practice

♦ Expanding a practice

♦ Managing a clinic

♦ Creating a budget request

♦ Leadership in state and national professional associations

♦ Selling a practice

♦ Negotiating a salary

♦ Running a practice on a daily basis

The chapter begins with an introduction to basic bookkeeping. The financial reports and financial ratios discussed in the later sections of this chapter will be easier to understand and more relevant to readers who must first understand where all the numbers are coming from and how those records are maintained. After the introduction to basic bookkeeping, this chapter addresses two accounting processes used for reporting and managing business income and expense: financial accounting and managerial accounting. A third process, tax accounting, addresses how the U.S. Internal Revenue Service (IRS) directs companies to calculate and report taxable income for the purpose of assessing taxes. This chapter does not cover tax accounting in detail. However, no chapter on practice accounting can entirely omit the IRS. Relevant points regarding the IRS tax code are made where appropriate throughout the chapter. The chapter is not intended to be a source for specific tax advice, but rather to orient the novice to accounting terminology and practices that will enhance communication with those people who do provide specific advice. It provides an overview of basic bookkeeping, financial accounting, and managerial accounting for audiology practice management.

♦ Basic Bookkeeping

Before the sections on financial reports and financial ratios, it is helpful to begin with some basic accounting record keeping so readers know where to get the numbers for financial reports and ratios and how to record those numbers. It is not rocket science, but it does require a strict routine. Financial reports address five basic accounts: assets, liabilities, equity, revenues, and expenses. Dollar amounts are added and subtracted from those accounts in the process of daily bookkeeping. It is imperative to set up the accounting system so that all transactions are recorded and data are entered in the right place. The daily accounting routine is a task that can and should be delegated to someone who has the requisite ability if the practice manager does not want to undertake the responsibility.

Except when starting a new business from scratch, the accounting system is likely already in place. Regardless of the work setting or employment arrangement, the professional audiologist will want to see that the daily bookkeeping system is sufficiently detailed for practice managers to make good decisions about salaries, raises, bonuses, equipment purchases, price changes, budget requests, and so on.

Special Consideration

- For the purposes of tax reporting, a company must choose an accounting period, or "tax year." Most small companies use the calendar year (ending December 31) as the tax year; they need IRS approval to elect an alternate fiscal year (any period that ends on the last day of any month except December).

Cash versus Accrual

The first step in setting up an accounting system is to determine whether to use a cash or accrual method of reporting taxable income and deductible expenses. The cash or accrual method is a tax accounting issue. It is perfectly legal and ethical to use a cash method for tax accounting and the accrual method for financial accounting. Cash and accrual methods differ in when income and expenses are recognized. Businesses that maintain inventory are required by the IRS to use the accrual method.

For the cash method, expenses are deducted in the tax year they are actually paid, and income is reported in the tax year in which it is received. In other words, the cash method simply corresponds to the date when cash has exchanged hands in transactions.

Using the accrual method, revenue is reported in the period in which goods or services are delivered and it is established that income is due to the company. The expense associated with that revenue is reported in the same accounting period that the revenue is reported.

For the following examples, assume a tax year that is the same as the calendar year (ending December 31).

Example 1: You fit and dispense two custom hearing aids on December 20, 2006. You receive payment for the hearing aids on January 15, 2007.

Cash method: You report income in 2007, the year you received payment.

Accrual method: You report the income in 2006, the year it was established that the payment was due to you.

Example 2: You order and receive two hearing aids from a manufacturer in December 2006, and you pay for them in January 2007.

Cash method: You deduct the expense in 2007, the year you paid for them.

Accrual method: You deduct the expense in 2006, when your liability for the hearing aids was established.

The preceding examples do not include inventory—ordering custom hearing aids from a manufacturer on a case-by-case basis does not constitute holding inventory. Cash-based accounting is generally used by small companies that provide services rather than goods; therefore, they do not have any inventory. Companies that produce or sell goods, in contrast, must account for inventory, and they must use the accrual method of accounting for tax purposes.

Accrual accounting is associated with inventory because a company could have a very large expenditure for the purchase or production of inventory in one accounting period followed by relatively small increments of revenue that are generated from that inventory over many subsequent accounting periods. Cash accounting would allow an inventory expense to be deducted in a period far removed from the period in which the revenue would be reported. Accrual accounting keeps the inventory expense in the same accounting period that the revenue from the inventory is generated. With accrual accounting, sale of merchandise always produces two events in the same period: (1) a revenue (increase in retained earnings) and (2) an expense (decrease in an asset). The net effect of these two events is income. The purpose of the accrual method is to match the revenue with the expense associated with that revenue in the same accounting period.

Example 3: A hearing aid manufacturer produces and pays for all the materials needed to produce 2000 behind-the-ear hearing aids in 2006. At the end of 2006, the company has 1850 hearing aids remaining in inventory. The IRS requires that the company use the accrual method because the production of inventory results in income. When the company reports income to the IRS using the accrual method, it reports the revenue and the expense associated only with the 150 hearing aids sold in 2006. If the company could use a cash basis, it would be able to deduct the expense for the entire cost of producing 2000 hearing aids in 2006. The accrual method requires that companies match the revenue of an accounting period with the expense associated with that revenue in the same period, not when the expense is incurred.

Current tax code is beyond the scope of this chapter. However, when production, purchase, or sale of merchandise produces income, companies must account for inventory and use the accrual method for sales and purchases of merchandise. There may be an exception to the requirement to use the accrual method rule if a company's principal activity is the provision of services, with the sale of property incident to those services. A tax professional ought to be consulted to determine if a business entity is required by the IRS to account for inventory and use the accrual method.

Chart of Accounts

When establishing an accounting system in a new business, it is necessary to set up a naming and numbering system for all the transactions and balances of the five basic accounts (assets, liabilities, equity, revenues, and expenses). This list of transaction categories is called the "chart of accounts." **Figure 15–1** is a sample chart of accounts, showing some of the subaccounts that would be included in a typical audiology practice. A real practice would include a more comprehensive chart of accounts. In this example, under the asset account there are many subaccounts, such as cash, accounts receivable, and diagnostic equipment. A typical audiology practice income account would include all of the revenue sources broken down by each service. Most revenue-generating services are associated with Current Procedural Terminology (CPT) codes, but it is not necessary to restrict the income accounts to services with CPT codes. Expense accounts will include

---

Audiology Practice Example
Chart of Accounts

Account #	Description		Account #	Description
1000.00	**ASSETS**		5000.00	**INCOME**
1001.00	Current Assets		5001.00	Sales
1003.00	Cash		5001.01	Hearing Aids - Digital
1004.00	Non Refundable Deposits		5001.02	Hearing Aids - Other
1005.00	Accounts Receivable		5001.03	Assistive Devices
1007.00	Total Current Assets		5001.04	Batteries
2000.00	Fixed Assets		5002.00	Audiologic Diagnostics
2001.00	Office Equipment		5002.01	92552 - Pure Tone Audiometry
2002.00	Diagnostic Equipment		5002.02	92557 - Comprehensive Audiometry
2003.00	Building		5002.03	92587 - Evoked Acoustic Emissions
2010.00	Total Fixed Assets		5003.00	Vestibular/Balance
2015.00	Accumulated Depreciation		5003.01	92541 - Spontaneous Nystagmus
2050.00	TOTAL ASSETS		5003.02	92543 - Caloric Vestibular Test
			5004.00	Rehabilitative Services
3000.00	**LIABILITIES**		5004.01	92591 - Hearing Aid Selection, binaural
3005.00	Current Liabilities		5004.02	92594 - Hearing Aid Selection, binaural
3007.00	Property Taxes		5050.00	TOTAL INCOME
3008.00	Property Insurance			
3009.00	Accrued Wages		6000.00	**EXPENSES**
3011.00	Accounts Payable		6002.00	Rent
3025.00	Total Current Liabilities		6015.00	Payroll
3030.00	Long Term Liabilities		6020.00	Fringe Benefits
3030.01	Bank Loan		6021.00	Payroll Taxes
3050.00	TOTAL LIABILITIES		6022.00	Workers Compensation Insurance
			6023.00	Health Insurance
4000.00	**EQUITY**		6028.00	Utilities
4001 00	Retained Earnings		6031.00	Postage/Mail Services
4030.00	Total Equity		6035.00	Professional Fees
4050.00	TOTAL LIABILITIES AND EQUITY		6035.01	ABA Dues
			6035.02	AAA Dues
			6036.00	Continuing Professional Education
			6040.00	Total Professional Fees
			6042.00	Magazine Subscriptions
			6043.00	Professional Journal Subscriptions
			6046.00	Coffee Service
			6047.00	Safe Deposit Box
			6050.00	Promotion and Advertising
			6051.00	Referral Development
			6061.00	Accounting Expense
			6070.00	TOTAL EXPENSE

Figure 15–1 Sample chart of accounts. Account-based record keeping forms the basis for generating financial reports and allows the audiology practice manager to analyze practice trends.

utilities, payroll, cost of goods sold, office supplies, and so on. Every transaction will be assigned to an account, enabling the manager to analyze thousands of business transactions within the framework of a discrete number of categories.

As the **Fig. 15–1** sample shows, the chart of accounts has a short descriptive name of the account and a number. The numbers are somewhat arbitrary, meaning any number may be assigned to individual accounts. It is wise to leave some available numbers for adding accounts, if needed, at a future date.

Most audiologists will never set up a new accounting system, but it could be beneficial to review a company's chart of accounts to identify what information is being tracked. An audiology program's fiscal records can be essential, for example, to salary negotiations, budget requests, and equipment justification; therefore, even audiologist-employees are wise to understand the details of the audiology program's financial record-keeping system.

The chart of accounts is used in every business transaction, and it is essential that the person who enters the data assigns various transactions to their proper accounts. In practice, if a check is written to pay a balance due to a supplier on accounts payable (a liability account), the details of the transaction, including the amount, the supplier, and the expense account associated with the payment, are also recorded. To complete the transaction, the reduction in accounts payable (a liability account) is associated with a reduction in cash (an asset account). This two-part transaction is the basis of the "double-entry" record-keeping system.

Double-Entry Bookkeeping

It is a basic tenet of accounting that every financial transaction affects the balance of two accounts. The double-entry system requires the entry of a debit and a credit for every transaction. The sum of these two entries must equal zero. This sounds like twice as much work as necessary, but it is a system that incorporates built-in checks and balances that allow a company to maintain accurate records. The use of double-entry bookkeeping is restricted to the balance sheet accounts: assets, liabilities, and equity. These three accounts have balances that go up and down as a result of doing business. The expense and income accounts move in one direction (increase) during the course of business (with the exception of returns for credit).

Table 15–1 suggests that accounting students learning how to assign debits and credits may suffer as much as audiology students learning how to mask properly. Fortunately, accounting software makes it possible to keep transactions records without having to decide if the transaction is a debit or credit.

Accounting Software

The days of paper ledgers and handwritten records with two entries for every transaction are almost a thing of the past. Today's accounting software does the double entry "behind the scenes." One of the first steps in customizing any accounting software for a business is to set up the chart of accounts. A typical software program will have a basic

Table 15–1 Breakout of Debits and Credits*

Account Category	Dollar Value	
	Increases	Decreases
Asset	Debit	Credit
Liabilities	Credit	Debit
Equity	Credit	Debit
Income	Credit	Debit
Expenses	Debit	Credit

* Debits and credits will increase or decrease the dollar value depending on the type of account. Double-entry bookkeeping requires a debit and a credit to be applied to at least one asset, liability, or equity account for every business transaction.

chart of accounts for several types of business, so the user selects the best general type of business, then modifies the chart of accounts to reflect the company's real activities. In addition, the setup of new accounting software requires an input for current assets (e.g., checking account balance, savings account balance, and money market balance), fixed assets (e.g., equipment purchase price and building value if owned), current liabilities (accounts payable, taxes payable, etc.), long-term liabilities (e.g., bank loan), and owner's equity. The chart of accounts in **Fig. 15–1** demonstrates some detail in the sales (5001.00 account) category, but users can modify their own chart of accounts to incorporate more detail as needed for an individual company's purposes.

Accounting software, with a sufficiently detailed chart of accounts, can be a tremendous tool for managers. For example, if there is more than one audiologist in the practice, tracking can include a record of hearing aid sales by audiologist, as well as by digital or analog, monaural or binaural hearing aid categories. Accounting software can also enable the manager to easily track sales by referral source, an essential ingredient in marketing efforts. By defining a comprehensive chart of accounts up front, there will be sufficient detail to perform valuable analyses. It is crucial that someone is continually and accurately maintaining the company's bookkeeping records.

Pitfall

- The garbage in, garbage out concept certainly applies to accounting software. If you are not entering data yourself, make periodic forays into your bookkeeper's world. Make sure the cost for electrodes you want recorded under diagnostic supplies is not being put under hearing aid laboratory supplies. Accurate financial records enable sound managerial decisions. Think about what you need to track, and make sure those details are recorded correctly.

Summary of Basic Bookkeeping

Summarizing the information presented so far, practice accounting begins with a systematic method of recording business transactions. Every business transaction results in a change (credit or debit) in two accounts. There are five main categories of accounts: assets, liabilities, equity, income, and expense. Each company should have a customized comprehensive chart of accounts that accurately records the company's activities in detail. Accounting software simplifies the task of maintaining records, but effort is needed at the outset of implementing a new software system to customize accounts and record existing assets and liabilities. Ongoing attention to detail and careful record keeping are essential.

It is the role of basic bookkeeping to record the numbers (dollar values) for every business transaction into a systematic set of accounts. The next section addresses how those numbers are reported.

♦ Financial Accounting

Many parties are interested in the details of a company's finances, and financial accounting is the process used to generate the financial statements for review within a company and by outside parties. The principal objective of financial reporting is to provide information to external users who make investment, credit, and related decisions (Mautz, 2005). The Securities and Exchange Commission (SEC) requires that publicly traded companies file quarterly and annual financial reports for review by the SEC, stockholders, and potential stockholders. In creating those financial reports, companies adhere to generally accepted accounting principles (GAAP) established by a nongovernmental organization, the Financial Accounting Standards Board (FASB). These accounting principles are the foundation of a systematic method that can be used by any business entity to communicate complex financial information. By defining standards for reporting financial information, the FASB ensures that financial reports are meaningful to the reader of those reports. Any business can use this well-defined and standardized method of financial reporting. The three financial statements that make up the conventional financial portfolio of a company are the balance sheet, the income statement (also called the profit and loss statement), and the statement of cash flows.

Pearl

- Financial statements might be viewed as the accounting equivalent to audiograms and audiologist's reports. Both use standardized methods to summarize and communicate complex information that is easily understood by others who are initiated in those standardized methods.

Balance Sheet

Recall that a company's financial information is recorded in five basic accounts (assets, liability, equity, income, and expense). The balance sheet is a report of the assets, liability, and equity accounts. It is referred to as a "snapshot," because the information contained in the balance sheet changes on a continual basis with every business transaction. It would be impossible to report the entire dynamic life of a business, but the balance sheet provides a snapshot at specified intervals, such as the end of the month, end of the quarter, or end of the annual accounting period. Balance sheets reveal more about a company's financial health when balance sheets from more than one period are compared.

As shown in **Fig. 15–2**, the balance sheet is divided into two sides, left and right. On the left side of the balance sheet are the assets (resources that the company owns). The asset side of the balance sheet consists of current assets and fixed assets. Current assets are those assets that are readily converted to cash, including cash, bank accounts, and accounts receivable. Fixed assets are not as easy to liquidate; these include land, buildings, and equipment. Fixed assets typically will depreciate in value. They are purchased for the benefit of future periods but have a limited life. Depreciation is the

XYZ Audiology Associates
Balance Sheet
12/31/2007

Assets			Liabilities and Equity		
Current Assets			*Current Liabilities*		
Cash	12,800		Accounts Payable	7,600	
Accounts Receivable	4,200		Taxes Payable	3,200	
Inventory	8,600		Accruals	5,400	
Total Current Assets		25,600	Short-term Notes Payable	2,000	
Fixed Assets			Total Current Liabilities		18,200
Equipment	68,000		*Long-term Liabilities*		
Building	180,000		Bank Loan Payable	150,000	
Less: Accum. Depreciation	(13,600)		Total Long-term Liability	150,000	
Total Fixed Assets		234,400			
			Total Liabilities		168,200
			Capital/Equity		
			Owner's Equity	91,800	
Total Assets		**260,000**	**Total Liabilities and Equity**		**260,000**

Figure 15–2 The balance sheet. The left side of the balance sheet (assets) is always equal to the right side (liabilities and equity).

method of converting the cost of an asset to an expense as the asset is "used up."

GAAP require separate disclosure of the original cost and the accumulated depreciation of a depreciable asset. Accumulated depreciation is an item on the left side of the balance sheet that reveals how much of the original value of an asset has been reduced over time. There are several methods of depreciation, all of which rely upon the expected service life of the asset. For income tax purposes, the effect of depreciation is to reduce the taxable income of a business.

On the right side of the balance sheet are the sources that provided those assets. Sources of assets are liabilities (debts owed) and equity (paid-in capital, i.e., from investors, and the retained earnings or profit of the business). Current liabilities include any liability that is due within a year; these include accounts payable and payroll. Long-term liabilities are those debts such as mortgages or bank loans that take more than a year to pay off. The equity includes the initial investment, which may include investors' money, as well as any money that is retained through business operations and is put back into the business.

The left and right sides of the balance sheet must always be equal (hence the term *balance sheet*). In other words, increases or decreases in assets on the left side of the balance sheet have an associated increase or decrease on the liabilities or equity on the right side. The fundamental account equation for the balance sheet is

$$\text{Assets} = \text{Liabilities} + \text{Equity}$$

The equality on the left and right side does not reveal any insight about the entity's financial condition; assets will always be equal to the sum of the liabilities plus equity. Because the equity account is the difference between the assets and the liabilities, the equity balance does provide insight to the company's health. If assets are greater than liabilities, equity will be positive, and the business is healthy. If liabilities outweigh assets, equity is negative, and the business is not healthy.

The balance sheet reveals a single snapshot of the historical cost of the assets of a company and the sources of funds that provided those assets. One might consider the balance sheet akin to hearing aid 2 cc coupler measurement: it reveals what the hearing aid was doing at one moment in time.

Income Statement

The balance sheet is derived from the records of the asset, liability, and equity accounts, but two additional accounts are tracked in daily bookkeeping: revenue and expense accounts. The income statement, often referred to as the

XYZ Audiology Associates Income Statement For the Year Ended December 31, 2007	
Sales Revenues	368,000
Sales Expenses:	
Cost of Goods Sold	136,000
Gross Margin	232,000
Other Expense:	
Sales, General and Administrative	203,800
EBIT	28,200
Interest Expense	8,000
Income Taxes	7,500
Total Expense	219,300
Net Income (Loss)	12,700

Figure 15–3 The income statement (also known as the profit and loss statement). EBIT, earnings before interest and taxes.

profit and loss statement, is derived from revenue and expense records, and it reflects the profitability of operations over some period. It may be prepared for any time period, such as an annual statement or some smaller, or interim, time period. The equation for the income statement is

$$\text{Revenues} - \text{Expenses} = \text{Net Income}$$

Figure 15–3 shows a sample income statement in a common format, although there is no standard format. The income statement begins with sales revenue. For an audiology practice, the sales revenue includes products and services (less returns). It may not seem appropriate to refer to diagnostic and rehabilitative services as sales, but for accounting purposes, that is where all revenues generated by the business are recorded. From the sales revenue, deduct the cost of sales, which includes the price paid to manufacturers for products such as hearing aids and assistive devices (cost of goods sold). Although revenues from hearing evaluations are recorded under sales, do not subtract the cost of an audiometer under cost of sales. An audiometer is a fixed asset that is tracked under an asset account on the balance sheet.

When cost of sales is deducted from the sales revenue, gross margin, or gross profit, remains.

$$\text{Sales Revenue} - \text{Cost of Sales} = \text{Gross Margin}$$

Gross margin does not include operating expenses, interest expense, or taxes. Those are deducted along with all other expenses incurred during practice operations, such as utilities, office supplies, salaries, rent, and telecommunications services. Broadly, these expenses are referred to as sales, general, and administrative expenses, or simply SG&A. Operating expenses are deducted from the gross margin, leaving earnings before interest and taxes, or EBIT. Interest expense is treated separately from the other operating expense and is deducted next, followed by a provision for incomes taxes. The income statement should give an indication of the company's income tax liability, but the tax liability is derived in accordance with IRS regulations, not by the income statement. Recall that financial statements are prepared following GAAP, which require the accrual method, but the cash method might be used for tax reporting. After taxes are deducted, the "bottom line" is net income (or loss). Net income is the amount that is added to owner's equity as a result of profitable operations during a period (Anthony et al, 1999).

Statement of Cash Flows

The first two financial statements, the balance sheet and the income statement, were derived using all five of the basic accounts that are tracked in a company's daily bookkeeping. The statement of cash flows is derived from the balance sheet and the income statement, and it adds a few new items derived by comparing data from more than one balance sheet. The statement of cash flows is considered by many to be the most valuable financial report in valuing a company. To put the quality of a company's earning to the test, one needs to examine the cash flow statement (Tergeson, 2001).

Figure 15–4 illustrates a model that shows net changes in cash flow based on activity, although there are other models for presenting the statement of cash flow. The cash flow statement begins with income, taken from the income statement. Next, the dollar value for each item is derived by subtracting balance sheet items of period N from period $N + 1$. The cash flow statement is organized into three categories of cash flow activity. These cash flow activities are operations, investing, and financing.

Cash flow from operations mainly reflects changes in current assets and current liabilities, which move more or less spontaneously with sales. The change in cash flow from operations, for example, might indicate a decline in sales earnings by showing that a company is having trouble collecting on accounts receivable. This can occur when accounts receivable is rising at a faster pace than sales.

Cash flow from an investment activity may include the purchase of long-term (fixed) operating assets, such as buildings and equipment. The purchase of a fixed operating asset such as videonystagmography (VNG) equipment is an investment activity. Negative cash flow from investment activity such as equipment would indicate the company is converting cash into operating assets, and down the road one would expect to see positive cash flow from operating activity based on that equipment investment.

Cash flow from financing activities includes loan principle and interest expense. A 10-year start-up business loan would be a long-term debt under the category of financing activities.

The cash flow statement shows how the company makes and spends its cash. Is it making money from operations? Ideally, if cash is flowing in and being collected as it should be, a company will have positive cash flow from operations. If the company has positive cash flows from operations and negative cash flows to investment, that may mean it is using cash income to invest in additional operating assets. The statement of cash flows identifies the source of cash and the use of a company's cash and can identify if the company is reinvesting in operating assets or if the company is debt-ridden and using operating cash flow to satisfy financing activity.

◆ Managerial Accounting

We have said that financial accounting is completed primarily for the benefit of people and entities outside the company, such as creditors and investors. Managerial accounting is a process that is used internally by managers to evaluate the business and direct decisions. The primary tools for managerial accounting are financial accounting ratios.

Financial Accounting Ratios

Financial statements are much more than static documents; they provide the source information for financial accounting ratios that yield a wealth of information about a practice. Financial accounting ratios have been described by Freeman et al (2000) in two forms, cross-sectional and a time series analysis. A cross-sectional analysis involves comparing the practice with industry standards compiled by a trade organization. Using financial ratios, one can compare the performance of any size practice with an industry standard. Unfortunately, these cross-sectional analyses are not easy to complete for practices in audiology, as benchmarks and industry standards are not readily available.

XYZ Audiology Associates
Statement of Cash Flows
For the Year Ending December 31, 2007

Operating Activities	
Net Income	12,700
Noncash Expenses and Revenues Included in Income	
Depreciation	2,720
Increase in Accounts Receivable	(1,480)
Increase in Inventory	3,600
Increase in Accounts Payable	(3,600)
Increase in Taxes Payable	1,200
Cash Flow from Operating Activity	15,140
Investing Activities	
Acquisition of Equipment	(18,000)
Net Cash Used by Investing Activity	(18,000)
Financing Activities	
Proceeds on Short-term Debt	2,000
Payment to Settle Short-term Debt	(2,400)
Proceeds of Long-term Debt	0
Payment on Long-term debt	(9,600)
Net Cash Provided by Financing Activity	(10,000)
Net Increase (Decrease) in Cash and Cash Equivalents	(12,860)

Figure 15–4 The statement of cash flows.

Pitfall

- There are many successful audiology practices, but those financial records are not in the public domain to provide a road map to practice owners or managers. Benchmarks for success are based on a practice's own history when a comparison to other practices is not available.

Because it is difficult to compare individual practice performance to industry standards, it is the time series analysis that becomes the most important to audiology practice. These analyses compare the practice to itself over periods of time, usually month to month or year to year. Time series calculations also are conducted on financial statements, specifically the balance sheet and the income statement. The real information in financial statements, particularly the balance sheet, is unlocked by a comparison of the statements and a ratio analysis across other time periods. When numbers in current statements are compared with financial statements conducted at, for example, monthly or yearly intervals, they come alive with informative data that paint a true picture of how success or failure has developed.

Financial statements can reveal a wealth of information to the stakeholders about earnings over time, as in the comparison of first quarter 2006 with the first quarter of 2007, or year ending December 31, 2005 with year ending December 31, 2006. Analyses can reveal possible reasons for soaring or stagnated sales, and even the practice's capability to pay back a loan to the bank. The following relatively simple measures can be calculated and tracked over time to assist management in making decisions related to the strategic plan of a business practice.

Balance Sheet Calculations

The balance sheet provides information regarding whether the practice has the capability to meet its financial obligations to suppliers, employees, lenders, and other essential operating expenses. Although there are calculations that are of interest on the other statements, most of the important ratios are performed on the balance sheet.

There are three major ratios used to analyze the balance sheet that will demonstrate the strengths and weaknesses of a practice: liquidity, activity, and leverage. Liquidity ratios are used to measure the short-term ability of a practice to generate cash to pay current liabilities. Activity ratios reveal how quickly assets can be turned into cash, a measure of the effectiveness of the organization. Debt or leverage ratios reflect the long-term solvency of the practice and are of considerable interest to the investors and/or the bankers that have loaned or may be asked to loan money to the practice. These ratios are described in more detail in the following sections.

Liquidity Ratios

A common liquidity ratio is the current ratio (CR). The CR is sometimes called a working capital ratio, as it is a calculation of how many times the practice's current assets cover its current liabilities and if the practice has sufficient resources to meet those liabilities. In other words, the CR asks the question, Can the practice pay its bills or not? The CR is figured as follows:

$$\text{Current Ratio} = \frac{\text{Current Assets}}{\text{Current Liabilities}}$$

If the result of a CR calculation is less than 1, the practice will not be able to meet its current liabilities; if the CR is 2 or more, the practice can pay its bills with money left over. Most bankers and practice managers like to see this ratio at least between 1 and 2.

Using the balance sheet in **Fig. 15–2** as an example, the CR is 25,600/18,200 = 1.4. The CR includes prepaid expenses (insurance, etc.) and the inventory, which sometimes will present a cloudy view of the real picture for audiology practices. In these days of custom hearing instruments that are ordered upon demand, most audiology practices would have small inventories, perhaps consisting of some noncustom products such as assistive listening devices, hearing protection devices, hearing aid batteries, and possibly a few digital behind-the-ear devices. Thus, a very common modification of the CR is the quick ratio (QR), sometimes known as the acid test ratio (ATR). The QR evaluates the practice's liquidity without considering the inventory and prepaid expenses and presents a more accurate indication of the practice's liquidity. The QR is figured as follows:

$$\text{Current Ratio} = \frac{\text{Cash} + \frac{\text{Marketable}}{\text{Securities}} + \frac{\text{Accounts}}{\text{Receivable}}}{\text{Current Liabilities}}$$

As with the CR, QR values less than 1 demonstrate that the practice has serious difficulty meeting everyday expenses. Managers, bankers, stockholders, and other stakeholders also prefer to see this ratio between 1 and 2. Using the **Fig. 15–2** example again, the QR would be (12,800 + 4,200)/18,200 = 0.93. This number is not as healthy as the CR, but it should not signal concern by itself; the real picture of a practice's health is formed when comparing ratios over more than one time period.

Another useful liquidity calculation is the defensive interval measure (DIM), a ratio that measures the time span that the practice can operate without any external cash flow or how long the practice can operate if there is no business. As with personal finances, wise practice managers keep an emergency fund at hand in case business drops off or ceases for some reason. Accountants refer to these emergency funds as defensive assets (DA). By definition, the DA are those assets that can be turned into cash within 3 months or less, such as cash (savings), marketable securities, and accounts receivable. To figure the DIM, it is first necessary to know the projected daily operating expenses (PDOE), or how much it costs to keep the practice open each day. To find the PDOE, simply add up the cost of goods sold in a year, the selling and administrative expenses in a year, and other ordinary cash expenses for the year and divide by 365:

$$\text{Projected Daily Operating Expenses} = \frac{\text{Total Yearly Expenses}}{365}$$

Once the PDOE are known, the DIM is found by dividing the DA by the PDOE:

$$\text{Defensive Interval Measure} = \frac{\text{Defensive Assets}}{\text{Projected Daily Operating Expenses}}$$

The DIM calculation gives the practice manager the length of time the business could survive if revenue were substantially reduced or absent.

Using the sample income statement in **Fig. 15–3**, the PDOE is $(136,000 + 203,800)/365 = \$931$. The DIM is $25,600/931 = 27$, meaning the practice can theoretically operate for almost 1 month without revenue from external sources.

Activity Ratios

Activity ratios are calculations that allow the manager to review the efficiency of the practice in the use of its assets to generate cash. Although there are several activity ratios that can indicate the efficiency of the practice, the accounts receivable turnover (ART) ratio, the inventory turnover (IT) ratio, and the total assets turnover (TAT) ratio are useful to practice managers.

It is customary for professionals to expect patients to pay when services are delivered, but the reality is* that some patients and insurance companies pay slowly. Third-party payers sometimes delay payment for 60 to 120 days after the services are rendered and may often not pay the first time the claim is submitted. Every practice should have a policy for how and when credit is extended to patients, and managers can use activity ratios as a warning if the policy needs to be revised. The main point is that the receivable account should be closely monitored to determine how much is due to the practice and how long, on average, it takes to collect these credit sales. The ART ratio reveals how many times the receivable account is turned into cash each year. To obtain the ART ratio, it is first necessary to find the average amount that is due the practice from the receivable account or average accounts receivable balance (AARB). This is obtained by adding the accounts receivable balance at the end of last year to the balance of the accounts receivable at the end of the current year and dividing by 2:

$$\text{AARB} = \frac{\text{ARB(Year 1)} + \text{ARB (Year 2)}}{2}$$

Once the average accounts receivable balance is computed, the ART ratio, or the time it takes to convert this account into cash, can be obtained by taking the net sales (sales after cost of sales are subtracted) and dividing that amount by the AARB:

$$\text{Art Ratio} = \frac{\text{Net Sales}}{\text{Average Accounts Receivable Balance}}$$

Once known, the ART ratio tells the manager how long it takes, on average, to collect the amounts in the accounts receivable. The higher, the better for this calculation; for example, if the ART ratio = 5.3, the practice turns over the accounts receivable 5.3 times per year, or every 2.26 months. To obtain more detail, the calculation of the number of days it takes to turn over the accounts receivable can be obtained by dividing the average accounts receivable into 365, in this case 68.86 days.

As indicated earlier, audiology practices do not keep too much inventory: a few loaners, some demonstration instruments, batteries, accessories, and, possibly, some assistive listening devices. Although there is not much inventory for most practices, it still may be beneficial to understand how fast this inventory turns over. In accounting, there are specific methods of figuring inventory, such as first in, first out (FIFO) or last in, first out (LIFO), and determining the best one for a practice is complex and should be considered carefully with a professional assistance. Generally, the IT ratio is a calculation that measures how fast the inventory is sold. To arrive at the IT ratio, it is necessary to obtain the value of the average inventory on hand in the practice. Thus, the average inventory is found by adding the beginning inventory for the period to the ending inventory and dividing by 2.

$$\text{Average Inventory} = \frac{\text{Beginning Inventory} + \text{Ending Inventory}}{2}$$

Once the average inventory is known, the IT ratio is computed by dividing the cost of the goods sold by the average inventory. If, for the year, the IT ratio was 5.9, the inventory will turn over almost 6 times each year.

$$\text{Inventory Turnover Ratio} = \frac{\text{Cost of Goods Sold}}{\text{Average Inventory}}$$

As with other activity ratios, the turning of the inventory can be further delineated to reflect how long it takes the inventory to sell out in days by simply dividing 365 by the IT ratio. In this example, if the inventory turns over ~6 times per year, then it takes ~61 days for the inventory to sell out. These data assist the practice manager in planning product orders efficiently throughout the year, ensuring that there is always a fresh, sufficient supply as well as taking advantage of discounts.

An activity measure that presents how effectively assets are turned into cash is the TAT ratio. The TAT ratio looks at the sales for goods and services and divides by the total assets to arrive at how many times the practice's assets turn over per year.

$$\text{Total Asset Turnover Ratio} = \frac{\text{Sales}}{\text{Total Assets}}$$

Of course, the higher the ratio, the better, as this is an indication that the assets turn over more times per year, suggesting a practice that uses its assets efficiently. Using our sample company, to obtain the TAT ratio, take total sales revenue from the income statement (**Fig. 15–3**) and divide that by total assets from the balance sheet (**Fig. 15–2**). The calculation is as follows: 368,000/260,000 = 1.4. The number, of course, takes on more meaning when compared across several periods for one company, or if compared against a known industry average.

Debt or Leverage Ratios

Two ratios that are beneficial in providing the practice manager information as to how much the practice debt is relative to its assets are the debt to assets ratio (DAR) and the times interest earned (TIE) ratio. These ratios indicate whether the practice has the capability to support more debt for the purpose of adding equipment, opening another location, or other activities.

The DAR yields how much liability the practice has for every dollar of assets and provides the creditors with information about the ability of the practice to withstand losses without impairing the interest of the creditors. The DAR is simply the total liabilities divided by the total assets:

$$\text{Debt to Assets Ratio} = \frac{\text{Total Liabilities}}{\text{Total Assets}}$$

A low DAR is desirable because a higher number indicates that the practice is more dependent on borrowed money to sustain itself and suggests that small changes in cash flow could cause serious difficulties in the capability to repay debt.

Using our sample company in **Fig. 15–2**, the DAR is as follows:

$$168,200/260,000 = 0.65$$

Income Statement Calculations

Although most routine calculations are conducted on the balance sheet, sometimes the ratios that tell the most about a practice are the profitability ratios conducted on the income statement. A projected income statement prepared for a business proposal should have enough detail to support ratio analyses. These profitability ratios are clues as to how well the practice has performed and reviews if the practice's net income is adequate, what rate of return was achieved, and profit margin as a percentage of sales. The ratios routinely considered in this group are the profit margin on sales (PMOS) and the asset turnover (AT) ratio that incorporates information from both the income statement and the balance sheet.

The PMOS is a measure of overall profitability. To compute the PMOS, net income is divided by sales:

$$\text{Profit Margin on Sales} = \frac{\text{Net Income}}{\text{Sales}}$$

PMOS results are presented in a percentage that reflects the amount of each dollar that is profit. For example, if the calculation yields 20%, then 20 cents of every dollar collected is profit. These values can be tracked to determine if there are changes in profitability that require attention.

For **Fig. 15–3** values, the PMOS is 12,700/368,000 = 0.035. In our sample company, only 3 cents on the dollar is profit. Net profit (net income) is the money that is added to owner's equity at the end of the accounting period; this should not be confused with the owner's salary, which is an operating expense and is paid before net profit is distributed.

Tracking

An easy method of tracking these ratios can be the use of a spreadsheet. By simply creating a spreadsheet and entering data on a monthly or quarterly basis, the data can be analyzed at a glance. Maintaining a record of the various ratios and reviewing them over time allows practice managers to visualize problems and react to them in a timely manner. Although this information is of great benefit, it must be remembered that all financial statements and the ratios conducted upon them contain information from the past and may or may not be an accurate predictor of the health of the business in the future.

Practice Accounting and the Business Plan

When writing a business plan proposal, of course, financial statements do not exist. It does not make sense to "make up" a balance sheet, because the balance sheet is a device showing only one moment in time anyway. Two balance sheets are needed for comparison to create a statement of cash flows. The income statement, in contrast, shows the revenues and expenses over an entire period (e.g., month, quarter, or year), making it the perfect financial "report" to include in a business plan. At the minimum, lenders and investors will expect to see a projected income statement (also called the pro forma income statement) that shows the anticipated revenues and expenses over at least the first year of operations.

It is not enough to show a number on the "sales income" line of the pro forma income statement; investors and lenders need to see how the company will generate the revenue. For an audiology practice, define the products and services that will be provided and the contribution of each to the practice's bottom line.

In Chapter 5 in this volume, Staab discusses analysis tools that can be used to identify the potential market for a company's services. Revenue projections should be supported with evidence of the existence of a potential market for the services and by an ability to provide those services. The revenue-producing capacity of a professional practice depends on how many services the professional owner and employees can perform. Therefore, to get an accurate picture of the revenue capacity, it is essential to consider vacations, holidays, and meeting attendance that will result in lost potential revenue (Nolan and Bober, 1997). In addition to calculating the actual professional service hours available to the practice, further identify the revenue-generating capacity by applying a break-even analysis to the business plan.

Break-even Analysis

The break-even calculation can make a significant contribution to the manager's strategic plan and the decision making. The breakeven analysis can be particularly important in the area of investment activity where it is critical to understand the profit potential of a particular investment. This tool can also assist in establishing performance goals for a practice.

The break-even volume (BEV) is the minimum number of products or services that are required to meet the expense of providing those products or services. It is calculated as

$$\text{BEV} = \frac{\text{Fixed Costs}}{\text{Sales Margin}}$$

The fixed costs of a practice include all of the operating expenses listed in the income statement, except for the cost of goods sold. The sales margin is the price of the product (what the consumer pays), less the cost of the goods sold (what the seller pays to the supplier). **Figure 15–5** depicts the sales margin and variable cost as a proportion of the sale price. Variable costs are any costs directly related to the sale of goods (cost of goods sold). Fixed costs include salaries and utilities and can be thought of as the cost of keeping the doors of the business open. Fixed costs are incurred even if no product is sold.

From an accounting perspective, the fixed and variable costs represent the fundamental difference between providing products and services. The delivery of a product (hearing aid, battery, assistive device) will always have fixed and variable costs associated with it. The sales price is made up of the variable cost and the sales margin. A service (vestibular evaluation, audiometric evaluation, auditory rehabilitation session) provided by the owner or employee of a practice is delivered entirely on fixed costs. The fee received (sales price) for service is entirely sales margin; there no deduction for variable costs. Although human resource issues are covered in Chapter 4 and are beyond the scope of this discussion, recognize that if a practice contracts with an audiologist to perform on a fee-for-service basis (not as an employee), the practice would incur a variable cost in addition to the fixed costs associated with the service delivery.

For an example of a product-based break-even analysis, assume that XYZ Audiology Associates generates all of its revenue from hearing aid sales and that **Fig. 15–5** represents an average binaural sale. How many sales are needed to break even?

From the income statement in **Fig. 15–3**, we see the fixed cost for operating the practice is $219,300. The margin (from **Fig. 15–5**) is $1800. The BEV is calculated as follows:

$$\$219,300/\$1800 = 122$$

This means XYZ needs to have at least 121 sales in a year, or ~10 per month (if the average sale is binaural, this would be 20 hearing aids). At the BEV, XYZ will cover the variable costs of the products, the fixed costs of the operating the practice, and maintain a net income of zero (no profit or loss).

Of course, the vast majority of audiology practices deliver many more services beyond hearing aid sales. If a practice is considering the investment in a new fixed operating asset such as VNG equipment, the practice manager can support the decision to purchase (or not to purchase) the equipment by demonstrating the BEV (number of tests conducted) for the equipment to be considered profitable.

For this example, assume the VNG equipment costs $35,000, and the national average CPT reimbursement for the test(s) is about $500 per patient (American Speech-Language-Hearing Association, 2005). There are no variable costs for providing this service, so the BEV analysis is calculated as follows:

$$\$35,000/\$500 = 70$$

The BEV is 70, meaning it will take 70 tests being reimbursed at an average of $500 for the equipment costs to be met. From this figure, the practice manager can determine if there are sufficient human resources available to perform these services and if the market demand exists. There are also income tax considerations for equipment purchase, and IRS tax code is supportive of investment in fixed assets. By depreciating fixed assets over time, a practice is able to deduct the expense to offset earnings and potentially reduce its income tax liability. Consult with a tax professional regarding the tax advantages of investing in fixed assets, but be aware that there may be considerable advantages.

Managers might respond to a break-even analysis by making one or more strategic business decisions, including

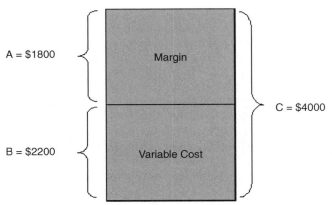

Figure 15–5 The sales margin (A) is the sale price (C) minus the variable cost of the sale (B).

investing in equipment, hiring new employees, performing a market analysis, or establishing new performance goals. On the other hand, rather than reacting to the BEV, the manager can change it.

Price Policy

Price is (mostly) a management/ownership decision. Audiologists need to be informed of the obligations and limitations for fees they charge when they become providers for third-party payers, including insurance companies, Medicare, and Medicaid. Those issues are discussed in Chapters 16 and 17.

This is a discussion of price from a practice management perspective. Price should never be a purely "bottom line" accounting decision. It is common for audiologists to seek a simple answer to the question of how to price their products and services, but establishing a price is a complex issue. Price policy should include a cost basis for establishing price of products and services. The managing audiologist can use a full cost basis for establishing price, where the fixed and variable costs are the basis for price. This is different from a variable cost basis, where only the costs associated with the product delivery are used in the pricing strategy. It might be tempting to set hearing aid prices by simply instituting a flat percentage over the variable cost, and many audiologists have done it that way. However, if the manufacturer changes its prices, a company will run into problems when its price to the consumer is based on the variable cost paid to the manufacturer.

Using a full cost basis, price is a real reflection of the financial needs of the practice. One can adjust prices as needed to meet the changing financial demands of the practice. To come up with a full cost basis price, a practice manager might use a break-even analysis: the fixed costs divided by the sales margin. Of course, the sales margin is based on price, and by manipulating price, the manager can come up with a BEV that suits the needs and capacity of a practice. Another full cost basis strategy would be to review the PMOS figure (which can be calculated based on a projected income statement). Recall that the PMOS is the net income divided by sales, and it reveals the percent of every dollar in sales that resulted in profit. One method of making a price decision is to formulate a PMOS goal and identify how much sales revenue needs to be generated to achieve that goal. From that sales goal figure, it is possible to identify how much prices need to increase to achieve the new sales goal. This can be calculated based on detailed records (or projections) of the company's sales. For example, assume total sales income was $200,000 and 80% ($160,000) was generated by the sale of hearing aids, and that 80 units were sold at an average price of $2,000. To increase the sales goal by $20,000 without changing fixed or variable costs, the price must be raised. An average unit price increase of $250 will generate $20,000 more revenue per year and will not affect cost of goods sold or fixed costs. Net income will increase, and the PMOS figure will increase accordingly.

It would be a big mistake to base any price policy entirely on some accounting solution. The fixed and variable costs of operating a practice are only one factor among several that should influence price strategy. Price has as much to do with market strategy as with the bottom line. The company's target market, product position, and differential advantage need to be considered in setting price policy. Accounting can identify the financial needs of a practice, but price policy should be part of the marketing strategy, helping to define how consumers view the practice. Winer (2000) states that market share is a function of the consumer's perceived value of the product or service and its price.

$$\text{Market Share} = f(\text{perceived value/price})$$

According to this equation, there are two things a practice manager can do to increase market share: increase perceived value or decrease price. Whether to increase perceived value or decrease price is a decision that is based on how the company defines its position in the marketplace. The company's price policy must be consistent with how the company wants to be perceived by consumers.

Competition is another factor that influences marketing strategy and may influence price policy. One of the five forces at work in a competitive environment is the threat of substitute products (Porter, 1980). Porter's theory of competitive forces tells us that when there are many alternative products available, competition becomes fierce, and prices tend to be forced downward as competitors struggle to retain market share. For example, it is common to see a lot of pizza options and very low pizza prices in areas near college campuses. Consider, too, metropolitan newspapers filled with advertisements for low-priced hearing aids. These advertisers are responding to the threat of the many available substitute products (other hearing aid offices) by offering even lower prices. How can a professional doctor of audiology respond to rampant price competition in a market where consumers have substitute products available? Audiologists have the opportunity to almost eliminate the threat of substitute products in their market by positioning themselves as unique professional identities. A marketing strategy that focuses on the identity or identifies of the professionals within the practice and the services they offer can never be substituted by the competition.

Controversial Point

- In hearing aid dispensing, price "bundling" refers to the practice of presenting the consumer with a price that includes the product and associated fitting and follow-up services. "Unbundled" prices separate the cost for the product and professional services. Historically, the costs for hearing aids and associated professional services have almost always been bundled into one price to the consumer. Separating professional service fees from products costs is gaining momentum, but the practice is not universally accepted or endorsed.

Good price policy decisions are not made by looking only at marketing objectives or financial goals. Price is a complex factor for consumers and businesses.

◆ Summary

Knowledge and understanding of how to maintain, report, and analyze the financial history of audiology practice should be viewed as the responsibility of the professional practitioner in any work setting. The information contained in this chapter will assist anyone who is, or who would like to be, responsible for some degree of practice management. An ability to understand the financial drivers of a successful practice is a fundamental and long-lasting skill set that will benefit any autonomous professional, regardless of the employment arrangement or work setting.

References

American Speech-Language-Hearing Association. (2005). Medicare fee schedule and hospital outpatient prospective payment system for audiologists. Retrieved from http://asha.org/members.issues/reimbursement/

Anthony, R. N., Hawkins, D. E., & Merchant, K. A. (1999). Accounting: Text and cases (10th ed.). Irwin/McGraw-Hill.

Freeman, B., Barimo, J., & Fox, G. (2000). Financial management of audiology practices and clinics. In H. Hosford-Dunn, R. J. Roeser, & M. Valente (Eds.), Audiology practice management (pp. 351–362). New York: Thieme Medical Publishers.

Mautz, D. (2005). Building a better understanding of financial reports. Commercial Lending Review, 20, 5.

Nolan, K. F., Jr., & Bober, C. R. (1997). Understanding the business of physician practice. Healthcare Financial Management, 51, 74–76.

Porter, M. (1980). Competitive strategy. New York: Free Press.

Tergeson, A. (2001, January 22). The ins and outs of cash flow. Business Week.

Winer, R. S. (2000). Marketing management. Upper Saddle River, NJ: Prentice Hall.

Chapter 16

The Evolution of Reimbursement for Audiology

Robert C. Fifer

There was a time in the United States when health care services were available without government oversight, with no established prices for each procedure and no predetermined reimbursement methodologies. Payment for medical services was not necessarily in the form of money. "Practice expense" had no meaning, except that the physician needed enough income to live on. House calls were common, and affiliation, referral, or service contracts were not. Audiologic services were also unheard of, and when they became available, they were found primarily only in large university settings and government facilities. (i.e., military). All of this began to change in 1935, with the establishment of Social Security (Social Security Online, 2006).

In the early 1900s, hospitals existed primarily by the largess of private agencies, philanthropists, or churches. It was also commonplace for a hospital to come into being through an initial arrangement between a university and a state department of health. But in 1935, the first rendition of the Social Security Act (SSA, 2007a) was passed, transferring much of the financial burden from the state departments of health to the federal government for operating hospitals and providing health care services. In exchange for federal money, the hospitals agreed to provide health care services to the poor and uninsured. The agreements between hospitals and the federal government resulted in a significant influx of money that was used to expand capacity and range of services provided by each hospital. The approval for adding new services evolved into a system of needs review and the granting of "certificates of need" (McGinley, 1995). The era of competition between hospitals had begun.

◆ Introduction of Medicare and Medicaid

Congress passed a broad revision to the Social Security Act in 1965 that resulted in a much larger change to the image of health care (42 u.s.c. 1395y, Section 1862). The Medicare portion of the 1965 update focused on two populations, individuals who were 65 years of age and older and those with severe disabilities. Physicians were permitted to evaluate those patients, prescribe diagnostic tests, and treat the patients, and Medicare paid the bills. There was no incentive for cost containment. All charges were based on what the physician or laboratory considered appropriate and were without analysis of delivery service costs. Medicare's primary criterion for reimbursement was whether each charge was "normal and customary" relative to what others in the same region charged for the same service (Social Security Online, 2006).

Medicaid also came into existence in the 1965 modification of the Social Security Act and is a combined federal–state program to provide health care to the indigent. In contrast to Medicare, state-level government has much input with regard to determining covered services and any service limitations. Each state legislature plays a significant role in determining reimbursement levels through the proportion of the state's general revenue budget that is allocated toward Medicaid expenditures (HHS, 2006). Although Medicaid has attracted much attention in recent years, the major influences on health care policy have originated with Medicare.

Soon after Medicare was established, the cost of health care increased at an alarming rate, much faster than predicted, because of the absence of a national payment policy and spending constraint incentives (GAO, 2004, May 15). In 1972, Congress authorized a study of service utilization relative to Medicare and Medicaid expenses. This resulted in establishing professional review organizations to determine the quality and quantity of services rendered. State and regional councils were also established to authorize specific procedures based on past utilization data. It was felt that if the availability and supply of services were controlled, programmatic costs could be contained more readily. Nothing of substance was accomplished, as reflected by the rise in Medicare spending from $3.2 billion in 1970 to $15.7 billion in 1985. The estimated outlays for Part B (physician services) and Part D (drug benefit) in 2006 were $216 billon (SSA, 2007b), of which $95.6 billion were payments for physician services (HHS, 2007b). The increases in health care spending far outpaced inflation, salaries, cost of living, and every other expense.

During the 1980s, significant changes were observed in insurance companies' and Medicare's reimbursement strategies. Prospective payment procedures were introduced to place caps on outpatient services. One of the principal elements of prospective payments was the diagnosis-related group (DRG) payments. DRGs represented fixed dollar amount fees based on a patient's primary diagnosis (Hoffman et al, 2006). If the cost of care was below the reimbursement level of the DRG, the hospital made money, but the hospital became the bearer of risk in the event that the cost of care exceeded DRG reimbursement. During this period, health maintenance organizations (HMOs) gained a strong foothold in various regions across the United States and became very popular as a model of controlling the quantity of services and subsequent costs (Morkovich, 2003). DRGs and HMOs forced all involved with health care to evaluate carefully the costs of providing services. The unlimited flow of reimbursement dollars common in the 1960s and 1970s no longer existed. Health care providers and hospitals had to weigh the costs of personnel, equipment, and disposable supplies to ensure that their financial outlays remained equal to or less than reimbursement levels.

The mid-1980s also found Congress asking a different question: How much does it cost to provide health care? At face value, this question represented a sea change from Congress's earlier attitude, which focused on either limiting the availability of services or capping reimbursement. Numerous studies had attempted to ascertain the reasons that health care spending increased so dramatically. Typically, each study focused individually on malpractice insurance, availability of services, new developments in treatments of various diseases, and the cost of pharmaceuticals. Because a clear, comprehensive answer was not forthcoming, Congress commissioned a study (Hsiao, Braun, Dunn, et al, 1988; Hsiao, Braun, Yntema, Becker, 1988) on the costs of delivering health care services by contracting with Harvard University's School of Public Health (AMA, 2007). The contract specified an extensive survey of physicians of every specialty and discipline as well as several nonphysician health care providers. The gathered data were relatively unrefined but represented a broad perspective of the elements of health care delivery: physician work (professional component), practice expense (technical component), professional liability insurance, and indirect costs for general office overhead. Based on the outcome of that study, a reimbursement model was developed to control health care costs: the Resource Based Relative Value System (RBRVS). The outcome of the survey and the development of the RBRVS brought in the American Medical Association (AMA) as a major participant in coding and reimbursement and solidified the relationship between the AMA, the Health Care Financing Administration (HCFA, now known as the Center for Medicare and Medicaid Services, CMS), and Congress. This relationship has had a major impact on the field of audiology's current status for coding and reimbursement in addition to influencing many of the current guidelines of how audiologists report procedures and submit claims.

♦ Current Procedural Terminology Codes

The Current Procedural Terminology (CPT) coding system was developed and copyrighted by the AMA. The first list of codes, published in 1966, encouraged a common terminology for designating medical procedures. Each code was assigned a unique four-digit identifier and a unique descriptor. The second edition, published in 1970, moved from four- to five-digit identifiers and divided codes into surgery, medicine, and a listing of procedures specific to internal medicine. Two more editions of the CPT listings were published in the 1970s. The cumulative number of new code additions for the 1977 fourth edition affirmed the need for regular updates based on the rapid growth in the number of CPT codes.

Pearl

- In 1983, HCFA formally adopted the CPT coding system as the preferred method of procedure identification (HHS, 2007b). In doing so, HCFA took the first step toward establishing the HCFA Common Procedure Coding System (HCPCS).

HCPCS was divided into levels based on purpose and availability. The AMA's CPT coding system was adopted to become level I HCPCS codes. Level II HCPCS codes were technical, equipment, and supply codes developed by HCFA and available nationally. Level III codes, developed by state and local entities serving primarily Medicaid patients, were local use codes not available nationally. They were eliminated when the Health Insurance Portability and Accountability Act (HIPAA) was adopted in October 2003. CMS required the use of HCPCS to report all procedures for Part B Medicare patients in 1986 and extended the requirement to outpatient hospital services in 1987.

Pearl

- Although many professionals think of CPT codes as useful only for billing and reimbursement, the primary purpose of the CPT system is to establish both descriptive and defining terms for all health care procedures.

Today, CPT is the most widely accepted health care procedure coding system in the United States. Each code is descriptive in the sense that it creates a common understanding of respective procedures. This is accomplished by standardizing nomenclature through which communication among various health care disciplines may be more effective. For example, a comprehensive audiologic test battery, know as CPT code 92557, originally was called a basic evaluation at one clinic, an audiological evaluation at another, and comprehensive diagnostic testing at yet another facility. Other names for this procedure were basic comprehensive evaluation, diagnostic audiological testing, and basic evaluation, among other terms. There were as many descriptions as there were facilities. To further complicate matters, some clinics included air conduction, bone conduction, speech reception threshold (SRT), and speech discrimination; others also included tympanometry and acoustic reflexes. Uniformity of terminology was an unknown concept. Today, CPT code 92557 is described as "[c]omprehensive audiometry threshold evaluation and speech recognition (92553 and 92556 combined)" and includes air conduction, bone conduction, SRT, and speech discrimination. Tympanometry and acoustic reflex measurements each have their own CPT codes. The language now describes the same procedure with the same terminology regardless of facility setting.

Definition of the procedure is distinct from the procedure descriptors and is also an essential concept for the universality of CPT codes. In contrast to a descriptor, the definition refers to the elements or components that comprise the overall procedure. For example, CPT code 92584 (electrocochleography) has a descriptor that offers a reasonable understanding of what the code represents. But the definition of the procedure involves more detail: a breakdown of the step-by-step elements and inclusion of a "typical" patient. For code 92584, the definition offered by the Health Care Economic Committee of the American Speech-Language-Hearing Association (ASHA) to the AMA coding panels is found in **Fig. 16–1**.

Most CPT codes since 1990 have such definitions as part of the "common language" concept to list the components of the procedure and, just as important, to convey what is not included in the procedure. These definitions may be found for some codes in the annual CPT manual (AMA, 2006a). However, for each new or significantly revised code, the AMA also publishes annual updates, the *CPT Assistant* (AMA, 1990–2006) and *CPT Changes: An Insider's View* (AMA, 2006b), including a typical patient and description of the procedure.

These publications are designed to assist professional coders, health care administrators, and insurers in understanding what each new code includes, what would be considered a "typical patient," and what is involved in the appropriate execution of the procedure. Neither publication carries the weight of authority as does the CPT manual, but both provide an excellent supplemental source of information for appropriate use and reporting of each procedure code.

Typical patient:

A 56-year-old female was referred for electrocochleography due to a three-month history of incapacitating vertigo, roaring tinnitus, and fluctuating hearing loss in the right ear. A previous audiogram revealed normal hearing sensitivity at all test frequencies for the left ear and a mild to moderate sensorineural hearing loss from 250 hertz through 6000 hertz in the right ear. Speech discrimination for the left ear was excellent whereas speech discrimination for the right ear was mildly reduced.

Description of procedure:

The audiologist greeted the patient in the waiting room and accompanied her to the audiometric test suite. Inside the suite was a gurney where the patient reclined. The audiologist prepped the skin for EEG electrode application using an electrolyte scrubbing solution and gauze pads. After mildly abrading the skin, the audiologist affixed EEG electrodes to the Al, A2, and FPz locations. The audiologist then checked the impedance of each electrode and adjusted them accordingly. After ensuring that the impedances were below 5000 ohms the audiologist prepared the tympanic membrane electrode. The tympanic membrane electrode has a sponge tip into which the audiologist must inject a conducting gel. Using a syringe with a 14-gauge needle, the audiologist injected the sponge with conducting gel to both saturate the sponge and create a crown of gel. The audiologist then gently inserted the electrode into the patient's ear canal until contact was made with the tympanic membrane. The electrode was then stabilized with tape and also through the use of an expanding sponge tip of an insert earphone. Clicks and tone bursts were presented to the test ear at a level of approximately 90 decibels. The evoked potentials were signal averaged for approximately 2000 repetitions. The resulting waveform was then stored in the computer's memory for later analysis. This procedure was repeated for both the non-involved ear and the involved ear. After data collection was completed for both ears, the audiologist recalled the averaged waveforms and analyzed the amplitudes of the summating potentials and the action potentials from the respective responses. A ratio was formed through the comparison of the amplitudes for the summating potential and the action potential for each ear. The ratios from each ear were compared to one another and to normative values in an effort to determine the presence of endolymphatic hydrops at the time of test. After the data were collected, stored, and analyzed, the audiologist removed the electrodes and cleaned the conducting paste from the patient's ear lobes and forehead. The patient was provided information regarding the outcome of the study. The audiologist called the referring physician immediately to convey the outcome of the evaluation and the interpretation of the ratio values. A written report was also prepared for the patient's medical records in both the audiologist's office and the physician's office.

Figure 16–1 The patient definition presented to the AMA CPT coding panels for CPT code 92584, Electrocochleography. CPT; Current Procedural Technology.

◆ Organization of the American Medical Association's CPT Coding Committees

CPT Editorial Panel

The CPT Editorial Panel is composed of 17 members (AMA, 2007c). Eleven members are nominated by the AMA; one physician is nominated respectively from the Blue Cross and Blue Shield Association, the Health Insurance Association of America, the American Hospital Association, and the CMS. In addition, two members of the panel represent nonphysician

(M.D./D.O.) health care specialties. One of the nonphysician members is also the cochair of the CPT Health Care Professions Advisory Committee. The other non-M.D./D.O. panelist is nominated and selected from the various nonphysician specialties that use CPT codes. The broad range of individuals who make up the editorial panel bring diverse experiences and perspectives to the table and represent sufficient expertise from clinical health care, insurance, government, and administration to permit an objective evaluation and critique of each code proposal. The panel requires a majority vote to decide whether to recognize the requested coding changes.

The decisions made by this panel have widespread influences on the fortunes of many. If medical equipment is integral to the procedure, industry may benefit. For health care professionals who provide the proposed procedures or services, the opportunity for reimbursement often hinges on the decisions made by this panel. Consequently, the panel considers each proposal very carefully according to established criteria before deciding whether to grant approval.

CPT Health Care Professions Advisory Committee

In 1991, concerns were expressed that nonphysician health care providers were being disadvantaged with regard to the review, development, and modifications of CPT codes used primarily by non-M.D./D.O. health care providers. In response to these concerns, the AMA invited organizations representing physician's assistants, nurses, occupational and physical therapists, optometrists, podiatrists, psychologists, social workers, audiologists, speech pathologists, and chiropractors to nominate representatives from their respective groups to form the CPT Health Care Professions Advisory Committee (HCPAC) (AMA, 2007b).

The original CPT HCPAC was developed only as an advisory group to the CPT Editorial Panel. The role and scope of the advisory committee were modified in 2001 to allow more active participation of nonphysician health care providers. At present, there are five major functions of the CPT HCPAC:

♦ To provide review of proposals concerning coding for procedures and services that may be provided by non-M.D./D.O.s

♦ To provide feedback and rationale to requesters of coding changes for nonphysician procedures

♦ To provide a recommendation to the CPT Editorial Panel for acceptance/rejection/modification of the items submitted to the panel via the CPT HCPAC

♦ To serve as liaison to any non-M.D./D.O. organization/association that may wish to submit coding proposals

♦ To serve as advocates for the CPT process

The CPT HCPAC currently consists of 13 members. The chair and two members of the committee are members of the CPT Editorial Panel, with one of these seats reserved for a representative of third-party payers, including CMS. The cochair of the committee is a representative of one of the 10 nonphysician health care representatives. The cochair also is a voting member of the CPT Editorial Panel. The 10 nonphysician health care providers are each nominated by their national associations and selected by the chair of the panel.

RVS Update Committee

Whereas the CPT Editorial Panel has primary responsibility for code development, the RVS Update Committee (RUC) has the primary responsibility for determining recommended values of each code. The RUC is made up of 29 members representing a variety of medical specialties (AMA, 2007b). The chair and the cochair of the RUC are appointed by the AMA. One member of the RUC represents the nonphysician health care providers and also cochairs the RUC HCPAC. One member serves as liaison with the CPT Editorial Panel. The remaining members are nominated by their respective medical societies and approved by the AMA. Representatives from CMS participate on the RUC panel in an advisory capacity. The primary functions of the RUC include

♦ Developing relative values for new or revised codes

♦ Enhancing the methodology of the relative value update process

♦ Making formal recommendations to CMS

♦ Notifying the CPT Editorial Panel of its actions as well as providing a report for future coding considerations

In addition to the RUC panel, there is an advisory committee to function as technical resources on the valuation issues pertaining to each specialty society. The advisory committee members are nominated by respective medical specialty societies and serve as formal liaisons between the RUC in the specialty society. The advisory committee is not a voting body but serves only to provide advice and technical expertise to the RUC panelists. At the present time, there are ~100 advisory committee members representing all aspects of medicine (AMA, 2005).

Another committee related to the RUC is the Practice Expense Review Committee (PERC). This committee is tasked with the responsibility of reviewing practice expense costs, including ancillary personnel, disposable supplies, and capital equipment. The information developed by this committee becomes an integral part of the overall RUC recommendation to CMS regarding the total recommended relative value of each procedure (AMA, 2005).

RUC Health Care Professions Advisory Committee

> **Controversial Point**
>
> • When the RUC HCPAC was organized in 1991, its only function was to advise the RUC panel. The RUC HCPAC was reorganized in 2001 with expanded responsibilities, including authority to send its recommendations directly to CMS (AMA, 2003).

Similar to the CPT HCPAC, the RUC HCPAC was formed to allow participation by nonphysician health care providers in the valuation process of CPT codes. The ability of the panel to make significant contributions has matured remarkably in recent years. Its current responsibilities include

♦ Commenting on proposed RVS changes

♦ Advising the RUC concerning the agenda for development of relative values for new and revised codes

- Identifying nonphysician providers affected by any relative value revision
- Assisting with the cooperative research agenda on the valuation process
- Providing advice on the update process
- Serving as liaison with the relevant national societies representing nonphysician providers

The RUC HCPAC is composed of 13 members; 3 are physician members of the RUC, with the remaining 10 members nominated from national organizations representing the same disciplines as the CPT HCPAC. The chair of the RUC HCPAC is one of the three physician members. The cochair of the committee is one of the 10 nonphysician health care providers. In addition, the RUC HCPAC selects an alternate cochair whose responsibility is to conduct the meeting in the absence of the cochair. Whereas the CPT HCPAC remains primarily in an advisory capacity, the RUC HCPAC has voting authority for its review of assigned CPT codes. Recommendations that come from the RUC HCPAC are transmitted directly to CMS for review and determination of payment policy.

◆ Development of New CPT Codes

New CPT codes are usually submitted for review by national organizations on the basis of members' needs surveys, development of new procedures, or changes in technology. However, proposals for new CPT codes may be submitted by individual practitioners. The appropriate forms for doing so are found on the AMA Web site (www.ama-assn.org). Regardless of its origin, each submission is initially reviewed by AMA staff to determine if the CPT Editorial Panel had previously addressed the issue. If AMA staff members determine that the proposal is for a new procedure or represents significant new information, the application is referred to members of the CPT advisory committee for a second-level review. If the advisory committee reviewers come to agreement that the proposal is appropriate, it is then referred to the full CPT Editorial Panel for review (AMA, 2007c).

The AMA has designated three types of CPT codes. A category I CPT code represents a procedure or service that reflects current, state-of-the-art practice and is designated by a unique five-digit identifier. The AMA has established five criteria for the development of new category I CPT codes. The first criterion is that each code describes a unique service and is not a significant component or an unbundling of another code. What this refers to is the ability to perform the service described by the code as a stand-alone procedure that is unique unto itself. It also means that the new procedure does not replicate any other procedure already in the CPT manual. The procedure or service must be approved by the Food and Drug Administration (FDA) if it incorporates medical equipment or pharmaceuticals. The procedure or service must be in widespread use across the United States and must not be investigational. Commensurate with this last requirement, the procedure must be supported by peer-reviewed literature appearing in U.S. published professional journals. Additionally, the procedure must not represent occasional extraordinary circumstances that would otherwise be reported using existing CPT codes. The physician members of the panel focus on the benefit to patients for diagnostic or treatment procedures and assurances that the procedure or service is in widespread versus local or regional use. Representatives of CMS and various insurers who sit on the panel will have a keen interest in the projected utilization of the procedure and its potential financial impact.

A category II CPT code is a supplemental tracking code that is used primarily for performance measurement. Use of this type of code minimizes the need for chart reviews and facilitates data collection for certain services or test results required for performance measures. These codes are optional, are not required for "correct coding," and may not be used as a substitute for category I codes. "Correct coding" refers to the requirement to report each procedure or treatment with the appropriate CPT code. Identifiers for category II CPT codes consist of four digits and an α character.

Category III CPT codes are designated for emerging technologies. The procedures described by this category of codes are reasonably new and may not be widely available across the country. They may also be part of the protocol for the study of the procedure being performed. However, as in category I CPT codes, they must have support among the specialties that use the procedure and must also be supported through U.S. published peer-reviewed literature outlining the efficacy of the procedure. These codes are assigned a numeric-α identifier and are found in their own section of the CPT manual. Category III codes will not be referred to the RUC or RUC HCPAC because no relative value units (RVUs) may be assigned to these codes. For Medicare purposes, CMS has stated that category III CPT codes serve a useful purpose and will not be categorically denied reimbursement. Although no RVUs are assigned to these codes, CMS has left it to the discretion of Medicare carriers whether reimbursement will be authorized for each code and for what amount. After 5 years, these codes must be converted to category I CPT codes, or they will be archived. If a category III code is archived, its designator will be retired and will not be reassigned to another category III code. There are occasions, however, when continuance of a category III code is necessary beyond 5 years. The AMA has made allowance for such appeals, which must be brought before the CPT Editorial Panel.

The CPT Editorial Panel meets three times per year to review up to 350 proposals. Two members of the panel are assigned to review and further investigate each application. Typically, the reviewers are from health care disciplines that have familiarity with the procedure. In addition to determining the appropriateness of each application, the reviewers read the submitted literature that came with the application and any other peer-reviewed journal articles with which they might have familiarity. It is of great benefit for the sake of expediting passage of the application for someone who is an expert in the proposed procedure to attend the meeting of the entire CPT Editorial Panel when the respective application is scheduled for panel discussion. The role of the expert is to answer questions, clarify issues, or provide background information not included in the application. Also, many or most members of the panel will have limited or no familiarity with the proposed procedure. As a consequence, the specialist sitting before the panel serves to educate each member in a thorough but short (2-minute) presentation or by answering questions. At the end of any discussion or debate, a secret vote is cast and tallied by AMA staff. A two-thirds vote of the panel is necessary for a positive outcome. Whether an application was approved is proprietary information until the Medicare Physician Fee Schedule (MPFS) or the next annual CPT manual is published.

Upon approval of an application, the AMA staff will forward a letter of interest (LOI) to all member organizations associated with the CPT process to determine their level of interest in either conducting or participating in the survey for valuing the code or providing commentary when the survey is completed. The purpose of the survey is to solicit the judgment of individuals who perform a procedure under consideration to determine the relative difficulty, skill level, and typical time to complete the procedure. The information that comes from the survey results forms the basis of the society's recommendation for the work RVU (also known as a professional component) of the reimbursement formula.

The surveys also determine the need for ancillary personnel to provide assistance to the physician in completing the procedure or providing a service to the patient. Most often this includes nursing staff or other technical support staff. The contribution of the ancillary personnel is determined by the number of minutes their services are required for a typical patient and their salary per minute as listed by the Bureau of Labor Statistics. Other elements of practice expense include the cost of disposable supplies and depreciation of capital equipment greater than $500 in value. Together, the ancillary staff, disposable supplies, and capital equipment depreciation comprise the practice expense RVU of the reimbursement formula.

The third element of the reimbursement formula is the professional liability insurance (PLI). At the present time, the RVU for this element is somewhat based on a dollar value of one RVU equals $6100. The actual RVU assignment, however, quickly moves away from that dollar value and is more often established on the basis of comparison to PLI values of other CPT codes of similar risk. As with other aspects of the RBRVS system, the PLI of each code ideally should reflect a rank-order compilation of relative risk as compared with all other CPT codes. That is, procedures of very low risk to the patient should have very small PLI RVUs, whereas procedures that expose the patient to great risk regarding health and welfare outcomes have large PLI RVUs.

There is yet a fourth, nonpublished element that is calculated and added to the three elements of the formula listed above to derive the final RVU. Whereas the RBRVS typically consists of physician work (professional component), practice expense (technical component), and PLI, CMS calculates an additional factor that is a percentage of the combined professional component and technical components to derive the indirect costs. Indirect costs include the salaries of administrative support personnel, the cost of scheduling appointments and verifying insurance, the cost of utilities and rent, and the cost of additional equipment necessary to maintain a viable health care practice. These nondirect

service components cannot be captured in survey estimates of direct service costs. However, they are essential to account for the total costs of a health care practice. It is noteworthy that to qualify for indirect cost calculations, the CPT codes must have both professional component and technical component reimbursement. Generally, codes that are only technical in nature and have no professional component or physician work associated with them are not eligible for calculation of indirect costs.

Modifiers

The AMA recognized that certain situations may arise whereby the standard use of CPT codes may not be appropriate. For that reason a variety of modifiers were created to account for unusual circumstances or situations (AMA, 2006a). Modifiers primarily applicable to audiology include "–52," which represents an abbreviated procedure or early termination of a procedure, and "–76," which represents repeated procedure performed by the same provider. For example, an auditory brainstem response (ABR) test that is terminated before completion would be reported as CPT code 92585–52. Patients with suspected endolymphatic hydrops often complete a glycerol or urea test requiring repeated diagnostic audiometry (92557). After completing a baseline audiogram and ingestion of the dehydration agent, a complete audiogram is repeated hourly for at least the next 3 hours. Under normal circumstances, code 92557 is eligible for reporting only once per date of service. However, using the modifier "–76," 92557 allows reporting for each hourly repeat test. Consequently, the audiologist would report 92557–76 for the baseline and 92557–76 for each repeat test for that date of service.

Another suffix that audiologists may use on occasion is "–53," which means a procedure that is terminated early based on the judgment of the provider for the safety and welfare of the patient. Examples for use of this suffix include a patient undergoing rotational chair evaluation who finds himself in an enclosed chamber, with goggles covering the eyes, immersed in darkness and experiencing a panic attack due to claustrophobia. Another example is a caloric electronystagmography (ENG) that is terminated following completion of the first ear due to patient reaction and resulting illness.

Unlisted Procedure

Within each health care discipline, certain procedures are performed for which CPT codes do not exist. Instead of trying to find a code that comes reasonably close to the procedure, clinicians are instructed to use a code for unspecified procedures. In the case of audiology and otolaryngology, this code is 92700. When 92700 is used, the report must include a complete description of the procedure, a justification why this particular procedure was performed, the time duration and equipment necessary for the procedure, the benefit to the patient, the information obtained, a clinical assessment of the outcome, and logical recommendations. The clinician should be prepared to submit a complete report with any claim using CPT code 92700, even if it is combined with other procedures having specific CPT code designators.

Advantages and Disadvantages of New Codes

The development of new CPT codes has advantages and disadvantages. The primary advantage is to recognize a clinical procedure that was not previously recognized. The primary disadvantage is an adverse effect upon the value of all previously existing codes within that family. In many cases, the effect is rather small for the addition of an individual code. However, if the family continues to grow with new codes that reflect state-of-the-art advancements, an additive influence with negative impact on the value of all codes may occur.

The basis of this effect originates with a congressional mandate that the annual Medicare budget will be a fixed amount of money established by calculated spending targets. The Medicare budget allocation is a fixed amount from which all health care costs will be paid under the Medicare program (GAO, 2004, May 15). The spending targets for Medicare come from the growth in the economy during the prior year. As a hypothetical example, if the economy grows at an annual rate of 2.3%, then the Medicare budget may also grow 2.3% compared with the previous year's budget. There are, however, caveats focused on the actual expenses for the prior year. Using the example of 2.3% growth for the prior year and increased Medicare spending of 5.0% during that same period, the expenditures in excess of the actual growth must be compensated for by reducing spending in the new calendar year. This is accomplished by decreasing the dollar multiplier used to convert RVUs to reimbursable amounts. In 2005, a procedure valued at 2.5 RVUs was reimbursed based on a dollar multiplier of $37.895 (HHS, 2007a), or $94.74. However, total Medicare spending for 2005 was in excess of the target amount. Therefore, the dollar multiplier for 2006 was initially reduced to $36.1770. The procedure that was worth $94.74 in 2005 would have been reimbursed at $90.44 in 2006. This methodology, called the sustainable growth rate (SGR), examines the number of patient visits, the utilization of all CPT codes, and the addition of new codes. However, Congress stepped in to negate the influence of the SGR and restored the 2006 dollar conversion factor to the 2005 value (HHS, 2007a). Consequently, new CPT codes have a tendency to increase utilization, which, by SGR calculations, decreases overall reimbursement. The conclusion is that if an audiologist performs the new procedure often and previously had no way to report it for reimbursement, that audiologist should do well. However, if the audiologist does not perform the new procedure, he or she may see the value of the current codes decrease somewhat. An overriding consideration is that new codes are necessary to reflect current, state-of-the-art patient care.

◆ ICD-9-CM Coding System

The diagnosis codes describing the outcomes of diagnostic evaluations come from the World Health Organization (WHO)'s *International Classification of Diseases* (9th ed., clinical modification; ICD-9-CM; 2006). This system has been in existence in one form or another since the 17th century. In its earliest period, it was known as the *London Bills of Mor-*

tality. In 1937, it became the *International List of Causes of Death*. Shortly after the United Nations was established, WHO adopted this coding system as an international classification of diseases. Although there have been updates and the submission of new diagnosis codes throughout the years, there have been no substantial changes among the code families for auditory symptoms, disorders, and audiologic findings since the early 1970s. In contrast to the CPT coding system, in which the audiologist must be very specific in the selection of CPT code, the ICD-9-CM coding system requires that the audiologist select the code that best fits the description of what was found as a result of a diagnostic evaluation. The audiologist encounters numerous circumstances where a diagnosis code that describes precisely the diagnostic findings does not exist. A classic example is the absence of a diagnosis code for degree of hearing loss (i.e., moderate sensorineural hearing loss).

> **Pitfall**
>
> • A patient is not allowed to be "normal" under the ICD-9 coding system. This system was developed on the assumption that anyone who was seen for health care services must have presenting symptoms and, therefore, the need for health care services (HHS, 2001b).

Similar to the CPT codes, the primary purpose of the ICD-9-CM coding system is to establish a uniform language of diagnoses that is common among all government officials, epidemiologists, third-party payers, and others. By virtue of this common language, this coding system also lends itself to statistical tracking of diseases and disorders and for standardized claims submissions for third-party payers.

The ICD-9-CM system is composed of three- to five-digit codes in which the first three digits represent the family of disorders, diagnoses, or symptoms, and the fourth and fifth digits increase the level of specificity for a more accurate diagnosis. For example, 389 is the family of hearing loss. Codes in the 389.1 family represent sensorineural hearing loss: 389.10 is "sensorineural hearing loss, unspecified"; 389.11 is "sensory hearing loss, bilateral"; 389.12 is "neural hearing loss, bilateral," and so on. Medicare has set forth a standard that one must code to the highest level of specificity (HHS, 2003). Therefore, if five digits are available to describe what was found diagnostically, the audiologist must use all five digits, or the claim will be rejected. Many private third-party payers have adopted the Medicare guidelines and require the highest level of specificity to process the claim.

How to select a diagnosis code for normal outcomes has been a source of tremendous frustration. Historically, audiologists have exercised options ranging from a "V" code found in the ICD-9-CM manual, selecting 389.9 (hearing loss, unspecified), to selecting a code representing a symptom. Medicine established a precedent years ago by selecting the family of codes that represented why the patient was seen and what was done (i.e., 389: hearing loss) and adding the ".9" suffix for "unspecified" (i.e., 389.9: hearing loss, unspecified). Numerous audiologists have expressed discomfort with this practice because of the perceived implication of hearing impairment when none existed.

In 2001, Medicare published a bulletin providing guidance to this vexing problem (U.S. Department of Health and Human Services [HHS], Centers for Medicare and Medicaid Services, 2001b). This bulletin, Transmittal AB-01-144, discusses the generalities of using the ICD-9-CM coding system and provides several examples focusing on what was found relative to what was done. Of particular importance, this bulletin provides guidance on code selection when the diagnostic outcome is normal.

Providing audiology examples that parallel the examples found in the bulletin: A patient with a presenting symptom of tinnitus is referred for an audiologic evaluation, and the audiologist affirms the presence of hearing impairment. Because hearing impairment was found, the primary diagnosis should be from the family of hearing loss codes. A secondary diagnosis could be the reason for referral, which, in this case, is the ICD-9-CM code corresponding to tinnitus. What happens, though, if the patient is referred for an audiologic evaluation with the presenting complaint of tinnitus, and the audiogram is consistent with normal auditory function? In this instance, the reason for referral, tinnitus, becomes the primary diagnosis. In a similar manner, if a patient is referred for an audiogram due to complaints of hearing loss, and the test results are consistent with hearing loss, the diagnosis code is selected from the 389 family of ICD-9-CM codes. However, if the patient is referred for an audiogram due to complaints of hearing loss, and the test results are consistent with normal hearing sensitivity, the diagnosis is still from the 389 family of ICD-9-CM codes. In this example, hearing loss was the presenting symptom.

Pearl

- The presenting symptom becomes the primary diagnosis when a diagnostic test is performed with normal outcomes on the basis that the presenting symptom was the reason for the test.

Within the 389 family of codes, 389.9 could be an appropriate diagnosis code because no particular information regarding type of hearing loss (conductive, sensory, or neural) is indicated by the audiometric test outcomes. Specifically, Medicare Bulletin AB-01-144 offers the following guidance: "If the diagnostic test did not provide a diagnosis or was normal, the interpreting physician should code the sign(s) or symptom(s) that prompted the treating physician to order the study" (HHS, 2001b, p. 2). This guidance is consistent with two key aspects of diagnoses coding. First, one assumes that if a patient seeks medical care, an abnormal condition, real or perceived, has influenced that patient to seek care. Second, if abnormal findings are found, the primary diagnosis code must match who you are, what you did, and what you found.

◆ ICD-9-CM V-Codes

The ICD-9-CM manual contains an additional chapter of supplementary codes that are alphanumeric (a letter combined with numbers) such as V72.19. Except under prearranged or special circumstances, these codes should not be used for reporting diagnostic procedures that were performed on the basis of medical necessity. This supplemental family of codes focuses on occasions and circumstances other than disease or injury (ICD-9-CM, 2006). Examples include a person who is not ill but seeks health care services; a person with known disease or injury seeks specific treatment or services for that disease or injury (e.g., cast change); a problem or circumstance arises that influences the person's health status but is not the current disease of concern (e.g., family history of cancer). In the third case, another example could include a patient who seeks follow-up medical care for high blood pressure and, while in the physician's office, desires a hearing test. V72.19 would be an appropriate code to report the hearing test to document the service rendered but also to convey that the service was not medically necessary relative to the primary reason for the patient's visit. In this example, there were no signs or symptoms to justify the audiologic evaluation.

Special Consideration

- Because virtually all of health care relies on the concept of medical necessity to justify the delivery of services, V72.19 generally is not a reimbursable code. For that reason, use of V72.19 and similar codes is not recommended with the exception of prior arrangements or a specific purpose as designated by the third-party payer.

For example, the state of Florida requires the use of V72.19 as the diagnosis code for all Medicaid-eligible babies who are tested under the state-mandated universal newborn hearing screening program. In this instance, the code identifies that child as a universal newborn screening baby, for which reimbursement within the state's Medicaid system is processed differently than reimbursement requests for older children and adults.

The ICD-9-CM V-codes are not to be confused with a different system coding under the CMS system, HCPCS, which also uses "V" codes. The HCPCS coding system was developed to meet the needs of Medicare and Medicaid. Within this system there are now two levels of codes. Level I HCPCS codes are the AMA CPT codes. Level II HCPCS codes focus on audiology procedures and are dominated by hearing aid and hearing aid procedure codes. Although these codes originated within CMS, the Department of Veterans Affairs (VA) has exerted significant influence in the development of new level II codes for additional designators for hearing aids, earmolds, and various types of repairs and services. Medicaid programs in states that offer hearing services are the main users of level II HCPCS. This system of reporting hearing aid–related procedures and equipment has also been adopted by the VA, the military, and an increasing number of third-party payers who offer some form of hearing aid coverage. Level III codes were developed by state and local Medicaid offices for hearing aid reporting but no longer exist because of HIPAA's requirements to use only nationally available code sets.

◆ The Influence of the Health Insurance Portability and Accountability Act

Besides addressing insurance portability or patient confidentiality, HIPAA focuses on national standards intended for electronic transactions of health care claims and electronic medical records. The HIPAA guidelines have impacted all aspects of health care in two ways: identification of required code sets and national professional identifiers (AMA, 2007c, 45 CFR 162.103, 45 CFR 162.1000).

The final rule dealing with code sets was issued in 2000 and specified that the CPT coding system would be the primary identifiers to describe all health care procedures (45 CFR 1002). This includes not only the CPT codes but also all the modifiers (i.e., "–52," "–53," and "–76") described above. It is important to note that these modifiers describe deviations from the standard provision of services or procedures due to specific circumstances and also serve to clarify that the procedure has not changed in definition or description despite the deviation from the standard.

HIPAA also designated the HCPCS code set for the following categories:

- ◆ Physician services
- ◆ Physical therapy and occupational therapy services
- ◆ Radiological procedures
- ◆ Clinical laboratory procedures
- ◆ Other medical diagnostic procedures
- ◆ Hearing and vision services
- ◆ Transportation services, including ambulance

In addition to use of the CPT coding system (level I HCPCS) and nationally available level II HCPCS, HIPAA designated the ICD-9-CM diagnosis coding system to describe the outcomes of diagnostic evaluations and patient status.

◆ Documentation

An extremely important element of coding is the supporting documentation. In the event of an audit or medicolegal action, the documentation justifies why the patient was seen and describes what was done, what was found, and what was recommended. Together these components of documentation support the respective selections of procedure and diagnosis codes. Including signature and service date, there are a minimum of six elements that must be included to comprise appropriate documentation (HHS, 1997). These requirements were initially developed for physicians using evaluation and management (office visit) codes. However, the documentation requirements are being applied universally to all health care providers to comply with all interpretations of the "medical necessity" requirement for patient visits.

History

The history section of a report must document why the patient is present. This should include the chief complaints, signs and symptoms, pertinent medical history, pertinent social history, pertinent family history, and the origin of the referral. The history section of the report should be sufficient to justify the medical necessity of the patient visit and to justify the procedures that were performed.

Procedures Performed

This portion of the report should document the procedures that were executed and the diagnostic outcomes for each individual procedure. The detail should be sufficient to include indications of outcome reliability, special circumstances, and noteworthy information that may influence the interpretation of the test results.

Clinical Assessment

This section of the report is an interpretation of the findings. Sufficient detail and discussion should be included such that the unfamiliar reader may understand not only what was found but also why it is important to the overall well-being of the patient.

Recommendations

This section should be a logical flow from the previous three sections and should contain specific recommendations for follow-up, referral, discharge, or a plan of care. The recommendations are influenced jointly by the history, the diagnostic outcomes, and the interpretation or clinical assessment.

The combination of all four sections of the report should permit an unfamiliar, naive reader to understand why the patient was present, why the audiologist performed the selected procedures, the significance of what was found, and the logical recommendations derived from the preceding three sections. In addition to the evaluation itself, all recommendations must be based on the principle of medical necessity (HHS, 1997; 2006f). Under this principle, it is no longer acceptable for an audiologist to bring the patient back for a routine follow-up audiogram or diagnostic testing without a change (real or perceived) in symptoms or condition. Exceptions to this could include conditions or etiologies for which a high probability exists that a change in auditory or balance status will occur. However, if a patient returns because the patient desires an annual follow-up audiogram or returns because the audiologist desires to recheck the individual, Medicare, Medicaid, and many third-party payers should not be billed for the services rendered. The patient must be notified that the services are not medically necessary and not covered for insurance payment unless the patient's policy permits such follow-up services and billing.

In addition to the narrative contained in each section as described above, each report must have an original signature and date, which must be the date of test or service delivery. Some hospitals or health care organizations allow for two additional dates: the date of dictation and the date of signing. These two dates are optional, but the date of service is obligatory. The electronic signature found within an electronic medical record system is acceptable in lieu of a handwritten signature on the basis that no one should be able to access that medical record except the health care provider identified in the report (HHS, 1997; 2001a).

In general, it is not acceptable to let the audiogram stand as the primary document for the report. This form of documentation is unacceptable because it violates the medical necessity principles of justifying why the patient was present and a narrative description of the procedures that were performed.

If errors are made in the chart notes or the formal report, do not remove and destroy the report if it was finalized and placed in the patient's chart. If a single-word error was discovered, generally a pen-and-ink correction is acceptable by drawing a single line through the incorrect word, writing the correct word, and placing the initials of the person making the correction adjacent to the sentence. If pieces of information are incorrect or information was discovered that changes the interpretation and recommendations, the audiologist should prepare an addendum report that is dated for the date that the report is prepared and place it in the patient's chart. The addendum must specify which elements of the previous report are incorrect and what the correct information should be. It is extremely important that the original report not be destroyed, rewritten, or replaced. Obviously, the moral of the story is to "get it right" the first time. However, errors will occur. When they do occur, they should be acknowledged and corrected in a manner that does not suggest malicious intent or cover-up (HHS, 2001a; 45 CFR 482.24 (c)).

Some special considerations exist for electronic medical records (EMRs). Because of HIPAA security requirements, the only individual authorized to log in and enter information under a provider's name is that provider. The computer assumes that the individual logging in to the EMR system is the owner of the user name and password and no one else. Another security feature focuses on the electronic signature. Each electronic signature identifies only one individual making an entry and is associated strictly with the provider that logged into the system.

EMRs also pose new considerations if errors are made. Because the medical record entry cannot be altered once the clinician closes the patient's medical record entry, the procedures described above for issuing corrections would be most difficult. If errors are discovered in the EMR, the provider must make a new entry into the patient's record identifying the error and offering the corrected information. Similar to a paper chart, discovery of information that changes the clinician's clinical assessment, interpretation of the test results, and recommendations essentially requires a new report/addendum referencing the original report and providing the corrected information.

There may also be occasions when the patient requests changes or amendments to the record. Under HIPAA, patients' requests do not automatically give them the right to remove or change information in their medical charts. The patient must petition the health care provider in writing with regard to the desired changes and an explanation for the rationale for the changes. The audiologist has the right to accept the request if incorrect information is in the record or deny the change request if the documentation is accurate and complete. Either decision requires independent documentation in the patient's chart and should include the specifics of the patient's request, the rationale on the part of the patient, whether the health care provider accepted or rejected the patient's request, and the rationale for doing so. A written denial must be forwarded to the patient explaining in plain language the reason for the denial. Conversely, if the request for amendment is accepted, the patient must be notified of such change in addition to any "business associates" as defined by HIPAA who may have received the original documentation (45 CFR 164.526).

◆ National Provider Identification

As part of the national standards requirements for code sets, HIPAA also required providers to adopt a single, unique national provider identifier (NPI) to supplant all other provider identification numbers (e.g., Medicare, Medicaid, Blue Cross/Blue Shield, Aetna, Humana, etc.) (NUCC, 2006; HHS, 2007c). This single identifier is specific to individual health care providers, identifying them professionally (e.g., audiologist) and personally (name, address, telephone number, etc.). It is an ongoing effort to simplify the designation process for individual providers, health care systems, employers, and payers of health care services.

Prior to the implementation of this HIPAA requirement, health care providers had identification numbers assigned by health plans for different business functions. At times, the provider numbers represented the actual health care provider. However, in other cases, the provider numbers represented the health care provider's employer, service locations, corporate headquarters, specialties, pay-to arrangements, or contracts. Under HIPAA, the designator and purpose of an identifying number must be standardized across all payers and facilities. As a result, each health care provider is assigned a unique alphanumeric descriptor that belongs to no one else.

The final rule, published in 2004 (HHS, 2004), describes the NPI as a 10 character alphanumeric identifier that is unique to each health care provider. Similar to a Social Security number, a provider's NPI number is assigned for life and cannot be used by another health care provider or other entity. The number is deactivated only upon the death of the provider. The only other allowance for deactivation and reapplication for the NPI is in the case of fraudulent use by another health care provider. In that instance, the affected health care provider may apply for a new NPI and request deactivation of the original identifier. The NPI continues with the provider regardless of the location, employment situation, or work status. There is a requirement to inform the National Provider System of address or employment changes within 30 calendar days.

Facilities such as hospitals, clinics, and group practices must also apply for an NPI. Similar to the individual NPI, the designator is unique to that facility and will remain in effect for as long as that facility exists. Changes in ownership, address, or even relocation to another state will not necessitate deactivation and reapplication for a new NPI. However, the file maintained at HHS must be updated within 30 days following a change in status. The only circumstance under which a facility NPI could be deactivated is the disbanding or dissolution of the entity.

A common question is Who is required to obtain an NPI? The answer, as a general rule, is any health care provider (individual, group, or facility) who transmits any health information in electronic form in connection with the provision of health care services. The formal definition in the NPI regulations includes a provider of medical or health services and any other person or organization who furnishes, bills, or is paid for health care in the normal course of business. Such a health care provider has been designated as a "covered entity." The provision of health care is defined in statute 42 CFR 160.103 as including but not limited to preventive, diagnostic, therapeutic, rehabilitative, maintenance, or palliative care, and counseling, service, assessment, or procedures with respect to the physical or mental condition, or functional status, of an individual or that affects the structure or function of the body. It also includes sale or dispensing of a drug, device, equipment, or other item in accordance with a prescription.

The NPI is designed to facilitate all types of electronic transactions involving health care. A list of NPI applications includes the following:

- Health care plans may use NPIs in their internal health care provider files to process transactions and communication with health care providers.

- Health care providers may use their own unique NPIs to identify themselves in nonstandard health care transactions and on related correspondence.

- Health care providers may use other health care providers' NPIs to identify those other health care providers in health care transactions and on related correspondence.

- The NPI may be used as a cross-reference in health care provider fraud and abuse files and other program integrity files.

- The NPI may be used to identify health care providers for debt collection under the provisions of the Debt Collection Improvement Act of 1996 (Pub. L. 104–134, enacted on April 26, 1996) and the Balanced Budget Act of 1997 (Pub. L. 105–33, enacted on August 5, 1997).

- Health plans may communicate NPIs to other health plans for coordination of benefits.

- Health care clearinghouses may use NPIs in their internal files to create and process standard transactions and in communication with health care providers and health plans.

- NPIs may be used to identify health care providers in patient medical records.

- NPIs may be used to identify health care providers that are health care card issuers on health care identification cards.

♦ Provider Classification System

The Health Care Provider Taxonomy Code List (NUCC, 2006) is a nonmedical listing of health care professions, specialty areas, and supply/equipment providers. This code series has 10-character alphanumeric identifiers similar to the NPI, but these identifiers are unique to each health care discipline or area of specialization. The code "hierarchy" is broken down into three distinct levels: provider type, classification, and area of specialization.

Level I, provider type, is a major grouping of services or occupations of health care providers. Examples include internal medicine, otolaryngology, and speech, language, and hearing service providers.

Level II, classification codes, defines a more specific service or occupation related to the provider type. For example, under internal medicine, one finds adolescent medicine, cardiovascular disease, gastroenterology, hematology, and sports medicine, to name a few. Under otolaryngology are listed facial plastic surgery, otology and neurotology, pediatric otolaryngology, and plastic surgery within the head and neck. And for speech, language, and hearing services providers, one finds audiologist and speech-language pathologist.

Level III codes represent area of specialization. At the time of this writing, this category is a work in progress. Within the realm of speech, language, and hearing services, the current level III codes include assistive technology practitioner, assistive technology supplier, audiology assistant, and speech-language pathology assistant. In the Provider Taxonomy Code List, however, many of the level III codes are not yet defined to describe the scope of activities. Until definitions are in place, the practical usefulness of level III codes will be limited. **Table 16–1** gives examples of the taxonomy listing for speech, language, and hearing services.

♦ General Coding and Reimbursement Guidelines

One Procedure, One Code

The first and most important guideline for procedure (CPT) code selection is One procedure, one code (AMA, 2006a). The temptation can be great at times to perform one procedure and attempt to describe it for billing purposes using two or three different codes. A variation of this theme is to perform one complete procedure and, in essence, include a "screening sample" of other procedures and bill multiple codes. In this context, a "screening sample" refers to a very small portion or percentage (timewise) of another procedure

Table 16–1 Health Care Provider Taxonomy of Descriptors for Provider Type, Classification, and Area of Specialization

Code Type: Level I Provider Type
Speech, Language, and Hearing Providers
A provider who renders services to improve communicative skills of people with language, speech, and hearing impairment.

Code 231H00000X
Type: Level II Classification
Audiologist
(1) A specialist in evaluation, habilitation, and rehabilitation of those whose communication disorders center in whole or in part in hearing function. Audiologists are autonomous professionals who identify, assess, and manage disorders of the auditory, balance and other neural systems. Audiologists provide audiological (aural) rehabilitation to children and adults across the entire age span. Audiologists select, fit, and dispense amplification systems such as hearing aids and related devices. (2) An audiologist is a person qualified by a master's degree in audiology, licensed by the state, where applicable, and practicing within the scope of that license. Audiologists evaluate and treat patients with impaired hearing. They plan, direct, and conduct rehabilitative programs with auditory substitutional devices (hearing aids) and other therapy.

Code: 231HA2400X
Type: Level III Area of Specialization
Assistive Technology Practitioner
Code: 231HA2500X
Type: Level III Area of Specialization
Assistive Technology Supplier

Code: 237600000X
Type: Level II Classification
Audiologist/Hearing Aid Fitter
An audiologist/hearing aid fitter is the professional who specializes in evaluating and treating people with hearing loss, conducts a wide variety of tests to determine the exact nature of an individual's hearing problem, presents a variety of treatment options to patients, dispenses and fits hearing aids, administers tests of balance to evaluate dizziness, and provides hearing rehabilitation training. This classification should be used where individuals are licensed as "audiologist/hearing aid fitters" as opposed to states that license individuals as "audiologists."

Code: 2355A2700X
Type: Level III Area of Specialization
Audiology Assistant
Code: 2355S0801X
Type: Level III Area of Specialization
Speech-Language Assistant

Code: 235Z00000X
Type: Level II Classification
Speech-Language Pathologist
A speech pathologist is a person qualified by a master's degree in speech-language pathology, and where applicable, licensed by the state and practicing within the scope of the license. Also, known as speech therapist, a speech pathologist evaluates patients with language and speech impairments or disorders, whether arising from physiological and neurological disturbances, defective articulation or foreign dialects, and conducts remedial programs designed to restore or improve their communication efficacy. Speech pathologists assess and treat persons with speech, language, voice, and fluency disorders.

Source: http://codelists.wpc.edi.com.

that is insufficient to reveal any clinically useful information, but was just enough of the procedure to say technically that it was done. The trouble with these methods of reporting codes (multiple code reporting and screening samples) is that both violate the principles upon which the CPT codes were established.

Recall that each code has a complete descriptor of all procedure components included in the code. Completing only a portion of the procedure, too little to obtain clinical meaning or interpretation, does not constitute sufficient execution of the procedure to report it and be reimbursed for the service. It also violates the requirement of "medical necessity" that is central to all services provided. However, this does not refer to an abbreviated procedure whereby only part of the protocol was completed, or the clinician intentionally terminated the procedure before completion for the welfare of the patient. In each of those instances, sufficient information to derive a partial or preliminary clinical assessment must be obtained to report the code with a "–52" or "–53" suffix.

> **Pearl**
>
> • To bill a CPT code, the clinician must have performed enough of the procedure whereby the results, albeit incomplete, may contribute to the final diagnostic status of the patient. If the procedure was terminated before any clinically useful information could be obtained, the procedure is not reportable and would not meet the standards of an audit.

Unbundling

The second general principle is Do not unbundle a procedure for the sake of increasing reimbursement (HHS,

2005b). This tends not to be as much of a problem for audiologists as for other specialties. Audiology has one primary code family that could represent unbundling, 92557. If one examines the values of 92553 and 92556, the components of 92557, the reimbursement of these two codes individually is greater than for 92557. The reason is that each individual code has a certain proportion of fixed overhead built in that should only be taken into account once per date of service. Medicare does not allow a service that is considered part of the basic allowance of another procedure to be billed separately (HHS, 2006c). In this example, CPT codes 92553 and 92556 are both part of 92557 and should not be billed independently of 92557.

Correct Coding Initiative Edits

Correct coding initiative (CCI) edits were developed by CMS as a fail-safe measure to prohibit overbilling or duplicative billing (HHS, 2006d). The edits focus on certain procedures (CPT codes) for which it would be illogical or inappropriate to bill certain other CPT codes on the same date. The CMS computers for Medicare billing are programmed with these edits to prohibit payment should they occur. An example of an illogical CCI edit is the prohibition of reporting CPT code 92601 (diagnostic analysis of cochlear implant, patient under 7 years of age; with programming) on the same date as CPT code 92602 (diagnostic analysis of cochlear implant, patient under 7 years of age; subsequent reprogramming). Code 92601 is the initial programming of a cochlear implant for younger patients. The expectation is that the initial programming will occupy an entire session on that date of service. Therefore, it is not logical to have a complete session of initial programming followed by a complete session of subsequent reprogramming on the same date.

An example of duplicative billing is the prohibition of reporting CPT code 92601 with codes

- 92506: Evaluation of speech, language, voice, communication, and/or auditory processing

- 92507: Treatment of speech, language, voice, communication, and/or auditory processing disorder; individual

- 92552: Pure-tone audiometry (threshold; air only)

- 97755: Assistive technology assessment (e.g., to restore, augment, or compensate for existing function, optimize functional tasks, and/or maximize environmental accessibility), direct one-on-one contact by provider, with written report, each 15 minutes

Elements of each of these other procedures are contained in the definition of 92601 and represent duplicative billing if reported on the same date. The complete list of CCI edits may be found at www.cms.hhs.gov/NationalCorrectCodInitEd/.

Advance Beneficiary Notice

The advance beneficiary notice (ABN) is used to inform a patient that the services he or she is about to receive are likely not to be covered by Medicare (HHS, 2006a). The ABN means that the patient agrees to be personally responsible for payment and to pay personally, either out of pocket or through other insurance, for any or all of the services listed on the ABN document. The signature of the patient or authorized representative is required to ensure assumption of liability for payment. An unsigned ABN is insufficient to transfer personal liability for payment of services to the patient or the patient's representative. In addition to maintaining the signed ABN form in the patient's chart or medical record, the provider of the service should document separately that the patient signed an ABN and specify for which services.

In general, ABNs are necessary when the patient is about to receive services under one or more of the following categories:

- Services and items found not to be reasonable and necessary for the diagnosis or treatment of illness or injury or to improve the functioning of a malformed body member

- Services and items that, in the case of hospice care, are not reasonable and necessary for the palliation or management of terminal illness

- Services and items that constitute research on outcomes of health care services and procedures

- Other services that are provided in excess of the guidelines rendered by Medicare

Medicare no longer excludes sensorineural hearing loss as a sole diagnosis, even when the diagnosis eventually results in a hearing aid fitting, on the condition that the hearing loss has not been previously diagnosed or the patient returns with new signs, symptoms, or a change in status. However, Medicare has a statutory list of categorical denials (HHS, 2005c), which, for audiology, include hearing aids and hearing examinations that are performed for reasons not associated with new symptoms or change in status (e.g., routine annual recheck of hearing for monitoring purposes). Also included in this list are services provided under an audiologist's private contract with the patient, services that are paid for by a government entity that is not Medicare, health care received outside the United States that is not covered by Medicare, and services provided by immediate relatives. An ABN is not necessary when the service or item falls under the categorical denial listing.

Pitfall

- The ABN must be signed by the beneficiary or authorized representative *before* services are rendered and, in the case of audiologic services, before the person leaves the waiting room/reception desk area.

Once the individual is in the audiometric sound booth, one could potentially interpret that service has already begun. Moreover, the provider of services is prohibited from obtaining the beneficiary's signature on a blank ABN. It must be completed describing the services included in the ABN and the reasons why these services are likely to be denied payment by Medicare.

Copies of ABNs in English may be obtained at http://cms.hhs.gov/medicare/bni/CMSR131G_June2002.pdf. The Spanish version may be found at http://cms.hhs.gov/medicare/bni/CMSR131G_Spanish_June2002.pdf. A good reference with guidelines on use of the ABN and associated coding requirements can be found in Medicare Bulletin AB-02-168 on the CMS Web site (www.cms.hhs.gov).

When clinicians download copies of the Medicare ABN form, it is important that the forms not be altered in any manner. The specific language of the ABN has undergone administrative and regulatory review with regard to meaning and intent. Alteration or editing of the language contained within the ABN automatically voids its usefulness.

Notice of Exclusion from Medicare Benefits

Whereas the ABN is designed to inform a beneficiary that the services *may* not be covered for payment, the Notice of Exclusion from Medicare Benefits (NEMB; HHS, 2006b) informs the patient that the items or services will not be covered for Medicare payment. An example would be a patient who is self-referred, desires a complete audiometric evaluation for a previously diagnosed sensorineural hearing loss, has no new signs or symptoms, and has no desire to see the primary care physician. Another example would be a Medicare patient who is seen for an auditory rehabilitation session given by an audiologist. In the first situation, the standard of medical necessity is not met due to the prior diagnosis and the absence of new symptoms. In the second situation, Medicare does not pay for auditory rehabilitation rendered by an audiologist. NEMB allows the patient to make an informed decision whether to receive the items or services listed for which he or she will pay out-of-pocket and is intended to make the patient a more interactive consumer of health care services. The NEMB may be used, on an entirely voluntary basis, by physicians, practitioners, suppliers, and providers to advise their Medicare patients of the services that Medicare never covers, and for which it is not appropriate to use ABNs. The English NEMB (CMS form 20007) is available at http://cms.hhs.gov/medicare/bni/20007_English.pdf; the Spanish version is found at http://cms.hhs.gov/medicare/bni/20007_Spanish.pdf.

Setting Charge Levels for Services

The Code of Federal Regulations (CFR) addresses setting charge levels for services; 42 CFR Chapter IV, sections 405.501–504 discusses charges for Medicare in view of equitable charges rendered to others for the same service or item: "(c) *Application of criteria.* In applying these criteria, the carriers are to exercise judgment based on factual data on the charges made by physicians to patients generally and by other persons to the public in general and on special factors that may exist in individual cases so that determinations of reasonable charge are realistic and equitable" (42 CFR Chapter IV, section 405.502, paragraph (10)(c)). Section 405.501–503 also discuss customary charges and are generally interpreted as

meaning that health care providers must have a single charge for each service that is consistent at all times. It is not appropriate to vary the charges for a particular service from one patient to the next. Section 405.503 and 405.511 are interpreted to mean that the most a provider may charge is the least that the provider charges. For example, if a "free hearing test" is advertised, implying that the equivalent of CPT code 92557 will be rendered at no charge, the audiologist rightfully should not charge for 92557 for any third-party payer. Token charges for charity patients or less than standard charges for indigent or low-income patients are not to be taken into consideration when evaluating the equitability of charges across payers and conditions. In other words, a provider must have a designated charge for each service that is billed the majority of the time to all payers and under all conditions with the exception of charity, indigent, or low-income patients. This does not refer to how much is reimbursed, only what would be considered an appropriate and "customary" charge. The customary charge may vary from one provider to the next and is justifiable to do so based on each provider's costs of service delivery.

How an audiologist establishes charge levels for specific services has often been a less than exact science. There are times when charge levels were chosen based on estimates of what others in the community are charging. At other times, the audiologist established charge levels blindly without any firm knowledge regarding the basis of the charge. Ideally, the charge level for each service should be justifiable on the basis of service delivery costs—the audiologist's fixed overhead for providing each service whether it is based on time or volume. Most importantly, the selected charge level must be consistent across all payers and all conditions except those described above. Of importance is that this policy does not reflect reimbursement levels. If an audiologist charges $120 for a given procedure, $120 becomes the charge for self-pay patients and all third-party payers. Reimbursement for that procedure may vary from $30 to $120 according to contract negotiations or payer status, but the charge for the service must remain constant.

Establishing a reasonable and customary charge may be accomplished using several techniques. One method is to determine the cost per hour of delivering all services. This is also known as the cost per hour to keep the doors open. Annualized costs of rent (or mortgage), salaries, benefits, utilities, insurance, supplies, equipment, maintenance, administrative tools, computers, software, and debt servicing can be broken down into a cost per hour for what must be collected to break even. A percentage increment may be added to that under the heading of "profit" to establish a capital reserve, program replacement equipment, anticipated growth, and so on. The audiologist then calculates or projects the number of procedures performed over a given time period, the time duration or other associated costs of the procedure, and derives a cost per hour for each procedure or item. It is good to then examine this cost per procedure with the MPFS as a basis of comparison. It is not uncommon that the procedure charge will exceed the MPFS for a variety of reasons. Typically, the charge per procedure does not exceed 2 to $2\frac{1}{2}$ times the MPFS. Exceptions can be made if the MPFS grossly undervalues a particular CPT code or if the costs of performing that procedure are justifiably higher than the $2^1/_2$ multiplier factor. The fee that is established, however, must be uniformly applied to all third-party payers to be considered "reasonable and customary." Again, that does not imply anything about reimbursement levels, only charge levels. This information also serves to guide the audiologist in making decisions whether to participate in a third-party payer's network based on the direct overhead cost for each service.

Prior Authorization

It is good practice to obtain a prior authorization for services rendered at the time the appointment is made. For many insurance and HMO systems, it is not sufficient to have a physician's prescription or written referral. Most often, this does not constitute authorization to see the patient, bill the third-party payer, and be reimbursed. As a matter of routine procedure, complete insurance information should be obtained from each patient, including Medicare patients, at the time he or she calls for an appointment. The information should include the patient's provider of insurance (typically the company he or she is employed by); the name, address, and contact telephone number listed on the patient's insurance card; the group number; the patient's identification number (also found on the insurance card) and date of birth; and the effective date of coverage. If there is a plan number on the insurance card, that should also be recorded. The insurance company or HMO will need this information to identify the patient and determine scope of coverage. It will be necessary to inform the company which CPT codes one expects to use and the anticipated diagnosis (ICD-9-CM code). The authorization to perform those services and the ability to bill the insurance company will depend in many cases on approval of the CPT codes that are provided. It is for this reason that the chief complaint(s) and/or presenting concerns are recorded at the time of the appointment.

If authorization is obtained for a particular list of procedure codes, but the audiologist discovers that he or she needs to do a more extensive evaluation as a result of the detailed case history or the outcomes of the testing performed thus far, it is often not appropriate to proceed without obtaining additional authorization for the expanded list of procedures. This can be handled by having an administrative assistant call the company for authorization while the patient waits, or schedule a follow-up visit while securing authorization before the patient returns.

The audiologist has grounds for an appeal for denied payment if authorized procedures were performed and billed to the insurance company or HMO accordingly. Insurance companies and HMOs have adopted the CMS philosophy of "medically necessary and reasonable" as the criterion for determining eligibility for payment. If payment is denied, it is the primary responsibility of the audiologist to affirm that what was done was both reasonable and medically necessary. The documentation once again becomes a critical factor in the entire process. As specified above, the justification for medical necessity will be contained in the history portion of the report, citing the primary symptoms or presenting complaints, and a complete history to describe the evolution of the signs and symptoms. The description of activities should consist of procedures selected on the basis of the signs, symptoms, and history and should have a specific reason for being included in the evaluation battery. Examples of such reasons include site of lesion investigation, standard of care for those signs and symptoms, and unexpected outcomes of other tests that require further investigation to assist the referring physician in deriving a diagnosis. Tests should not be performed simply because that was the battery that is used for each person. There should be a reason and justification for each procedure.

Audits

Medicare, Medicaid, and each private insurer/HMO have the right to inspect an audiologist's records to ensure that proper payment was made for medically necessary procedures. They have the right to conduct short notice, or even no notice, inspections of office facilities and the medical records of the patients that are covered under their respective plans. They do not have the right to look at the records of patients who are covered by other insurers, only their own. In particular, auditors will be examining the records for evidence of referrals (if referrals are required), documentation of medical necessity, a complete description of procedures, a clinical interpretation of the findings, and logical recommendations that were developed based on the combined factors of history, diagnostic outcomes, and clinical interpretations. The documentation must also contain assurances that the professional under whose name the billing went out was actually the one to see the patient. This does not rule out the role of the assistant except for payers that prohibit the use of assistants (e.g., Medicare). Both Medicare and Medicaid permit students to participate in the diagnostic process but require the licensed, supervising audiologist to have contact with the patient during the evaluation. Chapter 5, Part B of the *Medicare Claims Processing Manual* (HHS, 2005a) addresses the issue of student participation and specifies significant restraints upon students' ability to function independently. In a clarification letter to ASHA dated November 9, 2001, a senior Medicare administrator affirmed that those restrictions extend to audiology students (T. Kay, letter to ASHA, November 9, 2001). For Medicare patients, the licensed, supervising audiologist must maintain line-of-sight supervision of the student during the evaluation, must actively participate in all aspects of patient care, and must not care for another patient at the same time. The Medicaid standard is somewhat less strict and requires the supervising audiologist to see the patient at the beginning of and periodically throughout the evaluation process and have continued involvement through the period of care of that patient. The auditor will be looking for agreement with what was documented and the codes that were billed. He or she will want to see that only one CPT code was reported for each respective procedure, that the diagnosis code is justifiable based on the diagnostic outcomes, and that the individual responsible for billing was directly involved with the patient.

If violations are found in the form of insufficient documentation or inappropriate billing, each payer has the right to request repayment of overcharges (HHS, 2001a). Moreover, if the pattern of perceived overcharge appears to be intentional and pervasive, the third-party payer may add sanctions and fines to the request for repayment of overcharges.

The moral of the story is that the clinician should have authorization to perform the procedures when authorization is required; complete documentation such that someone from the outside may come in, read a report, and have a very good understanding of why specific procedures were done; and have assurances that all services performed were reasonable and medically necessary.

♦ Summary

The topic of coding and reimbursement is not of tremendous continuing educational interest to many individuals, but it is the lifeblood of what audiologists as health care professionals do in their everyday professional lives. A significant number of problems with reimbursement are attributable to inappropriate coding or inadequate supporting documentation. As the profession of audiology continues its journey into professional adulthood, learning and living by the rules of the larger health care community will be essential for professional acceptance, opportunities to contribute additional coding changes, and participation in reimbursement policy discussions. Learning and abiding by the rules of coding and documentation constitute a major first step toward professional maturity and acceptance.

Audiology has been given a voice in the coding process to establish new codes and to provide input for CMS valuation. Fourteen new procedure codes have been added to the audiology family since 1995, and three CPT codes have undergone editorial revision. The purpose of this chapter has been to provide foundational information regarding the process of developing and valuing CPT codes, appropriate use and selection of both CPT and ICD-9-CM codes, and the influence of various agencies, including HIPAA, Congress, CMS, and the AMA.

References

American Medical Association. (1990–2006). CPT assistant (16 vols.). Chicago: AMA Press.

American Medical Association. (2003). AMA/Specialty Society RVS update process: Structure and function of the RUC. Chicago: AMA Press.

American Medical Association. (2005). RVS update process. Chicago: AMA Press.

American Medical Association. (2006a). Current Procedural Terminology: CPT 2006. Chicago: AMA Press.

American Medical Association. (2006b). CPT changes: An insider's view. Chicago: AMA Press.

American Medical Association. (2006c). CPT process: How a code becomes a code. Retrieved May 16, 2006, from http://www.ama-assn.org/ama/pub/category/3882.html

American Medical Association. (2006d). RVS Updating Committee and members. Retrieved May 20, 2007, from http://www.ama-assn.org/ama/pub/category/3108.html

American Medical Association. (2007a). History of the RBRVS and the RUC. Retrieved May 20, 2007, from http://www.ama-assn.org/ama/pub/category/10559.html

American Medical Association. (2007c). RVS survey process: Instructions for specialty societies developing recommendations. Retrieved May 20, 2007, from http://www.ama-assn.org/ama/pub/category/3150.html

Code of Federal Regulations. 42 CFR 405.501–511. (2001). Retrieved May 16, 2006, from http://a257.g.akamaitech.net/7/257/2422/12feb20041500/edocket. access.gpo.gov/cfr_2004/octqtr/42cfr405.511.htm

Code of Federal Regulations. 45 CFR 164.526. (2002). Retrieved February 18, 2006, from http://www.access.gpo.gov/nara/cfr/waisidx_02/45cfr164_02.html

Code of Federal Regulations. 42 CFR 482.24(c). (2004). Retrieved March 20, 2006, from http://a257.g.akamaitech.net/7/257/2422/14mar20010800/edocket.access.gpo.gov/cfr_2002/octqtr/42cfr405.502.htm

Code of Federal Regulations. 45 CFR 162.103. (2007). Retrieved May 20, 2007, from http://a257.g.akamaitech.net/7/257/2422/05dec20031700/edocket. access.gpo.gov/cfr_2003/octqtr/pdf/45cfr162.103.pdf

Code of Federal Regulations. 45 CFR 162.1000. (2007). Retrieved May 20, 2007, from http://www.access.gpo.gov/nara/cfr/waisidx_03/ 45cfr162_03.html

Code of Federal Regolations, 45 CFR 162.1002. (2007). Retrived May 20, 2007, from http://www.access.gpo.gov/nara/cfr/waisidx 03/45cfr162_03.html

Hoffman, E.D. Jr., Klees, B.S., Curtis, C.A. (2006). Brief summaries of Medicare and Medicaid Title XIII and Title XIX of the Social Security Act. Center for Medicare and Medicaid Services (pp. 1–26). Baltimore, Maryland.

Hsiao, W.J., Braun, P., Dunn, D. Becker, E.R., DeNicola, M., Ketcham, T.R. (1988). Results and policy implications of the Resource-Based Relative-Value Study. N Engl J Med. 318:881–888.

Hsiao, W.J., Braun, P., Yntema, D., Becker, E.R. (1988). Estimating physicians' work for a resource-based relative-value scale. N Engl J Med. 319:835–841.

International Classification of Diseases (9th ed., clinical modification). (2006). Salt Lake City: Medicode.

Markovich, M. (2003). The rise of HMOs. Ph.D. dissertation, RAND Graduate School. Santa Monica, CA.

McGinley, P. J. (1995). Beyond health care reform: Reconsidering certificate of need laws in a managed competition system. Florida State University Law Review, 23, 1–46.

National Uniform Claim Committee. (2007). NPI codes. Retrieved May 20, 2007, from http://www.nucc.org

Office of the Assistant Secretary for Planning and Evaluation, U.S. Department of Health and Human Services. (2005). Effects of health care spending on the U.S. economy. Retrieved June 15, 2005, from http://aspe.hhs.gov/health/costgrowth

Rakich, J. S., Longest, B. B., & Darr, K. (1992). The health care delivery system. In K. Darr, B. B. Longest, & J. Rakich (Eds.), Managing health services organizations (3rd ed.). Baltimore: Health Professions Press.

Social Security Administration. (2006). History of SSA during the Johnson administration, 1963–1968. Retrieved May 15, 2006, from http://www.ssa.gov/history/ssa/lbjmedicare1.html

Social Security Online. (2006). Legislative history: Social Security Act of 1935. Retrieved May 15, 2006, from http://www.ssa.gov/history/35actpre. html

Social Security Administration (2007b). Status of the Social Security and Medicare programs. A summary of the 2007 annual reports. Retrived May 19, 2007, from www.ssa.gov/OACT/TRSUM/trsummary.html

United States Code. 42 U.S.C. 1395y Section 1862(a)(1)(A). Retrieved May 16, 2006, from http://www.ssa.gov/OP_Home/ssact/title18/1862. htm

U.S. Department of Health and Human Services, Centers for Medicare and Medicaid Services. (1997). Documentation guidelines for evaluation and management services. Retrieved March 15, 2006, from http://www. cms.hhs.gov/MLNProducts/Downloads/MASTER1.pdf

U.S. Department of Health and Human Services, Centers for Medicare and Medicaid Services. (2001a). Peer review organization manual: Transmittal 86. Retrieved March 16, 2006, from http://www.cms.hhs.gov/transmittals/downloads/r86pi.pdf

U.S. Department of Health and Human Services, Centers for Medicare and Medicaid Services. (2001b). Program memorandum intermediaries/carriers: Transmittal AB-01-144, September 26, 2001. Retrieved March 30, 2006, from http://www.cms.hhs.gov/Transmittals/downloads/AB01144.pdf

U.S. Department of Health and Humarn Services, Centers for Medicare and Medicaid Services. (2002). Program memorandum intermediaries/carriers: Transmittal AB-02-168, November 22, 2002, Retrieved March 30, 2006, from http://www.cms.hhs.gov/Transmittals/downloads/AB02168.pdf

U.S. Department of Health and Human Services, Centers for Medicare and Medicaid Services. (2003). Program memorandum intermediaries/carriers: Transmittal B-03-028, April 18, 2003. Retrieved March 30, 2006, from http://www.cms.hhs.gov/Transmittals/downloads/AB03028.pdf

U.S. Department of Health and Human Services, Centers for Medicare and Medicaid Services. (2004). HIPAA Administrative Simplification: Standard Unique Health Identifier for Health Care Providers. Federal Register. 69(15), 3434–3469.

U.S. Department of Health and Human Services, Centers for Medicare and Medicaid Services. (2005a). Medicare claims processing manual: Outpatient rehabilitation and CORF services (ch. 5, part B). Washington, DC: U.S. Government Printing Office.

U.S. Department of Health and Human Services, Centers for Medicare and Medicaid Services. (2005b). Medicare claims processing manual: Physicians/non-physician practitioners (ch. 12). Washington, DC: U.S. Government Printing Office.

U.S. Department of Health and Human Services, Centers for Medicare and Medicaid Services. (2005c). Medicare claims processing manual: Financial liability protections (ch. 30). Washington, DC: U.S. Government Printing Office.

U.S. Department of Health and Human Services, Centers for Medicare and Medicaid Services. (2006). The Medicare medical review program. Retrived May 20, 2007, from http://www.cms.hhs.goy/MLNProducts/downloads/MRFactSheetMay06.pdf

U.S. Department of Health and Human Services, Centers for Medicare and Medicaid Services. (2006a). FFS ABN-G and ABN-L. Retrieved May 16, 2006, from http://www.cms.hhs.gov/BNI/02_ABNGABNL.asp

U.S. Department of Health and Human Services, Centers for Medicare and Medicaid Services. (2006b). FFS NEMB. Retrieved May 16, 2006, from http://www.cms.hhs.gov/BNI/11_FFSNEMBGeneral.asp

U.S. Department of Health and Human Services, Centers for Medicare and Medicaid Services. (2006c). Medicaid Program General Information: Overview. Retrieved May 20, 2007, from http://www.cms.hhs.gov/MedicaidGenInfo/

U.S. Department of Health and Human Services, Centers for Medicare and Medicaid Services. (2006d). National Correct Coding Initiatives edits. Retrieved May 16, 2006, from http://www.cms.hhs.gov/NationalCorrectCodInitEd/01_overview.asp

U.S. Department of Health and Human Services, Centers for Medicare and Medicaid Services. (2006e). Understanding the remittance advice: A guide for Medicare providers, physicians, suppliers, and billers. Retrieved March 2, 2006, from http://www.cms.hhs.gov/medlearn

U.S. Department of Health and Human Services. Centers for Medicare and Medicaid Services. (2007a). Estimated sustainable growth rate and conversion factor. for Medicare payments to physicians in 2007. Retrieved May 20, 2007, from http://www.cms.hhs.gov/SustainableGRatesConFact/Downloads/sgr2007f.pdf

U.S. Department of Health and Human Services, Centers for Medicare and Medicaid Services. (2007b). HCPCS background information. Retrieved February 13, 2006, from http://www.cms.hhs.gov/MedHCPCSGenInfo/

U.S. Department of Health and Human Services, Centers for Medicare and Medicaid Services. (2007c). National provider identifier standard: Overview. Retrieved May 20, 2007, from http://www.cms.hhs.gov/NationalProvidentStand/

U.S. Government Accountability Office. (2007, February 15). Health care spending: Public payers face burden of entitlement program growth, while all payers face rising prices and increasing use of service. Retrieved May 20, 2007, from http://www.gao.gov/new.items/d07497t.pdf

U.S. Government Accountability Office. (2004, May 15). Medicare physician payments: Information on spending trends and targets. Retrieved June 15, 2005, from http://www.gao.gov/cgi-bin/getrpt?GAO-04-751T

U.S. Government Accountability Office. (2004, October 8). Medicare physician payments: Concerns about spending target system prompt interest in considering reforms. Retrieved May 16, 2006, from http://www.gao.gov/new.items/d0585.pdf

Chapter 17

Proposing Audiology Services to Group Providers

Kathy A. Foltner

Managed care organizations (MCOs) first emerged in limited regions of the United States in the late 1970s. At that time, health care focused primarily on treating disease and the acute care needs of the population, and health care costs were skyrocketing at rates greater than inflationary values. MCOs offered a new health care model that shifted the focus from treating disease and acute care needs to prevention, with a focus on wellness and health maintenance. In addition to shifting the focus of health care management, managed care was positioned as a possible cost-containing solution to the nation's rising health care costs. Pessis and Freint (2000) point out that managed care was structured "to limit access to health care and clamp down on spiraling costs." However, Managed Care On-line (MCOL, 2005a) reports average premium rate increases in 2005 for the various managed care health care products—health maintenance organizations (HMOs), preferred provider organizations (PPOs), point-of-service (POS) plans, and fee-for-service (FFS) plans—ranging from 8 to 15.2%. One could assume these average increases in health care premium rates correspond to continued increases in health care costs, which appear to far exceed inflationary values.

HMO enrollment grew slowly but steadily between 1985 and 1995. According to MCOL (2005a), "In 1985 there were approximately 20 million covered lives in HMOs, whereas in 1995 there were approximately 50 million covered lives." These data are consistent with an average growth in HMO enrollment in the United States of ~3 million covered lives per year between 1985 and 1995. HMO enrollment grew more rapidly after 1995 until it peaked at 80 million covered lives in 1999 (MCOL, 2005a). During that 4-year period, HMO enrollment increased by 30 million lives, or at an average rate of 7.5 million lives per year, over double the prior 10-year average increase in enrollment. However, following the peak in 1999, HMO enrollment began to decline and has declined each year since by just over an average of 2.2 million lives, reaching 68.8 million covered lives in 2004 (MCOL, 2005a). Although HMO enrollment has been declining since 1999, nearly 70 million lives continue to receive health care services through HMOs. In addition, another 109 million lives received health care services through PPOs, which further increased managed care penetration to 177.8 million covered lives in 2004 (MCOL, 2005a,b). This reported number of covered lives in the MCO system represents ~59% of the total population of the United States.

With the majority of the U.S. population participating in one of the managed care entities, it becomes increasingly more difficult for health care providers, including audiologists, to ignore MCOs. When deciding to participate or not with managed care entities, every audiologist must consider health care trends, professional autonomy, patient expectations, and the potential financial impact on the business.

♦ To Contract or Not with Managed Care and Other Third-Party Payers

Health Care Trends

As stated previously, managed care in the United States started in the late 1970s, and although enrollment has experienced a recent decline, MCOs are here to stay for the foreseeable future. It is becoming more and more difficult to find communities that have not been touched by MCOs. Even Medicare offers MCO options and incentives in the form of reduced costs or increased benefits for their beneficiaries in an attempt to shift traditional health care coverage to Medicare MCOs.

In November 2003, Congress passed the Medicare Modernization Act (MMA) of 2003. According to the Centers for Medicare and Medicaid Services (CMS 2005), "This law brings the most dramatic and innovative changes to the Medicare program since it began in 1965." An important concept to understand is the fact that the MMA "provides about $14 billion over 10 years in new federal funding to encourage private plans to participate in Medicare Advantage" (Williams, 2005). In essence Congress has approved funds that can be used by MCOs to encourage seniors to enroll in MCO health systems. Williams goes on to note that "the MMA renamed the Medicare+ Choice program the Medicare Advantage program and provided higher payments intended to stabilize and expand the Medicare private plan market." In this reference, the term *Medicare private plan market* actually refers to a managed care delivery system, not a traditional FFS health care model; therefore, it becomes clear the federal government is theoretically and financially supporting the MCO delivery system.

Goals for managed care have long included containing costs, improving benefits, and increasing plan participation and beneficiary enrollment in an effort to increase health care choices. Although traditional Medicare does not cover hearing tests completed for the purpose of fitting hearing aids or hearing aids, it does cover many auditory and vestibular services with a physician referral. In addition, a Medicare MCO might offer expanded care and include typically noncovered services or products, such as hearing aids, as an incentive for joining that MCO. This potential shift to Medicare MCOs could have a huge impact on the way hearing services and hearing aids are delivered in America.

Corporations with large established networks will have an edge in securing business from that Medicare segment of the population, especially if those covered by Medicare or other MCOs are contractually obligated or receive incentives to see those contracted providers for their hearing health care needs. MCO contracts can include financial incentives for their beneficiaries to obtain audiology services and hearing aids from a contracted or in-network provider, which means the beneficiaries' costs for services or products may be greater if they receive services outside of their contracted network. Reduced costs for services and products are a strong motivator for beneficiaries to seek services from within their contracted network. Therefore, being an in-network provider or part of the contracted network can be an important initial step in securing third-party business. However, it is the audiology provider's responsibility to understand both the benefits and the consequences of participating in any network or becoming an in-network provider.

Although a large population exists beyond those covered by Medicare, it is also a fact that many MCOs and traditional health insurers look to Medicare for their example. This can be both a benefit and a detriment for the field of audiology. It is a benefit in that Current Procedural Terminology (CPT) codes do exist for the majority of auditory and vestibular procedures, which provides credibility for those as legitimate health care procedures. This reliance on Medicare is also a detriment in that the documented reimbursement levels are bleak for most procedures within an audiologist's scope of practice, which can place the audiologist in a difficult negotiating position when it comes to establishing reasonable contracted reimbursement levels.

Another problem is that audiologists have not secured limited license practitioner status and therefore are not considered as physicians when it comes to Medicare reimbursement policy. Access to audiology procedures for Medicare beneficiaries still requires a written physician referral and sets a questionable precedent for accessing audiology care, because such physician referral is not in the best interests of patients seeking audiology services or of audiology providers. It is well documented that only 10 to 15% of those diagnosed with hearing loss require medical intervention from a physician, yet this current policy limits access to audiology care and increases costs unnecessarily by mandating every Medicare beneficiary first see a physician and receive a referral for a medically necessary hearing evaluation. It should be far more cost-effective for the health care system to allow patients direct access to audiology care and rely on audiologists' ability to diagnose hearing loss as stated in their scope of practice. Although the federal government has not yet embraced this premise for Medicare, not all private health insurers require physician referral as a requirement for reimbursement for auditory testing.

Professional Autonomy

Audiology made huge strides in the 1990s and early 2000s with the introduction, establishment, and acceptance of the doctor of audiology (Au.D.) degree. According to Susan Paarlberg, executive director of the Audiology Foundation of America, as of 2005, 2928 audiologists had earned their Au.D. degree. Another 1800 are expected to earn the degree through distance-learning programs by the end of 2009; most distance-learning programs are expected to be phased out by 2010. The number of residential Au.D. graduates is also on the rise, with an anticipated additional 2000 graduates by

Table 17–1 State Statutes and Rules Governing Licensure of Audiologists

State	Minimum Degree*	Effective Date
Ohio	Au.D.	1/1/06
Indiana	Au.D.	1/1/07
New Mexico	Au.D.	1/1/07
Oklahoma	Au.D.	1/1/07
Montana	Au.D.	1/1/07†
Alaska, Arkansas, Colorado, Connecticut, Florida, Georgia, Idaho, Illinois, Iowa, Kentucky, Louisiana, New Hampshire, Maryland, Michigan, Minnesota, Missouri, Nevada, Rhode Island, South Carolina, South Dakota, Tennessee, Utah, Vermont, Virginia, Washington, and Wisconsin	Master's degree or doctoral degree (Ph.D., Au.D., Sc.D., etc.) with clinical practice	
Alabama, Arizona, Delaware, California, Hawaii, Kansas, Maine, Massachusetts, Mississippi, Nebraska, New Jersey, New York, North Carolina, North Dakota, Oregon, Pennsylvania, Texas, West Virginia, and Wyoming	Master's degree with clinical practice	

* Minimum licensure standards for new career entrants. Those previously licensed are generally grandfathered under older standards.
† Rule revision pending, expected to be adopted during 2006.
Au.D., doctor of audiology; Ph.D., doctor of philosophy; Sc.D., doctor of science.
Source: Research completed January 2006 by Emily Yoder, law clerk, at Goldman & Rosen, Ltd., Akron, OH, Robert M. Gippin, Esq., supervising. Courtesy of Audiology Foundation of America.

2010. Currently, 68 universities offer Au.D. programs, but that number changes regularly and is down from a high of over 110 master's-level programs (S. Paarlberg, personal communication, September 15, 2005). Although these numbers are relatively small in comparison to other health care professions, the U.S. Department of Labor has determined that the job outlook for audiologists is expected to grow faster than the average for all occupations through 2012 (U.S. Department of Labor, 2005). This faster-than-average growth prediction is based on the aging population demographic and increasing incidence of hearing, vestibular, and neurological pathology associated with an aging population. The mandates for newborn infant screening programs in many states are cited as another reason for a positive job outlook for audiologists.

According to Barry Freeman, 49 states require licensure for the practice of audiology, and 1 state (Colorado) requires registration (B. Freeman, personal communication, September 12, 2005). State licensure laws are being rewritten to remove the obsolete requirement for certification, and several states include the Au.D. as the entry-level degree to practice the profession of audiology **(Table 17–1)**. The Audiology Foundation of America, the Academy of Doctors of Audiology (formerly the Academy of Dispensing Audiologists), and the American Academy of Audiology support the Au.D. as the entry-level degree and have collaborated in an effort to prepare a model licensure law. The fact that audiology is becoming designated as a doctoring profession that is now regulated in all 50 states and that those regulations define audiologists' scope of practice are important and positive steps not only for autonomy but also for third-party payer contracting and reimbursement.

Limited license practitioner status not only would allow direct access to audiology care for Medicare beneficiaries but also would set precedence for direct access for audiology care for other third-party payers. Currently, four groups

of professionals are classified as limited license practitioners: optometrists (O.D.), oral surgeons (D.D.S. or D.M.D.), chiropractors (D.C.), and podiatrists (D.P.M.). Although not physicians, Medicare considers these limited license practitioners as physicians when it determines access and reimbursement. Specifically, consumers can access these services without a referral from a physician, and limited license practitioners are reimbursed from Medicare based on their training, state license, and scope of practice as defined in their license.

Historically, the Hearing Health Accessibility Act (HR 2821) was first introduced in the House of Representatives in July 2003 with the Senate companion bill S-1647; however, the 108th Congress passed neither bill. The act was reintroduced as HR 415 in the House of Representatives in January 2005, with the Senate companion bill S-277 being introduced in February 2005. Direct access legislation remains an important and appropriate goal in the areas of access, reimbursement, and autonomy for the field of audiology. The passage of such legislation will set a positive precedent for direct access and reimbursement for audiology care for all third-party payers.

Patient Expectations

Unfortunately, *hearing health care* has become a generic term that includes the services of audiologists, ear, nose, and throat (ENT) physicians, hearing aid dispensers, hearing technicians, speech pathologists, and others. It is often difficult for the public to differentiate the services provided by these various professionals as unique and distinct from one another. Licensing laws that define scope of practice often overlap, which contributes to public confusion about the profession of audiology. In many states, although an audiologist must complete diagnostic hearing testing, it remains legal for technicians or nurses to complete hearing tests under the supervision of a physician. It is also legal for those licensed to sell hearing aids to complete hearing tests for that purpose. In essence, licensing laws do not provide a clear and distinct line regarding scope of practice between hearing professionals.

In addition to licensing regulations, marketing tactics have contributed to the public confusion associated with audiology care. It is not uncommon to see both audiologists with substantial educational credentials and hearing aid dispensers with far fewer credentials depicted in marketing pieces or newspaper advertisements dressed in white coats. Although quite different, to the consumer those professionals look the same. Another marketing tactic highlighted in an advertisement in the *Orlando* (Florida) *Sentinel* in 2005 included the introduction of an evaluation called "diagnostic audiobiologic testing." No CPT code exists for such a procedure, but the average consumer is not likely to understand CPT coding or procedural definitions. Such local attempts to attract consumers through supposedly innovative marketing have actually contributed to the confusion surrounding audiology care.

As a group of professionals, audiologists have not been consistent in their pursuit of autonomy or recognition. In many parts of the country, audiologists have followed the lead of hearing aid salespersons by offering free hearing tests rather than distinguishing audiology services as something distinct and with value for which payment is clearly justified. This marketing strategy has generated several conflicts for audiologists, including the following:

♦ Medicare does cover diagnostic hearing tests and will pay for air, bone, and speech audiometry under CPT code 92557 as long as the audiologist has a written referral from a physician. However, that same 92557 completed for the purpose of fitting hearing aids and without a written physician referral is not a covered benefit under the current Medicare system. This third-party reimbursement issue goes beyond direct access. Advertising a Medicare-covered service as free will withstand a Medicare audit only if the audiologist is not billing Medicare for that same service in other cases. In other words, audiologists should not bill Medicare for a covered service (i.e., 92557) in some cases and also give away that same service at no charge in other cases.

♦ By offering audiology services inconsistently at no charge, audiologists not only may be violating Medicare policy and other laws but at the same time are devaluing those audiology services. In addition, it is not appropriate to call a covered service by another name to usurp the Medicare regulations. CPT code 92557 is clearly defined as "comprehensive audiometry threshold evaluation and speech recognition 92553 and 92556 combined" (Medicode, 2001). If the completed tests look like an audiogram or records thresholds and speech testing results in some format, it will be considered a 92557 regardless of what it is labeled by the audiologist.

♦ Patients' experiences with audiologists should be clearly unique and distinct when compared with their experience with others who compete for those patients. A diagnostic evaluation must include a comprehensive health case history; otoscopic evaluation; complete audiometric assessment of the outer, middle, and inner ear; and patient counseling, which includes not only test results but also recommendations for treatment. The experience of audiology care must be separate and unique and not mimic that of any other hearing care provider. This becomes increasingly important with third-party payers. After all, why would any third-party payer, or individual, choose to pay for the same service that is offered for free?

Controversial Point

- All audiologists must recognize the value associated with the services they provide and consistently charge for those services.

Most patients desire quality audiology and vestibular care at a reasonable price. The same is true for third-party payers. In other words, the "value" of the services and products must be clearly identified and differentiated. Third-party payers will evaluate the costs associated with contracted audiology services, but rarely will a contract be secured based on cost or price alone. Just as most patients will judge the cost of services and products based on their value and perceived benefit, so too will third-party payers seek value. Quality of services and products, access, qualifications of providers, and ease and consistency of service are important variables for third-party payers when assessing value.

Pearl

- MCOs and other third-party payers want access, credentials, ease of administration, continuous quality monitoring, high value, and reasonable cost. Most third-party payers prefer turnkey operations where care is consistent across the service area.

Financial Impact

Some audiologists feel they cannot afford to participate with MCOs, whereas others maintain they cannot afford to not participate with MCOs. With nearly 60% of the U.S. population participating with MCOs for their health care, far more audiologists are choosing to participate than not. Whatever the decision, there is no doubt that an audiologist's decision regarding participation with any of the various group provider organizations will have a financial impact on the business. The luxury of a private pay caseload is long gone for most audiologists. The key is to balance one's caseload between private pay patients and the various third-party payers.

As a general rule, no one source of patients should represent more revenue generation than an audiologist is willing to lose. Why? Because third-party entities change ownership, discontinue member benefits, file bankruptcy, and cancel provider contracts with as little as 60 days' notice. Building a business based on referrals from one source or with one third-party payer is risky. It is a far better business decision, regardless of practice setting, to secure patients from a balance of referral sources and third-party payers with no one entity representing more than 10 to 15% of the total business revenue. No audiologist would like the fact that a third-party payer canceled a contract that represented 15% of his or her total business, but the business should survive that 15% loss. The same may not be true if that same business lost 30 to 40% of its business with short notice.

Pitfall

- Contracting with third-party payers is both beneficial and risky. No one referral source or third-party entity should represent more than 10 to 15% of an audiologist's total business or the amount of business one is willing to lose with short notice.

◆ The Hearing Industry and National Networks

History of Existing National Networks

The landscape of the hearing industry, especially the hearing aid industry, has changed dramatically over the past quarter century. It has become one of substantial consolidation. In 1980, some 60 manufacturers of hearing aids did business in the United States and offered their products for sale though various professionals. In 2005, there were fewer than 15 international vendors of hearing aids, and many of these international vendors did business under multiple names. For example, Siemens, a German-based company, not only manufactures hearing aids under that name, but also owns Rexton and Electone. William Demant, a Danish company, owns Oticon and Bernafon, as well as Maico Diagnostics, Interacoustics, Phonic Ear, and Sennheiser Communications (Smriga, 2005). Great Nordic, another Danish company, owns GNReSound, Interton–American Hearing Systems, and the Beltone brand. Starkey, an American company, acquired NuEar, Omni, Microtech, and Qualitone, among others. Phonak, a Swiss company, purchased Unitron (Smriga, 2005). This is a far different landscape than that which existed 25 years ago, and it is one that will continue to change, as evidenced by the announcement in July 2006 that the GN Group (GNReSound, Beltone, and Interton) was up for sale (Granholm, 2006) and the announcement in October 2006 that Phonak had agreed to acquire ReSound Group from GN Store Nord A/S (Phonak, 2006). Products, choices, and professional options have been homogenized in today's market.

The current major manufacturers of hearing aids have purchased market share through their acquisitions. According to Carole Rogin, president of the Hearing Industries Associations (HIA), "HIA tracks and reports quarterly accumulated hearing aid sales data in the United States by type of circuitry, model of hearing aid, and shipment by destination. Specific data regarding hearing aid manufacturer market share in the USA is not tracked or available" (C. Rogin, personal communication, September 8, 2005). With minimal reportable published data regarding U.S. market share, one can only speculate regarding the distribution of market share across today's manufacturers of hearing aids in the United States. In addition, speculation regarding market share within the United States versus worldwide would yield different numbers.

Regardless of market share, there is no doubt that the sales of many manufacturers of hearing aids financially support their international parent organizations. Several manufacturers of hearing aids have also entered the retail market or informally partnered with large distribution networks to better control their distribution and to gain market share. This strategy, although smart for the parent organizations, often places the manufacturer of hearing aids in direct competition with dispensing audiologists at the retail level.

Controversial Point

- Several hearing aid manufacturers, their parent companies, and some networks are purchasing retail hearing aid centers to secure market share. When choosing with whom to do business, should audiologists not only consider product quality, customer service, software programming features and ease, potential referrals, and product costs, but also each company's business practices?

In addition to manufacturer consolidation, the move to consolidate the retail distribution channels for hearing aids emerged in the mid-1980s in Florida. Approximately 20 retail hearing aid offices on the east and west coasts of Florida merged to become Hearing Centers of America (HCA). Shortly thereafter, in 1988, Sound Resources, a private audiology practice with 14 locations in the Chicago area, was sold to Maryland-based Integrated Health Services (IHS). Prior to that acquisition, IHS specialized in long-term health and rehabilitative care, but in 1989, IHS purchased Florida-based HCA to expand its market share in the hearing industry (News, 1989). However, in the early 1990s, IHS transitioned its newly acquired hearing division to Pennsylvania-based Hearing Health Services, Inc. (HHS), a sister company of NovaCare. HHS entered the hearing industry with about 30 locations in Florida, 15 offices in Illinois, and 1 office in Indiana, and continued its acquisition strategy by buying audiology private practices in Illinois and Michigan (Audio-Vestibular Testing Center, Inc.) through 1994. However, not even the power, wisdom, and money behind HHS's parent company rehab giant NovaCare could save the

Florida hearing care offices. In late 1994, all of the HHS Florida offices were sold to HEARx, leaving HHS with around 15 financially sound Midwest offices operating under multiple names.

The name Sonus was introduced in the Midwest at one office in Indiana, five offices in Michigan, and approximately a dozen offices in Illinois in 1995 following a long and expensive market analysis and name search. That name change marked the birth of Sonus and the introduction of the Sonus name into the American hearing health care market. In 1996, those midwestern offices were sold to Healthcare Capital, a Canadian-based publicly traded corporation that later incorporated in the state of Washington and established the name SonusUSA. From 1996 to 2001, Sonus experienced substantial growth through the purchase of some 80 offices in multiple states and the affiliated provider network, HearPO. In addition, the Sonus Network was started during that time. In 2002, Italian-based Amplifon purchased Sonus USA and its affiliated networks, the Sonus Network and HearPO.

Although the roots of Sonus can be traced to the mid-1980s, the primary growth of Sonus has occurred since 1994. In 2005, Sonus claimed to "have grown into the largest professional hearing care network in North America ... with more than 1600 locations in the United States and Canada, including company-owned clinics and independent providers who are licensed Sonus Network affiliates" (Sonus, 2005). In addition, Amplifon, the Sonus parent company, "operates in several countries, including Austria, Canada, Egypt, France, Hungary, Italy, the Netherlands, Portugal, Spain, Switzerland, and the United States. With an international network of more than 3000 locations, Amplifon has become the largest distributor of hearing aids in the world" (Sonus, 2005).

During nearly the same time in the late 1980s, HEARx also entered the American hearing care market with offices primarily on the East Coast. After over 20 years in operation under various names, including HEARx, HearUSA, and HEARx West, plus the sale and acquisition of many offices, HearUSA, the current parent company of HEARx, has some 157 corporately owned offices in 11 states and the province of Ontario (HearUSA, 2005) and an affiliated provider network of 1400 audiologists. Although these are the published numbers, it is generally known that several HearUSA stores were sold, and Cindy Beyer, Au.D., senior vice president of

professional services for HearUSA, reported in 2005 that HearUSA owned 136 corporate offices. In addition, HearUSA had close to 1000 payers or benefit sponsors (C. Beyer, personal communication, September 12, 2005).

Helix, another company with Canadian roots, also entered the American hearing care market in 1997 with ~120 offices on the East Coast and in the Midwest and Canada. Its inclusion in the American hearing care market proved to be relatively short-lived, however, when it was purchased by HearUSA in 2001 (News, 2001). Helix had already acquired National Ear Care Plan (NECP), another national network of audiology providers, and the acquisition of Helix also included NECP, which was later renamed The Hearing Care Network.

In 2005, Smriga attempted to calculate current hearing aid market share based on an estimated 11,000 outlet base in the United States. He determined that

> Amplifon, the Italian-based marketing company that owns Miracle Ear, Sonus, and National Hearing Centers (also known as Wal-Mart's retail distribution), owns 23.7% of the U.S. retail distribution. William Demant, which owns Oticon and Bernafon, has secured 21.48% of the U.S. retail distribution through their Avada and AHAA retail affiliates. HearUSA reported in their annual report 173 corporately owned stores in 11 states plus 1400 affiliated network providers that represent 14.3% of US distribution. Audibel, a Starkey affiliated network, and Beltone, which is owned by Great Nordic (Great Nordic also owns GNResound), have secured ~15.5% of U.S. retail distribution combined. (Smriga, 2005)

See **Fig. 17–1** for a breakout of the top companies in 2005 in terms of retail market share.

These percentages can vary based on definitions of total hearing (aid) market universe, provider, and retail outlet. In addition, there is a flaw associated with including affiliated network members in any organization's market share because the majority of those members are independent practitioners that may belong to multiple networks. Also, the retail outlet universe does not necessarily tie directly to market share in terms of hearing aid units sold. Overall, these numbers represent a dramatic shift in the retail delivery of hearing health care services and products in the United States to large corporations and corporate consolidators. This primary and substantial shift has occurred in less than 15 years.

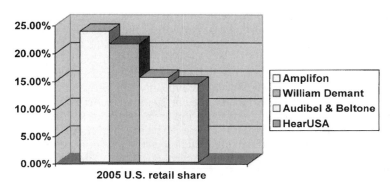

Fig. 17–1 Breakout of top companies in 2005 in terms of U.S. retail market distribution.

The Amplifon-Sonus and HearUSA distribution networks have secured substantial market share in a relatively short period of time. Although they are not the only national hearing care networks, they are among the largest. At some point in their careers, audiologists will have to decide whether or not they will join and support a national network, and if so, which network(s) they will join. On the surface, this can appear to be an easy decision, but in reality, the results of this decision will affect not only the individual audiologist and his or her patients, but also the profession and the practice of audiology as a whole. It is important to identify the parent company of any provider network with which one might affiliate and understand its management and clinical strategies, including any affiliation it might have with a manufacturer of hearing aids or providers other than audiologists. This decision will impact not only referrals and reimbursement but also how one practices audiology and fulfills contract obligations.

The strategy of manufacturers' controlling or owning their own distribution networks is not a new one. It has existed for many years and is one that more manufacturers of hearing aids are embracing. It is likely this movement will change the landscape of the hearing aid industry once again by generating new competitive challenges for reimbursement and third-party contracting. As the manufacturers of hearing aids secure retail market share, it is likely they too through their hearing care employees will participate with third-party payers as contracted providers. It will be very difficult for dispensing audiologists regardless of practice setting to compete on a cost basis with manufacturer-owned stores due to the manufacturer's innate cost-of-goods advantage.

Pros and Cons of Delegating Third-Party Contracting

There are several obvious and good reasons for audiologists to support national networks and to allow these networks to secure third-party contracts on the audiologist's behalf. Some of the benefits include the upfront costs associated with contracting, legal and liability issues, credentialing, record keeping, and logistical contracting requirements, including record keeping and quality management. The process of contracting can be a long, detailed, and tedious one. Contracts are binding and should either be prepared by an attorney or be reviewed by an attorney. Credentialing is an ongoing and essential process, and licenses to practice and malpractice expiration dates must be updated on a regular basis. No longer can an audiologist rely on manual tracking, reporting, and financial systems. Information technology plays an important role in quality management, billing, and record keeping. Joining a national network to fulfill these requirements certainly is appealing and appears smart on the surface, but there are also downsides to such arrangements:

♦ When a network negotiates and secures a third-party contract, it is the network that "owns" that contract. The formal relationship and contract are between the network and the third-party payer, with the understanding that the network represents the group of affiliated providers. Even though the provider has little if any say about the terms of that contract, the provider is bound by the terms of that contract. For example, the provider may not agree with the negotiated fees for audiology and vestibular services or hearing aids, but if the provider wants to participate with that network, he or she has no choice but to accept those negotiated fees.

♦ A provider's continued participation in the third-party contract is dependent upon the network's ability to manage and maintain the contracted relationship with the third-party payer. If the network fails to maintain that contract, the provider could lose his or her ability to service the third-party payer's beneficiaries as a result of the network's inability to do its job, not because the provider failed to meet patients' needs. Many audiologists have already experienced the loss of a contract not because they did anything wrong, but because the national network in which they are a preferred provider lost the third-party contract.

♦ In any business, the timing of payments for services and products is crucial. Delays in payments to providers for services completed or products sold can be devastating for cash flow and the health of an audiology practice. National networks often hold payments to providers until after they receive payment from the third-party payer, which can delay payments to providers for many months. It is important to identify not only the reimbursement levels for services and products, but also the timing of those payments from any network with which one might participate.

♦ To rely on the revenue generated from participation in network contracts is risky if that revenue represents anything more than 10 to 15% of the total practice revenue. On the one hand, the additional revenue is welcome; on the other, a future potential purchaser of that practice could discount any revenue generated as a result of participation in a network if the purchaser knows he or she cannot belong to the network from which those referrals are generated. The result would be reduced gross revenue, reduced net profit, and therefore a corresponding practice devaluation.

Joining multiple networks and being included in the provider databases of those networks could be viewed as a way to participate in and receive referrals from multiple plans. Although this strategy can result in patient referrals, there is also risk beyond not receiving referrals. By allowing their names to be included in a network database, audiologists are supporting that network's ability to cover and promote access locally, regionally, and nationally. Access is one of the more important components in third-party negotiations. By law, MCOs must have sufficient access to the various health care specialties, typically, but with some exception, access within 20 miles or 20 minutes. Access presents a challenge for both small and large networks. Regardless of credentials, without sufficient access, it is difficult for both networks and individual audiologists to negotiate contracts with third-party payers. Audiologists must know to whom they are providing access.

Special Consideration

- Most health care administrators rank access as one of the most important contracting requirements. Access can be one advantage large networks have over independent providers. Independent providers can refer potential contracts to a network for negotiation or formally and legally unite as independents to fulfill access requirements.

Another consequence of being a credentialed provider in multiple networks or allowing one's name to appear on the provider roster of multiple networks is that in doing so, audiologists are in essence competing with themselves. In the hearing industry, there are only a few national networks that have the capability of offering national audiology coverage, and those national networks often bid for the same third-party contracts. Belonging to multiple networks may result in increased referrals from one of those networks, but those competing networks often lower their proposed reimbursement levels to win the contract in a competitive market. When the negotiated reimbursement drops, so too does the reimbursement to the provider, and both the network and the provider accept less money. The winner in terms of cost is often the third-party payer.

Although it is certainly easier to leave contract negotiation to the larger networks, it puts audiologists in the position of accepting the contract terms and reimbursement levels that are negotiated by their network representatives. In some cases, terms and reimbursement levels are reasonable and consistent with an individual audiologist's practice needs, but in other cases, reimbursement can be unreasonable and barely worth the audiologist's effort.

There are potential benefits to participating in local, regional, and national networks that negotiate with third-party payers, but there are also consequences to such participation (**Table 17–2**). Audiologists have a professional responsibility to know the facts about each network before they allow their names to be included on the membership rosters of any network. Allowing one's name to be included

in the database of a network provides negotiating power to that network by increasing that network's appearance of access. If audiologists desire to give networks that power, they should choose one organization and allow that organization to negotiate on their behalf to eliminate the issue of self-competition that results from belonging to multiple networks. If audiologists do not want to give national networks the negotiation power associated with access, they should request that their name be removed from all membership rosters of networks with which they do not participate.

As with many things in life, balance is often the key to success. Achieving a balance among referral sources, including participation with national networks and contracting directly, may be the best decision when it comes to contracting with third-party payers. To achieve such balance, audiologists must understand the processes of becoming a preferred provider as well as how to negotiate third-party payer contracts.

◆ Negotiating Third-Party Payer Contracts

Although it may be beyond most audiologists' capabilities to fulfill access requirements for national contracts, many regional and local contracting opportunities exist. Obtaining approved provider status for a specific third-party payer can be as easy as completing a credentialing application and securing a provider number. In these cases, the provider agreement typically stipulates covered and noncovered services and products, service and billing requirements, and reimbursement levels. By signing the provider agreement, the audiologist agrees to abide by the terms stipulated in that agreement. There is very little if any negotiation in such cases. Medicare, Blue Cross Blue Shield (BCBS), and United Healthcare are examples of third-party payers that have implemented such a system with some of their health care plans or for some covered employer groups.

Other third-party payers do not have a preestablished open panel provider credentialing process, but rather prefer to contract with individual specialty providers or groups of

Table 17–2 Pros and Cons of Network Participation

Pros	Cons
Potential for patient referrals with minimal effort on the part of the audiologist	There is no guarantee of referrals.
The network assumes the cost, time, and effort associated with negotiation, legal, and contract implementation.	The network owns the contract; therefore, such contracts cannot be considered a business asset.
The network assumes responsibility for continuous quality improvement, credentialing, billing, and tracking.	Audiologists must accept the negotiated fees for services and products and monitor billing and payment, which can be delayed.
Utilization management and marketing falls to the network, not the audiologists.	Although utilization management falls to the network, it will affect the audiologists in ways with which they may not agree.
The network assumes responsibility for provider credentialing.	Membership in multiple networks puts audiologists in the position of competing with themselves.
Overall, the network is responsible for all aspects of contract management, which allows audiologists to focus on patient care.	The network could lose the contract and by default the audiologists also lose the contract, possibly through no fault of the audiologists.

providers. In these cases, contract negotiation can be a time-intensive process that requires substantial effort to finalize; however, negotiating and securing third-party contracts are possible for any audiology business. In brief, the process includes these steps:

♦ Identify opportunities with key third-party payers.

♦ Identify the appropriate contact people and decision makers.

♦ Research the organization's needs regarding audiology and vestibular care, hearing aids, assistive listening devices (ALDs), and other hearing-related products.

♦ Understand the payer's current system for the delivery of audiology services and related care. If the payer is currently under contract, research the terms of that contract. Ask questions regarding satisfaction levels with current providers and areas of desired improvement. Listen for perceived gaps, problems, and dissatisfaction, which represent potential contract opportunities.

♦ Prepare and submit a comprehensive proposal that not only addresses and meets the payer's needs but also adds value for the payer. This proposal must comply with established quality standards and the financial goals for both the payer and the provider.

♦ Negotiate to secure the contract.

♦ Secure the contract.

♦ Implement the terms of the contract.

♦ Track and report activities, using total quality management and continuous quality improvement (CQI) programs.

Identify Opportunities with Third-Party Payers

Identifying opportunities with key third-party payers can be applicable on a local, regional, or national scale. One of the best sources of information about third-party payers at a local level is patients seeking services. An audiologist should ask patients that enter his or her office about their insurance coverage, including not only the name and location of the third-party payer but also benefit details. Initial contact information for third-party payers can be found on patients' insurance cards, in local phone directories, via the local chamber of commerce, in managed care directories or books, and on Web-based health care sites.

As with the hearing industry, the trend in the health insurance industry has been one of consolidation. Many small local carriers have been purchased and merged to form large national groups. Third-party organizations with which one can contract include insurance companies, MCOs (including HMOs and PPOs), independent physician associations (IPAs), workers' compensation carriers, federal and state governments, and employer groups. **Table 17–3** summarizes examples of third-party payers that offer hearing health care plans under one or more of the various third-party payer categories on either a regional or national basis.

Table 17–3 is not meant to be inclusive of every third-party payer, and certainly far more payers exist than are listed. In addition, some third-party payers offer only one type of health care plan, whereas others offer a complete family of plans from which the consumer can choose. Therefore, when contracting to be a provider for a third-party payer, it is important to identify the specific plan for which one is negotiating. Not only can reimbursement levels vary by plan type, but so too can the mandatory management procedures. One obvious example: those patients covered under PPO plans are usually free to seek services from any participating preferred provider without a written referral from their primary care physician (PCP); however, those patients covered under HMO plans are required not only to remain in network but also to secure a referral from their PCP for all health care services. Provider reimbursement is dependent upon that PCP referral in the HMO system, but not the PPO system.

A less traditional but fast-growing segment of the health benefit industry is ancillary health care plans. Ancillary health care plans typically do not cover major medical care for hospitalization or physician visits but usually do include health care services that are not covered by major medical policies. Those services can include dental, nutraceuticals, chiropractic, vision testing including eye glasses, and hearing care including hearing aids. Most ancillary health care plans function as discounted private pay plans, meaning patients pay for the services they receive, but those services are offered at discounted levels by participating providers. A funded benefit is typically not a part of ancillary health care plans.

Examples of national ancillary health care plans include Affordable Health and Benefits, Complementary Care Company, and Countdown USA. Under these plans, providers are credentialed by either the plan or the contracting network

Table 17–3 Sample Third-Party Payers Covering Hearing Services

Insurance companies	Blue Cross Blue Shield (BCBS; each state has its own BCBS affiliate), United HealthCare, CIGNA HealthCare, CareAmerica, Edlerplan, and Providence Health System
Managed care organizations	Home First, Health Central, and Sharp Health Plan
Preferred provider organizations	Physician's Health Plan, United Payors and United Providers, and Admar
Workers' compensation carriers	Pharmacy Management Services, Inc. (PMSI) and the Washington Self-Insurers Association (WSIA)
Federal or state government	Department of Veterans Affairs, Medicare, and Medicaid
Employer/labor groups	Joint Benefit Trust of the Teamsters, Operating Engineers, and Fort James Corporation

and are considered preferred providers. Patients typically go directly to a preferred provider for services, and a prior authorization is not usually required. The patient pays the provider directly at the negotiated discounted rate, which can be a flat rate or a percent off usual and customary fees. Although services and products must be provided at a discounted rate, participation in such ancillary health care plans can be beneficial if the plan directs new patients to the audiologist's office and does not require discounts beyond that which a practice can afford.

Identify Decision Makers at the Third-Party Payer

In some cases, all that is required to become an approved provider is the completion of a provider application; however, in those cases, the audiologist must also accept the predetermined reimbursement schedule for that third-party payer and all of the established contract terms. For example, an audiologist can become a Medicare provider by completing an application; when submitting that application, though, the audiologist is contractually obligated to follow Medicare policy and accept Medicare's reimbursement levels. Violating Medicare policy can be considered fraud and result not only in a loss of provider status but also in substantial monetary fines. The same is true of some BCBS and United Healthcare plans that cover auto workers. Under these plans, the audiologist agrees to participate and follow the contract terms, which are stipulated by the third-party payer. By signing the agreement to become a participating provider, the audiologist can be held liable for noncompliance. This alone is not a reason to not participate in these plans; however, an audiologist must understand the terms of any application or contract before signing the same.

In the case of Medicare, the audiologist should contact the third-party intermediary for the region in question to secure the appropriate applications. In the case of other third-party payers, one would contact the local representative for the specific payer to request a provider application.

There are also many third-party payers that do not have established hearing care programs or an established credentialing process for audiology providers. Many do not cover hearing services or hearing aids, but that lack of coverage presents an opportunity for audiologists. Identifying the appropriate contact people and decision makers at third-party payer organizations can be challenging; however, it can usually be accomplished with a phone call to the organization. Provider contracting might be handled in one of many departments, including marketing, provider relations, contracting, operations, and legal. Typically, the person answering the phone will be able to direct the audiologist wishing to become a preferred provider to the appropriate department, contact people, and decision makers. Start the process by identifying the name, title, and contact information of the contract decision maker.

Research the Third-Party Payer Organization

To effectively negotiate with third-party payers, one must first understand the organization. The following is a list of questions to consider when beginning the research phase of the negotiation process. The specific answers to these questions will determine not only if the audiologist's business is qualified to fulfill the contract requirements but also if the third-party payer is one with which it would be worth contracting. It is also important to be familiar with third-party payer terminology (see Appendix 17–1).

Third-Party Payer Organization

- What is the complete and formal name of the organization? If it is a corporation, in which state is it incorporated?
- What structure is the organization (e.g., HMO, PPO, IPA)?
- How many lives does the organization cover?
- What geographic area does the organization cover?
- Does the organization prefer to contract locally, regionally, or nationally?
- Does the organization prefer capitated or FFS payment arrangements?
- Does the organization currently contract with or include audiologists in its panel of providers? If so, will the organization share the details regarding its current panel of providers and current contract terms for audiology and related services and products?
- If the organization currently has a contract that covers audiology or vestibular services, does that contract include exclusivity language?
- Does the organization have an unmet need regarding audiology services and products? Is it satisfied with its current arrangement for audiology care and hearing aids?

Providers

- What are the mandated credentials and qualifications for preferred provider status?
- How often and at what time interval does the organization have open enrollment?
- Does the organization restrict its provider panel?

Benefits

- Does the organization currently provide a benefit for audiology services?
- Does the organization currently provide a benefit for hearing aids?
- Are there other benefits for services or products that would fall under this agreement (e.g., vestibular testing, ALDs)?
- Are benefits funded? If so, what are those funded levels?
- Are all group participant benefits the same, or are there multiple and varying benefit plans that differ by employer group?

♦ What are the various employer groups that participate with this third-party payer, and what are the various benefit plans for each group?

The answers to the above questions provide some of the necessary information to determine whether or not the particular third-party payer is a candidate for contracting. For example, a third-party payer may have a need for audiology providers, but that need might be across numerous counties or even states. The payer may prefer to negotiate with one entity that can meet its need across the entire service area and be unwilling to negotiate with multiple providers. In this example, a national network may have a contracting advantage over a local provider. Local providers could either legally unite to cover the service area or refer this third-party payer to one of the national networks for negotiation. Another example would be an HMO that confirms the need for audiology services but prefers capitation arrangements to FFS. In this case, although the third-party payer will provide some data, it will be the provider who must determine a reasonable per member per month (pmpm) fee. Without experience with capitation, the provider could have substantial risk.

Prepare the Proposal

Preparing the third-party payer proposal can be the most time-consuming and tedious part of the contracting process. Armed with the specific facts about the third-party payer, it is now the audiologist's responsibility to provide a proposal that will meet the needs of the third-party payer while at the same time meeting the needs of the audiologist's business. It makes no sense to secure a long list of contracts that discount audiology services and products to the point that it becomes detrimental to the business. It is important to determine that fine line between the business's ability to survive and thrive while offering a discount on services and products and a discount that burdens the business and forces it into financial ruin or bankruptcy.

A third-party proposal should include, at a minimum, the following:

♦ Vendor overview with a brief description of the practice, primary contact information, when the company was established, tax identification number, company ownership, state of incorporation, mission statement, and other pertinent identifying company information

♦ Personnel and services, including job descriptions of those providing services and management staff, number of personnel, key personnel, list of services and products available and an overview of those services, professional staff competencies with provider credentials, examples of other similar contracts, customer service support, and service location details

♦ Information technology and capabilities, including patient record keeping, authorization tracking, and claims processing

♦ Reporting system, including available format for communicating test results, time to process reports, and associated costs (Sample reports can also be provided.)

♦ Credentialing for all providers, with specific credentialing details (educational degree, license number, malpractice insurance with amount of coverage, continuing education hours, etc.), including a maintenance process

♦ Quality management with a description of a CQI program, quality audit results, outcome measurements, and grievance policy

♦ Clinical management detailing clinical protocols and co-ordination of patient care

♦ Financial information, including usual and customary pricing with proposed discounts or a pmpm capitation rate

In addition and depending upon the type of third-party payer and whether or not the contract includes a funded benefit, a section on marketing with sample pieces and communications to consumers as well as referral sources and staff may be requested.

Larger organizations such as the Department of Veterans Affairs (VA), BCBS, and CIGNA HealthCare may require the completion of a request for proposal (RFP). An RFP includes a list of very specific questions that are given to any provider who desires to bid for the contract. All questions must be answered within the stated time period and submitted for consideration to the third-party payer. Although topic areas will not differ significantly from those already mentioned, it is more likely than not that the questions will require comprehensive written discussion about technical capability; managerial capability and approach; past performance; the qualifications of the providers, management staff, and the contracting organization; price, and backup documentation.

Large established networks often have teams of people to do the necessary research, format the proposal, and put in writing all that is required to sufficiently complete an RFP within the stated time period, in comparison to the independent practice owner, who also serves as a provider of services, human resources director, finance manager, general business manager, and so on. This fact is certainly a benefit of network participation; however, as an alternative to network participation, independent audiologists could unite and contract with a consultant to complete the RFP on their behalf as long as they are fully informed about all applicable laws.

Negotiate the Contract

By the time an audiologist gets to the negotiation phase, he or she has already identified the opportunity and the key contact people as well as completed all of the necessary research. In some cases, especially if an RFP is involved, the written proposal serves as the negotiation tool. Although some final clarification and negotiation can occur, the audiologist must assess the overall contract proposal and usually presents his or her best offer as part of that RFP. In other circumstances, there is an opportunity for face-to-face negotiation before or after the written proposal is submitted. Regardless of the timing and the specific negotiation process, it is always in the audiologist's best interest to know his or her break-even point and the point below which it would not be financially responsible to become a preferred provider for a third-party payer.

As defined by Kasewurm (2000), a break-even analysis "provides a sales objective expressed in either dollar or unit sales at which the business will be breaking even." In other words, the break-even point could be represented by the amount of revenue it takes to cover all expenses without a resulting profit. For example, in an office with operational, clinical, cost of goods, and personnel expenses of $300,000 per year, the break-even point would be $144 per hour for one provider working full time, or 2080 hours per year ($300,000 in annual expenses ÷ 2080 annual hours worked = break-even hourly rate). In this example, any service that generates less than $144 per hour would be doing so at a loss, and any service that generates more than that amount would result in a profit. Specifically, if an air-bone-speech procedure (CPT code 92557) is scheduled for 30 minutes, the audiologist would have to collect $72.00 to break even on that service. If that same procedure is scheduled for 60 minutes, the audiologist would have to collect $144.00 to break even. If a particular service is generating a loss, the audiologist can either increase the charge for that service or reduce the time spent performing that service. Knowing the break-even point not only will provide the necessary information for establishing an appropriate fee schedule by CPT code, but also will identify the maximum discount that can be offered to a third-party payer.

Pearl

- Calculate the break-even point for all practice expenses and the minimum hourly revenue generation required to cover that point. Use that figure to identify the break-even number below which a practice cannot afford to offer services.

Calculating the break-even point for hearing aid sales is a bit more complicated if the audiologist bundles a service and product warranty into the initial cost for the hearing instruments, but it, too, can be calculated in basically the same way as long as the audiologist knows the actual dollars collected, cost of goods, and time involved with selling, evaluating, and maintaining hearing aid performance. If a pair of hearing instruments sell for $3500, and those same hearing aids cost the provider $1400, the resulting revenue from the sale of those hearing instruments is $2100, assuming the provider collects the $3500. To calculate a break-even point for this sale, one must consider how many hours of service will be associated with that sale, the resulting revenue, and any additional costs. The following would be a legitimate example: Assume it takes the provider 3 hours for the evaluation, sale process, and fitting with orientation.

In addition, assume that the hearing instruments were sold with a 3-year warranty, including a no-charge service plan, and that the hearing aids are covered by a 3-year manufacturer's warranty. Assume the patient returns for a 2-week postfitting check and one 30-minute check every 6 months for the life of the hearing instrument warranty. All totaled, the audiologist will provide ~6.5 hours of service for that $2100 of revenue, or generate $323 per hour. However, if that same audiologist spends more time over the life of that hearing instrument warranty than is stated in the example or must pay to repair the hearing aids, the hourly revenue generated per hour declines. (For further detail and discussion on this topic, see Chapter 15.)

When the amount of time spent on hearing instrument exchanges and returns, monaural fittings, difficult-to-fit patients, and dissatisfied patients reaches or exceeds the break-even calculation for a practice, it becomes very costly. In addition, when revenue declines as a result of a third-party reimbursement, it is essential that the audiologist-provider know exactly how many hours of service the negotiated fee will cover before the provider is in a losing financial situation. Unbundling fees associated with products and services may be one viable solution, but regardless of payment structure, there is much to be said financially for doing things right the first time and knowing that break-even number. In addition, when contracting for hearing instruments, it is important to consider the cost associated with any product warranty.

Some audiologists will argue that it is better to have at least some revenue coming to the practice rather than no revenue as a justification for accepting reduced fees for services and products that are often associated with third-party contracting. In addition, many audiologists feel they have an obligation to serve the needy and therefore choose to participate in the various states' Medicaid programs even though most Medicaid programs typically operate at far below most practices' break-even points. It is not this author's intent to suggest that audiologists do or do not have an obligation to serve the needy. In fact, this health care dilemma crosses all specialties. However, it can be fiscally irresponsible to the business and other paying patients to provide services and products on a regular basis at rates that fall below the break-even point of the practice. Practice owners must cover their expenses if they are to remain in business to serve all patients.

There are basically two methods of payment under which an audiologist can negotiate with a third-party payer: discounted FFS and capitation arrangements. Discounted FFS payment arrangements are exactly what the term implies. The audiologist offers a discount off usual and customary fees for services and/or products. This can be presented to the third-party payer on an encounter form that details the contracted services by CPT code showing usual and customary charges as well as negotiated fees. See **Table 17–4** for an example.

Using the break-even analysis previously explained, one can determine the greatest discount a provider can afford. Although the sample encounter form in **Table 17–4** portrays a 25% discount off usual and customary fees, that is not meant to suggest that 25% is a reasonable discount for

Table 17–4 Sample Encounter Form for Audiology and Hearing Aid Services

Audiology Services	Third-Party Price	CPT Code	Usual and Customary	Hearing Aids and Related Services	Third-Party Price	CPT Code	Usual and Customary
Screening (air only)	15.00	92551	$20.00	Hearing aid evaluation, monaural	67.50	92590	$90.00
Pure-tone threshold (air only)	22.50	92552	$30.00	Hearing aid evaluation, binaural	67.50	92591	$90.00
Pure-tone threshold (air and bone)	33.75	92553	$45.00	Hearing aid check, monaural	18.75	92592	$25.00
SRT or SDT	15.00	92555	$20.00	Hearing aid check, binaural	30.00	92593	$40.00
SRT and speech discrimination	26.25	92556	$35.00	Electroacoustic evaluation, monaural	18.75	92594	$25.00
Air, bone, SRT, and speech discrimination	60.00	92557	$80.00	Electroacoustic evaluation, binaural	30.00	92595	$40.00
Audiometric testing of groups	37.50	92559	$50.00	HPD attenuation measurement	56.25	92596	$75.00
Loudness balance	18.75	92562	$25.00	Hearing aid, monaural ITE/BTE		V5050–60	
Tone decay	18.75	92563	$25.00	Hearing aid, binaural ITE/BTE		V5130–40	
Stenger (pure-tone)	18.75	92565	$25.00	Dispensing fee: hearing aid delivery	N/C	V5090	$210.00
Tympanometry	22.50	92567	$30.00	Hearing aid repair, traditional (6 months)	93.75	V5014	$125.00
Acoustic reflex test	18.75	92568	$25.00	Hearing aid repair, traditional (1 year)	120.00	V5014	$160.00
Reflex decay test	18.75	92569	$25.00	Hearing aid repair, programmable (6 months)	142.50	V5014	$190.00
Filtered speech	37.50	92571	$50.00	Hearing aid repair, programmable (1 year)	180.00	V5014	$240.00
Staggered Spondee Word test	37.50	92572	$50.00	Hearing aid repair, digital (6 months)	176.25	V5014	$235.00
Lombard test	18.75	92573	$25.00	Hearing aid repair, digital (1 year)	225.00	V5014	$300.00
Sensorineural acuity level	18.75	92575	$25.00	Hearing aid repair (in warranty)	N/C	V5014	N/C
Synthetic Sentence Identification test	75.00	92576	$100.00	Hearing aid repair (in house, minor)	15.00	V5014	$20.00
Stenger (speech)	18.75	92577	$25.00	Hearing aid or earmold pickup	N/C	V5299	N/C
Visual reinforcement audio	60.00	92579	$80.00	Hearing aid replate (add to repair)	75.00	V5014	$100.00
Conditioning play audio	33.75	92582	$45.00	Hearing aid recase (add to repair)	75.00	V5299	$100.00
Select picture audiometry	26.25	92583	$35.00	Remote repair (6 months)	105.00	V5299	$140.00
ABR (threshold or complete)	262.50	92585	$350.00	Remote repair (1 year)	150.00	V5299	$200.00
OAE (limited or complete)	63.75	92587–88	$85.00	Earmold (1 or 2)	41.25ea	V5299	$55.00ea
Central testing	131.25	92589	$175.00	Swim mold or HPDs (1 or 2)	45.00pr	V5299	$60.00pr
Spontaneous nystagmus with gaze nystagmus	47.25	92541	$63.00	Musician noise plugs (1 or 2)	N/A	V5299	$75.00ea
Positional nystagmus (4)	42.00	92542	$56.00	Special handling and postage	N/A	V5299	
Caloric vestibular test (4)	84.75	92543	$113.00	**Other Services and Products**			
Optokinetic nystagmus	32.25	92544	$43.00	Unlisted service or procedure	N/A	92559	
Oscillating tracking	27.75	92545	$37.00	Assistive listening devices	N/A	V5299	
Sinusoidal vertical rotational	N/A	92546	N/A	Other products	N/A	V5299	
Use of vertical electrodes	24.75	92547	$33.00	Medical record copies	18.75	92599	$25.00
Posturography	N/A	92548	$550.00	Medical report	37.50	92599	$50.00
Electrocochleography		92584					
Cerumen removal	22.50	69210	$30.00	Home visit, new/established (per hour)	N/A	99341–47	$45.00
Weber test	18.75	92599	$25.00	**Speech/Language Services and Prosthetics**			
Tinnitus evaluation	N/A	92599	$100.00	Speech evaluation	N/A	92506	$95.00
Hearing therapy	N/A	92507	$75.00hr	Language evaluation	N/A	92506	$95.00
Special event consultation	N/A	92599	N/C	Speech/language therapy	N/A	92507	$75.00hr
Special event test	N/A	92599	N/C	Voice prosthetic evaluation	N/A	92597	
Office visit (new or established)	22.50	99201–11	$30.00	Modification of voice prosthetic	N/A	92598	

Diagnosis	Code	Diagnosis	Code	Diagnosis	Code
Acoustic neuroma	225.1	Hearing loss, mixed	389.2	Recruitment	388.44
Atresia	744.02	Hearing loss, noise-induced	388.12	Speech, delayed	315.39
Cerumen	380.4	Hearing loss, SN	389.10	Speech, disorder	784.5
Cleft lip and palate	749.20	Hyperacusis	388.42	TM perforation	384.2
Cleft palate	749.00	Ménière's	386.00	Tinnitus	388.31
Communication problem	388.43	Ossicular discontinuity	385.23	TMJ dysfunction	524.6
Eustachian tube dysfunction	381.81	Otalgia	388.70	Vertigo/dizziness	780.4
Hearing loss (central)	389.14	Otitis media	381.3	Other (must include code)	
Hearing loss (conductive)	389.0	Otosclerosis	387.9		

ABR, auditory brainstem response; BTE, behind the ear; CPT, Current Procedural Terminology; HPD, hearing protection device; ITE, in the ear; N/A, not applicable; N/C, no charge; OAE, otoacoustic emissions; SDT, speech detection threshold; SN, TK; SRT, speech reception threshold; TM, tympanic membrane; TMJ, temporomandibular joint.

any individual practice. Nor is the sample meant to suggest appropriate procedure charges or to imply that a 25% discount off usual and customary fees will be sufficient to secure a particular contract. Appropriate fees and discounts must be determined for each third-party payer and each individual practice. As mentioned previously, many third-party organizations look to Medicare as a standard for reimbursement; therefore, it would be wise for negotiating audiologists to be aware of Medicare reimbursement levels for each CPT code.

Discounted FFS arrangements can be lucrative as long as the provider identifies the actual breakeven and does not offer discounts beyond those that the practice can afford. The administrative costs associated with third-party approvals, billing, and CQI programs must also be considered in that break-even analysis. Although contracts usually stipulate terms for billing and payment, it is not unusual for some third-party payers to take 90 days from the date of billing or longer to pay providers. In addition, under a discounted FFS arrangement, it is very important that the provider adhere to the billing terms stated in the contract. Some third-party payers allow providers to bill for up to 1 year following the date of service, but others restrict payment to services completed and billed within 60 days. Electronic billing, although relatively new to audiology, can help to expedite billing and payment from some third-party payers. For others, electronic billing is not an option for audiology.

Capitation is another method of reimbursement used by some third-party payers, especially HMOs. Under a capitation arrangement, the provider agrees to offer the contracted services and products for a set monthly fee. This set monthly fee is usually stated as a pmpm fee to cover the third-party payer's member population. Although there can be exceptions, the set monthly fee is paid regardless of the number of actual services or products provided. Under a capitation agreement, there could be a perceived incentive to see fewer patients, to provide fewer services, or to reduce the time spent with individual patients because the provider will receive the same amount of money regardless of how many services are provided, how many patients are seen, or how much time is spent with individual patients. However, there are usually strict quality standards including patient satisfaction measures that must be monitored and reported to the third-party payer, which should deter abuse.

The benefits of capitation include the fact that the provider eliminates the need for costly billing procedures and staff and receives a known quantity of money on a given date each month. Providers are typically reimbursed more rapidly and administrative expenses are typically less when compared with FFS arrangements. The primary risk associated with capitation for the provider is underestimating utilization and therefore negotiating a pmpm fee that does not cover the actual expenses that are incurred. According to Managed Care On-Line (2005a), a capitation rate survey in 2003 showed average HMO capitation rates for physicians to be $53.35 pmpm under commercial plans and $209.43 under Medicare. However, those pmpm rates are substantially lower for audiology care and hearing aids.

According to Cindy Beyer, Au.D., senior vice president of professional services for HearUSA, $0.015 to over $2.00 pmpm is "more typical for the hearing industry and is dependent upon the benefit structure, the volume, and the type of agreement" (C. Beyer, personal communication, September 12, 2005). A $2.00 pmpm for a third-party payer covering 5000 lives would result in a $10,000 monthly payment to the contracted provider regardless of the number of patents served.

There are benefits and risks associated with both discounted FFS and capitation agreements when contracting with third-party payers. It is important that contracting audiologists have a clear understanding of both those benefits and risks.

Secure the Contract

In some remote areas of the United States, access to health care may be limited, but in most areas, competition does exist and therefore must be considered during negotiation. A good third-party administrator will be aware of the providers that can meet their third-party specialty needs and the local, regional, or national fees for various audiology services and products. As mentioned previously, third-party payers often look to Medicare as a guide for covered services and products, which represents both a detriment and a benefit for audiologists. On the one hand, using Medicare as a guide means a third-party payer could require a physician referral for audiology services and not cover hearing aids as a benefit. On the other hand, in an HMO, where the PCP is the gatekeeper, there is a valid cost containment rationale to support referring directly to an audiologist for audiology testing versus initially referring all patients to an otolaryngologist. The fact that many diagnostic hearing and vestibular procedures are a covered service under Medicare also provides credibility, which can help with negotiations.

Under an FFS contract, utilization can be a concern for the third-party payer because the higher the utilization, the greater their cost. It is not uncommon for administrators of funded FFS arrangements to limit provider marketing and provider access to plan members. However, under a capitation arrangement, the third-party payer's costs are contractually fixed. Although the contracted rate may require adjustment over time based on utilization, there is less cost risk for the third-party payer. Funding or lack thereof also impacts utilization. Although a funded benefit usually increases utilization, the fact that hearing aids are not a covered benefit under Medicare and other third-party plans does not mean patients who are seen for hearing evaluations are not candidates for hearing aids. Those who do not have a hearing aid benefit under their health plan become private pay patients for those noncovered products, in essence increasing a provider's access to patients who are hearing aid candidates. Although reimbursement for these noncovered products increases as patients pay out of pocket for those products, a nonfunded hearing aid benefit will also reduce utilization when compared with a funded benefit.

Once the terms of the contract are decided, it is essential that all terms be documented in writing. Large third-party payers may prefer to provide the written contract, but some smaller organizations may request that the contracting audiologist provide the contract. With the former, it is advisable to have an attorney who specializes in health care contracting review the contract, whereas with the latter, it is advisable to have an attorney who specializes in health care contracting prepare the contract.

At a minimum, the contract with a third-party payer should include the formal name of the business and the third-party payer, detail the covered services and products, mention required credentials, detail exact billing and payment terms, and include a statement that if the contract is terminated, all rendered services will be paid, including those initiated before the contract termination but completed after the termination date of the contract. Automatic renewal statements are recommended and make contract administration much easier than annual renewal requirements. It is suggested that third-party payer contracts for audiology services and/or hearing instruments not include statements that reference 7 days a week, 24 hours a day service capacity, statements that reference hospitalizing patients, notification of institutional services, catastrophic case management, guarantees that the negotiated fees are the provider's lowest fees, malpractice "tail" policies, statements that prohibit the provider from marketing the benefit, statements with less than a 90-day billing period, or statements that do not allow the provider to assign the agreement. Although these are fairly common inclusions in health care contracts, they are either not applicable to audiology or not in the best interest of the audiologist's business.

Implement the Contract: Utilization of Third-Party Payer

One might think that the steps to finding and securing a third-party contract represent the majority of the associated work; however, there can be even more work associated with managing the contract. Just because a contract is signed at the administrative level does not mean that physicians will refer in an HMO or that patients will seek services in PPO or ancillary health care systems. With a funded discounted FFS arrangement, the payer may place marketing restrictions on the provider because increased utilization will result in increased costs for the third-party payer. However, in a capitated or nonfunded discounted FFS arrangement, the third-party payer's costs are stable even with increased utilization. Whether or not one can market and how one can market the covered benefit can differ with every third-party payer. It is essential that marketing limits and details be identified.

As with any referral source, that first referral will come from education. The audiologist-provider must educate physicians not only about the benefit but also about the diagnosis of hearing and vestibular disorders and the associated treatment. Most current physician gatekeepers in a managed care system have received very little training in otology and audiology, yet many are eager to learn about these specialties, especially when their patients present with auditory or vestibular disorders. The audiologist who gains the respect of PCPs will receive far more referrals regardless of the payer than will the audiologist who does not earn that respect.

Pearl

- To increase physician referrals, be recognized as a leader in the field of audiology and as a resource for current information regarding the diagnosis and treatment of auditory and vestibular disorders.

Marketing directly to the consumer patient will be important in any ancillary third-party health care system, and such marketing will likely be approved by administration because increased utilization will not mean increased costs to the organization. Even though most of these programs are discounted FFS and do not offer a funded benefit, it is important to inform the third-party beneficiaries not only of the discounts for which they qualify but also about the importance of audiology care and services. As is true in the general population, educating consumers about audiology care and hearing aids will positively impact utilization.

Track and Report: Total Quality Management and Continuous Quality Improvement Programs

Many third-party payers will require providers to have a CQI program. It is not acceptable simply to say that one is compliant with quality standards. At a minimum, structure, process, and outcome indicators should be identified, monitored, and reported. These indicators are typically measured on a percent basis and tracked for a given period of time against a stated minimum compliance threshold.

Structure indicators typically include variables that relate to the business's or professional's foundation or structure. In an audiology practice, structure indicators could include statements about barrier-free facility, diagnostic audiometer calibration, audiologist credentials, and test environment in compliance with standards established by the American National Standards Institute. Process indicators typically relate to compliance with clinical, support, or legal processes and procedures. In an audiology practice, process indicators could include specifics about audiologic reports, recommendations for treatment, coordination of services between professionals, and confirmation of medical clearance or signed waiver with hearing aid sales. Outcome indicators tie to results and could include follow-up and performance measures regarding hearing aids, improved communication abilities, and patient satisfaction.

The benefits of a CQI program and total quality management (TQM) far exceed the third-party payer requirements. TQM, as a management strategy, emphasizes the importance of quality maintenance in all organizational processes. The four fundamental principles of TQM are

Table 17–5 Sample Continuous Quality Improvement Report for a Dispensing Audiology Practice

Indicators Measured	Prior Compliance (%)	Target Threshold (%)	Current Compliance (%)	Improved/ Stable/Declined (select one)	Evaluation Period	Month/Year Evaluated
Structure Indicators						
1. Barrier-free facility		100%				
2. Diagnostic audiometer		100%				
3. Immittance testing instrumentation		100%				
4. Audiometer daily calibration		90%				
5. Audiometric test environment complies with ANSI standards.		90%				
6. Audiologist licensed		100%				
7. All reports are signed by responsible audiologist.		100%				
Process Indicators						
1. Evaluation tools and procedures are appropriate for the disorder, age, and abilities of patient.		100%				
2. Diagnostic reports include a statement regarding type and severity of communication disorder.		100%				
3. Diagnostic reports contain clinical impressions, including diagnosis.		100%				
4. Diagnostic reports specify recommendations for treatment.		100%				
5. Appropriate follow-up after fitting with new hearing instruments		90%				
6. Case records indicate coordination between the audiologist, physician, speech pathologist, school system, family, and other significant persons or services.		100%				
7. Medical clearance or medical waiver is present in the file and dated within 6 months of the hearing instrument fitting.		100%				
8. Case records contain the name, address, phone number, billing information, and parent or guardian name if patient is under 18 years of age.		90%				
9. The patient's PCP is on the general information form.		100%				
10. Hearing aid evaluation forms are complete and used appropriately.		90%				
Outcome Indicators						
1. Audiologic follow-up after hearing aid fitting indicates:						
a. Frequency of hearing instrument use is consistent with expectations.		80%				
b. Parents/caregivers/patients are able to operate and care for hearing instruments.		90%				
c. Patient demonstrates optimal aided auditory abilities.		90%				
d. Patient does not indicate frequent adverse reaction to loud sounds.		90%				
2. Final recommendations indicate continued management of auditory disorder.		100%				
3. Patient reports satisfaction with services and hearing instruments.		90%				

ANSI, American National Standards Institute; PCP, primary care physician.

delighting the customer, improving processes, empowering all employees, and management by fact. As W. Edwards Deming, one of the original proponents of TQM, said, "94% of all problems can be tracked to a system and only 6% of all problems are special in nature or caused due to people or equipment failure" (SkillPath, 1992).

Table 17–5 offers one example of a CQI report that can be used to fulfill the quality requirements of some third-party payer contracts. Specific indicators can be adjusted to meet the individual needs of each contract; however, because the data-gathering stage of the process can be timely, consistency across contracts is strongly suggested when that is within the audiologist's control. Privacy regulations dictated by the Health Insurance Portability and Accountability Act and all federal or state laws that relate to patient privacy must be honored. For maximum benefit, it is suggested that the data be used not only to fulfill contract obligations but to identify practice weaknesses and to implement changes that result in practice improvement. CQI should be an improvement process for a business, not only something that must be fulfilled by contract. (For further information on CQI, see Chapter 3.)

♦ Summary

The hearing industry continues to experience substantial changes in terms of cost management that represent both challenges and opportunities. Audiologists must understand how these changes will affect the practice of audiology. Although audiology care is necessary for all ages and demographics, clearly the expanding senior population is increasing the need for and awareness of audiology care on a national scale. Audiologists, regardless of work setting, must make informed decisions regarding how they practice, participate in health care networks, and contract with third-party payers based on demographics, competition, reimbursement, and the overall healthcare delivery system in their communities. Individual decisions regarding how one chooses to practice audiology today will influence the profession as a whole and determine how audiology is positioned in the future. As autonomous licensed professionals, audiologists will be held accountable for individual business decisions and must take responsibility for the future of audiology practice.

Appendix 17–1

Managed Care Glossary

The following selected terms are a subset of the complete *MCOL e-Dictionary*, which includes almost 750 terms of interest to health management professionals. Additional information about the *e-Dictionary* can be found at https://www.managedcarestore.com/ymcol/swdict.htm.

accreditation Involves a rigorous on-site review, according to comprehensive standards, by a recognized independent specialized agency that certifies an organization.

actuary An insurance industry–based individual who performs statistical calculations/analysis and establishes policy rates.

adjudication Processing provider claims in accordance with terms of agreement between provider and health plan.

assignment of benefits When a member requests to have his or her claim benefits paid directly to the provider of service.

average wholesale price Usually used in determining pharmaceutical charges based on average price of a given drug.

beneficiary The person(s) eligible to receive insurance benefits under a specific policy.

carve-out Separate purchase of specific services that generally are part of a managed care benefits package (e.g., vision, chiropractor benefits). These services are then typically provided by a specialty managed care organization or provider organization.

case management Involves having a nurse or other health care professional assigned to specific catastrophic cases to intensively monitor, coordinate, and proactively work toward improving their outcomes and monitor resources used.

catastrophic case A medical case involving a serious illness or accident that is typically complex, often life threatening, and consumes significant health resources and costs.

Centers for Medicare and Medicaid Services (CMS) The federal agency under the Department of Health and Human Services responsible for the Medicare and Medicaid programs. Formerly called the Health Care Financing Administration (HCFA).

concurrent review Utilization review conducted during the course of actual treatment, usually for the purpose of monitoring the length and level of treatment provided; most often applies to an inpatient review after admission.

credentialing A review process, using specific criteria, of a provider to determine if the provider meets requirements to participate in a health plan. This review process also outlines the conditions the provider must meet to remain in good standing on an ongoing basis. The purposes of the credentialing process are to provide a formal process for deciding provider participation, to maintain quality standards in provider membership, and potentially to provide some legal safeguards.

days per 1000 A utilization performance ratio measuring the annual number of inpatient days per 1000 members. The calculation is (Annual Inpatient Days/Annualized Members) × 1000.

demand management A program administered by managed care or provider organizations to monitor and process many types of initial member requests for clinical information and services. The program may involve operating an extended hours' nursing telephone triage service for members and patient education materials and resources.

disease management Involves aspects of case and outcomes management, but the approach focuses on specific diseases, looking at what creates the costs, what treatment plan works, educating patients and providers, and coordinating care at all levels: hospital, pharmacy, physician, and so on.

eligibility A process used by the plan and providers to determine if a person is a covered member of the plan at the time provider services are to be rendered. If so, the person is determined to be an eligible member. If not, the person is determined to be ineligible.

enrollment area The geographic area that an individual must live in to be eligible for health plan coverage.

exclusivity clause A section in a provider's contract with a health plan stating that the provider cannot contract with more than one managed care organization.

freedom of choice A benefits option for health maintenance organizations or other prepaid organizations where plan members can select the provider of choice; benefits are not limited to an established panel of physicians.

grievance procedure The procedure stipulated by the health plan for resolving health plan or provider complaints.

group contract A health insurance contract between an employer and a health plan where the employer or other entity purchases health care for groups of individuals.

Health Insurance Portability and Accountability Act (HIPAA) of 1996 A federal law that makes several changes that have the goal of allowing persons to qualify immediately for comparable health insurance coverage when they change their employment relationships. Title II, Subtitle F, of HIPAA gives the Department of Health and Human Services the authority to mandate the use of standards for the electronic exchange of health care data; to specify what medical and administrative code sets should be used within those standards; to require the use of national identification systems for health care patients, providers, payers (or plans), and employers (or sponsors); and to specify the types of measures required to protect the security and privacy of personally identifiable health care information. Also known as the Kennedy-Kassebaum bill and Public Law 104–191.

Health Plan Employer Data and Information Set (HEDIS) A standard protocol for reporting of specified data by health plans and providers.

health reimbursement arrangements Qualified employer-funded health care accounts for covered employees or retirees designated by an Internal Revenue Service ruling that allow for rollover from year to year of unspent funds on a tax-free basis. Such accounts may be included as a feature of a consumer-driven health plan.

hold harmless clause A clause in most managed care contracts between the provider and the health plan stating that each party does not hold the other responsible in the event of malpractice or financial insolvency.

individual contract The health benefits agreement between an individual and health maintenance organization.

managed care A type of health care delivery that emphasizes active coordination and arrangement of health services. Managed care usually involves three key components: oversight of the medical care given, contractual relationships with and organization of the providers giving care, and the covered benefits tied to managed care regulations.

managed care organization (MCO) An insurance organization arranging benefits through managed care. Sometimes the term is used more broadly to also include provider organizations that enter into managed care subcontracts with insurance organizations. The most common types of MCOs are health maintenance organizations and preferred provider organizations.

member months The total membership each month is cumulated for a given time period; for example, 100 members served each month for 6 months equals 600 member months.

National Committee for Quality Assurance A nonprofit organization dedicated to assessing and reporting the quality of care delivered by managed care organizations.

network model HMO A health care arrangement where a health maintenance organization (HMO) secures contracts with several physician groups. The physician group in turn may also provide health care services to non-HMO members.

open-ended HMO A health maintenance organization that allows its members to seek medical services outside of its contracted provider panel.

out-of-area Services rendered outside a predefined service area.

per member per month (pmpm) A measurement ratio for utilization of various clinical or administrative services, or for various financial applications, including revenue, expenses, and margins. The ratio takes the average units per each applicable member used on a monthly basis. Calculations are made as follows: Total Units for Entire Time Period/Member Months.

point-of-service (POS) plan A health maintenance organization (HMO) arrangement where the health plan covers out-of-network providers like preferred provider organizations (PPOs) under POS (open-ended) plans. Unlike PPOs, when the HMO/exclusive provider organization (EPO) system is used, the plan continues to be a regular HMO or EPO, both for members and providers.

quality management (also quality assurance) Involves ensuring members are getting accessible and available care, delivered within community standards; ensuring a system exists to identify and correct problems and to monitor ongoing performance. Tools include profiling of data, audits of health plan and provider records and facilities, surveys of providers and members, and recording of problem incidents as they occur.

referral A request by a provider for a patient under his or her care to be evaluated and/or treated by another provider.

retrospective review An assessment of medical care given after service has been performed.

risk pool This term can be used in two different ways: (1) A pool of money that providers set aside, according to the terms of their contract with the health plan, for excess payment of ancillary and/or referral services. The amount of money remaining in the risk pool at the end of the contract year is either given to the provider or split between the provider and the health plan, depending on the provider agreement. Provider risk pools are designed for providers to render cost-effective health care services. (2) The expected patient population within a defined geographic location and their anticipated claims costs/utilization, which is then used to determine expected revenue and expenses. Once established, the risk pool is used to determine anticipated claims liability.

shared risk fund Physician groups share in a portion of the financial risk and potential profit of hospital or other facility expenses, or other items such as prescription costs.

traditional care Traditional health care could be defined as "lacking a system." In traditional health care, the patient–physician relationship is the focal point. Purchasers are mostly passive third parties, paying for all the services a physician orders, at the provider's usual charges. Traditional health care is most identified with freedom of choice for patients and physicians. Patients can choose whatever provider they want to see, and physicians can choose to order whatever services they feel are necessary.

utilization In managed care, utilization refers to how often specific services are being used.

utilization management Involves coordinating how much or how long care is given for each patient, as well as the level of care. The goal is to ensure care is delivered cost-effectively, at the right level, and does not use unnecessary resources. Tools include authorization requirements to approve services before they occur, concurrent review for continuing cases, and profiling of cases after they occur for analysis.

wellness Programs offered by managed care organizations promoting preventive medicine and improvements in health-related lifestyle, including smoking cessation, nutrition, weight and stress management, and fitness programs.

References

Advertisement. (2005, July 6). Orlando Sentinel, p. J3.

Centers for Medicare and Medicaid Services. (2005). Medicare Modernization Act of 2003. Retrieved October 3, 2005, from http://www.cms. hhs.gov

Granholm, L. (2006). GN Store Nord: Takeover price dented by deteriorating profitability [analyst's report]. Enskilda, Denmark: Telecom Equipment, SEB.

HearUSA. (2005). Web site. Retrieved October 9, 2005, from http:///www.hearusa.com/company/about_us/index.asp

Kasewurm, G. (2000). The business plan and practice accounting. In H. Hosford-Dunn, R. J. Roeser, & M. Valente (Eds.), Audiology practice management (pp. 313–336). New York: Thieme Medical Publishers.

Managed Care On-Line. (2005a). Managed care fact sheets: Managed care national statistics. Retrieved September 14, 2005, from http://www.mcareol.com/factshts/factnati.htm

Managed Care On-Line. (2005b). MCOL e-dictionary. Retrieved October 10, 2005, from http://www.mcareol.com/inmcodic.htm

Medicode. (2001). 2001 national fee analyzer: Charge data for evaluating fees nationwide. Salt Lake City: Ingenix Publishing Group.

News. (1989). Hearing Instruments, 40(10), 47.

News. (2001, June). Hearing Review, 14.

Pessis, P., & Freint, A. (2000). Managed care and reimbursement. In H. Hosford-Dunn, R. J. Roeser, & M. Valente (Eds.), Audiology practice management (pp. 363–382). New York: Thieme Medical Publishers.

Phonak. (2006). Web site. Retrieved October 5, 2006, from http://www.phonak.com

SkillPath. (1992). The fundamentals of total quality management. Mission, KS: Author.

Smriga, D. (2005). Are we asleep at the wheel? Feedback, 15(4), 8–15.

Sonus. (2005). Web site. Retrieved October 9, 2005, from http://www.sonus.com/about sonus/sonushistory.asp

U.S. Department of Labor, Bureau of Labor Statistics. (2005). Occupational outlook handbook. Retrieved October 6, 2005, from http://www. bls.gov/oco/ocos085.htm

Williams, R. (2005). Payment and participation: A renaissance for Medicare's private health plans? National Academy of Social Insurance. Retrieved October 7, 2005, from http://www.nasi.org/publications2763/publications_show.htm?doc_id=275191

Chapter 18

Computer Principles and Applications

Robert R. De Jonge and J. Mark Goffinet

The past 3 decades have been exciting times for people interested in microcomputers. Originally, computers were large, arcane devices, housed in their own special rooms and attended to by professionals trained in a highly technical field. These large computers were mysterious, vaguely distrusted, and portrayed by science fiction writers as dark, foreboding devices designed to dominate and control the world. Then, in the 1970s, small computers were sold, at first in kit form to hobbyists who controlled them by writing their own programs in the BASIC (acronym for Beginner's All-Purpose Symbolic Instruction Code) programming language. Virtually no commercial software was available. Microcomputers, personal computers (PCs), home computers—no one was quite sure what to call them, or even what niche they would occupy. Some envisioned the computer as a device for controlling the home environment: turning lights on and off, adjusting the ambient temperature, and making appliances "intelligent." Soon, preassembled computers were marketed by such companies as Apple, Commodore, and Atari. People used these computers for scientific investigation as well as playing games.

Early business systems were powerful for their time, having dual floppy drives, 64 kilobytes (KB) of random access memory (RAM) powered by the 2 megahertz (MHz) Z80 processor. The success of word-processing software helped define the PC as something more than a game machine or household appliance. In the mid-1980s, IBM introduced its own PC, and now the microcomputer was viewed as a legitimate, serious tool for business. Several work-likes (IBM PC–compatible systems) soon entered the market. Shortly after IBM's entry, Apple introduced the Macintosh (Mac); its graphical interface set a new standard for how the user could easily interact with the machine. Improvements in hardware occurred at a remarkable pace as each new generation of microprocessor replaced the previous; toward the turn of the century, computers with 300+ MHz processors, 128 megabytes (MB) of RAM, and 8 gigabyte (GB) hard drives made the most sophisticated computers of only a few years before seem quaint and underpowered.

Today, these "impressive" statistics are no longer impressive. The steady, inexorable increases in computing power (and hard-drive storage capacity) allow more sophisticated programs to be developed with an ever-increasing array of useful features. Meanwhile, a global network of computers, the Internet, was being developed. E-mail was replacing the standard mail service, software was being downloaded, and people were getting instant access to information from their homes via telephone lines. Attitudes about computers were changing. Although some people were, and still are, intimidated, many more became excited about the possibilities for working smarter and more efficiently, and new markets opened. Computers filled schools as well as businesses, government offices, hospitals, and clinics. Now, computers are widely used for study (attending university classes), recreation (downloading music and games), accessing information (from where to vacation to evaluating the scientific literature for evidence-based practice), financial transactions, and a myriad of other uses great and small.

The issues of interest in this chapter are what is available for audiology and how the practice of our profession might be enhanced by computer applications. The general focus of this chapter is to identify programs useful for audiology and to describe their features. When used in a computing context, the term *application* is a synonym for *computer program*. But application can be considered in a broader context: how can computers facilitate work that is typically performed by audiologists? There are programs (e.g., Microsoft Office), designed for the general computing public, that have useful features for audiologists. So these applications, generally referred to as "integrated office suites," will be briefly described.

The purpose of this chapter is to make audiologists and students in training to be audiologists aware of how computers have been and might be integrated into their practice. Toward that end, the chapter is structured with the following guidelines:

* Emphasis is on general, guiding principles that help readers better understand computing and its relevance to audiology. Material covered in this chapter is expected to still be relevant 5 years hence. This chapter is not a review of the most current versions of applications and software specifics.

* The prevailing attitude is nonjudgmental. The intent is to inform readers about useful features offered by applications, without providing a critical review of different software packages or recommending one program over another.

* The chapter does not include user manual–type descriptions of each program. Nor does the mention of a program imply an endorsement of its features or its appropriateness for a particular task.

Special Consideration

* Software is constantly evolving. What is true about a program one day may change entirely the next. Be skeptical about "expert advice." Before buying, ask questions to make sure the software is compatible with your hardware and the programs you run.

◆ General Computer Issues and Applications

The following sections briefly describe important issues for understanding how programs run, the major computer applications, and how these programs may be used by audiologists. Computers are often sold with bundled software. Frequently, new users are unfamiliar with these software packages and their potential professional application.

There are many references readily available for those seeking additional information. Microcomputing is a popular subject, with many magazines devoted to the topic. Major bookstores have a large section devoted to microcomputing. People find the practical *Dummies* series (e.g., *Networking for Dummies, Windows XP for Dummies, QuickBooks for Dummies,* etc.) a useful introduction.

Running Computer Programs

To have an overall appreciation of what computers do, it is extremely useful to have a good understanding of exactly what a computer program is. The only activity computers perform is running, or executing, programs. To understand what the computer is doing at any point in time, know the programs the computer is running, identify the features those programs have to offer, and learn how to control those features. From the user's perspective, a program appears as a file stored on a disk drive. From a programmer's perspective, the program exists as a series of statements that are written according to the syntax of a programming language. There are many programming languages (BASIC, FORTRAN, C++, Pascal, Java, Pearl, etc.), and each language can have variations, such as Microsoft's version of Visual BASIC. Each language has a highly structured set of rules (syntax) for expressing statements. Program users do not need to know anything about the details of the programming language to use programs effectively. Usually, programs have a main event loop; the program continuously cycles through this main loop looking for an event to react to: a key being pressed, a button being clicked, or an event from a piece of hardware attached to the computer (e.g., modem, printer, Hi-Pro box, etc.). When an event is detected, the program branches to a subroutine designed to respond to the event, like calculating and displaying a target real ear insertion gain (REIG) curve when the "NAL" menu item is selected. Collectively, the features that the program offers are the sum of all the subroutines and events the programmer has built into the program—and nothing more.

Programs and Microprocessors

Once the computer program is written, it must be converted into a format that the microprocessor (AMD Athlon, Intel Pentium, etc.) of the computer understands. Other programs, called compilers or interpreters, convert the (usually) English-like syntax of the programmer's statement into a series numbers that set switches in the microprocessor, which allows the computer to perform the actions requested by the program. It is fortunate that neither the user nor the programmer needs to be concerned with this level of detail, but there are consequences that should be appreciated. The main one is that programs will run only on a particular platform, Mac or PC, because the coding is specific to the particular family of microprocessor (e.g., Intel, Pentium, or Motorola PowerPC). Although it is possible for a program to be cross-platform, that requires the development of different versions of the program. In larger markets, developers often produce software that runs on both the Mac and PC, or different developers will produce equivalent products for each platform. Software manufacturers in small, vertical markets (like audiology) usually focus on a single platform. In the hearing health care industry, almost all software is developed only for the PC.

Operating Systems, Program Versions, and File Formats

The computer's operating system (OS) is a significant factor influencing whether a program will execute on a computer. Currently, Microsoft's Windows is the dominant operating system, and virtually all software for audiology runs under it. The Mac OS is a distant competitor. The Linux OS is popular among many of the more technically oriented users, but it is mainly used "behind the scenes" running servers on the Internet. The OS itself is a sophisticated program that controls the computer's basic hardware (monitor, keyboard, disk and universal serial bus [USB] drives, etc.) and provides an environment within which the user's applications run. It also catalogs and allows the user to manipulate files stored on the computer's hard drive(s) or floppy disk drives. Microsoft developed an early disk operating system (DOS) for the PC. By today's standards, DOS is primitive, and its use is almost nonexistent; the user is presented with a blank screen, and commands are typed, one line at a time, with a very specific syntax. The user needed to memorize quite a few commands to control the computer effectively. From the programmer's perspective, DOS did very little to help him or her develop a user interface. Each programmer built the user interface from scratch, and each program was likely to have a unique method for controlling how it worked. Learning how to use one program often did not carry over to helping one use another. By contrast, in the 1980s, the Macintosh OS provided a rich "toolbox" to help the programmer develop the user interface: menus, window, buttons, and so on, provided a consistent look and feel from one program to another. This trend was repeated for the PC platform in Windows 3.x, 95, NT, 98, 2000, Me, and XP. The important point to realize is that modern programs are not self-contained. Significant portions of the code needed to run a program are part of the OS. As with microprocessors, OSs are often backwardly compatible, but not always. A DOS program likely would run under Windows 3.1 (without the look and feel of Windows) or Windows 95, but a program designed to take advantage of the features in Windows 95 will not run under Windows 3.1. There is no guarantee that a Windows 95 program will run under XP, although most will, but with a caveat. There may be problems with how the program interacts with hardware (a software "driver" that communicates with hardware, like a printer or Hi-Pro box). Often, when upgrading to a new OS, the drivers will need to be upgraded. With older programs, there may be no drivers for the new OS. Upgrading to a new OS may mean no longer being able to use older programs (and foregoing access to the data they created). Alternatively, the audiologist may be forced to continue using an older computer because a critical program needs the drivers of an older OS. Therefore, when contemplating the purchase of a program or a new computer, the OS environment (and how it will affect running older, legacy programs) is a consideration. Microsoft's Windows XP Professional is the recommended operating system for most audiology software.

Pearl

- The computing requirements for running audiology software are not too demanding. A computer capable of running Windows XP Professional and Microsoft Office is adequate.

The version number of a program is also important. Many programs, especially popular ones, are constantly evolving. New features make the program more useful, but compatibility issues can arise. The format of the document file often is the problem. For example, a word-processing document saved under a newer program version may be unreadable by an older version. The file format of more recent versions of Word are compatible with older versions. Still, be careful when taking that important document to another (especially older) computer.

Major Productivity Tools

The major applications for office management are word processing, spreadsheet, database, presentation, and scheduling. These applications are generic, not developed specifically for any one profession, and there are many programs that fall into this category, but Microsoft Office is the de facto standard. There is a tendency for many users to learn only the basic features of one program, like a word processor, and use that tool to solve all problems, even when creating a database or spreadsheet would be much easier and more efficient. There are many different productivity tools, and the scope of this chapter permits only a superficial introduction to their main features. However, a general understanding or awareness may encourage audiologists to learn and implement more of these programs in their own practice setting.

Pitfall

- New computers are often sold with a great deal of useful software. Few people take the time to learn the applications, seldom moving beyond the basic features. Consequently, work is done less efficiently, and more time is lost in the long run.

The following are some examples of how these productivity tools can be adapted to audiology. The Virtual Audiogram (Zapala, 1998) plots air- and bone-conduction thresholds along with the "speech banana." The pure-tone average (PTA) and percent hearing loss are calculated, and tympanograms are plotted with normative data for immittance parameters. The articulation index (AI) is used to derive performance-intensity functions to which the patient's actual intelligibility can be compared. Hearing aid prescriptions are made for real ear and coupler gain, and patient information can be stored in a database. Other audiologists have used spreadsheet programs for tracking audiology patients or calculating prescriptive targets for hearing aid fitting. REIG, coupler gain, and output are determined. The AI is used to determine the effect on speech intelligibility. The *Educational Audiology Handbook* (Johnson et al, 1997) comes with a disk that contains a variety of forms, checklists, profiles, letters, and fact sheets for use with word-processing programs for the Mac and PC. Newman et al (1997) explain how to use macro statements (described later in this chapter) with a word processor for rapidly generating hearing disability and handicap profiles.

Word-Processing Programs

Word processing is one of the most popular activities, and most computer users are familiar with at least one program, Microsoft Word, which has become a standard. So many features are offered that few people manage to learn them all. There is a tendency to achieve a basic level of competency and a resistance to exploring more complicated features. The main purpose of a word processor is to facilitate the creation, editing, formatting, and printing of documents. Word processors, however, do more than just manipulate text. They can create tables and combine text with graphics in a variety of useful layouts, or templates, to create basic forms, reports, brochures, receipts, contracts, and newsletter-style documents. Blocks of frequently used phrases can be defined and automatically inserted. Short sequences of keystrokes can be associated with a complex graphic, such as a tympanogram or letterhead logo. Complicated clinical reports can be built easily and rapidly. Graphics, such as line and bar graphs, scatter plots, and pie charts, and even a spreadsheet can be added to a word-processing document. A template could be created for a monthly report that automatically adds and summarizes hearing aid–related expenses.

The mail merge function is used in marketing to create form letters personalized for each recipient. Most of the letter is the same for each person, but certain segments of the letter, such as the person's name, title, and address, are inserted automatically by the program. The inserted information is exported from a database or entered from the word-processing program. Marketing activities are enhanced by making correspondence more specific and meaningful to the individual. Mailing labels can be printed for envelopes, or labels can be made for any other purpose, such as labeling drawers for bins containing parts, such as tubing or loaner hearing aids.

Spreadsheet Programs

The main purpose of a spreadsheet is to perform calculations on numerical data, but a spreadsheet can also function as a simple database. A spreadsheet is a matrix of horizontal rows and vertical columns labeled by numbers and letters. A rectangular cell appears at the intersection of each row and column. For example, the cell forming the intersection

between the third row and first column would be A3. Cells contain three types of entries: text, numbers, and mathematical/logical formulas. Text is usually entered as a label, to identify the values in a row or column. Numerical data entered by the user are used to perform calculations. When a cell contains a formula, the spreadsheet uses the numerical data in the rows and columns to calculate a value, which is displayed in the cell. Spreadsheet programs were originally developed to simulate the pencil-and-paper spreadsheets that were used to display business-related calculations. However, spreadsheets are useful for displaying and performing calculations on any types of data that fit into a tabular format. Spreadsheets have the ability to visualize data by quickly creating charts. A chart is drawn, complete with legends and title, by selecting a block of cells and choosing a format (pie chart, bar graph, scatter plot, etc.).

Figure 18–1 is a simple illustration of how an Excel spreadsheet might be used by an audiologist. The percent hearing loss is calculated from the PTA (500, 1000, and 2000 Hz) using a 25 dB fence and a 1.5% increase in hearing loss for each decibel the PTA exceeds the fence. The percent binaural hearing loss is calculated by weighting the better ear to the poorer ear using a 5:1 ratio. Audiogram thresholds are entered in cells B5 to H6, and the percentage hearing loss is automatically calculated according to formulas entered in E10 to E12. Text can be styled with different fonts, sizes, and justification (centering, left, or right), and borders with single and double lines can be added to ranges of cells. A chart showing the audiogram is displayed at the bottom of the spreadsheet. When numerical values in the audiogram are changed, the percent hearing loss is automatically recalculated, and the audiogram is automatically redrawn. The proportions of the audiogram (aspect ratio) are roughly accurate. Excel provided a proper X symbol for the left ear. The default circle was too small, so a larger circle was created using the drawing tools. Creating different audiometric symbols (e.g., bone conduction, no response) proceeds in a similar fashion.

Database Programs

Database applications are the major tools for storing, sorting, organizing, cataloging, and retrieving information. A custom database allows great flexibility for managing data unique to a practice. Audiologists might include special information about their patients, such as interests or hobbies, difficulties in certain environments, or primary method of communication (oral or sign). Fausti et al (1993) describe how database software was used to store and collect data from a multisite study of ototoxicity.

A database is essentially a collection of records. Each record contains fields that are the objects where the information is stored. Fields can store text or numeric data, the results of calculations (like the cell in a spreadsheet), or even graphic objects or sounds. Typical fields include the patient's first and last name, street address, city, state, zip code, insurance carrier, and so on. Additional audiometric information could include audiogram thresholds (air and bone, separately for each ear), speech thresholds, word recognition scores, peak admittance, auditory brainstem response (ABR) waveforms, otoacoustic emissions (OAE), images from video

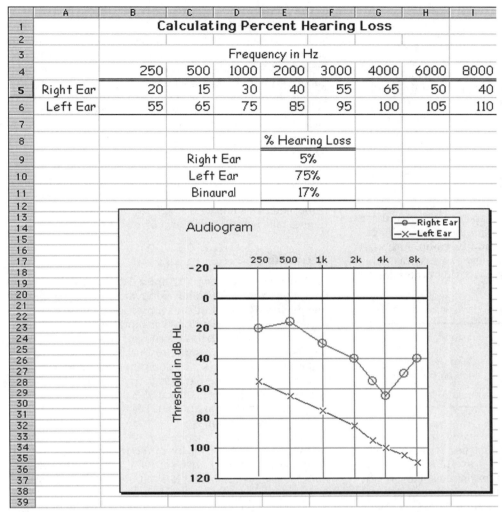

	A	B	C	D	E	F	G	H	I
1				**Calculating Percent Hearing Loss**					
2									
3					Frequency in Hz				
4			250	500	1000	2000	3000	4000	6000	8000
5	Right Ear	20	15	30	40	55	65	50	40
6	Left Ear	55	65	75	85	95	100	105	110
7									
8					% Hearing Loss				
9				Right Ear	5%				
10				Left Ear	75%				
11				Binaural	17%				

Figure 18–1 An example of how an Excel spreadsheet can be used to calculate percent hearing loss. The audiogram is illustrated by a chart that is automatically drawn from the threshold data. HL, hearing level.

otoscopy—when one stops to consider the potential amount of data that can be generated from an audiologic evaluation, the quantity seems endless. Hearing aid information includes date of purchase, purchase price, balance due, make/model, serial number, ear(s) fitted, warranty expiration date, battery club membership, programmable hearing aid session data, and journal entries. Databases can contain all information in a single file (flat file database), or the information can be split into different files (relational database). As the amount of information increases, it is easier to manage data if they are divided into smaller logical units. Patient demographic data could be stored in one file, audiometrics in another, hearing aid information in a third. The master file organizes and displays a subset of the information.

Databases allow different displays, or layouts, of information in each record. Each layout is analogous to a report on a subset of the data. Layouts can arrange the data in different orders and incorporate graphical backgrounds to achieve the desired appearance. For example, the audiometric data could be used to automatically generate a standard audiologic report. Another use for a custom layout is to produce cells of demographic information to fit on a standard sheet of mailing labels. Yet another layout could be similar to a mail merge form letter. The database could sort the information according to whether patients have PTAs greater than a particular value or have a hearing aid older than a particular value, and a mailing could go out describing the features of a new power aid.

Databases generally allow data import or export for sharing between applications. Data from a word processor or spreadsheet can be imported into the database. Information from the database could be exported to a spreadsheet. Data are not locked into a particular database. If a newer, more useful database program appears on the market, the old data could be exported to it. A database program may reside on a computer connected to a network, and the program may allow users at other computers on the network to run the program remotely, accessing data or entering information. Managing all data from the same database guards against fragmenting information over several different computers.

Presentation Programs

Presentation software helps convey ideas and images to people. Sometimes ideas are best expressed in writing. At other times pictures, diagrams, charts, or line drawings are more useful. Short video clips, animation, and sound can get points across. Presentation software facilitates the creation of multimedia. Many individuals find themselves in the role of presenter: classroom instructors giving lectures and trying to stimulate discussion, salespeople trying to present a product, members of work groups attempting to persuade managers or inform about the level of progress being made. Audiologists need to explain results of diagnostic evaluations, counsel and enable patients to understand their impairment and disability; create motivation for patients to try hearing aids or assistive devices, and explain what those devices are and how they work. Audiologists may be explaining the profession to a community group. Although putting a presentation together is never an easy task, this software is very useful for quickly creating professional-looking results.

Special Consideration

- Presentation software is not only for groups. Counseling patients, explaining a product line, and unattended waiting room kiosk viewing are other uses.

Virtually all of the computer-assisted presentations shown at conventions and workshops use Microsoft PowerPoint. The familiar slide show is a useful metaphor for understanding this application. At its simplest, PowerPoint creates a computerized version of a slide show, each computer screen being analogous to a slide. Slides can have different backgrounds with different colors and shading. Layouts define different formats for how text and graphics appear on the slides, and several templates come with the program to help design an attractive display. Different presentations have different purposes, for example, recommending a strategy, selling a product, or training in the use of a technique. A setup Wizard helps create a sample presentation based upon the purpose. A variety of media can be incorporated on the slide. Charts can be created from numerical data entered in a spreadsheet-like display and automatically placed on the slide. Pictures, photographic images, or clip art can be imported. Movies and sounds can be played from within the slide. Slide transitions and other special effects animate the presentation and help hold audience interest. Lecture notes help the speaker remember main points, and handouts can be made for the audience that contain thumbnails (miniature pictures) of the slides and room for written notes. The presentation can be printed on paper, overhead transparencies, or sent to a processing laboratory for 35 mm slides. A presentation can be made to only one or two individuals watching the computer monitor, or the computer's video out can be connected to a liquid crystal display (LCD) projector and displayed in large format for larger audiences.

The slides can be advanced manually by the presenter or in a timed mode suitable for unattended viewing, say, in a waiting room as an information kiosk. Such presentations could explain how to insert a battery, put on a hearing aid, or clean wax from a receiver tube, or offer helpful hints about communicating with persons who are hearing impaired. Audiologists may become bored with repetitive tasks or move quickly through an explanation that has been given hundreds of times. Computers are patient, don't inadvertently leave out important points, and document that a particular point (e.g., battery ingestion) was covered. A generic presentation can easily be personalized by including a digital snapshot of a patient, including the patient's name and the make/model of hearing aid. Presentations can be burned to a compact disc (CD) or printed out for the patient to take home, review, or show to family members.

Networking

The term *personal computer* aptly described early microcomputers that were stand-alone machines controlled by one person. The system's resources were not shared with anyone else. This situation has advantages (simplicity, control, and security) and disadvantages. The major disadvantage is the inability to share resources, such as programs and printers. By connecting computers in a network, data stored in a file on the hard drive of one computer can be accessed from another computer. A program on one computer can be run from another. For audiologists, this can offer significant advantages in certain situations. For example, imagine a busy dispensing office with four fitting rooms that can be used by different audiologists. Each room has a computer with software used to fit programmable hearing aids. Patient X is initially seen by audiologist A in fitting room 1. Without a network, all patient information is stored on the computer in room 1. On the next visit, patient X sees audiologist B (because audiologist A is at a satellite office) in room 2. But X's records are nowhere to be found, and unless some mechanism is in place to keep track of who is fitted where, the records could be in any one of the four fitting rooms. The situation becomes even more complicated if X decides to occasionally drop in at the satellite office. With a network, all data and fitting programs can be stored in one central location (on one computer), and each audiologist can access patient records from any one of the fitting rooms. The network can be accessed from a computer at a remote location, such as the satellite office. In an ideal situation, all pertinent information is available anywhere, anytime.

Network Topology

The original operating system for PCs, DOS, did not permit functional networking. Early network operating systems, such as Novell NetWare and LANtastic, evolved to fill this need. Microsoft's later OSs support networking, and most recent networks are Windows based. Windows XP has built-in capability for networking and conforms to the Ethernet standard. Ethernet is fast, so even though data are located on a remote computer, the illusion is that it is present on one's own computer. Physically, each computer sends a cable out to a device called a hub or router, creating a star topology, which routes the signals out to each computer. Programs and files located on other computers appear on one's own desktop, just as if they were stored locally on the hard drive. This is a basic description of what is referred to as a local area network (LAN).

Running Software over Peer-to-Peer Networks

One type of network is peer-to-peer; another uses a client–server model. In a client–server model, one computer is designated as the server, the main repository of programs and data files. The other computers (clients) access the server. Usually, the server is dedicated to supplying files and running programs for other users; the server is not for personal use. In a peer-to-peer network, all computers share the role of client or server. However, if many users are trying to access a single PC, that PC's performance slows considerably. On the positive side, a Windows XP peer-to-peer network is relatively easy to set up and practical.

Network software poses significant challenges to software developers. Problems that exist on a single computer are often multiplied when programs are run over a network. Many applications run simultaneously on a network. Programs might run fine by themselves, but an attempt to access the same resources when running at the same time may cause the system to freeze or crash. Consider several issues when running a program over the network. First, will the application accept multiple users? A multiuser database program will permit more than one person to access its information at one time. Another issue is access to individual records. The program may allow only one user access to a record at one time, or it may permit many users to read the information, but only one user (usually the first to access the record) can change the information. Security involves deciding who has privileges to access what information and restricting access by others. Scheduling information may be available to all, but sensitive financial information needs to be restricted. Only authorized personnel should have remote access privileges.

Pitfall

- Networking computers offers great possibilities. However, running software over a network poses significant challenges to software developers, especially as the network becomes more complex. Don't necessarily assume everything will run smoothly. It probably won't.

It is a challenge to keep larger networks running. Yet they have become indispensable, and critical services, such as revenue generating and programming hearing aids, require them. Large organizations hire people solely to ensure a smoothly running network. Who will administer and troubleshoot the network in a smaller office? A paid consultant? Should one or more audiologists attempt to take on the responsibility of learning network management? Will these audiologists have the time to devote to this task? Will lost productivity make the cost justifiable?

Wired versus Wireless Networks (Wi-Fi)

Wireless networks are not difficult to set up. They function in the same way as those wired with Ethernet cable. With wireless, there is no need to string wires through the office or drill holes in walls. Also, computers can be easily repositioned within a room or moved to a different office.

A wireless network has a router identical to the router used with Ethernet cable, but in addition the router has an antenna (the access point [AP]), which transmits information to any computer within a maximum distance of 100 m (300 m outside). Practically, the maximum distance can be much less due to signal attenuation by walls, metal ducts, water heaters, interference with other electronic devices, and so on. Each computer on the network needs to have a wireless adapter to detect the transmission. Most notebook computers have the adapter built in, and desktop computers can be fitted with a USB adapter. Generally, the adapter detects the transmission from the AP automatically, and connection is largely transparent to the user. A wireless network can be a mixed combination of Ethernet wired and wireless connections. Replace the existing router in a wired network with a wireless router and add PCs with wireless adapters to create a mixed network.

The current wireless standard (802.11g) operates at 2.4 gigahertz (GHz) and transmits information at 54 megabits per second (Mbps), which, although half the speed of Ethernet cable (100 Mbps), is still very fast, at least under ideal conditions. With walls and other metal obstacles separating the AP from the computer, signal strength will diminish, and reliability and connection speed are reduced, perhaps to the point of being functionally useless. One of the frustrations in setting up a wireless network is finding out that the ideal location for a computer is in a "dead spot."

Security is the other main concern. The default is for wireless routers to ship with security features disabled. This means that anyone with a wireless adapter (even outside the office) could connect to your network, with the risk of your data being compromised. Plus, the original security methods (Wi-Fi protected access [WPA]) were not particularly robust and were easily cracked by skillful hackers. However, more recent methods (WPA-2) are more secure, but most individuals find enabling the security features confusing. It is useful to consult with a knowledgeable technician when setting up a Wi-Fi network.

The Internet

The Internet has become a major force affecting how information is stored, made available to users, and accessed. The Internet, especially the World Wide Web, is growing at a very rapid pace, and with new developments occurring so quickly, it is difficult to envision what it will be like 5 years from now. However, it is extremely likely that Internet applications will continue to profoundly influence how computers are used in many professions, including audiology. It is likely that accessing the Internet will become the primary use for computers. **Table 18–1** illustrates the diversity in audiology-related information by describing a variety of Web sites.

A Brief History

What was destined to be the Internet was created in 1969 by the U.S. Defense Department's Advanced Research Projects Agency (DARPA). It was an experimental computer network (ARPAnet) connecting the campuses of the University of California at Los Angeles (UCLA), the University of California at Santa Barbara (UCBS), and the University of Utah with the Stanford Research Institute at Stanford University (now the independent nonprofit SRI International). The computers (Honeywell 516 minicomputers) were connected via high-speed (at the time, 56 kilobits

Table 18–1 Web Sites that Illustrate the Diversity of Information Available on the Internet about Audiology

Web Site/Web Page	Description
http://www.audiology.com http://www.asha.org	Web sites for the American Academy of Audiology and the American Speech-Language-Hearing Association contain information regarding issues for professionals and consumers.
http://www.mnsu.edu/comdis/kuster2/welcome.html	Judith Kuster has compiled links to a variety of audiology sites.
http://www.audiologyonline.com/	Continuing education opportunities, journal articles, and links to Web sites of interest to audiologists and consumers
http://www.audiologynet.com/	Get links to Web sites that provide information about tinnitus, Meniere's disease, acoustic neuroma, cholesteatoma, and other medical conditions.
http://www.google.com/	Search for Web sites by typing words that might appear on those Web sites.
http://www.boystownhospital.org	Boys Town National Research Hospital posts information about genetics, hearing loss, and cochlear implants.
http://www.gnresound-group.com/ http://www.starkey.com http://www.phonak.com	Get information about hearing aid products and services. Most manufacturers maintain a presence on the Web.
http://www.gnotometrics.com/products/fitting_testing/fitting/aurical.htm	Read a description of the Madsen Aurical system by GN Otometrics. Download a brochure for further information.
http://www.pubmed.gov	Do an audiology peer-reviewed literature review by searching Medline.
http://www.himsa.com/	Find out which products are NOAH certified. Get more information about NOAHlink (wireless replacement for Hi-Pro).
http://www.rcsullivan.com/www/ears.htm	Get access to hundreds of video-otoscopy images illustrating the pathology of the external and middle ear.
http://www.uwo.ca/nca/	Visit the National Centre for Audiology at the University of Western Ontario. Find out more about the desired sensation level (DSL) [i/o] procedure and where it was developed.
http://www.gennum.com	Visit Gennum Corp.'s Web site and find out more about the company's Bluetooth products and products for hearing instruments.
http://www.hearingoffice.com/	Download Hearing Office Lite, office management freeware written by an audiologist.
http://www.frye.com/	Find out about Frye Electronics Inc.'s products; also get free CD/DVDs about topics relating to hearing aid measurement.
http://www.earmold.com/	See what earmold products are available from Westone Laboratories Inc. Show the pictures to patients.
http://www.bio.net/hypermail/AUDIOLOGY/	Read postings to the bionet.audiology newsgroup.
http://www.ugr.es/~atv/web_ci_SIM/en/ci_sim_en.htm	Download an application that simulates listening through a cochlear implant.
http://www.howstuffworks.com/	Interested in finding out how technical things work? Type in "Bluetooth" for more information about this wireless technology.
http://www.infanthearing.org/	Issues involving universal newborn hearing screening, software for database management

per second [Kbps]) leased telephone lines. Researchers exchanged e-mail and data files over the network. The networking software, NCP (Network Control Protocol), was developed by Bolt, Beranek and Newman (BBN) in Cambridge MA. This "packet switching network" was able to route packets around a damaged line (e.g., the network could survive a bomb attack), and in this respect it was like the interstate highway system. For over a decade the ARPAnet grew slowly, by adding a computer every 20 days. In 1983, NCP was changed to TCP/IP (transmission-control protocol/ Internet protocol), and this is considered to be the beginning of the Internet. At this time, the military portion (Milnet) split off to form a separate network. In 1987, the National Science Foundation (NSF) expanded ARPAnet, creating the NSFnet, a high-speed "backbone" to connect five supercomputer centers across the nation (e.g., from the Massachusetts Institute of Technology to the University of San Francisco to the University of Illinois). The NSFnet charter supported research and education as appropriate uses for the Internet. Commercial use of the backbone was forbidden. Meanwhile, commercial organizations were creating similar networks (AlterNet, PSInet, etc.). In 1991, Commercial Internet Exchange (CIX), an interconnection point, was created. It merged the commercial and noncommercial networks. This was a great benefit to audiologists, considering their close interaction with hearing aid manufacturers and equipment vendors.

Tim Berners-Lee and others in 1989 at CERN (the European Particle Physics Laboratory in Geneva, Switzerland) developed HTML (hypertext markup language) and HTTP (hypertext transfer protocol), and the World Wide Web and hypermedia were born. The Web permits the transfer of rich media (i.e., text, graphics, and sound) from a host computer (running Web server software) to a remote computer running client software, a Web browser such as Internet Explorer. In 1991, the first Web server and browser went online. In January 1993, there were 50 Web servers, increasing to 4500 in May 1994. Since then, growth has been exponential. Although the Internet has been around for some time, the Web is a fairly recent development. Web access accounts for most Internet use.

HTML, HTTP, Web Sites, and Web Pages

HTML is largely responsible for the popularity and ease of use of the Internet. HTML (and its successor, extensible markup language, or XML) is a language that formats Web pages. HTTP is one of the Internet's software protocols that transport Web pages between computers. A Web site is a collection of files, in directories (folders), on the hard drive of a computer connected to the Internet. The computer hosts the Web site and runs a Web server program that serves these files to a client when requested to do so. The client software (e.g., Internet Explorer) is a Web browser program running on another Internet-connected computer. The client requests a Web page from the server, and (via HTTP) the server sends a text file (HTML document) to the client. The HTML document contains hidden tags (HTML code) that tell the browser how to format the document

(font size, centering, boldface, etc.). HTML code can also instruct the browser to request a graphics file from the server. The server downloads the picture, and the browser integrates it with the text. The Web page can look like any page out of a magazine containing colorful, stylized text and graphics.

More significantly, HTML defines hypertext, the (usually) blue, underlined text in the Web page. Click on the hypertext, and a link is invoked (in the HTML code) to another place on the Web page, another Web page, a movie or sound file (which will download), a Java applet or ActiveX control (small programs), which will download and run on your computer. HTML and HTTP allow for an interesting, interactive experience. The real possibility exists that the Internet can become a virtual extension of one's computer. The vast collection of resources existing on all the Internet-connected computers appears as though located on each individual's computer.

Viruses, Spyware, and Online Threats

With the advantage of connectivity comes intrusion in the form of viruses, Trojan horses, worms, spyware, browser hijackers, adware, and similar threats. Although each of these rogue programs causes damage, performance decline, or mere annoyance, users need to protect themselves from malicious software designed to destroy data, collect personal information and passwords, or direct browsers to Web sites of questionable content. Fortunately, Norton Antivirus (www.symantic.com) and Spy Sweeper (www.webroot.com) software are mostly effective in neutralizing these threats. Install these (or similar) products immediately when purchasing a computer that is going to be connected to the Internet, especially if using a persistent connection.

Special Consideration

- It's not too difficult to envision a time when all the computing resources of the Internet will appear to be simply an extension of one's own computer. With that advantage comes the disadvantage of viruses and spyware.

URLs, DNS, and TCP/IP

The Internet is a vast network of networks, consisting of millions of computers spread out across the world and present in most countries. The domain naming system (DNS) is responsible for keeping track of all the computers. DNS assigns a value to each computer in the form of four, 8-bit numbers separated by dots. This allows for 256^4 or ~4.3 billion unique addresses. A universal resource locator (URL) is also used to help users remember domain names. For example, the domain "205.242.230.2" is equivalent to "www.iland.net" and represents the Web server software running a Web site for an Internet service provider (ISP). The Web site could be accessed by the address "http://www.iland.net." URLs are so commonly used that it is useful to be able to decipher them. The "http:" portion of the URL indicates that the hypertext transport protocol is being used to transfer information from a Web site. There are other protocols, such as ftp, telnet, gopher, mailto, and news. The "ftp:" protocol is used for downloading files. The "telnet:" protocol is used for running programs on a remote computer, "mailto:" for sending e-mail, and "news:" for accessing a newsgroup. A gopher is a menu-based system developed at the University of Minnesota (home of the Golden Gophers) for finding and retrieving information.

The domain portion of the URL is "www.iland.net" and references the Web site. Government Web sites end in ".gov," commercial sites are ".com," organizations are ".org," and networks are ".net." Different countries have unique designations, such as ".dk" (for Denmark) and ".ca" (for Canada). The URL "http://www.frye.com/products/analyzers/ansi96-03.html" references an HTML document (a Web page) called "ansi96-03.html" located in a directory called "analyzers" embedded in the directory "products" in Frye Electronics Inc.'s Web site. Differences between the ANSI-1996 and ANSI-2003 standards of the American National Standards Institute (ANSI) are described in "ansi96-03. html."

Computers exist on the Internet for different purposes. Host computers run Web server programs accessed by client software. Other computers, routers, calculate the best route for the packets of information to reach their destination. Some of these routes are high-speed digital lines (150 Mbps), others are slower (e.g., a 28.8 Kbps modem line). Internet use is tedious when computers do not respond quickly to our requests. A brief understanding of the protocols, TCP/IP, helps to understand why this can happen. A large file sent over the Internet is disassembled at the source and reassembled at the destination. TCP divides the file into smaller parts, packets of ~1500 bytes each. Each packet has header information, information about where the packet came from and where it is going—like splitting a document into individual pages and placing each page within an addressed envelope. IP is responsible for determining the best route for the packet to reach its destination, and each packet may take a different route. Packets are analogous to cars moving down highways; heavy rush-hour traffic (a large number of packets) or a slow highway (a low-speed transmission line) can cause delays and frustration while waiting. Connecting to the Internet at high speed is a big advantage.

Connecting to the Internet

For most individuals, there are three ways to make the connection from home or work: via a dial-up, modem-based telephone connection over the lines used to place voice calls or send faxes; from a digital subscriber line (DSL), which also uses the phone lines, or from the cable (or satellite connection) used for television/video. It is also possible to connect from a network administered by a business, university, or hospital. For dial-up, the basic hardware needs are a computer, a modem, and an ordinary telephone line. The modem allows your computer to "speak" and "listen" over telephone lines. Establish an Internet account with an ISP like EarthLink which, for a monthly fee, provides a gateway to the Internet, e-mail accounts, and often space for a

small Web site. Online services (e.g., America Online [AOL] and the Microsoft Network [MSN]) provide this in addition to other services. The ISP will supply whatever software its users need to connect to the Internet and access its services. Most of this software is included with the OS. Dial-up software establishes a connection to the ISP or online service, the TCP/IP stack enables data transmission over the Internet, an e-mail program (Eudora and Pegasus Mail are free and popular, in addition to Microsoft Outlook) sends and receives messages, and a Web browser (Netscape Navigator or Microsoft Internet Explorer) downloads Web pages.

Dial-up is fairly slow. Downloading large amounts of information becomes tedious. DSL and cable are popular alternatives, offering speeds 50 times or more faster than dial-up. Exactly how fast DSL and cable are, and how they compare with one another, depends on many factors. For DSL, noisy phone lines and distances greater than 3 miles will reduce performance. Cable, though theoretically faster, shares bandwidth with other users. Performance may suffer if too many people in your "neighborhood" are active online. Both DSL and cable require special modems that make the final connection to the computer. Modem output sent to a router creates a computer network. Other computers share the Internet connection (more about networking later). In addition to the speed advantage, DSL and cable are always-on (or persistent) services. The user is constantly/instantly connected to the Internet. Dial-up users typically must take time to log on, work, then terminate the connection to free up the phone line.

E-mail and Mailing Lists

E-mail is one of the Internet's most useful activities. There is no charge for each message sent or received. Each ISP sets up an e-mail account for its users and provides an application (e.g., Eudora) that sends and receives e-mail from each address (e.g., JaneDoe@iland.net). Sending e-mail is extremely simple. Enter the address of the recipient, type a message, and click a button. The message is routed, usually in a manner of seconds, to the mail server of the recipient's ISP, where it waits to be downloaded and read. E-mail can contain styled text or appear like an HTML document. Other files can be attached (e.g., a graphics image or word processor document). E-mail can be sent to a single person or a group of people. A message can be forwarded to another person (or group of people). This flexibility enables virtually instantaneous communication with one or more people, all over the world.

People with similar interests subscribe to mailing lists to engage in the equivalent of "town hall" meetings, such as the audiology forum of the American Speech-Language-Hearing Association (ASHA). Each e-mail message sent to the forum's e-mail address is copied and sent to each other subscriber. Participants choose to actively participate in the discussion or merely observe. Any topic is possible, and discussions cover a wide range of topics, from professional issues to clinical interests. For example, an audiologist could post a message relating to a difficult case, requesting advice from forum members. Job openings and continuing education activity can be publicized. Usenet is another network dedicated to newsgroups, which are similar to mailing lists. There are over 12,000 newsgroups devoted to a variety of interests; some are audiology related: deafness, tinnitus, and so on. Bionet.audiology is the newsgroup devoted specifically to audiology issues.

Audiology-Related Web Sites and Web Logs (Blogs)

Several Web sites provide information for audiologists (see **Table 18–1**). Judith Kuster's Web page (see ASHA's Web site at www.asha.org) catalogs links to URLs covering a range of topics on hearing loss, support groups for the hearing impaired, anatomy and physiology of the hearing mechanism, disorders, diagnosis, and treatment relating to hearing loss, acoustic neuromas, Ménière's disease, inflammatory disease of the ear—the list is almost endless, a virtual library of information consisting of anything that someone wishes to make public. Some Web sites are maintained by professional organizations, such as ASHA and the American Academy of Audiology (AAA; www.audiology.org), to serve their members. Other Web sites are primarily informative or educational in nature, such as www.rcsullivan.com/www/ears. htm on video-otoscopy. Web sites devoted to commercial endeavors are a mix of marketing and educational material, or demonstration software for downloading.

"Blogging" is a fairly recent development that may interest audiologists who want to easily maintain a presence on the Internet and who may want to use the blog to remain in touch with patients. The term *blog* is a contraction of "Web log." These are essentially Websites that function like an online journal, personal diary, a collection of links, a daily pulpit, a collaborative space where people can respond to your postings, and so on. Software is freely available for easily creating and maintaining these Web sites. See www.blogger. com for an explanatory tour and how to create a blog.

Searching the Internet

There is no master directory for the Internet, but search engines help locate information, and the leading one is Google. Search engines operate by periodically visiting a very large number (millions) of Web pages, cataloging and indexing their contents, and building a large database about the contents of the Web. Sites are located by typing words or phrases into a field and searching the database; "hits" (i.e., URLs to pages containing the key words) are returned. For example, the words *syndromes Treacher-Collins bone conduction hearing aid* might produce a useful Web site about amplification for atresia. Some search engines allow Boolean search operators such as *and* and *or,* so hits would be returned on a Web page that contains all of the search terms or any of them. Searching the Internet is an art. The basic idea is to anticipate those words that are likely to appear on a Web page of interest, then search for those terms. Search engines offer "intelligent" searches, sophisticated algorithms using artificial intelligence to increase the probability of identifying useful information.

Google is an efficient tool for finding information on the Internet, even more useful than a listing of constantly changing Web sites. Have trouble remembering a URL for

Boys Town genetics information? Google "boystown genetics." More information about virtual private networks or Bluetooth technology (referred to later in this chapter) can be found in the same way.

Challenges and Opportunities

When confronted with boring, repetitive tasks, the question often arises, Can a computer program be written to do this? In theory, the following is true:

- If the program has access to all the relevant information needed to achieve an outcome, and

- If the methods necessary to achieving the desired outcome are understood well enough so that each step in the process can be stated explicitly,

- Then it is possible to write a program to accomplish the task.

Most often the answer to the question above is yes, but how much in the way of resources is one willing to commit? The reality is that practical limitations (money, time) may make it unfeasible to implement some solutions. Computerization offers great opportunities, but be aware of the challenges.

Pearl

- Don't ask, Can the computer do *this*? The answer is almost always yes. The real question is, How much time, money, and effort are you willing to spend?

Learning the Terminology

Effective computer use demands familiarity with a whole new set of concepts and ideas. Just as every little bump, curve, and crevice on the pinna has a name, hardware devices, the OS, and user interface all have names: scroll bars, menus, menu items, combo boxes, tabbed dialogs, control panels, and so on. Take the time to learn the correct names and what the objects do. The benefits become apparent when problems arise that require troubleshooting and the user finds that he or she cannot begin to explain to an expert exactly what happened. The statement "I can't 'pull up' my file" is not nearly as informative as "When I click the Start button and go to All Programs, I cannot find the Microsoft Word application." It is difficult to diagnose the problem without an accurate description of the symptoms. Imagine trying to describe a hearing loss without using the terms *frequency, decibel,* and *threshold* accurately.

Pearl

- Make an effort to learn the terminology used to describe the computer and the operating system. When things go wrong, nobody can help unless you can accurately describe the problem.

Attitudes about Computers

Attitudes bias how computers are used. Some people are vaguely fearful and mistrust computers; some openly admit to being intimidated. Others embrace the computer with the trusting abandon of a child discovering a new toy. The first group finds many reasons, which are little more than excuses, for not using computers, even if the benefits are compelling and obvious. The latter group finds computers fascinating devices. However, they may develop complex, time-consuming, computer-based systems when a manual solution is more efficient. Analyze the practical impact the computer will have on completing the task with the ultimate goal of improving patient service. Will it be accomplished sooner, more efficiently, reduce the number of errors, save money, free personnel from boring or repetitive tasks, and allow personnel to engage in other, more productive activities?

Feasible Solutions?

Is computerization an appropriate solution to a problem? To answer this question, adopt a global perspective of how this solution fits into the overall work flow in the clinic. Make a detailed analysis of how the job is performed, where it is performed, which steps are taken in what sequence to complete the job, and see if there are any major problems. The task can be more complex than initially anticipated. The issue may be whether or not to automate audiologic report writing. Clinical data used to generate a report come from many sources and separate pieces of equipment, often spread out in different physical locations. Case history information may begin with written comments from the patient (or the patient's chart) entered on a paper form. Answers to additional questions are jotted down by the audiologist on another piece of paper. Or perhaps the computer is located where the case history information is taken, and the patient's comments are entered directly into the computer. Data from the audiometer may be manually transferred to a paper audiogram, speech thresholds and word recognition scores may be written on a form, tympanograms and acoustic reflex data may be printed directly from the tympanometer, OAE may be stored in a data file and printed on paper, and images from a video-otoscope are archived on paper from the video printer. And the list could go on.

A custom database could hold all this information. Fields store demographic information, numerical values for test results, and text describing patient history, impressions, and recommendations. Graphics, such as the audiogram, can be created from the numerical data, or a scanner can create a digital representation of the paper image for insertion in the database. To search the database for a graphic, a field with a text description could accompany the image. The database should be flexible enough for entry of all relevant information, perhaps even a self-report questionnaire on hearing aid satisfaction, or the results and accompanying letter from an outside referral source. Otherwise, patient information would have to be maintained in two separate locations, a paper file and an electronic file. If the audiology clinic is part of a larger organization, all information may have to be output to paper anyway.

This situation poses significant challenges to creating a comprehensive system of electronic records. Modest goals are more reasonable. Data are generated at different locations, and computers are not located at each location. Most audiometric equipment does not generate information in the proper format. Too much information comes from outside sources, and there is no control over the format in which the data are received. It would take an inordinate amount of time to type, or retype, information, scan images, and create one's own custom database software, assuming that an off-the-shelf program does not exist to integrate all information. Devising a system that is flexible enough for even present needs, and capable of anticipating future needs, is a daunting task. Analyze why all this information needs to be collected: To what practical use will it be put? Will there be a future savings in time and efficiency by storing this information, or will the data never be accessed again?

The Ideal Computer-Based System

It is very likely that comprehensive computer-based systems will evolve for managing the flow of information through the audiology clinic. The following are some ideas that may prove useful for evaluating programs.

♦ Consider the amount and type of data the practice generates and how the software will accommodate them. Visualize all the information that appears in the charts, and think of how the application will deal with it. Even something audiologists regard as simple, such as an audiogram, is complex when viewed from a programmer's perspective. Sixteen different symbols can be generated for each frequency for air- and bone-conduction thresholds for each of two ears, masked and unmasked, response and no response. Convention dictates our expectations of how information will be displayed (e.g., in a table, graph, or narrative form).

♦ Automate data entry from external equipment (e.g., audiometers, immittance devices, and hearing aid analyzers) into the database application. A considerable time savings can be realized if data can be sent directly to the computer via a network connection or a USB port.

♦ Integrate data from different devices, or applications. For example, audiogram information should be available to probe-microphone verification systems.

♦ Organization and reporting of data should be flexible. Will the software allow user-defined fields? Can field names be changed? For example, if there is a field labeled "Word Discrimination," can it be changed to "Word Recognition"?

♦ Consider the scope of the practice in terms of all the procedures that are performed and what software solutions are available for each. Does software integrate well with other packages, such as scheduling and accounting? Ideally, these applications will exchange information. Otherwise, time will be wasted in retyping data. Hosford-Dunn et al (1995) provide a detailed description of procedures that could be automated in a hypothetical audiology practice: patient and customer care activities (including audiologic testing), scheduling, record keeping, planning, correspondence, hearing aid fitting, maintaining product logs and reports, accounting and billing, marketing, and communications.

◆ The same information should be entered only once. The software should be "smart" enough to find information already stored (e.g., a name and address) so the user does not waste time repeatedly providing the system with information it already knows. Minimizing redundancy reduces chances for making errors, as well as saves time.

Pearl

• "Smart" software does not waste your time asking for the same information twice. Minimizing redundancy also reduces chances for making errors.

• The application should automate tasks and not require the audiologist to perform calculations easily made by the computer, such as categorizing degree of hearing loss based on PTA.

• The potential exists for more complex data analysis, the application of artificial intelligence, based on results from the literature. As examples, the likelihood of middle ear effusion is predictable from a combination of the peak admittance and tympanogram slope; the probability that an ABR's wave V latency being outside the normal range can be calculated, based on the patient's age.

• The program should give feedback if unusual or erroneous conditions exist. Audiometry is a repetitive task, and people tend to make errors. A message could alert the audiologist to a discrepancy between the speech reception threshold (SRT) and the PTA, an interoctave frequency that should be tested, or an air–bone gap that suggests masking.

• Does purchase of the program force the clinic to continue with a system long past its usefulness? Once a system is running smoothly, people are loath to change for fear the change will cause errors. Updating to a new system always creates major and minor glitches. Companies go out of business, and product support may no longer exist. An application that dominates the market one year may be obsolete a few years later. An ideal system allows for exporting and importing data, the ability to choose among vendors, and flexibility to purchase new modules without compromising the integrity of the entire system.

◆ Dispensing and Office Management

The previous sections of this chapter discussed computer usage for audiology in a general sense. Computer and computer applications are an essential part of the audiology practice. From the time a patient makes the first contact with the practice, computers and the information entered into the applications provide the audiologist with the tools to assure the highest quality patient care.

The Patient Database

Key to efficient patient management is an effective patient database. This database stores all aspects of patient information. For the database to be useful, the data need to be easily accessible and the procedures for using the data easy to implement. The following sections describe the general features of databases.

Patient Information

The database consists of a record for each patient. Each record contains many fields of information. Most databases are relational. That means certain data are stored in a separate file for each patient. An example: Patient A has a specific record; A's hearing aid information is stored in one file, and his insurance information is stored in another. Both of these files relate to A's patient record. Relational databases manage data more efficiently.

Each record contains basic patient information, such as name, address, phone number, date of birth, Social Security number, and spouse's name. The related files of this record could contain information about insurance, type of hearing aid, audiometrics, contact numbers, and other pertinent information. The key is to have this information readily available for each patient at the click of a mouse.

Pitfall

• The client database is the heart of a practice. Before investing time and money in an office management system (OMS), be sure that it meets the clinic's needs. Ask specific questions, and find out if a demonstration is available.

Standardized Data Entry

Another key component of an efficient database is data entered consistently into each field, no matter who enters the data. A search or query is done to retrieve information from the database. The information in the search field determines if a particular patient record is selected from the query. Therefore, each field's data must be consistent from record to record for the search to be valid. An example would be a field containing a referral source, for example, "Yellow Pages." One patient's file had the entry "YP," another's had "Yellow Pages." The entries need to be consistent so that a search will locate all files. The database manager establishes the data entry protocol from the beginning.

Available Database Systems

There are specific OMSs available for the audiology practice. A system that works fine in one practice, however, might not be practical for another. A good online resource is www.audiologysoftware.com. This site provides a review of available audiology software programs, current costs, and pros and cons of each system.

Manufacturer-Supported Systems

Currently, there are two hearing instrument manufacturers that offer and support OMSs. Starkey Laboratories Inc. (Eden Prairie, Minnesota) offers the ProHear OMS. Siemens Hearing Instruments Inc. has Practice Navigator OMS. Both of these systems have been available for several years, and both companies are well established in the industry. The Web site www.audiologysoftware.com reviews these products; information is also available on the manufacturers' Web sites. Most hearing instrument manufacturers do not offer OMSs because of the cost of development and ongoing support.

Independently Supported Software

There are three programs that are offered and supported by independent companies. TIMS (Total Information Management System) for audiology is a NOAH integrated system that has been available for several years. The company also offers systems for other professions. HearForm from HearForm Software LLC (Caldwell, Idaho) was written by practitioners specifically for the audiology/hearing aid industry.

The third independent system is new and unique to the industry. Sycle.net is a Web-based OMS that was also developed with a lot of input from industry practitioners. Because it is Web-based, the user does not purchase any software but pays a monthly subscription fee. This eliminates the need for software upgrades.

Other Systems

Some practitioners have taken it upon themselves to develop their own systems. Unless a professional is well versed in programming, a programmer must be employed to write the code and provide upgrades. These programs are usually not offered for sale because the private practice developer does not want the commitment of supporting the product. Hearing Office Lite (www.hearingoffice.com) is an example.

Another approach is to purchase off-the-shelf software and adapt it to the audiology practice. ACT! by Sage Software is a contact database management system that is used by many sales and service organizations. The program is very flexible and can be easily adapted. Because it is so widely used, there is very good support available. Several medical OMSs are available. However, although these programs are very good for third-party billing, they are not readily adaptable for audiology specifically.

Considerations for Selecting a System

In selecting a database system, you must first determine what you want the system to do in your practice setting, Then you must determine the budget available for the

system. Select a program that is flexible enough to fit your specific needs. Consider the ongoing costs of support and upgrades to the system. Also, be certain that the company and the support will be there when needed.

Uses of the Patient Database

After establishing the database, the information can be used for a variety of marketing, patient care, and storage operations. Information retrieved from the database can be customized to facilitate such operations.

Scheduling

Most OMSs feature built-in scheduling, eliminating the need for an additional scheduling program. The patient's name is pulled from the database and inserted into the schedule. Many of these systems automatically record an appointment history for each patient. Multiple scheduling is needed if the practice has several professionals.

Marketing

Marketing to current patients and prospects is essential to retaining patients and increasing patient referrals. This effort, referred to as internal marketing, provides improved patient care by keeping patients informed of new technologies, updating the status of hearing needs, and generating follow-up care reminders. One common internal marketing effort is sending patient reminders for yearly follow-up visits. Lists can be generated using "last visit" or "last test" fields. Patients are sent a personalized letter or card to remind them of the service offered, or office personnel can phone patients as a reminder. Other internal marketing efforts, such as offering new technology information and special savings on accessories, are easily done using patient databases.

Data Analysis

Patient databases prove to be essential management tools, allowing the generation of customized reports. For example, searches of a database can be done to generate reports on such focuses as repair information on hearing aids, hearing aid models, degree of hearing loss, and most recent visits.

Financial Management

Financial management is another important aspect of excellent patient care. All practices, whether private or otherwise, must be profitable to remain in business and continue to provide patient services. There are many accounting and bookkeeping applications.

Most of the previously mentioned OMSs contain or integrate with a financial package, and QuickBooks by Intuit Software (Mountain View, CA) is the application of choice. It is easy to implement and provides all the financial information necessary to manage a practice; additionally, the company provides excellent support. Other applications are available; consult with your accountant to select the most appropriate system for the practice.

Another aspect of financial applications is third-party billing. Many professionals choose to contract with a billing service to do insurance billing. If you choose to do in-house billing, there are several software packages available. Considerations in choosing a billing package are integration with the practice's bookkeeping system and meeting Health Insurance Portability and Accountability Act (HIPAA) privacy regulations.

Programmable Hearing Aids

Programmable hearing instruments currently represent ~90% of the market in the United States (Strom, 2005). One industry solution is a proprietary, stand-alone device—for example, Widex's LP2 (Widex A/S, Vaerloese, Denmark) or GN ReSound's P3 (GN ReSound, Bloomington, Minnesota)—that connects to individual manufacturers' hearing aids. Programmable hearing aids from Micro-Tech Hearing Instruments (Eden Prairie, Minnesota) interface to a PC card. This credit card–sized device inserts into a PC slot on a personal digital assistant (PDA). A PDA is an interesting choice for an interface because it offers so much extra functionality: converting handwritten notes to typed reports, faxing, drawing, word processing, spreadsheet, address book, appointment calendar, and other features. Unfortunately, audiologists dispensing from several manufacturers collect several functionally redundant devices. Another approach is for the manufacturer to develop programming software to run on an industry-standard PC. An interface box connecting the hearing aid to the PC is still required, but the box can be used with many brands of hearing aids.

Even with such a universal programming solution, practical problems exist. Hearing aid dispensing happens within a broader context of office management (patient records, scheduling, billing, accounting, marketing, etc.), and audiologists do not want their patient data spread out among several different databases. So it would be burdensome and inefficient for each manufacturer to create a complete suite of applications. NOAH and Hi-Pro (hearing instrument programmer) were developed as solutions to these problems.

NOAH

NOAH is a software integration platform, a Windows application developed by the Hearing Instrument Manufacturers' Software Association (HIMSA) that runs on standard PCs. NOAH is purchased through the manufacturers who sell NOAH products. HIMSA's Web site (www.himsa.com) maintains a current list of manufacturers, compatible (certified) software applications, and instruments. The Hi-Pro universal programming interface from GN Otometrics (Taastrup, Denmark) connects to the PC's serial port. NOAHlink is a wireless (Bluetooth) version of Hi-Pro. Programmable hearing aids connect to Hi-Pro (or NOAHlink) via proprietary cables supplied by manufacturers. The Hi-Pro box programs any hearing aid from a NOAH-compatible manufacturer. NOAH provides rudimentary database functions, but it mostly serves as a gateway to software modules written by

other manufacturers. These software modules have access to the NOAH database, and NOAH allows the modules from different manufacturers to share information. The software modules fit the general categories of audiologic equipment, hearing aid fitting, and OMSs. Most software development has occurred in the hearing aid fitting category, and NOAH is currently functioning primarily as a tool for fitting programmable hearing aids. It is important to stress that NOAH's potential is not limited to just this function. NOAH software modules can be developed for controlling or communicating with any type of device: clinical audiometer, immittance audiometer, video-otoscope, evoked potential, or otoacoustic emission (OAE) equipment. Software modules written for comprehensive office management functions can have direct access to data generated by the audiologic equipment. A manufacturer would be free to focus on one aspect of audiologic management, develop hardware and software for meeting a need, yet still have its product fit into a broader context of data management.

<table>
<tr><td>**Pitfall**</td></tr>
<tr><td>• Although some audiologic equipment interfaces with the computer via a USB port, most use the serial port. Typical computers have only one or, at most, two available ports. An AB switch can be attached to a serial port so that different devices can be selected manually. These devices cannot provide information to the computer simultaneously, for example, when a hearing aid is programmed at the same time real ear measures are taken.</td></tr>
</table>

NOAH has five basic modules. The client module collects demographic information, such as name, address, phone number, birth date, and referral source. The audiometry module allows point-and-click entry of audiogram thresholds and entry of numerical values, such as speech audiometric and immittance data. Audi-Link permits installation of audiometer drivers for data to be sent directly to NOAH. The selection of New Hearing Instrument Module displays a screen showing all the installed manufacturers' software fitting modules. Clicking a manufacturer's logo launches that software. A NOAH fitting module collects general information (make, model, battery, earmold, etc.) from manufacturers that have not developed fitting software. Patients fit with these aids can still be included in the database. The measurement selection module is where software is launched for controlling any audiologic equipment modules that are installed (audiometers, probe-microphone systems, etc.). Once a client has been selected, the journal module provides basic word-processing tools for storing written comments. The NOAH 2.0 version is no longer supported by HIMSA. The current version, NOAH 3.6, is written for the Windows platform and is the only version supported by HIMSA.

Electronic Transmission of NOAH Actions (eTona) and iScan

The NOAH eTona system is an emerging technology HIMSA developed to expedite the process of ordering hearing aids.

Traditionally, an ear impression and paper order form were mailed to the hearing aid manufacturer. Siemens introduced iScan at the 2005 AAA convention. With iScan, the impression is placed in a chamber and laser scanned, and its digitized dimensions are transmitted to the manufacture via the Internet. The order form is replaced by eTona, and each manufacturer develops its own software version as a NOAH module (Ingrao, 2005).

There are several potential advantages to using this system, a major one being improved turn-around time, because the ear impression does not need to be physically shipped. Additionally, earmold remakes do not require a new impression (unless the reason for the remake was a poor initial impression), and paper order forms, with their inherent tendency to be filled out inaccurately, are eliminated. The software checks to make certain incompatible options have not been selected, for example, ordering a completely in the canal (CIC) hearing aid with a telecoil. Also, there is no issue about the order form being out of date. The status of an order can be tracked online, and the order can be integrated with inventory and accounting functions.

Fitting Software

Manufacturers update software each time a new instrument is introduced. Programming software is typically developed to run under the NOAH platform as well as a stand-alone version. Software must meet the needs of various countries as well as different levels of user sophistication. New software should be backward compatible with older hearing aid models.

The Windows' graphical user interface provides a consistent, easily understood, virtual control panel for adjusting programmable hearing aids. There are a number of options for how this control panel may appear because there are many manufacturers and even more programmable hearing aids. Each hearing aid has different electroacoustic characteristics, so each instrument has different parameters to adjust. Instruments have different numbers of bands, channels, and memories. Compression thresholds, compression ratios, attack and release times, overall gain, output, gain in the band or channel, crossover frequency—all of these have the potential for being variable. Virtual controls (push buttons, trim pots, sliders, etc.) are created in software to manipulate these parameters. With well-designed software, the function of the control is obvious by its appearance. Frequency responses, input-output functions, conventional audiograms, and sound pressure level (SPL) audiograms may be used to illustrate the effects of manipulating the controls.

Pearl

- Applications for fitting programmable hearing aids use Windows to create a virtual control panel. How to use the controls should be obvious with well-designed software.

Software will often give a picture of the hearing aid and a brief description of its important features. An audiogram may display the current patient's hearing loss superimposed over the fitting range of the instrument. Some software will suggest a particular model of hearing aid. The software may proceed in a series of ordered steps, helping the dispenser follow a logical sequence. Once a particular aid is selected, usually there are several different prescriptive procedures to choose from; NAL-R and DSL[i/o] are popular options, but the manufacturer may have custom algorithms. The target (or level-dependent targets) may be displayed along with the simulated output of the hearing aid, either in 2 cc coupler or real ear terms. Changing the parameters typically produces a change in the aid's gain, and it is easy to visualize how closely the target is met. There may be an "autofit" option to automatically adjust the aid's parameters to achieve a best match to the target. The manufacturer may provide other tools for visualizing the effect of the chosen frequency response. The audible and inaudible areas of the ACL speech spectrum may overlay the audiogram thresholds, or an AI value could be calculated.

Some fitting software permits loudness scaling so that the patient's subjective preferences are factored into the target. Categorical loudness scaling methods are popular, similar to those used with the Independent Hearing Aid Fitting Forum (IHAFF) contour procedure or the loudness growth in half-octave bands (LGOB) test. Loudness matching may require a software interface to external hardware that is capable of generating stimuli, such as an audiometer or a real ear measurement system, but some hearing aids generate their own signals for in situ measurements. Another option is for calibrated signals to be presented in the sound field while the gain (within the channel) of the hearing aid is adjusted to reach an appropriate loudness level relative to normal. If the fitting system is interfaced with a probe-microphone system, then real ear verification of targets can be performed. The actual, rather than simulated, effect of manipulating the hearing aid's controls can be visualized directly on the computer screen. Similarly, connecting a hearing aid test box will permit adjusting the aid to 2 cc targets, as is recommended for children with the desired sensation level procedure. The software may permit real ear unaided gain (REUG) and real ear-to-coupler difference (RECD) to be determined for the individual, thereby customizing conversions.

Several fitting systems take advantage of the computer's multimedia capability to play digitized sound from a CD-ROM, or stored as MP3 files on the hard drive. Listening environments are simulated using low- or high-level speech, dishes clattering, traffic noise, or music to help the new hearing aid user judge the appropriateness of the fitting. Adjustments can be made to the hearing aids while the patient responds to the selected sounds. Other applications provide objective documentation of aided improvement in speech intelligibility. The Hearing in Noise Test for Windows (HINT/Windows) is a PC-based application distributed by Starkey in CD-ROM format. HINT presents sentences in speech-spectrum noise to simulate typical listening in noisy environments where sound is coming from spatially separated sources. The software enables automatic test administration, scoring, and reporting. HINT/Windows, with a proprietary sound-processing card, can also perform audiometry and data management (see the discussion in Telehealth below).

Self-report questionnaires, such as the Abbreviated Profile of Hearing Aid Benefit (APHAB) and Client-Oriented Scale of Improvement (COSI), may be part of the fitting software. The computer collects, archives, analyzes, and displays data. Multimedia computers enable Clear Speech, a training technique for improving intelligibility through modifying speaking style. A fitting program can play recorded materials that demonstrate this technique and print instructions and practice exercises that family members can take home (Schum, 1997). A variety of other material can be printed. Journal entries are maintained in the database or printed for inclusion in a paper file. The patient can take home a printed custom user manual to reinforce points made during counseling. Even an order form can be printed.

The fitting software may have special features, such as an automatic feedback test. The instrument's gain is automatically increased until feedback is present, allowing a hearing aid with an automatic volume control feature to "know" its limits for increasing gain. Troubleshooting user complaints is another process that is automated by some fitting software. A series of multiple-choice questions are asked, and the program recommends specific changes in the aid's parameters based on the nature of the complaint. Some software detects unusual or improbable combinations of settings and warns the dispenser. The software may be compatible with another manufacturer's database, allowing those aids to be fitted. Binaural corrections can be applied, automatically reducing gain by a fixed amount (usually 4–6 dB). The effect of earmold acoustics may be simulated and entered into the display of the frequency response. Because so many different features are offered by different manufacturers, and because these features are likely to change with software updates, it is important for audiologists to comparison shop to make sure the fitting software offers the right mix of features.

◆ Other Applications

There are other applications for audiology that do not deal with hearing aid fitting or managing the dispensing office. Some do not fit neatly into any major category. The computer-based tinnitus evaluation system is an example (Lay and Nunley, 1996). This system consists of a PC, digital audio board, patient headphones, and a module for mixing, attenuating, and amplifying. It can be used for matching the pitch and loudness of tinnitus and for generating noise bands to mask tinnitus. Initially, computer-assisted audiometry was just an automated system for determining threshold. Kunov et al (1997) describe a system that combines five devices: a clinical audiometer, immittance, evoked responses, and transient and distortion product OAE equipment. Data generated from the different

modules can be stored in a database and shared over a network.

Computer-Assisted Audiometry

Currently, computer-assisted audiometry systems, such as Siemens' Unity, Affinity and Equinox from Interacoustics A/S(Minneapolis, Minnesota), and the Avant system from MedRx Inc., represent the state of the art. Typically, they combine several common functions: audiometry, otoscopy, hearing instrument testing, and conventional real ear probe-microphone measures, along with visible speech displays in real time. The technology behind these systems, surprisingly, is not new. In 1987, as part of Project Phoenix, Nicolet developed the first true digital hearing aid, and the Aurora test system was designed as a necessary component to a comprehensive fitting protocol. Aurora's main modules contained an audiometer, real ear measurement device, hearing aid analyzer, and database. A PC-based middle ear analyzer was able to send data to the database via a serial port. A PC ran disk operating system (DOS) applications. There are several possible reasons why the audiologic community did not accept the system, but soon after its introduction, the project folded. Perhaps rumors of its demise became a self-fulfilling prophecy, or perhaps, for its time, it was "too far ahead of the curve."

Most manufacturers now offer audiometers with an RS-232 serial or USB interface. Software is available for data transfer from the audiometer to the computer. An example is DSL/Fonix Link software that integrates Frye Electronics Inc. (Tigard, Oregon) products to a standard PC. Thresholds from the audiometer are available to the DSL software, and targets are shared with the hearing aid analyzer and probe-microphone system. Interacoustics manufactures a whole family of audiometers and a middle ear analyzer that are NOAH compatible (www.interacoustics.com).

Picard et al (1993) demonstrated that computer-assisted audiometry produced reliable thresholds in children as young as 7.5 years and adults up to age 80. This system had been in use prior to 1987. Despite its fairly long history, there are no ANSI standards for computerized audiometry, including automated procedures. An ANSI working group, S3:76, is dealing with this issue. The most common protocol to automate is the familiar Hughson-Westlake procedure "down 10 and up 5 dB." Computers can be more than just a virtual control panel for operating equipment. They also can be expert systems, where intelligent decision making is incorporated into the hardware/software.

The Audiometer Operating System

An excellent example of a system that offers helpful decision support is the Audiometer Operating System (AOS) developed at the Massachusetts Eye and Ear Infirmary (Thornton et al, 1993). AOS software, running on a PC in a DOS environment, controls all functions of an audiometer via the serial port. It supports several common, commercially available audiometers. The software is entirely aware of the state of the audiometer (i.e., which stimuli are set to be delivered to which ears). AOS can change the state of the audiometer and deliver signals, much as a human operator could. Unlike a human operator, however, AOS has instant access to the relevant audiologic literature. It "knows," for example, actual interaural attenuation values, rather than just the 40 dB value that is easy to remember. Two major areas that are addressed by AOS are masking and word recognition testing (Halpin et al, 1996). Masking has long been recognized as a concept that is both difficult to understand and technically challenging to administer. AOS turns masking on automatically when it is needed, adjusts levels properly according to available air and bone thresholds, and searches for a plateau. This frees the tester from having to recall the theory and memorize constants. The system records detailed information to prepare accurate reports for the computer-generated audiogram. Thornton (1993) maintains that this system is so successful that technicians can be employed for routine testing, without sacrificing quality. Audiologists can spend more time using their professional training for patient evaluation and management.

Special Consideration

- AOS intelligently assists the audiologist during masking and word recognition testing. It "knows" when peripheral hearing loss cannot account for poor speech understanding.

Speech recognition testing is a unique feature of AOS. The intelligibility of speech is calculated using the AI. Given the level of the speech (knowing its spectrum) and the amount of hearing loss, it is possible to compute intelligibility. A predicted performance-intensity function is derived, along with estimates of normal variability. The level where PB-max should occur is calculated, and words are presented at that level. Masking can be delivered to the contralateral ear, taking into account such variables as interaural attenuations for each frequency, air–bone gaps, and band sensation level of speech. A masking level can be selected that is just high enough to drive intelligibility to zero in the contralateral ear. The actual word recognition score can be compared with the predicted score to determine if a statistically significant difference exists. A difference would indicate that some factor, other than the audiogram's effect on audibility, is compromising the auditory system. Further investigation could rule out a possible central auditory processing disorder (CAPD) or retrocochlear lesion.

Automating Special Tests

CASRA (Computer-Assisted Speech Recognition Assessment) was developed to minimize problems associated with conventional speech testing (Gelfand, 1997). A major problem in speech recognition testing is that the limited number of words typically used (25 or 50 item lists) affects the practitioner's ability to interpret small differences in performance. For example, 92% correct would require a score less than 72% in the other ear to be significant at the

95% confidence level. CASRA solves this problem by presenting 450 items to the listener (150 words, 3 phonemes per word) in 50 three-word combinations. Each test item is displayed on the computer screen. The examiner simply clicks each incorrectly repeated phoneme; the computer keeps track of the errors and scores the test.

Bochner et al (1997) described the Speech Sound Pattern Discrimination test as a computerized, adaptive delivery system. A mathematical model is used to select test items that, based on the subject's previous responses, are appropriate in terms of level of difficulty. The system is useful for evaluating the auditory capabilities of the deaf. Using the virtual audiometer, McCullough et al (1994) described a multimedia approach to assessing word recognition for speakers of Spanish. Two monitors were used. In the control room, the computer displayed a list of words. The tester initiated a trial by selecting a word. In the test booth, a picture showing four test foils was drawn on the second monitor. By observing the patient's pointing behavior, the audiologist automatically scores the item by clicking a mouse. Myers et al (1996) used a computer-based system for presenting octave-band filtered sound effects. Such stimuli have been suggested as being more appropriate for testing children. CAST (Classification of Audiogram by Sequential Testing) is a computer-mediated form of visual reinforcement audiometry (Merer and Gravel, 1997). The technique uses a sophisticated mathematical model to predict a child's audiogram from fewer stimuli than are conventionally required. The technique appears to be useful for testing children aged 6 months to 5 years. Game audiometry is incorporated into the ProDigit 2000.

Using standard software that is part of both Windows and Apple Macintosh operating systems, it is fairly easy to present any type of sound recorded on audio CDs. Standard speech recognition materials and assessment of (CAPDs) can be performed using the CDs produced by the Department of Veterans Affairs. Sound effects and competing messages can be played from Micro Sound Products Party Noise CD. Auditec will produce custom-recordable CDs, potentially containing a wide variety of useful materials. Newby and Popelka (1992) described a system using an Apple Macintosh and HyperCard for presenting speech stimuli. In our clinic, speech recognition materials have been digitized and stored on the hard drive of a Mac or PC located in our test booth. Custom software was developed to play the words in sequence with a user-selectable time delay between presentations. Alternatively, any test item could be presented at random by clicking on the word. The audio output of the computer was inputted to the audiometer in the same manner as a tape deck. Standardized, recorded speech stimuli can be presented with the flexibility of live voice (de Jonge, 1992). Stach et al (1998) found that when a computer is used to manually present recorded speech, there is about a 22% time savings, when compared with delivering speech with a fixed time interval. Other software was developed to facilitate the administration of the frequency pattern test. One of six sequences of tones is randomly selected (hi-hi-lo, lo-hi-lo, lo-lo-hi, etc.). The tester presents the sequence by clicking the mouse, and correct-incorrect responses are tallied automatically by the software, which also contains material describing the test protocol and its interpretation.

Pearl

- Under computer control, digitized words are presented with the flexibility of monitored live voice and the standardization of recorded speech.

The SCAN-C and SCAN-A (available from Oaktree Products Inc.) are screening procedures for detecting CAPD in children and adults. Like many tests for CAPD, the audiologist must remember quite a bit of detail regarding test setup, administration, and norms for scoring. With the SCAN, responses must be tallied and raw scores converted to standard scores (based on the child's age), then converted to percentiles and age equivalents. There are many opportunities for mistakes to occur and results to be misinterpreted. ScanWare is a Windows program that, once raw data are entered, completes the scoring. Tables summarizing patient performance are displayed, and a narrative report is generated. The report can be printed directly or stored in a file to be read by a word-processing program. Considering the difficulty in administering and interpreting a CAPD test battery, it seems that this is one area ripe for computerization.

Managing Newborn Screening Programs

There are approximately 4 million children born in the United States each year, with hearing loss affecting an estimated 24,000. The goal of universal hearing screening is to test each child using automated ABR, transient evoked OAE (TEOAE), or distortion product OAE. As Albright and Finitzo (1997) have noted, however, "detection is a costly exercise if there is a poor design for follow-up services." Follow-up is essentially a matter of information management, and 4 million children would generate a prodigious amount of information. It is inconceivable for manual systems or paper logbooks to handle the job of managing screening of such a large population. In addition to the consequences of lost opportunity for early intervention, unidentified children with hearing loss pose the threat of litigation. Computerized screening programs are the perfect solution. They can be used to track which babies have been screened and which still need to be screened; schedule rescreening and diagnostic ABRs, along with behavioral and medical evaluations; and send reminders of upcoming appointments. Pediatricians and parents can be sent letters informing them of the results of the screen and subsequent diagnostic evaluation. People managing the program need data analyzed and reported in a useful manner for monitoring key quality indicators of the program (White, 1996).

In 1993, Rhode Island mandated the first comprehensive statewide universal newborn hearing screen. The Rhode Island Hearing Assessment Project (RIHAP) used RI-Track, a custom-designed DOS-based dBase IV database for managing its statewide TEOAE screening program. Using this information management system had a positive effect on the program. After implementing the computer tracking application, the percentage of successful rescreens increased from 77 to 94% (Johnson et al, 1993).

Finitzo and Diefendorf (1997), reporting the results of a national survey of infant screening programs, indicated that 50% of the programs used a computerized data management system. Of those using software, 47% indicated that it reduced the workload. Some of the programs were custom designed, such as RI-Track. Others used Hi-Track, Hi-Screen, and Hi-Data, which are offered by the National Center for Hearing Assessment and Management (NCHAM). Other programs include the Screening and Information Management System (SIMS) and eScreener Plus (ESP), sold by Oz Systems (Arlington, Texas; www.oz-systems.com). Bio-logic Systems Corp. (Mundelein, Illinois) developed another database management program, the Infant Screening Database. The Hi-Track software is a comprehensive package covering virtually all aspects of a screening program. The software, which originally ran in a DOS environment, now runs under Windows (as do all others); there is also a Web-enabled version that does not require software installation, so it can be run from any location with Internet access (ESP from Oz Systems is another Web-based product). The software links to state databases, interfaces with a variety of screeners, including their software, does scheduling, generates reports and physician letters, can be networked, and offers secure data transfer. NCHAM maintains an extensive Web site (www.infanthearing.org) providing useful information regarding all aspects of a newborn screening program.

Aural Rehabilitation and Hearing Conservation

Cochlear Implants, Aural Rehabilitation, and Computer-Assisted Interactive Video

The measurement and interpretation of an electrically evoked auditory response in the initial selection of candidates for cochlear implants require the use of computers. The subsequent fitting and follow-up fine tuning of the cochlear implant are facilitated by software and hardware very similar to that used in the fitting of programmable hearing aids. The computer screen becomes the control panel used to adjust implant parameters, so that a wide range of incoming sound is within the user's dynamic range, for as many channels as possible. SCLIN for Windows software is used to fit the Clarion cochlear implant. SCLIN is an example of how software can enhance fitting techniques for young children. To program a cochlear implant, ideally, thresholds and most comfortable levels (MCLs) would be obtained for all channels. This information, however, may be missing for young children. SCLIN allows channel settings to be interpolated from data obtained on only one or two other channels. Also, children can have difficulty with the concept of loudness, especially for tonal stimuli, so live-voice stimuli can be used to adjust MCLs. The software allows limits to be set for the volume control, and the memories of the processor can be programmed for different listening environments.

Aural rehabilitation, following implantation, is important for developing auditory skills such as sound detection, discrimination, identification, and comprehension. This is particularly true for children who are active in learning language and acquiring speech skills. Children often do not have the advantage of an extensive "auditory database" enjoyed by postlingually deafened adults. Cochlear Corp. (Englewood, Colorado) distributes a CD-ROM software program, Foundations in Speech Perception, for children with moderate to profound hearing losses, including those using cochlear implants. The program, for children aged 3 to 12 years, is designed to help with both speechreading and auditory training. Computer-assisted interactive video (CAIV) was first used in a system called DAVID (Dynamic Audio Video Interactive Device). DAVID consisted of a computer-controlled videotape player. The software would find video clips of sentences, which students were supposed to speechread. Responses were typed on the keyboard, or a selection was made using a multiple-choice format. Lessons progressed from easy to more difficult as fewer contextual cues were provided (Sims et al, 1979). As videodisc technology emerged, it was incorporated into DAVID, replacing the slower videotape system. Several CAIV systems, generally similar in concept to DAVID, were later developed. (See Sims and Gottermeier, 1995, for a review.) Laser videodisc technology, as described by Tye-Murray (1996), may help to encourage more time spent in aural rehabilitation activities. The high-quality video (and audio) images, which can be played via computer control, make videodiscs a natural medium for developing speechreading and auditory training exercises (Sims, 1988). The DVD format is capable of storing the equivalent of a full-length motion picture on a disk the size of a standard CD-ROM. It has largely replaced the older videodisc format and has become standard equipment in new PCs. A training station includes a video player, a computer, and speakers. A touch-screen monitor provides a more natural way for patients to interact with the computer, avoiding problems with typing commands or learning to use a mouse. The computer determines which items are presented and the sequence. The aural rehabilitation program described by Tye-Murray (1996) focused on training for audiovisual recognition of speech, practice in using conversational repair strategies, and communication strategies for patients' spouses and family members. The program provides a full range of analytic and synthetic activities designed to promote effective communication in a variety of natural listening environments. The therapy experiences can operate with the audiologist present or absent, and the software can track performance and display progress reports. While the hearing aid fitting is taking place, family members can receive instructions on appropriate and inappropriate speaking behaviors. Sweetow and Henderson-Sabes (2004) developed a system called Listening and Communication Enhancement (LACE). Distributed on CD, it is a home-based, interactive computer program designed to facilitate the development of auditory skills following hearing aid fitting. The underlying assumption is that the auditory system is plastic and can be modified to improve performance.

Therapy is done for 30 minutes a day over a period of 4 weeks. The patient listens to stimuli (e.g., speech in noise, time-compressed speech) and responds, and the computer adapts to the accuracy of the response. For example, if a word is correctly identified at $+2$ dB signal-to-noise ratio (SNR), the level is reduced, and another stimulus is presented. In addition to degraded speech, other areas of the program focus on cognitive skills and communication strategies. The program will graph daily performance, and the results are transmitted to a Web site where the audiologist can monitor and modify training.

> **Special Consideration**
>
> - Audiologists may use their time more productively with CAIV. Unattended aural rehabilitation therapy is possible for the patient. Also, while the patient is engaged in a hearing aid fitting, family members can receive instruction on appropriate communication behaviors.

Hearing Conservation Programs

The Occupational Safety and Health Administration (OSHA) is the federal agency charged with protecting workers' safety and health, including hearing in industrial environments. The Occupational Noise Exposure standard (29 CFR 1910.95) defines what is an effective hearing conservation program (HCP). The standard specifies virtually every aspect of an HCP, what measurements need to be made and when, the tests that must be given and the actions taken, and specific records that need to be kept for each worker. Since noise is so pervasive in industry, and millions of workers are in HCPs, the amount of data is very large. OSHA requires that specific records be maintained for each worker. For instance, noise exposure levels must be determined, and appropriate attenuation values for hearing protectors must be calculated. Calibration records for audiometers must be stored along with ambient noise levels within the test suite. Employees must be scheduled for baseline and annual audiograms. Each year the annual audiogram must be saved and compared with the baseline. Corrections for the effects of aging can be looked up from a table, and applied. Standard threshold shifts have to be calculated. Employees found to have hearing loss are rescheduled for follow-up audiometry or scheduled for diagnostic evaluations. The standard requires that employees receive timely, written documentation of changes in their hearing. Letters have to be written to referral sources. An OSHA form 300 must be filed depending on whether specific criteria are met. In short, a database must be maintained. There are several programs that are commercially available to handle this (**Table 18–2**).

HCP applications usually interface directly with an audiometer for direct data transfer and function in a networked environment. The programs are designed to automate paperwork and to lower administrative costs. They can record case history information, generate personalized employee notification letters and retest lists, schedule

Table 18–2 Hearing Conservation Software Programs and Manufacturers of Compatible Audiometers

Application	Manufacturer
Employee Audiometric Reporting System (EARS)	Digital Hearing Systems Corp. www.dhsc.com/ears.htm
Occupational Health Manager (OHM)	Unique Software Solutions Inc. www.ohmsoftware.com
HEAR/TRAK	HAWKWA Group Inc. hawkwa@mindspring.com
XM Network	Examinetics Inc. www.examinetics.com
CT (Computer Aided Testing) Audiometric Testing Software	TK Group Inc. www.tkontheweb.com/cat.htm
Audiometers with serial ports for direct input to hearing conservation industrial testing software	Micro Audiometrics Corp. www.microaud.com
Audiometric Surveillance software module	Workplace Group www.workplacegroup.net

employee hearing tests, analyze trends in audiometric data, measure program performance, create reports—in general, handle the requirements dictated by the occupational noise standard. Industrial hygienists are often responsible for monitoring and safeguarding workers from all sorts of hazardous exposures, including noise. Consequently, some applications, such as Occupational Health Manager (OHM) from Unique Software Solutions Inc. (Colorado Springs, Colorado), include hearing conservation as only one of several components of the program. OHM maintains information about all areas of each employee's health.

A key issue in selecting software involves giving the tester access to pertinent information at the time of the test. Ideally, programs should present the individual's baseline, the most recent annual audiogram, and expected thresholds for different gender and race groups. Programs should also be able to export data for special evaluations, such as the type of audiometric database analysis specified in ANSI S12.13 TR-2002. This is a standard offering guideline for evaluating the effectiveness of HCPs. Audiogram thresholds are tracked over time for a large number of employees who are exposed to noise. The standard identifies statistical procedures that can be used to compare the noise-exposed group to a control group. Audiometric variability (the year-to-year variability in a population's thresholds) is a valid indicator of the effectiveness of the HCP. Results for the noise-exposed group should not be greater than the control group.

Ford Motor Co.'s technical consultant to the National Institute for Occupational Safety and Health (NIOSH) tested the HEAR/TRAK software from HAWKWA Group Inc. (Grayslake, Illinois) with a public domain database of over 5000 people and 150,000 audiograms (over 8 serial tests). Ford purchased the software for use in 60 plants in the United States. The system was described as being complete, stable, networked to the company's mainframe, and capable of handling ~75 000 hearing tests each year.

Telehealth

Telehealth can be as simple as traditional correspondence by mailer or as complex as video compression available over the Web. Even remote surgery using robotics is a possibility. The major benefit of telehealth is improving access to health care, by linking people needing services with those professionals who are qualified to provide them. Telehealth involves removing barriers created by geography and improving the efficient use of providers' time.

Staab et al (1997) describe remote teleprogramming (RTP), a service that could potentially improve patient management. With RTP, a hearing aid's remote control acts as the instrument's programmer. The remote receives its instructions acoustically (dual-tone multifrequency), either from loudspeakers attached to a computer or from a standard telephone. The dispenser can change the aid's programming remotely by sending signals to the patient via a modem/telephone or broadband connection. Eliminating the need for an office visit could save both the patient and the audiologist time and money. Care could be given to patients who are less ambulatory or those who are experiencing problems with their hearing aid while on business trips or vacation. Also, the hearing aid could be programmed while the patient is at home or in a particularly troublesome listening situation.

Pearl

- In the future, audiologists may routinely use broadband connections to remotely program patients' hearing aids, perform diagnostic procedures, and counsel patients using real-time video and audio connections.

Video-otoscopy is another area where possibilities exist for remote patient management. Physicians, whether they are physically present or not, can visualize conditions of the external/middle ear. Images from a video-otoscope can be captured by computer, compressed, and transmitted to a remote location via the Internet. The images could be uploaded to a Web site or sent as attachments to an e-mail message. An audiologist testing in a remote area, using a portable video-otoscope, computer, and modem, could consult with a physician, either online or off.

Database software is available for storing images. TeleMedRx from MedRx is Windows software for database management: image acquisition from the video-otoscope, transmission, archiving, printing, and generating reports. Fields are set up so comments can be written to define the images, permitting database searches for images with particular characteristics (e.g., middle ear effusion, ventilation tube, or exostosis). Starkey's StarView includes a record-keeping system. Voice recognition software is controlled in a "hands-off" mode (see Kay, 1998, for a review of voice recognition software). Ear Vision is Windows software that performs similar database functions. Images can be resized or rotated, and written or live-voice comments are stored.

The possibilities for novel treatment paradigms are intriguing. Consider the following scenario. A host computer with high-speed access to the Internet, at a distant location (call-in location A), is running software that allows it to be controlled remotely by a computer at location B. The computer at location A has diagnostic equipment interfaced to it (video-otoscopy, audiometer, OAE, ABR, etc.), and a technician or aide is present to assist with speculum positioning, earphone placement, and similar physical activities. The computer at location A is also running conferencing software to transmit (and receive), in real time, audio and video images to (and from) location B. The audiologist at location B can control the diagnostic testing at location A, just as if he or she were operating the computer directly at location B. Moreover, the audiologist can hear, see, and speak to the patient. The patient (and technician) can also hear, speak, and listen to the audiologist.

Software and hardware currently exist to implement just such a virtual office (see the February 2005 issue of *Seminars in Hearing*). The ViGO system consists of a microphone, camera, and speaker. When interfaced with VCON Meeting Point software, two-way remote communication and computer control are possible. This system has been used for universal newborn hearing screening, testing speech in noise using the HINT, performing pure-tone audiometry, and diagnostic ABR. Results obtained off-site have been documented to be equivalent to those obtained on-site.

However, there are legal, technical, and reimbursement issues related to telepractice (Denton and Gladstone, 2005). The same standard of care should be provided regardless of the delivery method. Support personnel need to be trained and used appropriately, state laws for licensure must be respected, and privacy needs to be maintained. A virtual private network can ensure data privacy when transmitted over the Internet, so HIPAA guidelines can be met. Meeting licensure laws can be more difficult. Currently, the professional treating a patient must be licensed to practice in the state where the patient is physically located. Licensure boards have traditionally been reluctant to permit "outsiders" easy access to "their" patients. The issue is complicated by the possibility that the outsider may not be just an audiologist from an adjacent state, but a willing provider from another country.

◆ Summary

As recently as 1991, computers were not even mentioned as a basic equipment need in audiologic practice (Teter and Schweitzer, 1991). Since that time, there has been a steady increase in computer use. In a needs survey by AAA, over 65% of the academy's members indicated a desire for hands-on training with common computer systems and software (Van Vliet, 1997). ASHA's *Guidelines for Education in Audiology Practice Management* include the use of computers for office automation as one of six specific competency areas. Computer use competency includes diagnostic applications, data storage and access, tracking patient outcomes and consumer satisfaction, professional correspondence, scheduling and billing, and marketing applications. Computer use is becoming common in virtually all areas of audiology. The use of well-designed software holds the promise of allowing audiologists to work more effectively and productively. With computers handling more routine tasks, audiologists can spend more time helping their patients, thus making the practice of audiology even more satisfying.

References

Albright, K., & Finitzo, T. (1997). Texas hospitals' quality control approach to universal infant hearing detection. American Journal of Audiology, 6, 88–90.

Bochner, J., Garrison, W., Palmer, L., & MacKenzie, D. (1997). A computerized adaptive testing system for speech discrimination measurement: The speech sound pattern discrimination test. Journal of the Acoustical Society of America, 101(4), 2289–2298.

de Jonge, R. R. (1992). HyperCard: A tool for computer-aided instruction in audiology. Journal for Computer Users in Speech and Hearing, 8, 137–147.

Denton, D. R., & Gladstone, V. S. (2005). Ethical and legal issues related to telepractice. Seminars in Hearing, 26(1), 43–52.

Fausti, S. A., Schaffer, H. I., Olson, D. J., Frey, R. H., & Henry, J. A. (1993). Software for managing multi-site auditory research. Audiology Today, 5(3), 22–25.

Finitzo, T., & Diefendorf, A. O. (1997). The state of the information. American Journal of Audiology, 6, 91–94.

Gelfand, S. A. (1997). Essentials of audiology. New York: Thieme Medical Publishers.

Halpin, C., Thornton, A., & House, Z. (1996). The articulation index in clinical diagnosis and hearing aid fitting. Current Opinion in Otolaryngology and Head and Neck Surgery, 4, 325–334.

Hosford-Dunn, H., Dunn, D. R., & Harford, E. R. (1995). Audiology business and practice management (pp. 171–195, 235–261). San Diego, CA: Singular Publishing Group.

Ingrao, B. B. (2005). E-business: Connecting hearing care professionals and their suppliers. Hearing Review, 12(9), 18–22.

Johnson, C. D., Benson, P. V., & Seaton, J. B. (1997). Educational audiology handbook. San Diego, CA: Singular Publishing Group.

Johnson, M. J., Maxon, A. B., White, K. R., & Vohr, B. R. (1993). Operating a hospital-based universal newborn hearing screening program using transient evoked otoacoustic emissions. Seminars in Hearing, 14(1), 46–55.

Kay, R. (1998). Do you hear what I say? [software review]. Byte, 23(1), 115–116.

Kunov, H., Madsen, P. B., & Sokolov, Y. (1997). Single system combines 5 audiometric devices. Hearing Journal, 50(3), 32, 34.

Lay, J., & Nunley, J. (1996). Computer-based tinnitus evaluation system. Hearing Instruments, 47(3), 46.

McCullough, J. A., Wilson, R. H., Birck, J. D., & Anderson, L. G. (1994). A multimedia approach for estimating speech recognition of multilingual clients. American Journal of Audiology, 3(1), 19–22.

Merer, D. M., & Gravel, J. S. (1997). Screening infants and young children for hearing loss: Examination of the CAST procedure. Journal of the American Academy of Audiology, 8, 233–242.

Myers, L. L., Letowski, T. R., Abouchacra, K. S., Kalb, J. T., & Haas, E. C. (1996). Detection and recognition of octave-band sound effects. Journal of the American Academy of Audiology, 7, 346–357.

Newman, C. W., Jacobson, G. P., Weinstein, B. E., & Sandridge, S. A. (1997). Computer-generated hearing disability/handicap profiles. American Journal of Audiology, 6(1), 17–21.

Picard, M., Ilecki, H. J., & Baxter, J. D. (1993). Clinical use of BOBCAT: Testing reliability and validity of computerized pure-tone audiometry with noise-exposed workers, children and the aged. Audiology, 32, 55–67.

Radcliffe, D. (1996). The computer-enhanced office and clinic: Fitting technology to consumer needs. Hearing Journal, 49(9), 15–16, 19, 22, 24, 26.

Schum, D. J. (1997). The use of advance fitting software in the counseling process. Hearing Review, 4(2), 57–58, 62.

Shennib, A., Lanser, M., & Omidvar, F. (1994). Personal digital audiometry: A new dimension in testing. Hearing Instruments, 45(3), 17–18, 20, 39.

Sims, D. G. (1988). Video methods for speechreading instruction. Volta Review, 90, 273–288.

Sims, D. G., & Gottermeier, L. (1995). Computer-assisted interactive video methods for speechreading instruction: A review. In G. Plant & K. E. Spens (Eds.), Profound deafness and speech communication. London: Whurr Publishers.

Sims, D. G., Von Feldt, J., Dowaliby, F., Hutchinson, K., & Myers, T. (1979). A pilot experiment in computer assisted speechreading instruction utilizing the data analysis video interactive device (DAVID). American Annals of the Deaf, 124(5), 618–623.

Staab, W. J., Edmonds, J., & Garcia, H. (1997). Remote teleprogramming (RTP): Future directions to patient management. Hearing Review, 2(Suppl.), 50–52.

Stach, B. A., Davis-Thaxton, M. L., & Jerger, J. (1998). Improving the efficiency of speech audiometry: Computer-based approach. Journal of the American Academy of Audiology, 6, 330–333.

Strom, K. E. (2005). A look at the 2004–2005 hearing instrument market. Hearing Review, 12(3), 18.

Sweetow, R. W., & Henderson-Sabes, J. (2004). The case for LACE. Hearing Journal, 57(3), 32–35, 38.

Teter, D. L., & Schweitzer, H. C. (1991). Hearing aid dispensing. Audiology Today, 3(5), 32–35.

Thornton, A. (1993). Computer-assisted audiometry and technicians in a high-volume practice. American Journal of Audiology, 2(3), 11–13.

Thornton, A. R., Halpin, C., Han, Y., & Hou, Z. (1993). The Massachusetts Eye and Ear audiometer operating system. Unpublished manuscript.

Tye-Murray, N. (1996). Laser videodisc technology in the aural rehabilitation setting: Good news for people with severe and profound hearing impairments. In R. L. Schow & M. A. Nerbonne (Eds.), Introduction to audiologic rehabilitation (3rd ed., pp. 516–521) Boston: Allyn & Bacon.

Van Vliet, D. (1997). AAA member CE needs survey summary. Audiology Today, 9(3), 17.

White, K. R. (1996). Universal newborn hearing screening using transient evoked otoacoustic emissions: Past, present, and future. Seminars in Hearing, 17(2), 171–183.

Zapala, D. (1998). The virtual audiogram. Retrieved from http://www. concentric.net/~kellytc/viraud.htm

Appendix I

Three Professional Organizations' Codes of Ethics

American Academy of Audiology Code of Ethics

◆ Preamble

The Code of Ethics of the American Academy of Audiology specifies professional standards that allow for the proper discharge of audiologists' responsibilities to those served, and that protect the integrity of the profession. The Code of Ethics consists of two parts. The first part, the Statement of Principles and Rules, presents precepts that members of the Academy agree to uphold. The second part, the Procedures, provides the process that enables enforcement of the Principles and Rules.

◆ Part I: Statement of Principles and Rules

Principle of Ethics I

Members shall provide professional services and conduct research with honesty and compassion, and shall respect the dignity, worth, and rights of those served.

Rule 1a: Individuals shall not limit the delivery of professional services on any basis that is unjustifiable or irrelevant to the need for the potential benefit from such services.
Rule 1b: Individuals shall not provide services except in a professional relationship, and shall not discriminate in the provision of services to individuals on the basis of sex, race, religion, national origin, sexual orientation, or general health.

Principle of Ethics II

Members shall maintain high standards of professional competence in rendering services.

Rule 2a: Members shall provide only those professional services for which they are qualified by education and experience.
Rule 2b: Individuals shall use available resources, including referrals to other specialists, and shall not accept benefits or items of personal value for receiving or making referrals.
Rule 2c: Individuals shall exercise all reasonable precautions to avoid injury to persons in the delivery of professional services or execution of research.

Rule 2d: Individuals shall provide appropriate supervision and assume full responsibility for services delegated to supportive personnel. Individuals shall not delegate any service requiring professional competence to unqualified persons.
Rule 2e: Individuals shall not permit personnel to engage in any practice that is a violation of the Code of Ethics.
Rule 2f: Individuals shall maintain professional competence, including participation in continuing education.

Principle of Ethics III

Members shall maintain the confidentiality of the information and records of those receiving services or involved in research.

Rule 3a: Individuals shall not reveal to unauthorized persons any professional or personal information obtained from the person served professionally, unless required by law.

Principle of Ethics IV

Members shall provide only services and products that are in the best interest of those served.

Rule 4a: Individuals shall not exploit persons in the delivery of professional services.
Rule 4b: Individuals shall not charge for services not rendered.
Rule 4c: Individuals shall not participate in activities that constitute a conflict of professional interest.
Rule 4d: Individuals using investigational procedures with patients, or prospectively collecting research data, shall first obtain full informed consent from the patient or guardian.

Principle of Ethics V

Members shall provide accurate information about the nature and management of communicative disorders and about the services and products offered.

Rule 5a: Individuals shall provide persons served with the information a reasonable person would want to know about the nature and possible effects of services rendered, or products provided or research being conducted.
Rule 5b: Individuals may make a statement of prognosis, but shall not guarantee results, mislead, or misinform persons served or studied.

Rule 5c: Individuals shall conduct and report product-related research only according to accepted standards of research practice.

Rule 5d: Individuals shall not carry out teaching or research activities in a manner that constitutes an invasion of privacy, or that fails to inform persons fully about the nature and possible effects of these activities, affording all persons informed free choice of participation.

Rule 5e: Individuals shall maintain documentation of professional services rendered.

Principle of Ethics VI

Members shall comply with the ethical standards of the Academy with regard to public statements or publication.

Rule 6a: Individuals shall not misrepresent their educational degrees, training, credentials, or competence. Only degrees earned from regionally accredited institutions in which training was obtained in audiology, or a directly related discipline, may be used in public statements concerning professional services.

Rule 6b: Individuals' public statements about professional services, products, or research results shall not contain representations or claims that are false, misleading, or deceptive.

Principle of Ethics VII

Members shall honor their responsibilities to the public and to professional colleagues.

Rule 7a: Individuals shall not use professional or commercial affiliations in any way that would limit services to or mislead patients or colleagues.

Rule 7b: Individuals shall inform colleagues and the public in a manner consistent with the highest professional standards about products and services they have developed or research they have conducted.

Principle of Ethics VIII

Members shall uphold the dignity of the profession and freely accept the Academy's self imposed standards.

Rule 8a: Individuals shall not violate these Principles and Rules, nor attempt to circumvent them.

Rule 8b: Individuals shall not engage in dishonesty or illegal conduct that adversely reflects on the profession.

Rule 8c: Individuals shall inform the Ethical Practice Committee when there are reasons to believe that a member of the Academy may have violated the Code of Ethics.

Rule 8d: Individuals shall cooperate with the Ethical Practice Committee in any matter related to the Code of Ethics.

Courtesy of the American Academy of Audiology.

Academy of Doctors of Audiology Code of Ethics

◆ Preamble

The Code of Ethics of the Academy of Doctors of Audiology has as its purpose the assurance of the highest quality of professional service rendered to those served. Each member of the Academy shall abide by this Code of Ethics. The six fundamental principles of this Code relate to each member's responsibility to the welfare of those served, to professional standards, to products and services, to public information, and to professional growth and involvement.

Principle of Ethics I

To Protect the Welfare of Persons Served Professionally

Rules of Ethics

1. Academy members shall use all resources, including those of other professionals, to provide the best possible service.
2. Members shall fully inform clients of the nature and possible results of services rendered and products sold.

a. Members shall not misrepresent benefits of any therapeutic procedure of professional services.
b. Members shall not misrepresent benefits from use of hearing instruments or other assistive listening products.
c. Members may make reasonable statements of prognosis for both products and services, but particular care must be taken not to mislead clients to expect results that cannot be predicted or expected.
d. Members shall not prescribe, fit or recommend products or services which are known, or suspected to be harmful to the client's hearing or well being without full disclosure to the client.
3. Members shall inform clients of the recommended services or products and any reasonable alternatives in a manner which allows the client to become involved in, and make informed, treatment decisions.
4. Members shall evaluate services and products rendered to determine effectiveness.
5. Members shall not release professional and personal information obtained from the client without the written permission of the client in accordance with applicable state and federal law.

6. Members shall not discriminate in the delivery of professional services on the basis of sex, marital status, age, religious preferences, nationality or race, or handicapping condition.

Principle of Ethics II

To Maintain High Standards of Professional Competence, Integrity, Conduct and Ethics

Rules of Ethics

1. Members shall provide only those clinical services for which appropriate licensure, certification or special training has been obtained.
2. Members shall state their professional credentials and provide supporting documentation on request.
3. Members shall engage in continuing professional education activities throughout their careers.
4. Members shall not permit clinical services to be provided by any staff member who is not properly prepared nor delegate services requiring the direct supervision of an audiologist to anyone unqualified to provide such services.
5. Members' clinical judgment and practice must not be determined by economic interest in, commitment to or benefit from, professionally related commercial enterprises.
6. Members agree to govern their professional activities by this Code of Ethics. Unethical practice shall be any action that violates the spirit or letter of this Code of Ethics.
   a. Members shall report to the Board of Directors of the Academy of Doctors of Audiology® (or to its designees) and violation of this Code.
   b. Members shall cooperate with any authorized inquiry or action the Board may undertake.
7. Members shall conduct business affairs in a manner consistent with all applicable state and federal regulations.

Principle of Ethics III

To Maintain a Professional Demeanor in Matters Concerning the Welfare of Persons Served

Rules of Ethics

1. Products associated with professional practice must be dispensed to the client as part of a program of comprehensive habilitative care.
2. Members shall provide only those procedures, products and services that, according to the member's best professional judgment, are in the best interests of the client.
3. Members shall recommend products and services only after careful assessment and documentation of the client's physical, social, emotional and occupational needs.
4. Members must provide full disclosure of the fees/prices of products and services. This information must be disclosed by providing a comprehensive schedule of fees to the client, to the best extent possible, in advance of providing services and products.

Principle of Ethics IV

To Provide Accurate Information to Persons Served and to the Public about the Nature and Management of Auditory Disorders and about the Profession and Services Provided by Its Members

Rules of Ethics

1. Members must not misrepresent their training or competence.
2. Members' public statements about services or products must not contain false, deceptive or misleading information.
3. Promotional activities used by members shall comply with applicable state and federal laws, rules and regulations.

Principle of Ethics V

To Engage in Conduct Which Shall Enhance the Status of the Profession

Rules of Ethics

1. Members must honor their responsibility to the public, their profession and their colleagues.
2. Members shall educate the public about hearing, hearing loss, and services and products which can benefit affected individuals.
3. Members shall educate the public about matters related to professional competence.
4. Members shall strive to increase knowledge within the profession and share such knowledge with colleagues.
5. Members shall establish harmonious relationships with professional colleagues and must not injure by false criticism, directly or indirectly, the character, qualifications, services, fees or products of another professional.

Principle of Ethics VI

To Maintain Ethical Standards and Practices of the Academy of Doctors of Audiology

Rules of Ethics

1. Members agree to govern their professional activities by this Code of Ethics.
2. Members agree to report to the Board of Directors for the Academy of Doctors of Audiology® (or to its designees) any violations of the Code of Ethics, and to cooperate with any authorized inquiry or action the Board may undertake.

Reprinted with permission from the Academy of Doctors of Audiology.

American Speech-Language-Hearing Association Code of Ethics

◆ Preamble

The preservation of the highest standards of integrity and ethical principles is vital to the responsible discharge of obligations by speech-language pathologists, audiologists, and speech, language, and hearing scientists. This Code of Ethics sets forth the fundamental principles and rules considered essential to this purpose.

Every individual who is (a) a member of the American Speech-Language-Hearing Association, whether certified or not, (b) a nonmember holding the Certificate of Clinical Competence from the Association, (c) an applicant for membership or certification, or (d) a Clinical Fellow seeking to fulfill standards for certification shall abide by this Code of Ethics.

Any violation of the spirit and purpose of this Code shall be considered unethical. Failure to specify any particular responsibility or practice in this Code of Ethics shall not be construed as denial of the existence of such responsibilities or practices.

The fundamentals of ethical conduct are described by Principles of Ethics and by Rules of Ethics as they relate to the conduct of research and scholarly activities and responsibility to persons served, the public, and speech-language pathologists, audiologists, and speech, language, and hearing scientists.

Principles of Ethics, aspirational and inspirational in nature, form the underlying moral basis for the Code of Ethics. Individuals shall observe these principles as affirmative obligations under all conditions of professional activity.

Rules of Ethics are specific statements of minimally acceptable professional conduct or of prohibitions and are applicable to all individuals.

Principle of Ethics I

Individuals shall honor their responsibility to hold paramount the welfare of persons they serve professionally or participants in research and scholarly activities and shall treat animals involved in research in a humane manner.

Rules of Ethics

A. Individuals shall provide all services competently.
B. Individuals shall use every resource, including referral when appropriate, to ensure that high-quality service is provided.
C. Individuals shall not discriminate in the delivery of professional services or the conduct of research and scholarly activities on the basis of race or ethnicity, gender, age, religion, national origin, sexual orientation, or disability.
D. Individuals shall not misrepresent the credentials of assistants, technicians, or support personnel and shall inform those they serve professionally of the name and professional credentials of persons providing services.
E. Individuals who hold the Certificates of Clinical Competence shall not delegate tasks that require the unique skills, knowledge, and judgment that are within the scope of their profession to assistants, technicians, support personnel, students, or any nonprofessionals over whom they have supervisory responsibility. An individual may delegate support services to assistants, technicians, support personnel, students, or any other persons only if those services are adequately supervised by an individual who holds the appropriate Certificate of Clinical Competence.
F. Individuals shall fully inform the persons they serve of the nature and possible effects of services rendered and products dispensed, and they shall inform participants in research about the possible effects of their participation in research conducted.
G. Individuals shall evaluate the effectiveness of services rendered and of products dispensed and shall provide services or dispense products only when benefit can reasonably be expected.
H. Individuals shall not guarantee the results of any treatment or procedure, directly or by implication; however, they may make a reasonable statement of prognosis.
I. Individuals shall not provide clinical services solely by correspondence.
J. Individuals may practice by telecommunication (for example, telehealth/e-health), where not prohibited by law.
K. Individuals shall adequately maintain and appropriately secure records of professional services rendered, research and scholarly activities conducted, and products dispensed and shall allow access to these records only when authorized or when required by law.
L. Individuals shall not reveal, without authorization, any professional or personal information about identified persons served professionally or identified participants involved in research and scholarly activities unless required by law to do so, or unless doing so is necessary to protect the welfare of the person or of the community or otherwise required by law.
M. Individuals shall not charge for services not rendered, nor shall they misrepresent services rendered, products dispensed, or research and scholarly activities conducted.
N. Individuals shall use persons in research or as subjects of teaching demonstrations only with their informed consent.
O. Individuals whose professional services are adversely affected by substance abuse or other health-related conditions shall seek professional assistance and, where appropriate, withdraw from the affected areas of practice.

Principle of Ethics II

Individuals shall honor their responsibility to achieve and maintain the highest level of professional competence.

Rules of Ethics

A. Individuals shall engage in the provision of clinical services only when they hold the appropriate Certificate of Clinical Competence or when they are in the certification process and are supervised by an individual who holds the appropriate Certificate of Clinical Competence.
B. Individuals shall engage in only those aspects of the professions that are within the scope of their competence, considering their level of education, training, and experience.
C. Individuals shall continue their professional development throughout their careers.
D. Individuals shall delegate the provision of clinical services only to: (1) persons who hold the appropriate Certificate of Clinical Competence; (2) persons in the education or certification process who are appropriately supervised by an individual who holds the appropriate Certificate of Clinical Competence; or (3) assistants, technicians, or support personnel who are adequately supervised by an individual who holds the appropriate Certificate of Clinical Competence.
E. Individuals shall not require or permit their professional staff to provide services or conduct research activities that exceed the staff member's competence, level of education, training, and experience.
F. Individuals shall ensure that all equipment used in the provision of services or to conduct research and scholarly activities is in proper working order and is properly calibrated.

Principle of Ethics III

Individuals shall honor their responsibility to the public by promoting public understanding of the professions, by supporting the development of services designed to fulfill the unmet needs of the public, and by providing accurate information in all communications involving any aspect of the professions, including dissemination of research findings and scholarly activities.

Rules of Ethics

A. Individuals shall not misrepresent their credentials, competence, education, training, experience, or scholarly or research contributions.
B. Individuals shall not participate in professional activities that constitute a conflict of interest.
C. Individuals shall refer those served professionally solely on the basis of the interest of those being referred and not on any personal financial interest.
D. Individuals shall not misrepresent diagnostic information, research, services rendered, or products dispensed; neither shall they engage in any scheme to defraud in connection with obtaining payment or reimbursement for such services or products.

E. Individuals' statements to the public shall provide accurate information about the nature and management of communication disorders, about the professions, about professional services, and about research and scholarly activities.
F. Individuals' statements to the public—advertising, announcing, and marketing their professional services, reporting research results, and promoting products—shall adhere to prevailing professional standards and shall not contain misrepresentations.

Principle of Ethics IV

Individuals shall honor their responsibilities to the professions and their relationships with colleagues, students, and members of allied professions. Individuals shall uphold the dignity and autonomy of the professions, maintain harmonious inter-professional and intra-professional relationships, and accept the professions' self-imposed standards.

Rules of Ethics

A. Individuals shall prohibit anyone under their supervision from engaging in any practice that violates the Code of Ethics.
B. Individuals shall not engage in dishonesty, fraud, deceit, misrepresentation, sexual harassment, or any other form of conduct that adversely reflects on the professions or on the individual's fitness to serve persons professionally.
C. Individuals shall not engage in sexual activities with clients or students over whom they exercise professional authority.
D. Individuals shall assign credit only to those who have contributed to a publication, presentation, or product. Credit shall be assigned in proportion to the contribution and only with the contributor's consent.
E. Individuals shall reference the source when using other persons' ideas, research, presentations, or products in written, oral, or any other media presentation or summary.
F. Individuals' statements to colleagues about professional services, research results, and products shall adhere to prevailing professional standards and shall contain no misrepresentations.
G. Individuals shall not provide professional services without exercising independent professional judgment, regardless of referral source or prescription.
H. Individuals shall not discriminate in their relationships with colleagues, students, and members of allied professions on the basis of race or ethnicity, gender, age, religion, national origin, sexual orientation, or disability.
I. Individuals who have reason to believe that the Code of Ethics has been violated shall inform the Board of Ethics.
J. Individuals shall comply fully with the policies of the Board of Ethics in its consideration and adjudication of complaints of violations of the Code of Ethics.

Reprinted with permission from American Speech-Language-Hearing Association (2003). Code of ethics (revised). Available from www.asha.org/reference.

Appendix II

Three Professional Organizations' Scopes of Practice

American Academy of Audiology Scope of Practice

1. Statement of Purpose

The purpose of this document is to define the profession of audiology by its scope of practice. This document outlines those activities that are within the expertise of members of the profession. This Scope of Practice statement is intended for use by audiologists, allied professionals, consumers of audiologic services, and the general public. It serves as a reference for issues of service delivery, third-party reimbursement, legislation, consumer education, regulatory action, state and professional licensure, and inter-professional relations. The document is not intended to be an exhaustive list of activities in which audiologists engage. Rather, it is a broad statement of professional practice. Periodic updating of any scope of practice statement is necessary as technologies and perspectives change.

2. Definition of an Audiologist

An audiologist is a person who, by virtue of academic degree, clinical training, and license to practice and/or professional credential, is uniquely qualified to provide a comprehensive array of professional services related to the prevention of hearing loss and the audiologic identification, assessment, diagnosis, and treatment of persons with impairment of auditory and vestibular function, and to the prevention of impairments associated with them. Audiologists serve in several roles including clinician, therapist, teacher, consultant, researcher and administrator. The supervising audiologist maintains legal and ethical responsibility for all assigned audiology activities provided by audiology assistants and audiology students.

The central focus of the profession of audiology is concerned with all auditory impairments and their relationship to disorders of communication. Audiologists identify, assess, diagnose, and treat individuals with impairment of either peripheral or central auditory and/or vestibular function, and strive to prevent such impairments.

Audiologists provide clinical and academic training to students in audiology. Audiologists teach physicians, medical students, residents, and fellows about the auditory and vestibular system. Specifically, they provide instruction about identification, assessment, diagnosis, prevention, and treatment of persons with hearing and/or vestibular impairment. They provide information and training on all aspects of hearing and balance to other professions including psychology, counseling, rehabilitation, and education. Audiologists provide information on hearing and balance, hearing loss and disability, prevention of hearing loss, and treatment to business and industry. They develop and oversee hearing conservation programs in industry. Further, audiologists serve as expert witnesses within the boundaries of forensic audiology. The audiologist is an independent practitioner who provides services in hospitals, clinics, schools, private practices, and other settings in which audiologic services are relevant.

3. Scope of Practice

The scope of practice of audiologists is defined by the training and knowledge base of professionals who are licensed and/or credentialed to practice as audiologists. Areas of practice include the audiologic identification, assessment, diagnosis, and treatment of individuals with impairment of auditory and vestibular function, prevention of hearing loss, and research in normal and disordered auditory and vestibular function. The practice of audiology includes:

A. Identification

Audiologists develop and oversee hearing screening programs for persons of all ages to detect individuals with hearing loss. Audiologists may perform speech or language screening, or other screening measures, for the purpose of initial identification and referral of persons with other communication disorders.

B. Assessment and Diagnosis

Assessment of hearing includes the administration and interpretation of behavioral, physioacoustic, and electrophysiologic measures of the peripheral and central auditory systems. Assessment of the vestibular system includes administration and interpretation of behavioral and electrophysiologic tests of equilibrium. Assessment is accomplished using standardized testing procedures and appropriately calibrated instrumentation and leads to the diagnosis of hearing and/or vestibular abnormality.

C. Treatment

The audiologist is the professional who provides the full range of audiologic treatment services for persons with impairment of hearing and vestibular function. The audiologist is responsible for the evaluation, fitting, and verification of amplification devices, including assistive listening devices. The audiologist determines the appropriateness of amplification systems for persons with hearing impairment, evaluates benefit, and provides counseling and training regarding their use. Audiologists conduct otoscopic examinations, clean ear canals and remove cerumen, take ear canal impressions, select, fit, evaluate, and dispense hearing aids and other amplification systems. Audiologists assess and provide audiologic treatment for persons with tinnitus using techniques that include, but are not limited to, biofeedback, masking, hearing aids, education, and counseling.

Audiologists also are involved in the treatment of persons with vestibular disorders. They participate as full members of balance treatment teams to recommend and carry out treatment and rehabilitation of impairments of vestibular function.

Audiologists provide audiologic treatment services for infants and children with hearing impairment and their families. These services may include clinical treatment, home intervention, family support, and case management.

The audiologist is the member of the implant team (e.g., cochlear implants, middle ear implantable hearing aids, fully implantable hearing aids, bone anchored hearing aids, and all other amplification/signal processing devices) who determines audiologic candidacy based on hearing and communication information. The audiologist provides pre and post surgical assessment, counseling, and all aspects of audiologic treatment including auditory training, rehabilitation, implant programming, and maintenance of implant hardware and software.

The audiologist provides audiologic treatment to persons with hearing impairment, and is a source of information for family members, other professionals and the general public. Counseling regarding hearing loss, the use of amplification systems and strategies for improving speech recognition is within the expertise of the audiologist. Additionally, the audiologist provides counseling regarding the effects of hearing loss on communication and psycho-social status in personal, social, and vocational arenas.

The audiologist administers audiologic identification, assessment, diagnosis, and treatment programs to children of all ages with hearing impairment from birth and preschool through school age. The audiologist is an integral part of the team within the school system that manages students with hearing impairments and students with central auditory processing disorders. The audiologist participates in the development of Individual Family Service Plans (IFSPs) and Individualized Educational Programs (IEPs), serves as a consultant in matters pertaining to classroom acoustics, assistive listening systems, hearing aids, communication, and psycho-social effects of hearing loss, and maintains both classroom assistive systems as well as students' personal hearing aids. The audiologist administers hearing screening programs in schools, and trains and supervises nonaudiologists performing hearing screening in the educational setting.

D. Hearing Conservation

The audiologist designs, implements and coordinates industrial and community hearing conservation programs. This includes identification and amelioration of noise-hazardous conditions, identification of hearing loss, recommendation and counseling on use of hearing protection, employee education, and the training and supervision of nonaudiologists performing hearing screening in the industrial setting.

E. Intraoperative Neurophysiologic Monitoring

Audiologists administer and interpret electrophysiologic measurements of neural function including, but not limited to, sensory and motor evoked potentials, tests of nerve conduction velocity, and electromyography. These measurements are used in differential diagnosis, pre and post operative evaluation of neural function, and neurophysiologic intraoperative monitoring of central nervous system, spinal cord, and cranial nerve function.

F. Research

Audiologists design, implement, analyze and interpret the results of research related to auditory and balance systems.

G. Additional Expertise

Some audiologists, by virtue of education, experience and personal choice choose to specialize in an area of practice not otherwise defined in this document. Nothing in this document shall be construed to limit individual freedom of choice in this regard provided that the activity is consistent with the American Academy of Audiology Code of Ethics.

This document will be reviewed, revised, and updated periodically to reflect changing clinical demands of audiologists and to keep pace with the changing scope of practice reflected by these changes and innovations in this specialty.

Courtesy of the American Academy of Audiology.

Academy of Doctors of Audiology Scope of Practice

◆ Statement of Purpose

The following Scope of Practice statement, jointly crafted by the Academy of Doctors of Audiology and the Audiology Foundation of America, is intended to be used by audiologists, allied professionals, consumers of audiological services, and the general public. It serves as a reference for issues of service delivery, third-party reimbursement, legislation, consumer education, regulatory action, state and professional licensure, and inter-professional relations. The document is not intended to be an exhaustive list of activities in which audiologists engage. Rather, it is a broad statement of professional practice. Periodic updating of any scope of practice statement is necessary as technologies and perspectives change.

◆ Definition of an Audiologist

"Audiologist," any person who engages in the practice of audiology. An audiologist is a person who, by virtue of academic degree, clinical training, and license to practice is uniquely qualified to provide a comprehensive array of professional services related to the identification, diagnosis and treatment of persons with auditory and balance disorders, and the prevention of these impairments. Audiologists serve in several roles including primary service provider, clinician, therapist, teacher, consultant, researcher, and administrator. In addition, the supervising audiologist maintains legal and ethical responsibility for all assigned audiology activities provided by audiology assistants and audiology students.

◆ Audiology

(a) The application of principles, methods, and procedures related to the development and disorders of human audio-vestibular system, which disorders shall include any and all conditions whether of organic or functional origin, including, but not limited to, disorders of hearing, balance, tinnitus, central auditory processing, and other neural functions, as those principles, methods, and procedures are taught in doctoral programs in audiology at regionally accredited institutions of higher learning.

(b) Such principles, methods, or procedures include, without limitation, those of diagnosis, assessment, measurement, testing, appraisal, evaluation, treatment, prevention, conservation, identification, consultation, counseling, intervention, management, interpretation, instruction or research related to hearing, vestibular function, balance and fall prevention, and associated neural systems, or any abnormal condition related to tinnitus, auditory sensitivity, acuity, function or processing, speech, language, or other aberrant behavior resulting from hearing loss, for the purpose of diagnosing, designing, and implementing audiological treatment or other programs for the amelioration of such disorders and conditions.

(c) Engaging in the practice of prescribing, selecting, specifying, evaluating, assisting in the adjustment to, and dispensing of prosthetic devices for hearing loss, including hearing aids, and hearing assistive devices by means of specialized audiometric equipment or by any other means accepted by the board.

◆ Scope of Practice

The scope of practice of audiologists is defined by the training and knowledge base of professionals who are licensed to practice as audiologists. The audiologist is an independent practitioner who provides services in hospitals, clinics, schools, private practices, and other settings in which audiological services are relevant.

Areas of practice include identification, diagnosis and treatment of individuals with auditory and balance disorders, prevention of hearing loss, and research in normal and disordered auditory and balance function.

The central focus of the profession of audiology is concerned with all auditory impairments and their relationship to disorders of communication. Audiologists identify, diagnose, evaluate, and treat individuals with either peripheral or central auditory impairments, and strive to prevent such impairments. All professional activities related to this central focus fall within the purview of audiology. In addition, professional activities related to diagnosis and treatment of persons with balance disorders are within the scope of practice of audiologists.

Audiologists provide clinical and academic training to students in audiology. Audiologists teach physicians and medical students about the evaluation of hearing and balance disorders, prevention of hearing loss, and diagnosis and treatment of persons with hearing and balance impairment. They provide information and training on all aspects of hearing and balance to other professions including psychology, counseling, rehabilitation, education, and other related professions. Audiologists provide information on hearing and balance, hearing loss and disability, prevention of hearing loss, and rehabilitation to business and industry. They develop and oversee hearing loss prevention programs in industry. Further, audiologists serve as expert witnesses within the boundaries of forensic audiology.

Identification

Audiologists develop and oversee screening programs to detect individuals of all ages with hearing and balance disorders. Audiologists may perform speech or language screening, or other screening measures for the purpose of initial identification and referral of persons with other communication disorders.

Diagnosis

Diagnosis of hearing status includes the administration and interpretation of behavioral and electrophysiologic measures of the peripheral and central auditory systems. Diagnosis of disorders of balance includes administration and interpretation of clinical and electrophysiologic tests of equilibrium. Diagnosis is accomplished using standardized testing procedures and appropriately calibrated instrumentation, together with the audiologist's interpretation of these measures, case history exploration, and use of the audiologist's clinical judgment.

Treatment

The audiologist is the professional who provides services for persons with hearing impairment and balance disorders. The audiologist is responsible for the evaluation and fitting of amplification devices, including assistive listening devices. The audiologist determines the appropriateness of amplification systems for persons with hearing impairment, evaluates benefit, and provides counseling and training regarding their use. Audiologists conduct otoscopic examinations, clean ear canals and remove cerumen, take appropriate ear canal impressions including deep canal impressions for middle ear implantable amplification devices. They prescribe, fit, sell, and dispense hearing aids and other amplification systems. Audiologists diagnose and provide management for persons with tinnitus using techniques that include, but are not limited to, biofeedback, masking, hearing aids, education, counseling, and tinnitus retraining therapy.

Audiologists provide diagnostic evaluations and counseling for functional hearing loss or pseudohypacusis. Audiologists are also involved in the treatment of persons with balance disorders. They participate as full members of a team to prescribe and carry out goals of treatment of balance disorders including, for example, habituation exercises, balance retraining exercises, general conditioning exercises, and adaptation techniques.

Audiologists provide treatment services for infants and children with hearing disorders and their families. These services may include therapy, home intervention, family support, and case management.

The audiologist is the member of the evaluation team who determines candidacy based on auditory and communication information for implantable hearing devices. The audiologist provides pre- and post-surgical assessment, counseling, auditory rehabilitation, programming of devices, and maintenance of hardware and software.

The audiologist provides habilitation and rehabilitation to persons with hearing and balance impairments, and is a source of information for family members, other professionals, and the general public. Counseling regarding hearing loss, the use of amplification systems, and strategies for improving speech recognition are within the expertise of the audiologist. Additionally, the audiologist provides counseling regarding the effects of hearing loss on communication and psychosocial status in personal, social, and vocational arenas.

The audiologist administers identification, evaluation, and treatment programs to children of all ages with hearing impairment from birth and preschool through school age. The audiologist administers hearing screening programs in schools, and trains and supervises non-audiologists performing hearing screening in the educational setting. The audiologist is an integral part of the team within the school system, which manages students with hearing impairments and students with auditory processing disorders. The audiologist participates in the development of Individual Family Service Plans (IFSPs), 504's, and Individualized Educational Programs (IEPs), serves as a consultant in matters pertaining to classroom acoustics, assistive listening systems, hearing aids, communication, and psycho-social effects of hearing loss, and maintains both classroom assistive systems as well as students' personal hearing aids.

Hearing Loss Prevention Programs

The audiologist designs, implements and coordinates industrial, community, and recreational hearing loss prevention programs. This includes identification and amelioration of noise-hazardous conditions, identification of hearing loss, prescription of and counseling for the use of hearing protection, employee education, and the training and supervision of non-audiologists performing hearing screening in the industrial setting.

Neurophysiologic Monitoring

Audiologists administer and interpret electrophysiologic measurements of neural function including, but not limited to, sensory and motor evoked potentials, tests of nerve conduction velocity, and electromyography. These measurements are in differential diagnosis, pre- and postoperative evaluation of neural function, and neuro-physiologic monitoring of central nervous system.

Research

Audiologists design, implement, analyze, and interpret the results of research related to auditory and balance systems.

Reprinted with permission from the Academy of Doctors of Audiology.

American Speech-Language-Hearing Association Scope of Practice

♦ Statement of Purpose

The purpose of this document is to define the scope of practice in audiology to (a) describe the services offered by qualified audiologists as primary service providers, case managers, and/or members of multidisciplinary and interdisciplinary teams; (b) serve as a reference for health care, education, and other professionals, and for consumers, members of the general public, and policy makers concerned with legislation, regulation, licensure, and third party reimbursement; and (c) inform members of ASHA, certificate holders, and students of the activities for which certification in audiology is required in accordance with the ASHA Code of Ethics.

Audiologists provide comprehensive diagnostic and treatment/rehabilitative services for auditory, vestibular, and related impairments. These services are provided to individuals across the entire age span from birth through adulthood; to individuals from diverse language, ethnic, cultural, and socioeconomic backgrounds; and to individuals who have multiple disabilities. This position statement is not intended to be exhaustive; however, the activities described reflect current practice within the profession. Practice activities related to emerging clinical, technological, and scientific developments are not precluded from consideration as part of the scope of practice of an audiologist. Such innovations and advances will result in the periodic revision and updating of this document. It is also recognized that specialty areas identified within the scope of practice will vary among the individual providers. ASHA also recognizes that credentialed professionals in related fields may have knowledge, skills, and experience that could be applied to some areas within the scope of audiology practice. Defining the scope of practice of audiologists is not meant to exclude other appropriately credentialed postgraduate professionals from rendering services in common practice areas.

Audiologists serve diverse populations. The patient/client population includes persons of different race, age, gender, religion, national origin, and sexual orientation. Audiologists' caseloads include individuals from diverse ethnic, cultural, or linguistic backgrounds, and persons with disabilities. Although audiologists are prohibited from discriminating in the provision of professional services based on these factors, in some cases such factors may be relevant to the development of an appropriate treatment plan. These factors may be considered in treatment plans only when firmly grounded in scientific and professional knowledge.

This scope of practice does not supersede existing state licensure laws or affect the interpretation or implementation

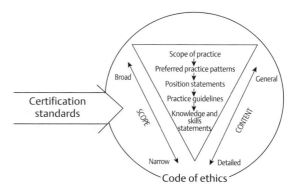

Figure AII–1 Conceptual framework of ASHA Standards and Policy Statements.

of such laws. It may serve, however, as a model for the development or modification of licensure laws.

The schema in **Fig. AII–1** depicts the relationship of the scope of practice to ASHA's policy documents that address current and emerging audiology practice areas; that is, preferred practice patterns, guidelines, and position statements. ASHA members and ASHA-certified professionals are bound by the ASHA Code of Ethics to provide services that are consistent with the scope of their competence, education, and experience (ASHA, 2003). There are other existing legislative and regulatory bodies that govern the practice of audiology.

♦ Framework for Practice

The practice of audiology includes both the prevention of and assessment of auditory, vestibular, and related impairments as well as the habilitation/rehabilitation and maintenance of persons with these impairments. The overall goal of the provision of audiology services should be to optimize and enhance the ability of an individual to hear, as well as to communicate in his/her everyday or natural environment. In addition, audiologists provide comprehensive services to individuals with normal hearing who interact with persons with a hearing impairment. The overall goal of audiologic services is to improve the quality of life for all of these individuals.

The World Health Organization (WHO) has developed a multipurpose health classification system known as the International Classification of Functioning, Disability, and Health (ICF) (WHO, 2001). The purpose of this classification system is to provide a standard language and framework for the description of functioning and health. The ICF framework is useful in describing the role of audiologists in the prevention, assessment, and habilitation/rehabilitation of auditory, vestibular, and other related impairments and restrictions or limitations of functioning.

The ICF is organized into two parts. The first part deals with Functioning and Disability while the second part deals with Contextual Factors. Each part has two components. The components of Functioning and Disability are:

Body Functions and Structures: Body Functions are the physiological functions of body systems and Body Structures are the anatomical parts of the body and their components. Impairments are limitations or variations in Body Function or Structure such as a deviation or loss. An example of a Body Function that might be evaluated by an audiologist would be hearing sensitivity. The use of tympanometry to access the mobility of the tympanic membrane is an example of a Body Structure that might be evaluated by an audiologist.

Activity/Participation: In the ICF, Activity and Participation are realized as one list. Activity refers to the execution of a task or action by an individual. Participation is the involvement in a life situation. Activity limitations are difficulties an individual may experience while executing a given activity. Participation restrictions are difficulties that may limit an individual's involvement in life situations. The Activity/Participation construct thus represents the effects that hearing, vestibular, and related impairments could have on the life of an individual. These effects could include the ability to hold conversations, participate in sports, attend religious services, understand a teacher in a classroom, and walk up and down stairs.

The components of Contextual Factors are:

Environmental Factors: Environmental Factors make up the physical, social, and attitudinal environment in which people live and conduct their lives. Examples of Environmental Factors, as they relate to audiology, include the acoustical properties of a given space and any type of hearing assistive technology.

Personal Factors: Personal Factors are the internal influences on an individual's functioning and disability and are not a part of the health condition. These factors may include but are not limited to age, gender, social background, and profession.

Functioning and Disability are interactive and evolutionary processes. **Figure AII–2** illustrates the interaction of the various components of the ICF. Each component of the ICF can be expressed on a continuum of function. On one end of the continuum is intact functioning. At the opposite end of the continuum is completely compromised functioning. Contextual Factors (Environmental and Personal Factors) may interact with any of the components of functioning and disability. Environmental and Personal Factors may act as facilitators or barriers to functioning.

The scope of practice in audiology encompasses all of the components of the ICF. During the assessment phase, audi-

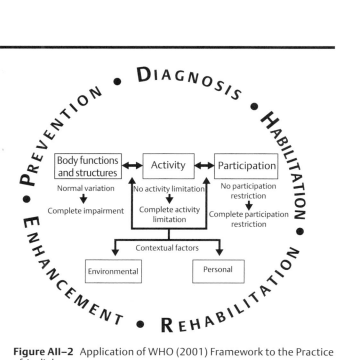

Figure AII–2 Application of WHO (2001) Framework to the Practice of Audiology.

ologists perform tests of Body Function and Structure. Examples of these types of tests include otoscopic examination, pure-tone audiometry, tympanometry, otoacoustic emissions measurements, and speech audiometry. Activity/Participation limitations and restrictions are sometimes addressed by audiologists through case history, interview, questionnaire, and counseling. For example, a question such as "Do you have trouble understanding while on the telephone?" or "Can you describe the difficulties you experience when you participate in a conversation with someone who is not familiar to you?" would be considered an assessment of Activity/Participation limitation or restriction. Questionnaires that require clients to report the magnitude of difficulty that they experience in certain specified settings can sometimes be used to measure aspects of Activity/Participation. For example: "Because of my hearing problems, I have difficulty conversing with others in a restaurant." In addition, Environmental and Personal Factors also need to be taken into consideration by audiologists as they treat individuals with auditory, vestibular, and other related impairments. In the above question regarding conversation in a restaurant, if the factor of "noise" (i.e., a noisy restaurant) is added to the question, this represents an Environmental Factor. Examples of Personal Factors might include a person's background or culture that influences his or her reaction to the use of a hearing aid or cochlear implant. The use of the ICF framework (WHO, 2001) may help audiologists broaden their perspective concerning their role in evaluating a client's needs or when designing and providing comprehensive services to their clients. Overall, audiologists work to improve quality of life by reducing impairments of body functions and structures, Activity limitations/Participation restrictions and Environmental barriers of the individuals they serve.

◆ Definition of an Audiologist

Audiologists are professionals engaged in autonomous practice to promote healthy hearing, communication competency, and quality of life for persons of all ages through the prevention, identification, assessment, and rehabilitation of hearing, auditory function, balance, and other related systems. They facilitate prevention through the fitting of hearing protective devices, education programs for industry and the public, hearing screening/conservation programs, and research. The audiologist is the professional responsible for the identification of impairments and dysfunction of the auditory, balance, and other related systems. Their unique education and training provides them with the skills to assess and diagnose dysfunction in hearing, auditory function, balance, and related disorders. The delivery of audiologic (re)habilitation services includes not only the selecting, fitting, and dispensing of hearing aids and other hearing assistive devices, but also the assessment and follow-up services for persons with cochlear implants. The audiologist providing audiologic (re)habilitation does so through a comprehensive program of therapeutic services, devices, counseling, and other management strategies. Functional diagnosis of vestibular disorders and management of balance rehabilitation is another aspect of the professional responsibilities of the audiologist. Audiologists engage in research pertinent to all of these domains.

Audiologists currently hold a master's or doctoral degree in audiology from a program accredited by the Council on Academic Accreditation in Audiology and Speech-Language Pathology (CAA) of the American Speech-Language-Hearing Association. ASHA-certified audiologists complete a supervised postgraduate professional experience or a similar supervised professional experience during the completion of the doctoral degree as described in the ASHA certification standards. Beginning January 1, 2012, all applicants for the Certificate of Clinical Competence in Audiology must have a doctoral degree from a CAA-accredited university program. Demonstration of continued professional development is mandated for the maintenance of the Certificate of Clinical Competence in Audiology. Where required, audiologists are licensed or registered by the state in which they practice.

◆ Professional Roles and Activities

Audiologists serve a diverse population and may function in one or more of a variety of activities. The practice of audiology includes:

A. Prevention

1. Promotion of hearing wellness, as well as the prevention of hearing loss and protection of hearing function by designing, implementing, and coordinating occupational, school, and community hearing conservation and identification programs

2. Participation in noise measurements of the acoustic environment to improve accessibility and to promote hearing wellness.

B. Identification

1. Activities that identify dysfunction in hearing, balance, and other auditory-related systems;
2. Supervision, implementation, and follow-up of newborn and school hearing screening programs;
3. Screening for speech, orofacial myofunctional disorders, language, cognitive communication disorders, and/or preferred communication modalities that may affect education, health, development or communication and may result in recommendations for rescreening or comprehensive speech-language pathology assessment or in referral for other examinations or services;
4. Identification of populations and individuals with or at risk for hearing loss and other auditory dysfunction, balance impairments, tinnitus, and associated communication impairments as well as of those with normal hearing;
5. In collaboration with speech-language pathologists, identification of populations and individuals at risk for developing speech-language impairments.

C. Assessment

1. The conduct and interpretation of behavioral, electroacoustic, and/or electrophysiologic methods to assess hearing, auditory function, balance, and related systems;
2. Measurement and interpretation of sensory and motor evoked potentials, electromyography, and other electrodiagnostic tests for purposes of neurophysiologic intraoperative monitoring and cranial nerve assessment;
3. Evaluation and management of children and adults with auditory-related processing disorders;
4. Performance of otoscopy for appropriate audiological management or to provide a basis for medical referral;
5. Cerumen management to prevent obstruction of the external ear canal and of amplification devices;
6. Preparation of a report including interpreting data, summarizing findings, generating recommendations and developing an audiologic treatment/management plan;
7. Referrals to other professions, agencies, and/or consumer organizations.

D. Rehabilitation

1. As part of the comprehensive audiologic (re)habilitation program, evaluates, selects, fits and dispenses hearing assistive technology devices to include hearing aids;
2. Assessment of candidacy of persons with hearing loss for cochlear implants and provision of fitting, mapping, and audiologic rehabilitation to optimize device use;
3. Development of a culturally appropriate, audiologic rehabilitative management plan including, when appropriate:
   a. Recommendations for fitting and dispensing, and educating the consumer and family/caregivers in the use of and adjustment to sensory aids, hearing assistive devices, alerting systems, and captioning devices;

b. Availability of counseling relating to psycho social aspects of hearing loss, and other auditory dysfunction, and processes to enhance communication competence;

c. Skills training and consultation concerning environmental modifications to facilitate development of receptive and expressive communication;

d. Evaluation and modification of the audiologic management plan.

4. Provision of comprehensive audiologic rehabilitation services, including management procedures for speech and language habilitation and/or rehabilitation for persons with hearing loss or other auditory dysfunction, including but not exclusive to speechreading, auditory training, communication strategies, manual communication and counseling for psychosocial adjustment for persons with hearing loss or other auditory dysfunction and their families/caregivers;

5. Consultation and provision of vestibular and balance rehabilitation therapy to persons with vestibular and balance impairments;

6. Assessment and non-medical management of tinnitus using biofeedback, behavioral management, masking, hearing aids, education, and counseling;

7. Provision of training for professionals of related and/or allied services when needed;

8. Participation in the development of an Individual Education Program (IEP) for school-age children or an Individual Family Service Plan (IFSP) for children from birth to 36 months old;

9. Provision of in-service programs for school personnel, and advising school districts in planning educational programs and accessibility for students with hearing loss and other auditory dysfunction;

10. Measurement of noise levels and provision of recommendations for environmental modifications to reduce the noise level;

11. Management of the selection, purchase, installation, and evaluation of large-area amplification systems.

E. Advocacy/Consultation

1. Advocacy for communication needs of all individuals that may include advocating for the rights/funding of services for those with hearing loss, auditory, or vestibular disorders;

2. Advocacy for issues (i.e., acoustic accessibility) that affect the rights of individuals with normal hearing;

3. Consultation with professionals of related and/or allied services when needed;

4. Consultation in development of an Individual Education Program (IEP) for school-age children or an Individual Family Service Plan (IFSP) for children from birth to 36 months old;

5. Consultation to educators as members of interdisciplinary teams about communication management, educational implications of hearing loss and other auditory dysfunction, educational programming, classroom acoustics, and large-area amplification systems for children with hearing loss and other auditory dysfunction;

6. Consultation about accessibility for persons with hearing loss and other auditory dysfunction in public and private buildings, programs, and services;

7. Consultation to individuals, public and private agencies, and governmental bodies, or as an expert witness regarding legal interpretations of audiology findings, effects of hearing loss and other auditory dysfunction, balance system impairments, and relevant noise-related considerations;

8. Case management and service as a liaison for the consumer, family, and agencies to monitor audiologic status and management and to make recommendations about educational and vocational programming;

9. Consultation to industry on the development of products and instrumentation related to the measurement and management of auditory or balance function.

F. Education/Research/Administration

1. Education, supervision, and administration for audiology graduate and other professional education programs;

2. Measurement of functional outcomes, consumer satisfaction, efficacy, effectiveness, and efficiency of practices and programs to maintain and improve the quality of audiologic services;

3. Design and conduct of basic and applied audiologic research to increase the knowledge base, to develop new methods and programs, and to determine the efficacy, effectiveness, and efficiency of assessment and treatment paradigms; disseminate research findings to other professionals and to the public;

4. Participation in the development of professional and technical standards;

5. Participation in quality improvement programs;

6. Program administration and supervision of professionals as well as support personnel.

♦ Practice Settings

Audiologists provide services in private practice; medical settings such as hospitals and physicians' offices; community and university hearing and speech centers; managed care systems; industry; the military; various state agencies; home health, subacute rehabilitation, long-term care, and intermediate-care facilities; and school systems. Audiologists provide academic education to students and practitioners in universities, to medical and surgical students and residents, and to other related professionals. Such education pertains to the identification, functional diagnosis/assessment, and non-medical treatment/management of auditory, vestibular, balance, and related impairments.

References

American Speech-Language-Hearing Association. (1996, Spring). Scope of practice in audiology. ASHA, 38(Suppl. 16), 12–15.

American Speech-Language-Hearing Association. (2003). Code of ethics (revised). ASHA Supplement, 23, 13–15.

World Health Organization (WHO). (2001). ICF: International classification of functioning, disability and health. Geneva: Author.

Resources General

American Speech-Language-Hearing Association. (1979, March). Severely hearing handicapped. ASHA, 21.

American Speech-Language-Hearing Association. (1985, June). Clinical supervision in speech-language pathology and audiology. ASHA, 27, 57–60.

American Speech-Language-Hearing Association. (1986, May). Autonomy of speech-language pathology and audiology. ASHA, 28, 53–57.

American Speech-Language-Hearing Association. (1987, June). Calibration of speech signals delivered via earphones. ASHA, 29, 44–48.

American Speech-Language-Hearing Association. (1988). Mental retardation and developmental disabilities curriculum guide for speech-language pathologists and audiologists. Rockville, MD: Author.

American Speech-Language-Hearing Association. (1989, March). Bilingual speech-language pathologists and audiologists: Definition. ASHA, 31, 93.

American Speech-Language-Hearing Association. (1989, June/July). AIDS/HIV: Implications for speech-language pathologists and audiologists. ASHA, 31, 33–38.

American Speech-Language-Hearing Association. (1990). The role of speech-language pathologists and audiologists in service delivery for persons with mental retardation and developmental disabilities in community settings. ASHA, 32(Suppl. 2), 5–6.

American Speech-Language-Hearing Association. (1990, April). Major issues affecting delivery of services in hospital settings: Recommendations and strategies. ASHA, 32, 67–70.

American Speech-Language-Hearing Association. (1991). Sound field measurement tutorial. ASHA, 33(Suppl. 3), 25–37.

American Speech-Language-Hearing Association. (1992). 1992 U.S. Department of Labor definition of speech-language pathologists and audiologists. ASHA, 4, 563–565.

American Speech-Language-Hearing Association. (1992, March). Sedation and topical anesthetics in audiology and speech-language pathology. ASHA, 34(Suppl. 7), 41–42.

American Speech-Language-Hearing Association. (1993). National health policy: Back to the future (technical report). ASHA, 35(Suppl. 10), 2–10.

American Speech-Language-Hearing Association. (1993). Position statement on national health policy. ASHA, 35(Suppl. 10), 1.

American Speech-Language-Hearing Association. (1993). Professional performance appraisal by individuals outside the professions of speech-language pathology and audiology. ASHA, 35(Suppl. 10), 11–13.

American Speech-Language-Hearing Association. (1994, January). The protection of rights of people receiving audiology or speech-language pathology services. ASHA, 36, 60–63.

American Speech-Language-Hearing Association. (1994, March). Guidelines for the audiologic management of individuals receiving cochleotoxic drug therapy. ASHA, 36(Suppl. 12), 11–19.

American Speech-Language-Hearing Association. (1995, March). Guidelines for education in audiology practice management. ASHA, 37(Suppl. 14), 20.

American Speech-Language-Hearing Association. (1997). Preferred practice patterns for the profession of audiology. Rockville, MD: Author.

American Speech-Language-Hearing Association. (1997, Spring). Position statement: Multiskilled personnel. ASHA, 39(Suppl. 17), 13.

American Speech-Language-Hearing Association. (1998). Position statement and guidelines on support personnel in audiology. ASHA, 40(Suppl. 18), 19–21.

American Speech-Language-Hearing Association. (2001). Scope of practice in speech-language pathology. Rockville, MD: Author.

American Speech-Language-Hearing Association. (2002). Certification and membership handbook: Audiology. Rockville, MD: Author.

American Speech-Language-Hearing Association. (2003). Code of ethics (revised). ASHA (Suppl. 23), 13–15.

Joint Committee of the American Speech-Language-Hearing Association (ASHA) and the Council on Education of the Deaf (CED). (1998). Hearing loss: Terminology and classification: Position statement and technical report. ASHA, 40(Suppl. 18), 22.

Joint Audiology Committee on Clinical Practice. (1999). Clinical practice statements and algorithms. Rockville, MD: American Speech-Language-Hearing Association.

Paul-Brown, D. (1994, May). Clinical record keeping in audiology and speech pathology. ASHA, 36, 40–43.

Amplification

American Speech-Language-Hearing Association. (1991). Amplification as a remediation technique for children with normal peripheral hearing. ASHA, 33(Suppl. 3), 22–24.

American Speech-Language-Hearing Association. (1998). Guidelines for hearing aid fitting for adults. American Journal of Audiology, 7(1), 5–13.

American Speech-Language-Hearing Association. (2000). Guidelines for graduate education in amplification. ASHA (Suppl. 20), 22–27.

American Speech-Language-Hearing Association. (2002). Guidelines for fitting and monitoring FM systems. ASHA Desk Reference, 2, 151–172.

American Speech-Language Hearing Association (2004). Technical report: Cochlear implants. ASHA (Suppl. 24).

Audiologic Rehabilitation

American Speech-Language-Hearing Association. (1981, April). On the definition of hearing handicap. ASHA, 23, 293–297.

American Speech-Language-Hearing Association. (1984, May). Definition of and competencies for aural rehabilitation. ASHA, 26, 37–41.

American Speech-Language-Hearing Association. (1990). Aural rehabilitation: An annotated bibliography. ASHA, 32(Suppl. 1), 1–12.

American Speech-Language-Hearing Association. (1992, March). Electrical stimulation for cochlear implant selection and rehabilitation. ASHA, 34(Suppl. 7), 13–16.

American Speech-Language-Hearing Association. (2001). ARBIB: Audiologic rehabilitation—basic information bibliography. Rockville, MD: Author.

American Speech-Language-Hearing Association. (2001). Knowledge and skills required for the practice of audiologic/aural rehabilitation. Rockville, MD: Author.

Audiologic Screening

American Speech-Language-Hearing Association. (1988, November). Telephone hearing screening. ASHA, 30, 53.

American Speech-Language-Hearing Association. (1994, June/July). Audiologic screening [executive summary]. ASHA, 36, 53–54.

American Speech-Language-Hearing Association Audiologic Assessment Panel 1996. (1997). Guidelines for audiologic screening. Rockville, MD: Author.

(Central) Auditory Processing Disorders

American Speech-Language-Hearing Association. (1979, December). The role of the speech-language pathologist and audiologist in learning disabilities. ASHA, 21, 1015.

American Speech-Language-Hearing Association (1990). Audiological assessment of central auditory processing: An annotated bibliography. ASHA, 32(Suppl. 1), 13–30.

American Speech-Language-Hearing Association. (1996, July). Central auditory processing: Current status of research and implications for clinical practice. American Journal of Audiology, 5(2), 41–54.

Business Practices

American Speech-Language-Hearing Association. (1987, March). Private practice. ASHA, 29, 35.

American Speech-Language-Hearing Association. (1991). Business, marketing, ethics, and professionalism in audiology: An updated annotated bibliography (1986–1989). ASHA, 33(Suppl. 3), 39–45.

American Speech-Language-Hearing Association. (1991). Considerations for establishing a private practice in audiology and/or speech-language pathology. ASHA, 33(Suppl. 3), 10–21.

American Speech-Language-Hearing Association. (1991). Report on private practice. ASHA, 33(Suppl. 6), 1–4.

American Speech-Language-Hearing Association. (1994, March). Professional liability and risk management for the audiology and special-language pathology professions. ASHA, 36(March, Suppl. 12), 25–38.

Diagnostic Procedures

American Speech-Language-Hearing Association. (1978). Guidelines for manual pure-tone threshold audiometry. ASHA, 20, 297–301.

American Speech-Language-Hearing Association. (1988, March). Guidelines for determining threshold level for speech. ASHA, 85–89.

American Speech-Language-Hearing Association. (1988, November). Tutorial: Tympanometry. Journal of Speech and Hearing Disorders, 53, 354–377.

American Speech-Language-Hearing Association. (1990). Guidelines for audiometric symbols. ASHA, 32(Suppl. 2), 25–30.

American Speech-Language-Hearing Association. (1991). Acoustic-immittance measures: A bibliography. ASHA, 33(Suppl. 4), 1–44.

American Speech-Language-Hearing Association. (1992, March). External auditory canal examination and cerumen management. ASHA, 34(Suppl. 7), 22–24.

Educational Audiology

American Speech-Language-Hearing Association. (1991). Utilization of Medicaid and other third party funds for covered services in the schools. ASHA, 33(Suppl. 5), 51–59.

American Speech-Language-Hearing Association. (1995, March). Acoustics in educational settings: Position statement and guidelines. ASHA, 37(Suppl. 14), 15–19.

American Speech-Language-Hearing Association. (1997). Trends and issues in school reform and their effects on speech-language pathologists, audiologists, and students with communication disorders. ASHA Desk Reference, 4, 317–326.

American Speech-Language-Hearing Association. (1997, Spring). Position statement: Roles of audiologists and speech-language-pathologists working with persons with attention deficit hyperactivity disorder: Position statement and technical report. ASHA, 39(Suppl. 17), 14.

American Speech-Language-Hearing Association. (2002). Guidelines for audiology service provision in and for schools. Rockville, MD: Author.

American Speech-Language-Hearing Association. (2002). Appropriate school facilities for students with speech-language-hearing disorders: Technical report. ASHA (Suppl. 23), 83–86.

Electrophysiological Assessment

American Speech-Language-Hearing Association. (1987). Short latency auditory evoked potentials. Rockville, MD: Author.

American Speech-Language-Hearing Association. (1992, March). Neurophysiologic intraoperative monitoring. ASHA, 34(Suppl. 7), 34–36.

American Speech-Language-Hearing Association. (2003). Guidelines for competencies in auditory evoked potential measurement and clinical applications. ASHA (Suppl. 23), 35–40.

Geriatric Audiology

American Speech-Language-Hearing Association. (1988, March). Provision of audiology and speech-language pathology services to older persons in nursing homes. ASHA, 772–774.

American Speech-Language-Hearing Association. (1988, March). The roles of speech-language pathologists and audiologists in working with older persons. ASHA, 30, 80–84.

American Speech-Language-Hearing Association. (1997, Spring). Guidelines for audiology service delivery in nursing homes. ASHA, 39(Suppl. 17), 15–29.

Occupational Audiology

American Speech-Language-Hearing Association. (1996, Spring). Guidelines on the audiologist's role in occupational and environmental hearing conservation. ASHA, 38(Suppl. 16), 34–41.

American Speech-Language-Hearing Association. (1997, Spring). Issues: Occupational and environmental hearing conservation. ASHA, 39(Suppl. 17), 30–34.

American Speech-Language-Hearing Association. (2004). The audiologist's role in occupational hearing conservation and hearing loss prevention programs: Technical report. ASHA (Suppl. 24).

Pediatric Audiology

American Speech-Language-Hearing Association. (1991). Guidelines for the audiological assessment of children from birth through 36 months of age. ASHA, 33(Suppl. 5), 37–43.

American Speech-Language-Hearing Association. (1991). The use of FM amplification instruments for infants and preschool children with hearing impairment. ASHA, 33(Suppl. 5), 1–2.

American Speech-Language-Hearing Association. (1994, August). Service provision under the Individuals with Disabilities Education Act-Part H, as amended (IDEA-Part H) to children who are deaf and hard of hearing—ages birth to 36 months. ASHA, 36, 117–121.

Joint Committee on Infant Hearing. (2000). JCIH year 2000 position statement: Principles and guidelines for early hearing detection and intervention programs. American Journal of Audiology, 9, 9–29.

Vestibular

American Speech-Language-Hearing Association. (1992, March). Balance system assessment. ASHA, 34(Suppl. 7), 9–12.

American Speech-Language-Hearing Association. (1999, March). Role of audiologists in vestibular and balance rehabilitation: Position statement, guidelines, and technical report. ASHA, 41(Suppl. 19), 13–22.

Reprinted with permission from American Speech-Language-Hearing Association (2001). Scope of practice in speech-language-pathology. Available from www.asha.org/reference.

Index

Note: Page numbers followed by *n, f,* and *t* indicate footnotes, figures, and tables, respectively.